Gastrointestinal

PHILADELPHIA

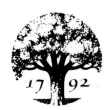

J. B. Lippincott Company

GASTROINTESTINAL
RADIOLOGY

Radiology

A Pattern Approach

Ronald L. Eisenberg, M.D.

Professor and Chairman, Department of Radiology
Louisiana State University School of Medicine, Shreveport, Louisiana

The author and publisher have exerted every effort to ensure that drug selection and dosage set forth in this text are in accord with current recommendations and practice at the time of publication. However, in view of ongoing research, changes in government regulations, and the constant flow of information relating to drug therapy and drug reactions, the reader is urged to check the package insert for each drug for any change in indications and dosage and for added warnings and precautions. This is particularly important when the recommended agent is a new or infrequently employed drug.

1989–Due Aug 1989

Acquisitions Editor: William Burgower
Sponsoring Editor: Darlene D. Pedersen
Manuscript Editor: Martha Hicks-Courant
Art Director: Maria S. Karkucinski

Designer: Ronald Dorfman
Production Assistant: Barney Fernandes
Compositor: Monotype Composition Company, Inc.
Printer/Binder: Halliday Lithograph

5 7 9 8 6

Library of Congress Cataloging in Publication Data

Eisenberg, Ronald Lee.
  Gastrointestinal radiology.

  Includes index.
    1. Gastrointestinal system—Radiography—Atlases.
2. Gastrointestinal system—Diseases—Diagnosis.
I. Title. [DNLM: 1. Gastrointestinal system—Radiography. 2. Gastrointestinal system—Radiography—Atlases. WI 141 E36g]
  RC804.R6E37   616.3′0757 82-7202
  ISBN 0-397-52113-8   AACR2

To Alex Margulis,
Teacher, Inspiration, Friend

CONTENTS

Preface   xi

Acknowledgments   xiii

PART ONE   ESOPHAGUS

1   Abnormalities of Esophageal Motility   3
2   Extrinsic Impressions on the Cervical Esophagus   27
3   Extrinsic Impressions on the Thoracic Esophagus   30
4   Esophageal Ulceration   47
5   Esophageal Narrowing   66
6   Esophageal Filling Defects   89
7   Esophageal Diverticula   106
8   Esophageal Varices   111
9   Esophagorespiratory Fistulas   118
10   Double-Barrel Esophagus   128
11   Diffuse Finely Nodular Lesions of the Esophagus   134

PART TWO   DIAPHRAGM

12   Elevation of the Diaphragm   141
13   Diaphragmatic Hernias   150

PART THREE   STOMACH

14   Gastric Ulcers   171
15   Superficial Gastric Erosions   197
16   Narrowing of the Stomach (Linitis Plastica Pattern)   201

17 Thickening of Gastric Folds — 219

18 Filling Defects in the Stomach — 238

19 Filling Defects in the Gastric Remnant — 267

20 Gastric Outlet Obstruction — 279

21 Gastric Dilatation Without Outlet Obstruction — 291

22 Intrinsic/Extrinsic Masses of the Fundus — 296

23 Widening of the Retrogastric Space — 309

24 Gas in the Wall of the Stomach — 313

25 Simultaneous Involvement of the Gastric Antrum
and Duodenal Bulb — 316

PART FOUR   DUODENUM

26 Postbulbar Ulceration of the Duodenum — 325

27 Thickening of Duodenal Folds — 332

28 Widening of the Duodenal Sweep — 342

29 Extrinsic Pressure on the Duodenum — 356

30 Duodenal Filling Defects — 363

31 Duodenal Narrowing/Obstruction — 385

32 Duodenal Dilatation (Superior Mesenteric Artery
Syndrome) — 403

PART FIVE   SMALL BOWEL

Introduction to Diseases of the Small Bowel — 411

33 Small Bowel Obstruction — 413

34 Adynamic Ileus — 433

35 Dilatation with Normal Folds — 446

36 Dilatation with Thickened Mucosal Folds — 459

37 Regular Thickening of Small Bowel Folds — 463

38 Generalized, Irregular, Distorted Folds — 476

39 Solitary Filling Defects in the Jejunum and Ileum — 492

40 Multiple Filling Defects in the Small Bowel — 505

41 Sandlike Lucencies — 516

42 Thickened Small Bowel Folds with Concomitant
Involvement of the Stomach — 522

43 Separation of Small Bowel Loops   526
44 Small Bowel Diverticula and Pseudodiverticula   538

PART SIX ILEOCECAL VALVE AND CECUM

45 Abnormalities of the Ileocecal Valve   553
46 Filling Defects in the Cecum   566
47 Coned Cecum   584

PART SEVEN COLON

48 Ulcerative Lesions of the Colon   597
49 Narrowing of the Colon   640
50 Single Filling Defects in the Colon   681
51 Multiple Filling Defects in the Colon   711
52 Large Bowel Obstruction   740
53 Toxic Megacolon   759
54 Thumbprinting of the Colon   765
55 Double Tracking in the Sigmoid Colon   775
56 Enlargement of the Retrorectal Space   779

PART EIGHT BILIARY SYSTEM

57 Nonvisualization of the Gallbladder   795
58 Alterations in Gallbladder Size   803
59 Displacement or Deformity of the Gallbladder   807
60 Filling Defects in an Opacified Gallbladder   811
61 Filling Defects in the Bile Ducts   825
62 Bile Duct Narrowing / Obstruction   835
63 Cystic Dilatation of the Bile Ducts   851
64 Enlargement of the Papilla of Vater   861
65 Gas in the Biliary System (Pancreaticobiliary Reflux)   868
66 Gas in the Portal Veins   876

PART NINE MISCELLANEOUS

67 Bull's-Eye Lesions in the Gastrointestinal Tract   883
68 Nondiaphragmatic Hernias   888
69 Gas in the Bowel Wall (Pneumatosis Intestinalis)   898
70 Pneumoperitoneum   910
71 Extraluminal Gas in the Upper Quadrants   921
72 Fistulas Involving the Small or Large Bowel   935
73 Abdominal Calcifications   953

Index   1021

PREFACE

With all the available books on gastrointestinal radiology, why should there be yet another one? Essentially all textbooks in gastrointestinal radiology (as well as other specialties in radiology) are disease-oriented, demonstrating and discussing all the radiographic manifestations of a specific disorder. Although this is an excellent approach for a large reference work, it is often of little value to the radiologist faced with the reality of daily film reading. The practicing radiologist is usually unaware of the underlying disease and is presented with a specific finding for which he or she must suggest a differential diagnosis and rational diagnostic approach. To address this problem, the gamut concept has been developed. Unfortunately, a book consisting only of gamuts is difficult and dull reading and still requires that a second textbook be consulted to aid in differentiating among the various diagnostic possibilities listed in the gamut. The "pattern" approach to gastrointestinal radiology presented here is an attempt to combine the best features of a list of gamuts and an extensive disease-oriented textbook. For each radiographic finding, an extensive gamut is presented, divided into subsections for convenient use. Textual material and a wealth of illustrations are then presented to aid the radiologist in arriving at a reasonable differential diagnosis.

I must stress that this book in no way intends to supplant the current excellent textbooks in gastrointestinal radiology. Rather, it is designed to complement these works by providing a handy reference for the practicing radiologist and resident faced with the daily challenge of interpreting gastrointestinal examinations.

Ronald L. Eisenberg, M.D.

ACKNOWLEDGMENTS

I want to offer special thanks to the following radiologists, who gave me free run of their extensive files and without whose case material this book could not have been compiled.

John R. Amberg, M.D.
Henry I. Goldberg, M.D.
Alexander R. Margulis, M.D.
Peter C. Meyers, M.D.
Hideyo Minagi, M.D.

The following colleagues have graciously permitted me to use radiographs from their unpublished cases.

Jose M. Alba, M.D.
Marvin S. Belasco, M.D.
Alan J. Davidson, M.D.
Michael Davis, M.D.
Herbert Y. Kressel, M.D.
Rajendra Kumar, M.D.
Marc S. Lapayowker, M.D.
Catherine V. Netchvolodoff, M.D.
Steven H. Ominsky, M.D.
Alphonse J. Palubinskas, M.D.
Sanford A. Rubin, M.D.
Melvin H. Schreiber, M.D.
McClure Wilson, M.D.
Justin J. Wolfson, M.D.

And, of course, I am grateful to the many physicians who have kindly allowed me to use their published material as illustrations in this book.

I would also like to express my thanks to Betty DiGrazia and Mary Smith for the many hours they spent in the arduous task of typing and retyping the manuscript. I gratefully appreciate the efforts of James Kendrick of George Washington University, Howard Miller of M. D. Anderson Medical Center, and the Medical Communications Department at Louisiana State University School of Medicine in Shreveport for skillfully photographing the many illustrations. Thanks should also go to the radiology residents at LSU, who continuously had eagle eyes trained to find appropriate case material. Finally, I acknowledge the unceasing encouragement and support of William Burgower, Senior Editor, and the entire staff at J. B. Lippincott Company, who have made the immense technical problems of preparing a book as painless as possible.

PART ONE

ESOPHAGUS

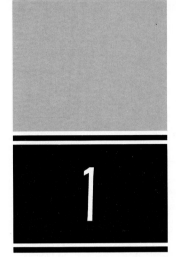

ABNORMALITIES OF ESOPHAGEAL MOTILITY

The esophagus is a muscular tube approximately 20 cm to 24 cm in length that begins at the level of the cricoid cartilage in the neck. The esophagus is lined predominantly by squamous epithelium, and its wall is composed of an outer longitudinal and an inner circular muscle layer. In the proximal one-third of the esophagus, there is mainly striated muscle; the distal two-thirds consist predominantly of smooth muscle. The point of demarcation between the striated and smooth muscle portions appears radiographically at about the level of the aortic knob.

There are two esophageal sphincters, areas that maintain a relatively high resting pressure compared with adjacent segments. The upper esophageal sphincter is about 1 cm to 3 cm in length and represents the zone of demarcation between the pharynx and esophagus. It is composed of the cricopharyngeus muscle proximally and intrinsic esophageal elements distally. The lower esophageal sphincter (1 cm to 4 cm in length) is located partially in both the thorax and the abdomen and straddles the diaphragmatic hiatus. It separates the positive intra-abdominal pressure from the esophagus, where pressure is negative with respect to the atmosphere.

The act of swallowing is a complex mechanism, mediated by several cranial nerves, that results in the well-ordered transport of a bolus from the mouth to the upper esophageal sphincter. Swallowing consists of posterior movement of the tongue, elevation of the soft palate with resultant closure of the nasopharynx, and closure of the respiratory passage by contraction and elevation of the larynx, which abuts the epiglottis. Relaxation of the cricopharyngeus muscle (upper esophageal sphincter) normally occurs at the precise moment at which the bolus reaches the uppermost part of the esophagus.

3

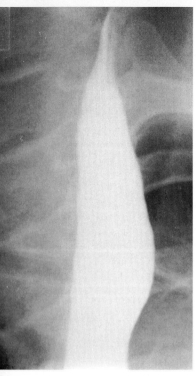

Fig. 1-1. Primary peristalsis. The upper end of the barium column has an inverted V-shaped configuration.

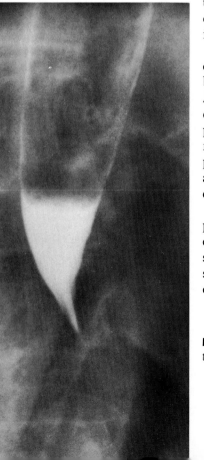

There are three phases of normal esophageal peristaltic activity. Primary peristalsis is the major stripping wave that is initiated by the act of swallowing and that propels ingested material through the entire length of the esophagus into the stomach. The primary wave begins with an inhibitory impulse that passes down the esophagus and relaxes the lower esophageal sphincter before the bolus reaches it.

Secondary esophageal peristalsis consists of stripping waves similar to primary peristalsis but elicited by different stimuli. Rather than beginning with swallowing, as in primary peristalsis, the secondary peristaltic wave occurs in response to distention or irritation anywhere along the esophagus. It begins at the level of the focus of stimulation and propels esophageal contents distally. In effect, secondary peristalsis is a mechanism for ridding the esophagus of refluxed gastric contents or material left from a previous swallow.

The primary and secondary esophageal contraction waves depend on a complex control mechanism composed of a succession of reflex arcs, each of which must function without fault. Sensory receptors located in the mucosal, submucosal, and muscular layers of the esophagus send afferent impulses to the vagal nuclei in the medulla, from which motor impulses pass downward to the myenteric plexuses of Auerbach in the esophageal wall. Integration of segmental motility into an orderly peristaltic contraction is mediated by synaptic connections between the vagal fibers and ganglion cells in the myenteric plexus.

Tertiary contractions (nonperistaltic) are uncoordinated, nonpropulsive, segmental esophageal contractions, the function of which is unknown. Whether tertiary contractions are abnormal is a controversial question. They can be found in many asymptomatic persons and increase in incidence in patients of advanced age.

The three phases of esophageal peristalsis can be well demonstrated on barium swallow. During primary peristalsis, the upper end of the barium column assumes an inverted V-shaped configuration (Fig. 1-1). As the peristaltic wave progresses, the inverted V-shaped tail moves down the esophagus. If the barium column reaches the distal esophagus prior to relaxation of the lower esophageal sphincter, there can be a momentary delay before it enters the stomach. This results in the lower part of the barium column (adjacent to the closed sphincter) assuming a V-shaped configuration, with the proximal margin of the lower esophageal sphincter beginning at the point of the V (Fig. 1-2).

Secondary peristalsis has the same radiographic appearance as a primary contraction wave except that it arises in the body of the esophagus in response to local distention or irritation. The nonpropulsive tertiary waves are seen as annular or segmental contractions that simultaneously displace barium both orally and aborally from the site of contraction, resulting in a to-and-fro motion of the barium.

Fig. 1-2. Closed lower esophageal sphincter causing the V-shaped configuration of the lower part of the barium column.

Disorders of esophageal motility can be conveniently divided according to the component of the process that is involved. There can be abnormalities of (1) striated muscle and the upper esophageal sphincter, (2) smooth muscle or innervation of the body of the esophagus, or (3) the lower esophageal sphincter.

ABNORMALITIES OF STRIATED MUSCLE AND THE UPPER ESOPHAGEAL SPHINCTER (CRICOPHARYNGEAL ACHALASIA)

Disease Entities

Normal variant
Minor, nonspecific neuromuscular dysfunction
Total laryngectomy (pseudodefect)
Primary muscle disorders
    Myasthenia gravis
    Myotonic dystrophy
    Polymyositis
    Dermatomyositis
    Amyotrophic lateral sclerosis
    Steroid myopathy
    Thyrotoxic myopathy
    Oculopharyngeal myopathy
Primary neural disorders
    Peripheral or cranial nerve palsy
    Cerebrovascular disease affecting the brain stem
    High unilateral cervical vagotomy
    Bulbar poliomyelitis
    Syringomyelia
    Huntington's chorea
    Familial dysautonomia (Riley–Day syndrome)
    Multiple sclerosis
    Diphtheria
    Tetanus

Cricopharyngeal achalasia is the failure of pharyngeal peristalsis to coordinate with relaxation of the upper esophageal sphincter. This condition, which occurs without mechanical obstruction or esophageal stenosis, is the result of any lesion that interferes with the complex neuromuscular activity in this region. When relaxation of the cricopharyngeus is incomplete, the characteristic radiographic appearance is that of a hemispherical or horizontal, shelflike posterior protrusion into the barium-filled pharyngoesophageal junction at approximately the C5-6 level (Fig. 1-3). Although the presence of this cricopharyngeus impression indicates the existence of some physiologic abnormality, lesser degrees of it may not be associated with clinical symptoms. More significant neuromuscular abnormalities can result in dysphagia by acting as obstructions to the passage of the bolus (Fig. 1-4). In severe disease, swallowing can result in an overflow of ingested material into

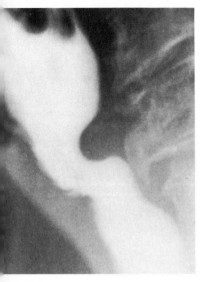

Fig. 1-3. Cricopharyngeal achalasia. A moderate posterior impression is visible on the esophagus of this 60-year-old man who had a cerebrovascular accident.

Fig. 1-4. Cricopharyngeal achalasia. There is a severe posterior impression on the esophagus.

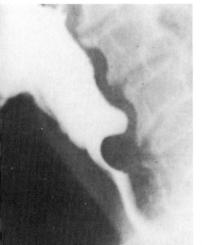

the larynx and trachea and pulmonary complications of aspiration. This severe incoordination of pharyngeal peristalsis and upper esophageal sphincter function can appear on cinefluoroscopy as dilatation and atony of the pyriform sinuses, retention of barium in the valleculae, aspiration into the trachea, regurgitation into the nasopharynx, and apparent obstruction at the level of the cricopharyngeus muscle. When cricopharyngeal achalasia is accompanied by severe dysphagia, cricopharyngeal myotomy can relieve the obstruction created by the nonrelaxing cricopharyngeus muscle.

Cricopharyngeal achalasia has been suggested as an important factor in the development of posterior pharyngeal (Zenker's) diverticula. If relaxation of the cricopharyngeus is inadequate or if the upper esophageal sphincter closes too soon, the elevated intraluminal pressure created by an oncoming peristaltic wave may be responsible for mucosal protrusion through the anatomic weak spot between the oblique and transverse fibers of the cricopharyngeus (Killian's dehiscence), resulting in a Zenker's diverticulum.

TOTAL LARYNGECTOMY (PSEUDODEFECT)

An appearance identical to the posterior cricopharyngeal impression can be demonstrated in patients who have undergone a total laryngectomy for carcinoma (Fig. 1-5). Although total laryngectomy involves removal of the cricoid cartilage, which acts as the anterior fixation point of the cricopharyngeal muscle and should therefore theoretically lead to a patulous cricopharyngeus, the muscle bundles tend to bunch posteriorly when a nerve impulse reaches them, resulting in a characteristic posterior impression. The radiologist must avoid the error of misdiagnosis of recurrent neoplasm in patients who have undergone total laryngectomy and demonstrate a prominent cricopharyngeal muscle defect. Clinically, the patient complains of dysphagia on the way down and dysphonia with esophageal speech on the way up. Because of the substantial incidence of cricopharyngeal problems postoperatively, some surgeons routinely perform a posterior cricopharyngeal myotomy at the time of laryngectomy.

PRIMARY MUSCLE DISORDERS

Primary striated muscle disease can cause failure to develop a good pharyngeal peristaltic wave. Difficulty in swallowing in patients with myasthenia gravis is due to muscular fatigability resulting from the failure of neural transmission between the motor end-plate and muscle fibers. On the initial swallow of barium, peristalsis may appear normal. During repeated swallows, however, peristalsis in the upper esophagus becomes feeble or disappears completely. In patients with myasthenia gravis, peristalsis in the upper esophagus can be demonstrated to improve after the administration of neostigmine or Tensilon (edrophonium).

Myotonic dystrophy is an uncommon hereditary disease in which an anatomic abnormality of the motor end-plate in striated muscle leads to atrophy and inability of the contracted muscle to relax (myotonia). Associated findings include swan neck, frontal baldness in men, testicular atrophy, cataracts, and a characteristic facial expression (myopathic facies). In addition to severely disturbed pharyngeal peristalsis, patients with myotonic dystrophy have reduced or absent resting pressure of the cricopharyngeus muscle. Because a major function of the upper esophageal sphincter is to prevent esophageal contents from refluxing into the pharynx, the diminished resting tone in patients with myotonic dystrophy permits easy regurgitation from the esophagus into the pharynx and leads to a high incidence of aspiration. Reflux across the cricopharyngeus results in the characteristic radiographic pattern of a continuous column of barium extending from the hypopharynx into the cervical esophagus (Fig. 1-6) even during the resting phase, when the patient is not swallowing.

Polymyositis and dermatomyositis are inflammatory degenerative diseases of striated muscle. Weakness and incoordination of the voluntary muscles of the soft palate, pharynx, and upper esophagus in patients with these conditions lead to dysphagia, regurgitation, and a propensity to develop aspiration pneumonia. Similarly, loss of motor-neuron function in patients with amyotrophic lateral sclerosis (Lou Gehrig's disease) results in ineffective pharyngeal peristalsis. Other causes of the inability to develop a good pharyngeal wave and clear the barium meal from the pharynx include (1) myopathies secondary to steroids and abnormal thyroid function and (2) oculopharyngeal myopathy, an extremely rare disease (occurring as a dominant trait especially in families of French-Canadian ancestry) that presents relatively late in life with ptosis and dysphagia.

PRIMARY NEURAL DISORDERS

Diseases of the central and peripheral nervous systems can lead to profound motor incoordination of the pharynx and upper esophageal sphincter. This can be due to peripheral or central cranial nerve palsy or to cerebrovascular occlusive disease affecting the brain stem. A high unilateral cervical vagotomy during extensive head and neck surgery for resection of neoplastic disease can also result in incoordination of upper esophageal motility and sphincter function. Other neurologic causes include bulbar poliomyelitis, syringomyelia, Huntington's chorea, familial dysautonomia (Riley–Day syndrome), multiple sclerosis, diphtheria, and tetanus.

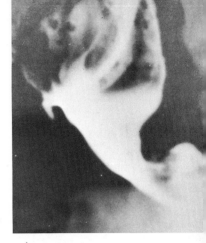

Fig. 1-5. Posterior cricopharyngeal impression following total laryngectomy for carcinoma.

Fig. 1-6. Myotonic dystrophy. A continuous column of barium extends from the hypopharynx into the cervical esophagus, caused by reflux across the level of the cricopharyngeus muscle. (Seaman WB: Functional disorders of the pharyngo-esophageal junction. Radiol Clin North Am 7:113–119, 1969)

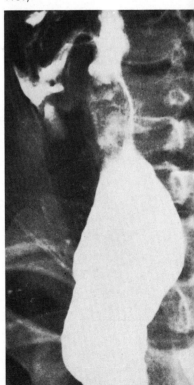

ABNORMALITIES OF SMOOTH MUSCLE AND INNERVATION OF THE BODY OF THE ESOPHAGUS

Disease Entities

Scleroderma
Other connective tissue disorders
   Systemic lupus erythematosus
   Rheumatoid arthritis
   Polymyositis
   Dermatomyositis
Disorders of myenteric plexus
   Achalasia
   Chagas' disease
   Metastases
Esophagitis
   Corrosive
   Reflux
   Infectious
   Radiation-induced
Alcoholic neuropathy
Diabetic neuropathy
Presbyesophagus
Anticholinergic medication
Myxedema
Amyloidosis
Muscular dystrophy

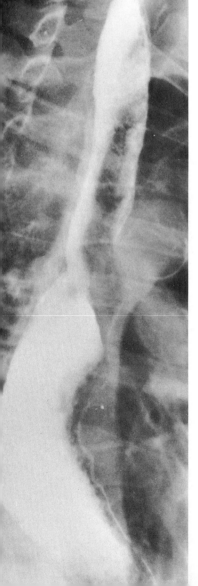

Fig. 1-7. *Scleroderma. There is dilatation of the esophagus with failure of peristaltic activity.*

SCLERODERMA

Atony of the esophagus with failure of peristaltic activity can result from atrophy or cellular disruption of esophageal smooth muscle. In this disorder, the muscular layer of the esophagus is unable to respond to motor impulses transmitted by the vagus nerve.

This mechanism of disordered esophageal motility is best illustrated by scleroderma (Fig. 1-7). The disease frequently (in up to 80% of cases) involves the esophagus, sometimes even before the characteristic skin changes become evident. In scleroderma, there is degeneration and atrophy of smooth muscle in the lower half to two-thirds of the esophagus with subsequent replacement of esophageal musculature by fibrosis. Neural elements, including ganglion cells, are normal.

The patient with diminished esophageal peristalsis due to scleroderma is often asymptomatic. Because the lower esophageal sphincter tone is severely decreased, eating or drinking in the sitting or erect position allows the bolus to be squirted well down the esophagus by the pharyngeal constrictors (striated muscle) and carried by gravity into the stomach. The incompetence of the lower esophageal sphincter, however, permits reflux of acid-pepsin gastric secretions into the distal esophagus. In about 40% of patients, this reflux leads to peptic esophagitis and stricture formation, resulting in heartburn and severe dysphagia.

Because the upper third of the esophagus is composed primarily of striated muscle infrequently affected by scleroderma, a barium swallow demonstrates a normal stripping wave that clears the upper esophagus but stops at about the level of the aortic arch. In early stages of scleroderma, some primary peristaltic activity and uncoordinated tertiary contractions can be observed in the lower two-thirds of the esophagus. However, these contractions are weak and infrequent and tend to disappear as the disease progresses. With the patient in the recumbent position, barium will remain for a long time in the dilated, atonic esophagus (Fig. 1-8). Multiple radiographs obtained several minutes apart can be effectively superimposed on each other. In contrast to the case in achalasia, however, when the patient with scleroderma is placed in the upright position, barium flows rapidly through the widely patent region of the lower esophageal sphincter (Fig. 1-9).

OTHER CONNECTIVE TISSUE DISORDERS

A similar pattern of esophageal atony can be demonstrated in patients with other connective tissue diseases, such as systemic lupus erythematosus (Fig. 1-10), rheumatoid arthritis, polymyositis, or dermatomyositis (in which the proximal, striated muscle esophageal segment is also involved). Regardless of the underlying disease, almost all of these patients with esophageal dysfunction have Raynaud's phenomenon, suggesting that a vasospastic neurogenic abnormality may be responsible for the esophageal aperistalsis.

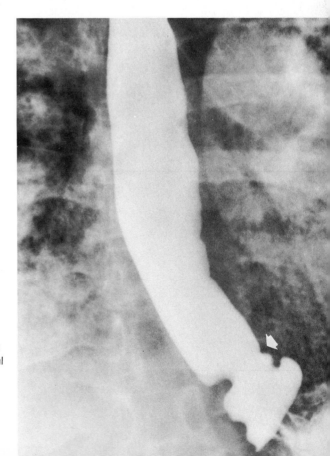

Fig. 1-8. *Scleroderma. There is dilatation of the esophagus with almost no peristalsis to the level of the moderate hiatal hernia* **(arrow).** *Severe pulmonary interstitial changes of scleroderma may be seen bilaterally in the lower lobes.*

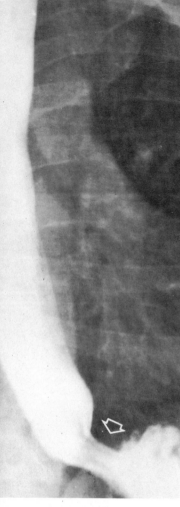 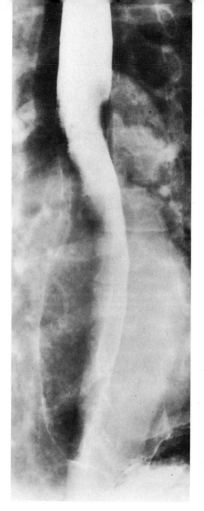

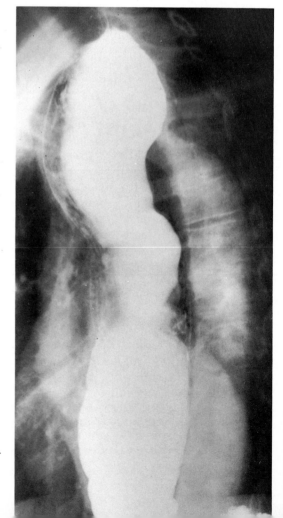

Fig. 1-9. Scleroderma. The esophagus is dilated and atonic, and the esophagogastric junction is patulous **(arrow)**. Surgical clips are from a cervical sympathectomy for Raynaud's phenomenon.

Fig. 1-10. Systemic lupus erythematosus. Esophageal dilatation and atony simulate scleroderma.

Fig. 1-11. Achalasia. There is esophageal dilatation and decreased peristalsis.

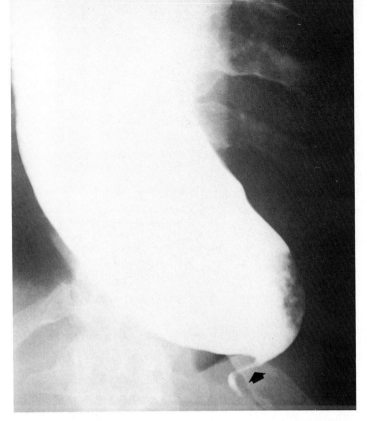

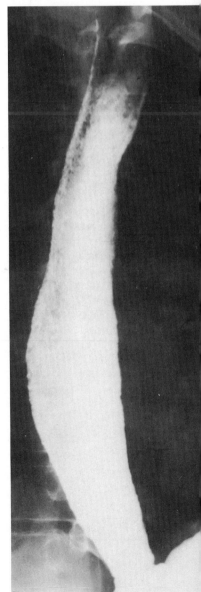

Fig. 1-13. Candidiasis. Aperistalsis and esophageal dilatation are associated with diffuse ulceration.

Fig. 1-12. Achalasia. Severe esophageal dilatation and aperistalsis are apparent. Note the narrowed distal esophagus **(arrow),** which contrasts with the patulous esophagogastric junction in scleroderma.

DISORDERS OF THE MYENTERIC PLEXUS

Failure of peristalsis and a markedly dilated esophagus are typical findings in patients with achalasia (Fig. 1-11). However, this appearance should cause no diagnostic difficulty, since patients with achalasia characteristically have a narrowed distal esophagus because of failure of relaxation of the lower esophageal sphincter (Fig. 1-12), in contrast to patients with scleroderma and other connective tissue disorders, who have a widely patent distal esophagus that frequently permits free gastroesophageal reflux. Destruction of ganglion cells in the myenteric plexus can lead to esophageal aperistalsis simulating achalasia. This can be caused by an inflammatory process, such as Chagas' disease, or by the invasion of tumor cells from a metastatic malignancy.

ESOPHAGITIS

In patients with esophagitis, whether secondary to corrosive agents, reflux, infection, or radiation injury, the earliest and most frequent radiographic abnormality is disordered esophageal motility (Fig. 1-13). Initially, there is failure of primary peristalsis to progress to the stomach, with interruption of the stripping wave in the region of the esophageal inflammation. Repetitive, nonperistaltic tertiary contractions often occur distal to the point of disruption of the primary wave. If the esophagitis is severe, complete aperistalsis can result.

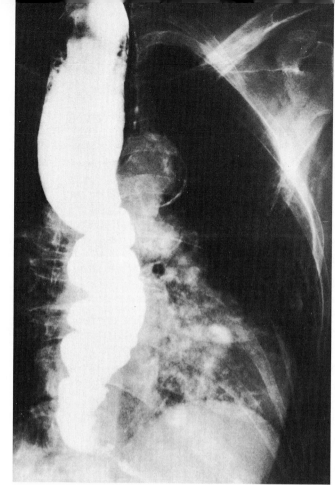

Fig. 1-14. Presbyesophagus. Esophageal dilatation is prominent. Tertiary contractions involve the lower esophagus. When there were no tertiary contractions, esophageal dilatation was relatively uniform. (Zboralske FF, Dodds WJ: Roentgenographic diagnosis of primary disorders of esophageal motility. Radiol Clin North Am 7:147–162, 1969)

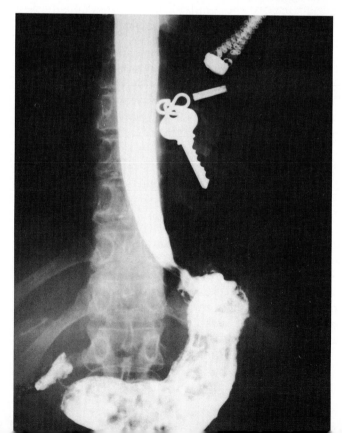

Fig. 1-15. Amyloidosis. Dilatation and weak motor activity of the esophagus are associated with a considerable amount of material retained in the stomach. (Legge DA, Carlson HC, Wollaeger EE: Roentgenologic appearance of systemic amyloidosis involving gastrointestinal tract. AJR 110: 406–412, 1970. Copyright 1970. Reproduced by permission)

An esophageal motor abnormality can often be demonstrated in chronic alcoholics. It is characterized by selective deterioration of esophageal peristalsis, most pronounced in the distal portion, with preservation of sphincter function. The precise mechanism for this disordered motility, though unclear, probably represents a combination of alcoholic myopathy and neuropathy.

In diabetics, especially those with neuropathy of long duration, there is a marked diminution of amplitude of pharyngeal and peristaltic contractions as well as a decreased percentage of swallows followed by progressive peristalsis in the body of the esophagus. This results in a substantial delay in esophageal emptying when the patient is recumbent.

OTHER CAUSES

Presbyesophagus is an esophageal motor dysfunction associated with aging (Fig. 1-14). It is characterized by an inability to initiate and propagate primary peristalsis and by an increase in nonpropulsive tertiary contractions. Concomitant failure of the lower esophageal sphincter to relax produces moderate and even pronounced dilatation of the esophagus.

Anticholinergic agents, such as atropine and Pro-Banthine (propantheline), can cause aperistalsis and dilatation of the esophagus, which mimic the esophageal dysfunction seen in patients with scleroderma. Myxedema can produce a similar pattern. Symptoms of dysphagia and the radiographic appearance of a dilated esophagus with decreased peristalsis are rarely the result of a massive deposition of amyloid in the muscular layers of the esophagus (Fig. 1-15) or a complication of muscular dystrophy.

FAILURE OF RELAXATION OF THE LOWER ESOPHAGEAL SPHINCTER (ACHALASIA PATTERN)

Disease Entities

> Achalasia
> Chagas' disease
> Central and peripheral neuropathy
> > Cerebrovascular accident
> > Postvagotomy syndrome
> > Diabetes mellitus
> > Chronic idiopathic intestinal pseudo-obstruction
> > Amyloidosis
> Malignant lesions
> > Destruction of myenteric plexus
> > Metastases to midbrain vagal nuclei
> > Direct involvement of vagus nerve
> Stricture secondary to reflux esophagitis

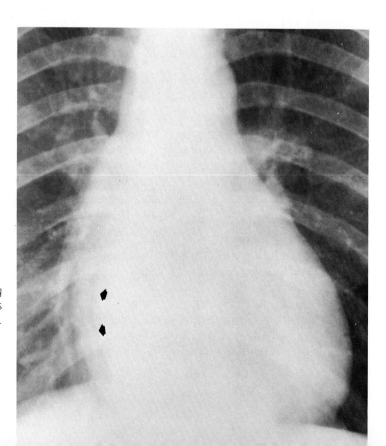

ACHALASIA

Achalasia is a functional obstruction of the distal esophagus with proximal dilatation caused by incomplete relaxation of the lower esophageal sphincter combined with failure of normal peristalsis in the smooth muscle portion of the esophagus (Fig. 1-16). Failure of sphincter relaxation can be defined radiographically as barium retention above the lower esophageal sphincter for longer than 2.5 sec after swallowing. Although the precise pathogenesis of achalasia is not known, the most accepted explanation is a defect in the cholinergic innervation of the esophagus related to a paucity or absence of ganglion cells in the myenteric plexuses (Auerbach) of the distal esophageal wall. This theory is supported by the demonstration in patients with achalasia of a denervation hypersensitivity response of the body of the esophagus to Mecholyl, a synthetic acetylcholine.

In addition to classic achalasia, generalized or localized interruption of the reflex arc controlling normal esophageal motility can also cause failure of relaxation of the lower esophageal sphincter. Thus, diseases of the medullary nuclei, an abnormality of the vagus nerve, or the absence or destruction of myenteric ganglion cells from any cause can produce a similar radiographic pattern.

Most cases of classic achalasia occur in persons between the ages of 20 and 40. Dysphagia is produced by ingestion of either solids or liquids and becomes worse during periods of emotional stress or when the patient is trying to eat rapidly. Regurgitation of retained material is common (it is often provoked by changes in position or by physical

Fig. 1-16. Achalasia. There is failure of relaxation of the region of the distal esophageal sphincter **(arrow)** with severe proximal dilatation.

Fig. 1-17. Plain chest radiograph demonstrating the margin of the dilated, tortuous esophagus **(arrows)** parallel to the right heart border.

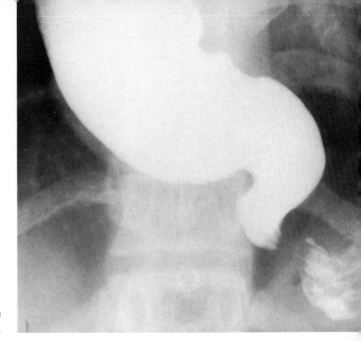

Fig. 1-18. Achalasia. Esophageal dilatation with multiple tertiary contractions is apparent.

exercise) and can result in aspiration and frequent attacks of pneumonia or, in combination with a reduction in food intake, can lead to significant weight loss and nutritional deficiencies.

Radiographic Findings

Plain chest radiographs are frequently sufficient for diagnosis of the achalasia pattern of failure of relaxation of the lower esophageal sphincter. Large amounts of retained food and fluid can be seen in the esophagus. Dilatation and tortuosity of the esophagus can present as a widened mediastinum, often with an air-fluid level, primarily on the right side adjacent to the cardiac shadow (Fig. 1-17). Associated aspiration frequently leads to chronic interstitial pulmonary disease or intermittent episodes of acute pneumonia. The air bubble of the gastric fundus on upright films is small or totally absent.

After the ingestion of barium, the esophagus usually demonstrates weak, nonpropulsive, dysrhythmic peristaltic waves (ripple like activity) that are ineffective in propelling the bolus into the stomach. This disordered esophageal motility is not secondary to distal obstruction related to failure of relaxation of the lower esophageal sphincter; it can antedate the radiographic appearance of distal narrowing and persists even after the narrowing has been successfully overcome by surgery or balloon dilatation. In some cases, multiple tertiary contractions move the bolus up and down the esophagus in an uncoordinated fashion (hyperactive achalasia) (Fig. 1-18). As the disease progresses, marked esophageal distention, elongation, and tortuosity develop (Fig. 1-19).

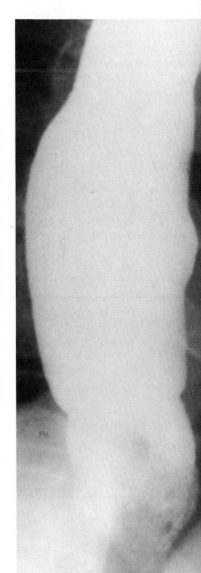

Fig. 1-19. Achalasia. There is marked esophageal dilatation and elongation.

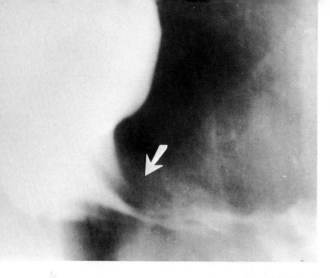

Fig. 1-20. Achalasia. Note the "rat-tail" narrowing of the distal esophageal segment **(arrow).**

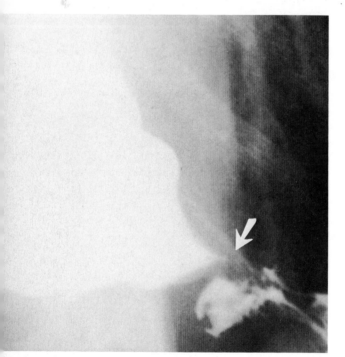

Fig. 1-21. Achalasia. There is characteristic narrowing of the distal esophageal segment ("beak" sign) **(arrow).**

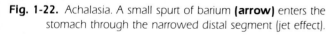

Fig. 1-22. Achalasia. A small spurt of barium **(arrow)** enters the stomach through the narrowed distal segment (jet effect).

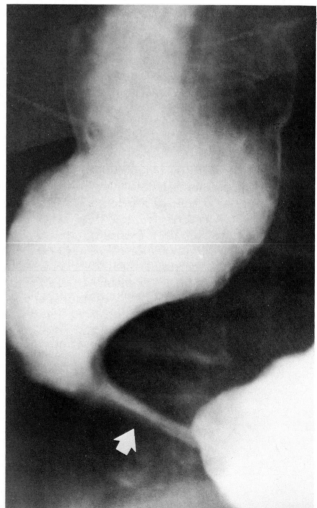

The hallmark of the achalasia pattern is a gradually tapered, smooth, conical narrowing of the distal esophageal segment that extends some 1 cm to 3 cm in length ("rat-tail" or "beak" appearance) (Figs. 1-20, 1-21). Sequential radiographs, especially when the patient is in the erect position, demonstrate small spurts of barium entering the stomach through the narrowed distal segment (Fig. 1-22).

It is essential that the patient suspected of having achalasia be examined in the recumbent position. If the patient is in the erect position, gravity can simulate the effect of peristalsis and hide subtle abnormalities. The upright position is also necessary for the barium column to be high enough to provide adequate hydrostatic pressure to force even small amounts of contrast into the stomach. In patients with achalasia, complete emptying of the esophagus does not occur even in the erect position, a differential point from scleroderma, in which emptying is usually normal when the patient is upright.

CHAGAS' DISEASE

An achalasia pattern is often observed in patients with Chagas' disease, in which destruction of the myenteric plexuses is due to infection by the protozoan *Trypanosoma cruzi* (Fig. 1-23). Trypanosomiasis develops from the bite of an infected reduviid bug and the resultant contamination of the punctured skin by the insect's feces. These blood-sucking insects usually acquire the trypanosomes by feeding on the armadillo, the chief host for the organism. In addition to changes in the esophagus, Chagas' disease can also result in megacolon with chronic constipation, dilatation of the ureters, acute or chronic myocarditis, and infestation of numerous body organs. The effects of Chagas' disease on the esophagus are most likely due to a neurotoxin that attacks and destroys ganglion cells in the myenteric plexuses of the affected organ.

CENTRAL AND PERIPHERAL NEUROPATHY

Central and peripheral neuropathy can result in the achalasia pattern. Brain stem abnormalities due to cerebrovascular accidents or infiltrating processes, such as amyloidosis or malignant lesions, can disrupt the reflex arc and result in failure of relaxation of the lower esophageal sphincter. A similar appearance can reflect a relatively infrequent postoperative complication of bilateral vagotomy. Dysphagia in patients who show this pattern typically occurs with the first ingestion of solid foods on the 7th to 14th postoperative day; the clinical symptoms and radiographic findings usually disappear spontaneously and completely within 2 months. An achalasia pattern can also occur in patients with diabetes, probably because of an arteritis of the vaso vasorum that interferes with the blood supply to the myenteric plexus. In patients with chronic idiopathic intestinal pseudo-obstruction, a radiographic

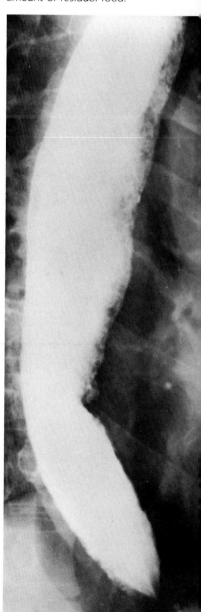

Fig. 1-23. Chagas' disease. There is esophageal dilatation and aperistalsis with a large amount of residual food.

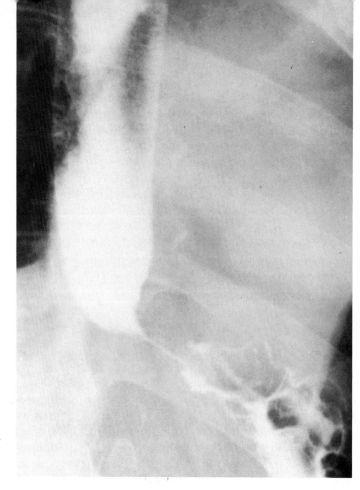

Fig. 1-24. Achalasia pattern (esophageal dilatation with distal narrowing) caused by the proximal extension of carcinoma of the fundus of the stomach.

appearance resembling achalasia has been reported as one of the manifestations of widespread congenital or acquired degeneration of innervation of the entire gut.

MALIGNANT LESIONS

Malignant lesions can produce an achalasia pattern by several mechanisms. Metastases to the midbrain or vagal nuclei, or direct extension of tumor to involve the vagus nerve, can result in failure of relaxation of the lower esophageal sphincter. A similar pattern can be produced by a carcinoma of the distal esophagus or a malignant lesion in the gastric cardia that invades the esophagus and destroys ganglion cells in the myenteric plexus (Fig. 1-24). Carcinoma-induced achalasia has also been reported in patients with pancreatic and bronchogenic carcinoma and in patients with lymphoma of the distal esophagus. Successful removal of the tumor by surgery or irradiation (as in the case of lymphoma) can result in restoration of normal esophageal function.

ESOPHAGITIS

Stricture formation secondary to reflux esophagitis can simulate the narrowed distal esophagus of the achalasia pattern. However, patients with this condition usually have a demonstrable hiatal hernia and a long history of heartburn and regurgitation, facilitating the diagnosis.

DIFFERENTIATION BETWEEN BENIGN AND MALIGNANT CAUSES

Clinical and Radiographic Findings

The major problem in differential diagnosis is to distinguish between nonmalignant causes of the achalasia pattern and carcinoma of the distal esophagus or gastric cardia. This is made especially difficult because of the occurrence of esophageal carcinoma in about 5% to 10% of patients with long-standing achalasia. These squamous cell tumors usually develop in the middle third of the esophagus and are presumed to be induced by chronic irritation of the mucosa caused by constant stasis and the retention of food and fluid secretions. Patients with achalasia who develop carcinoma are generally younger than the average patient with esophageal malignancy. The lesions are often masked by large amounts of residual food and fluid in the esophagus that can obscure the mucosal pattern and produce confusing filling defects on barium examination.

Both clinical and radiographic features can aid in differentiating between benign and malignant causes of the achalasia pattern. Patients with classic benign achalasia are usually less than 40 years old and have symptoms of more than 1 year's duration; those with carcinoma of the esophagus or gastric cardia are generally older (average age, > 60), and a majority have had symptoms for less than 6 months. Melena is unusual in achalasia but common in patients with carcinoma. Radiographically, there is persistence of the normal mucosal pattern in achalasia, in contrast to mucosal destruction or nodularity in carcinoma. The zone of transition in achalasia tapers gradually, unlike the sharply defined, more rapid transition zone between normal esophagus and neoplasm. Severe neuromuscular disturbance of the entire esophagus is common in achalasia but is rarely seen in patients with carcinoma. The distal segment in achalasia has some degree of pliability, in contrast to rigidity and lack of changeability in carcinoma. The presence of a mass in the gas-filled fundus, a deformity of fundal contour, irregular streaming of barium as it flows from the esophagus into the stomach, or an increase in the soft-tissue thickness between the fundus and the diaphragm suggests malignancy.

Pharmacologic Tests

Two pharmacologic tests can aid in establishing the diagnosis of achalasia. In the Mecholyl test, 5 mg to 10 mg of the parasympathomimetic drug is injected subcutaneously. In patients with achalasia, denervation hypersensitivity (Cannon's law) results in a substantial increase in peristaltic activity, though the waves are still ineffective in propelling barium into the stomach. The Mecholyl test is associated with numerous complications, including nausea and vomiting and severe chest pain, and should never be performed in a patient with a history of significant heart disease.

The Seidlitz test, though not infallible, can be helpful in differentiating achalasia from a malignant neoplasm or stricture and has the advantage of being far less uncomfortable for the patient than the Mecholyl test. The ingestion of Seidlitz powder or a carbonated beverage causes the rapid release of carbon dioxide in the esophagus. The resultant acute increase in intraluminal esophageal pressure momentarily distends the contracted distal segment in the case of achalasia but has no effect on the fixed stenosis resulting from a malignant tumor or postinflammatory fibrotic stricture.

TREATMENT OF ACHALASIA

Fig. 1-25. Pneumatic bougie for balloon dilatation of the esophagus in a patient with achalasia.

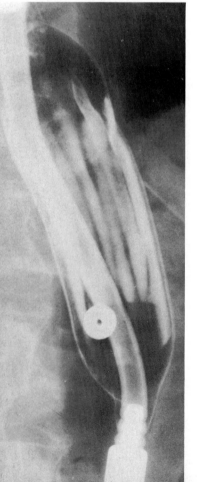

Balloon dilatation or surgery can be used to treat achalasia. Balloon dilatation consists of the placement (under fluoroscopic control) of a pneumatic bougie so that its midportion is positioned at the narrowest level of the gastroesophageal junction (Fig. 1-25). With brisk, rapid dilatation, the radiopaque margin of the balloon is seen to expand the narrowed gastroesophageal segment to the desired degree of dilatation. This "bloodless myotomy" tears the circular muscle fibers of the lower esophageal sphincter in a graded manner, with the operator stopping just short of mucosal penetration. After the procedure, up to 75% of patients can eat a normal diet without dysphagia and have decreased retention of barium in the dilated esophagus.

The most serious, albeit uncommon, complication of balloon dilatation of the lower esophageal sphincter is esophageal rupture. It must be emphasized that esophageal perforation may not be radiographically detectable on a barium swallow obtained immediately after dilatation. Persistent or increasing symptoms in a patient who has undergone this procedure should suggest the possibility of delayed esophageal perforation and the need for a repeat radiographic evaluation.

Surgical therapy of achalasia (Heller myotomy) is designed to disrupt the lower esophageal sphincter from the outside of the esophagus. The operation involves incising the circular muscle fibers down to the mucosa and allowing the mucosa to protrude through. Heller myotomy results in a good clinical and radiographic remission in about 80% of cases. Unfortunately, disruption of the lower esophageal sphincter leads to a substantial incidence of gastroesophageal reflux, which can cause esophagitis and stricture.

Disease Entities

Presbyesophagus
Diffuse esophageal spasm
Esophageal inflammation
   Reflux esophagitis
   Ingestion of corrosive agents
   Infectious esophagitis (*e.g.,* candidiasis)
   Radiation injury
Hyperactive achalasia
Neuromuscular disorders (*e.g.,* diabetes mellitus)
Obstruction of the cardia
   Malignant lesion
   Distal esophageal stricture
   Benign lesion
   Postsurgical repair of hiatal hernia

Tertiary contractions are multiple, irregular, ringlike contractions that occur in the lower two-thirds of the esophagus. These nonpropulsive contractions appear and disappear rapidly, following each other from top to bottom with such speed that they appear to occur simultaneously. This phenomenon appears radiographically as asymmetric indentations of unequal width and depth along the esophagus, with pointed, rounded, or truncated projections between them (Fig. 1-26).

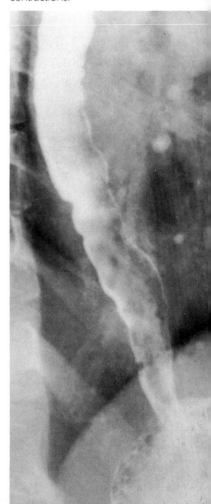

Fig. 1-26. Tertiary contractions.

PRESBYESOPHAGUS

Nonpropulsive tertiary contractions are most commonly seen in patients with presbyesophagus, an esophageal motility disturbance associated with aging (Fig. 1-27). The cause of the disordered motor activity is probably interruption of the reflex arc, which in some cases may be the result of a minor cerebrovascular accident affecting the central nuclei. Most patients with presbyesophagus are asymptomatic; occasionally, a patient experiences moderate dysphagia when eating solid food. The radiographic appearance varies from occasional, mild, nonpropulsive contractions to frequent, strong, uncoordinated ones. Concomitant failure of relaxation of the lower esophageal sphincter can produce moderate dilatation of the esophagus.

DIFFUSE ESOPHAGEAL SPASM

Diffuse esophageal spasm is a controversial entity with a classic clinical triad of massive uncoordinated esophageal contractions, chest pain, and increased intraluminal pressure. Most patients, however, do not manifest all three components. Chest pain is characteristically intermittent and is usually substernal and moderate, though it can be colicky

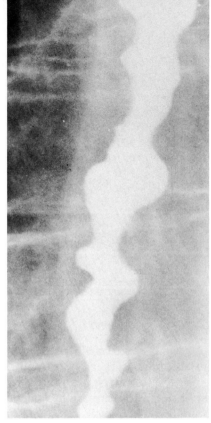

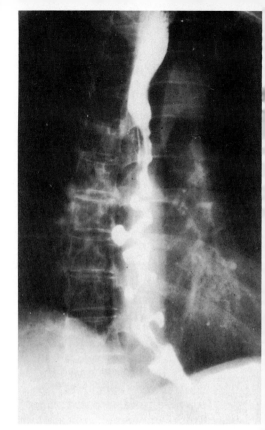

Fig. 1-27. Presbyesophagus. Tertiary esophageal contractions are apparent in this elderly man.

Fig. 1-28　　　　　　　　　　**Fig. 1-29**

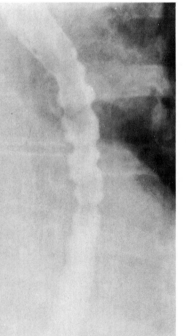

or mimic angina. Symptoms are frequently caused or aggravated by eating but can occur spontaneously and even awaken the patient at night.

Radiographically, peristalsis in the upper esophagus is initiated in response to some and occasionally all swallows, though the wave tends to break at about the level of the aortic arch. In the lower two-thirds of the esophagus, tertiary contractions of abnormally high amplitude can obliterate the lumen and cause compartmentalization of the barium column (Fig. 1-28). These segmental, nonpropulsive contractions can be accompanied by pain and result in barium being displaced both proximally and distally from the site of spasm, producing a corkscrew radiographic appearance of transient sacculations or pseudodiverticula ("rosary bead" esophagus) (Fig. 1-29).

ESOPHAGEAL INFLAMMATION

Reflux esophagitis causes continuous excitation of esophageal sensory receptors, and this can lead to the spillover of impulses to the motor ganglia in the myenteric plexus and result in uncoordinated contractions. These contractions range from mild fasciculations to severe segmental spasms that can be continuous and simulate a fixed stricture. In a similar manner, the ingestion of corrosive agents can act as an irritant and produce strong tertiary contractions. Nonpropulsive waves are also one of the manifestations of abnormal esophageal motility in patients with candida esophagitis (Fig. 1-30), amyloidosis (Fig. 1-31), or postirradiation inflammatory changes in the esophagus (Fig. 1-32).

◀ **Fig. 1-28.** Diffuse esophageal spasm. High amplitude contractions irregularly narrow the lumen of the esophagus.

◀ **Fig. 1-29.** Diffuse esophageal spasm. Pseudodiverticula are in a corkscrew pattern.

Fig. 1-30. Candida esophagitis. Tertiary contractions are assocated with a deep, penetrating ulcer.

Fig. 1-31. Amyloidosis. Tertiary contractions are assocated with diffuse deposition of amyloid within the wall of the esophagus.

Fig. 1-32. Radiation injury. Tertiary contractions are secondary to esophageal motility disturbance due to radiation therapy for carcinoma of the lung. The disordered contractions begin at the upper margin of the treatment port. (Rogers LF, Goldstein HM: Roentgen manifestations of radiation injury to the gastrointestinal tract. Gastrointest Radiol 2:281–291, 1977)

Fig. 1-30

Fig. 1-31

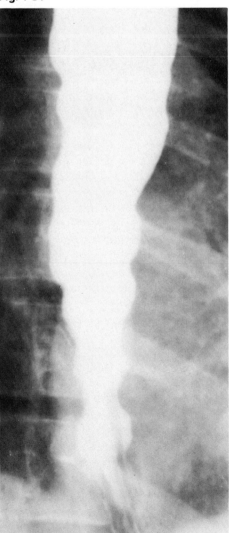

Fig. 1-32

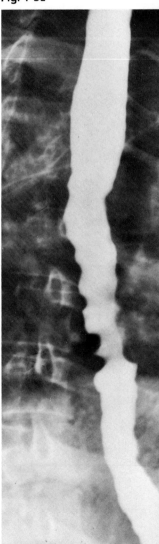

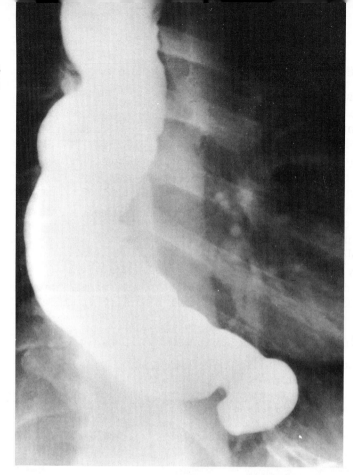

Fig. 1-33. Achalasia. Tertiary contractions are superimposed on a severely dilated esophagus.

Fig. 1-34. Diabetes mellitus. Note the diffuse tertiary contractions.

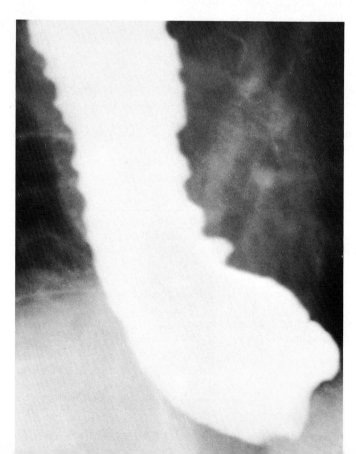

Multiple tertiary contractions can occur during the early stages of achalasia (Fig. 1-33). In this "hyperactive" phase of the disease, uncoordinated muscular activity can cause the bolus to move up and down the esophagus with a to-and-fro motion.

Neuromuscular abnormalities, especially diabetes mellitus, can produce tertiary contractions of the esophagus (Fig. 1-34). This radiographic pattern has also been reported in patients with parkinsonism, amyotrophic lateral sclerosis, multiple sclerosis, thyrotoxic myopathy, and myotonic dystrophy.

Obstruction of the cardia by a malignant neoplasm can result in repetitive, prolonged, high-pressure esophageal contractions. This pattern of tertiary contractions can also be observed in patients who have distal esophageal strictures or benign neoplasms of the cardia, or who have undergone the surgical repair of a hiatal hernia.

BIBLIOGRAPHY

Bennett JR, Hendrix TR: Diffuse esophageal spasm: A disorder with more than one cause. Curr Clin Concepts 59:273–279, 1970

Cohen S: Motor disorders of the esophagus. N Engl J Med 301:184–192, 1979

Davis JA, Kantrowitz PA, Chandler HL et al: Reversible achalasia due to reticulum-cell sarcoma. N Engl J Med 293:130–132, 1975

Dodds WJ: Current concepts of esophageal motor function: Clinical implications for radiology. AJR 128:549–561, 1977

Donner MW, Saba GP, Martinez CR: Diffuse disease of the esophagus: A practical approach. Semin Roentgenol 16:198–213, 1981

Mandelstam P, Siegel CI, Lieber A et al: The swallowing disorder in patients with diabetic neuropathy–gastroenteropathy. Gastroenterology 56:1–12, 1969

Margulis AR, Burhenne HJ: Alimentary Tract Roentgenology. St. Louis, C.V. Mosby, 1973

Margulis AR, Koehler RE: Radiologic diagnosis of disordered esophageal motility: A unified physiologic approach. Radiol Clin North Am 14:429–439, 1976

Ozonoff MB, Flynn FJ: Roentgenologic features of dermatomyositis of childhood. AJR 118:206–212, 1973

Reeder MM, Hamilton LC: Radiologic diagnosis of tropical diseases of the gastrointestinal tract. Radiol Clin North Am 7:57–81, 1969

Rogers LF: Transient post-vagotomy dysphagia: A distinct clinical and roentgenographic entity. AJR 125:956–960, 1975

Seaman WB: Functional disorders of the pharyngo-esophageal junction: Achalasia and chalasia. Radiol Clin North Am 7:113–119, 1969

Seaman WB: Pathophysiology of the esophagus. Semin Roentgenol 16:214–227, 1981

Shulze KS, Goresky CA, Jabbari M et al: Esophageal achalasia associated with gastric carcinoma: Lack of evidence for widespread plexus destruction. Can Med Assoc J 1:857–864, 1975

Simeone J, Burrell M, Toffler R: Esophageal aperistalsis secondary to metastatic invasion of the myenteric plexus. AJR 127:862–864, 1976

Simeone J, Burrell M, Toffler R et al: Aperistalsis and esophagitis. Radiology 123:9–14, 1977

Simpson AJ, Khilnani MT: Gastrointestinal manifestations of the muscular dystrophies. A review of roentgen findings. AJR 125:948–955, 1975

Stewart ET, Miller WN, Hogan WJ et al: Desirability of roentgen esophageal examination immediately after pneumatic dilatation for achalasia. Radiology 130:589–591, 1979

Winship DH, Calfish GR, Zboralske FF et al: Deterioration of esophageal peristalsis in patients with alcoholic neuropathy. Gastroenterology 55:173–178, 1968

Zboralske FF, Dodds WJ: Roentgenographic diagnosis of primary disorders of esophageal motility. Radiol Clin North Am 7:147–162, 1969

Zegel HG, Kressel HY, Levine GM et al: Delayed esophageal perforation after pneumatic dilatation for the treatment of achalasia. Gastrointest Radiol 4:219–221, 1979

2

EXTRINSIC IMPRESSIONS ON THE CERVICAL ESOPHAGUS

Disease Entities

Cricopharyngeus muscle
Pharyngeal venous plexus (postcricoid impression)
Esophageal web
Anterior marginal osteophyte
Anterior herniation of intervertebral disk
Thyroid enlargement
Parathyroid enlargement
Lymph node enlargement
Soft-tissue lesions
    Abscess
    Hematoma
Spinal lesions
    Neoplasm
    Inflammatory

CRICOPHARYNGEUS MUSCLE

Failure of the cricopharyngeus muscle to relax (cricopharyngeal achalasia) can produce a relatively constant posterior impression on the esophagus at about the C5-6 level (Fig. 2-1). A similar posterior impression on the barium-filled esophagus can often be observed after total laryngectomy, and some investigators have attributed this appearance to compensatory hyperactivity of the pharyngeal constrictor muscles.

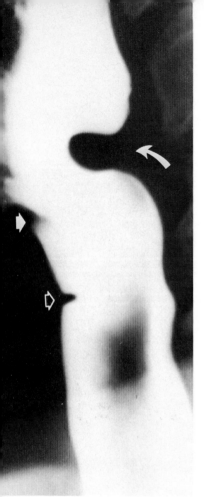

Fig. 2-1. Three impressions on the cervical esophagus: cricopharyngeal impression **(curved arrow)**, pharyngeal venous plexus **(short, closed arrow)**, and esophageal web **(short, open arrow)**. (Clements JL, Cox GW, Torres WE et al: Cervical esophageal webs: A roentgen–anatomic correlation. AJR 121:221–231,1974. Copyright 1974. Reproduced by permission)

PHARYNGEAL VENOUS PLEXUS

An anterior impression on the esophagus at about the C6 level can be caused by the prolapse of lax mucosal folds over the rich central submucosal pharyngeal venous plexus (Fig. 2-2). This "postcricoid impression" occurs as a small indentation just below the slight impression that may be produced by the posterior lamina of the cricoid cartilage. It sometimes has a weblike configuration or is so prominent that it suggests an intramural tumor. The appearance of the postcricoid impression may be seen to vary from swallow to swallow and even during a single swallow recorded on cine or videotape. The impression can frequently (in 70%–90% of adults) be demonstrated on careful study and is usually considered a normal finding.

ESOPHAGEAL WEB

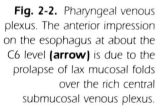

Fig. 2-2. Pharyngeal venous plexus. The anterior impression on the esophagus at about the C6 level **(arrow)** is due to the prolapse of lax mucosal folds over the rich central submucosal venous plexus.

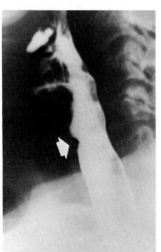

Esophageal webs can present as extrinsic impressions on the barium-filled esophagus (see Fig. 2-1). Although they usually appear as thin, delicate membranes that sweep partially across the lumen, especially at the level of the pharyngoesophageal junction, esophageal webs can produce rounded, masslike impressions. They can be multiple and, since they tend to arise from the anterior wall, are best seen on lateral projection. Esophageal webs never appear on the posterior wall, an important differential distinction from the prominent cricopharyngeus impression, which always arises posteriorly.

ANTERIOR MARGINAL OSTEOPHYTE

Anterior marginal osteophytes of the cervical spine can produce smooth, regular indentations on the posterior wall of the cervical esophagus (Fig. 2-3). Profuse osteophytosis from vertebral margins in diffuse idiopathic skeletal hyperostosis (DISH, or Forrestier's disease) is especially likely to interfere with pharyngoesophageal function. These extrinsic impressions are best seen during complete filling of the esophageal segment and disappear during active contraction. Although usually asymptomatic, osteophytes impinging on the cervical esophagus may produce pain or difficulty in swallowing solids, the sensation of a foreign body, or a constant urge to clear the throat. When a posterior impression on the esophagus is seen at a midcervical intervertebral disk space level, the possibility of the presence of anterior osteophytes must be closely evaluated. Rarely, a similar radiographic appearance is produced by anterior herniation of a cervical intervertebral disk.

THYROID ENLARGEMENT

Enlargement of the thyroid gland often causes compression and displacement of the cervical esophagus (Fig. 2-4). There is usually parallel displacement of the trachea, although, in some cases, a hypertrophic thyroid lobe can insinuate itself between the trachea and esophagus, displacing the trachea anteriorly and the esophagus posteriorly. A thyroid impression on the cervical esophagus can be caused by localized or generalized hypertrophy of the gland, inflammatory disease, or thyroid malignancy. Similarly, enlargement of a parathyroid gland can impinge upon the cervical esophagus. In a patient with symptoms of hyperparathyroidism due to a functioning parathyroid tumor, detection of an extrinsic impression on the cervical esophagus can be of great value in determining the site of the lesion.

OTHER CAUSES

Cervical lymph node enlargement, due to either inflammation or malignancy, can cause an extrinsic impression on the adjacent esophagus. Similarly, abscesses or hematomas in the periesophageal soft tissues can produce indentations on the barium-filled esophagus. The combination of a posterior esophageal impression and vertebral bone destruction suggests the presence of a spinal neoplasm or osteomyelitis.

BIBLIOGRAPHY

Clements JL, Cox GW, Torres WE et al: Cervical esophageal webs: A roentgen-anatomic correlation. AJR 121:221–231, 1974

Pitman RG, Fraser MG: The post-cricoid impression on the oesophagus. Clin Radiol 16:34–39, 1965

Resnick D, Shaul SR, Robins JM: Diffuse idiopathic skeletal hyperostosis (DISH): Forrestier's disease with extraspinal manifestations. Radiology 115:513–524, 1975

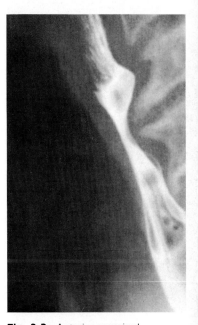

Fig. 2-3. Anterior marginal osteophytes of the cervical spine. A smooth, regular indentation may be seen on the posterior wall at the level of an intervertebral disk space.

Fig. 2-4. Enlargement of the thyroid gland. A smooth impression on the cervical esophagus is evident **(arrow).**

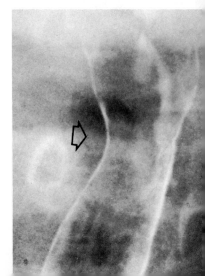

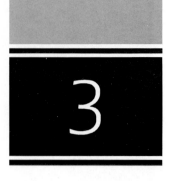

3

EXTRINSIC IMPRESSIONS ON THE THORACIC ESOPHAGUS

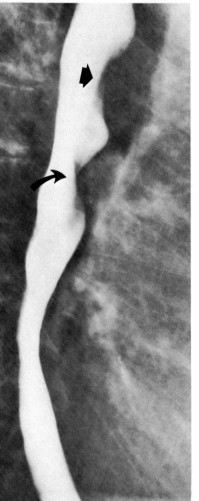

Fig. 3-1. Normal esophageal impressions caused by the aorta **(short arrow)** and left main stem bronchus **(long arrow).**

Normal structures
  Aortic knob
  Left main stem bronchus
  Left inferior pulmonary vein/confluence of left pulmonary veins
Vascular abnormalities
  Aortic lesions
    Right aortic arch
    Cervical aortic arch
    Double aortic arch
    Coarctation of the aorta
    Aortic aneurysm/tortuosity
  Nonaortic lesions
    Aberrant right subclavian artery
    Aberrant left pulmonary artery
    Anomalous pulmonary venous return (type III)
    Persistent truncus arteriosus
Cardiac enlargement
  Left atrium
  Left ventricle
Pericardial lesion
  Effusion
  Tumor
  Cyst
Mediastinal mass
  Tumor
  Duplication cyst
Pulmonary mass
  Tumor
  Bronchogenic cyst
Lymph node enlargement
Paraesophageal hernia
Apical pleuropulmonary fibrosis (pseudoimpression)

During its course through the thorax, the esophagus runs through the posterior portion of the middle mediastinum and is in intimate contact with the aorta and its branches, the tracheobronchial tree, the heart, the lungs, and the interbronchial lymph nodes. Abnormalities in any of these or other structures in the middle or posterior portion of the mediastinum can compress or displace adjacent segments of the esophagus.

NORMAL STRUCTURES

Two structures normally indent the anterior and lateral aspects of the thoracic esophagus (Fig. 3-1). The more cephalad normal impression, which is due to the transverse arch of the aorta (aortic knob), is more prominent as the aorta becomes increasingly dilated and tortuous with age. The more caudal impression is caused by the left main stem bronchus.

In about 10% of patients, the left inferior pulmonary vein or a common confluence of the left pulmonary veins near their insertion into the left atrium produces an extrinsic indentation on the anterior left wall of the esophagus about 4 cm to 5 cm below the carina (Fig. 3-2). This impression is best seen in a steep left posterior oblique horizontal position. The vascular nature of the indentation can be confirmed by Valsalva and Müller maneuvers, in which the impression becomes smaller and more prominent, respectively.

VASCULAR ABNORMALITIES

RIGHT AORTIC ARCH

Vascular lesions of the aorta and its branches, as well as of the pulmonary arteries and veins, can cause extrinsic impressions on the thoracic esophagus. The most common aortic anomaly is a right-sided aortic arch (Fig. 3-3). This condition is easily detected on plain chest radiographs by the absence of the characteristic left aortic knob and its replacement by a slightly higher bulge on the right. The trachea is seen to deviate to the left, and the barium-filled esophagus is indented on the right.

When the aortic arch is right-sided, the descending aorta can run on either the right or the left. If it descends on the right, the brachiocephalic vessels can originate in one of three ways. With the mirror-image pattern, no vessels cross the mediastinum posterior to the esophagus, and, consequently, there is no esophageal indentation on the lateral projection. This anomaly is frequently associated with congenital heart disease, primarily tetralogy of Fallot.

The other two anomalies associated with a right-sided aortic arch and right descending aorta differ with respect to the origin of the left subclavian artery. In the more common type, the left subclavian artery arises as the most distal branch of the aorta (reverse of the aberrant

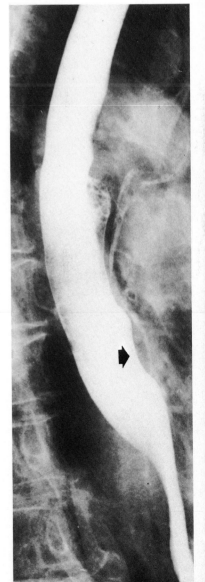

Fig. 3-2. Normal pulmonary venous indentation **(arrow)** on the anterior left wall of the distal esophagus, best seen in a steep left posterior oblique projection. (Yeh HC, Wolf BS: A pulmonary venous indentation on the esophagus—A normal variant. Radiology 116:299–303, 1975)

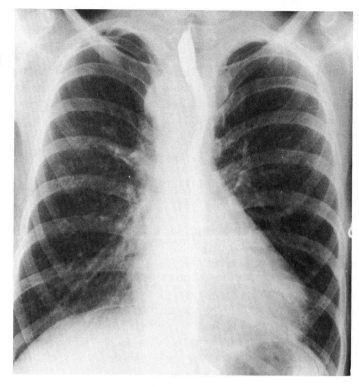

Fig. 3-3. Right-sided aortic arch (pseudotruncus).

Fig. 3-4. Aberrant left subclavian artery with right aortic arch. **(A)** A posterior impression on the esophagus is visible on the oblique view. **(B)** The right aortic arch is evident on the frontal view.

A B

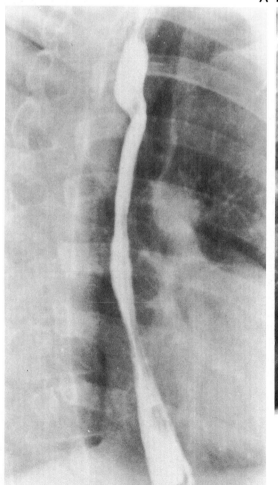

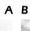

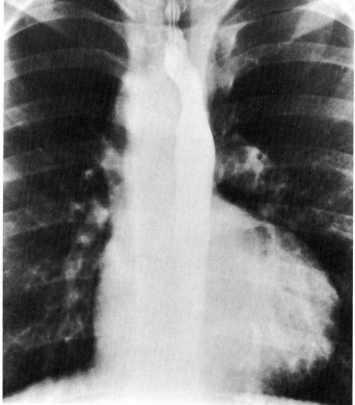

right subclavian artery, which originates from a left aortic arch). In order to reach the left upper extremity, the left subclavian artery must course across the mediastinum posterior to the esophagus, producing a characteristic oblique posterior indentation on the esophagus (Fig. 3-4). Almost all patients with this anomaly have no associated congenital heart disease.

In the second type of anomaly, the left subclavian artery is atretic at its base and totally isolated from the aorta (isolated left subclavian artery). In this rare condition, the left subclavian artery receives blood from the left pulmonary artery, or from the aorta in a circuitous fashion through retrograde flow by way of the ipsilateral vertebral artery (congenital subclavian steal syndrome). The tenuous blood supply in patients with this condition often results in decreased pulses and ischemia of the left upper extremity.

A right aortic arch with left descending aorta is an uncommon anomaly. Because the aortic knob is on the right and the aorta descends on the left, the transverse portion must cross the mediastinum. This usually occurs posterior to the esophagus, resulting in a prominent posterior esophageal indentation that tends to be more transverse and much larger than that seen with an aberrant left subclavian artery.

CERVICAL AORTIC ARCH

A posterior impression on the esophagus associated with a pulsatile mass above the clavicle suggests the diagnosis of a cervical aortic arch (Fig. 3-5). The pulsatile mass may be mistaken for an aneurysm of the subclavian, carotid, or innominate artery. No coexistent intracardiac congenital heart disease has been described in the few cases reported. The posterior esophageal impression is caused by the distal arch or proximal descending aorta as it courses in a retroesophageal position.

Fig. 3-5. Cervical aortic arch. **(A)** Posterior esophageal impression caused by the retroesophageal course of the distal arch or the proximal descending aorta. **(B)** Subtraction film from an aortogram demonstrating the aortic arch extending into the neck.

A B

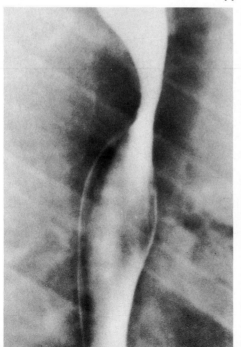
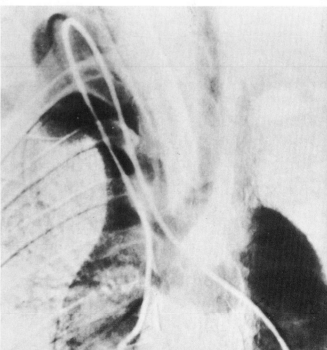

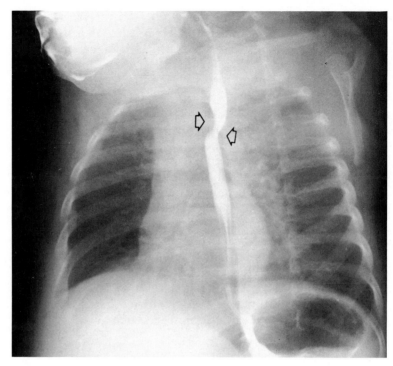

Fig. 3-6. Double aortic arch. Characteristic reverse S-shaped indentation on the esophagus **(arrows).** As usual, the right (posterior) arch is higher and larger than the left (anterior) arch. (Swischuk LE: Radiology of the Newborn and Young Infant. Baltimore, Williams & Wilkins, 1980)

DOUBLE AORTIC ARCH

In most patients with a double aortic arch, the aorta ascends on the right, branches, and finally reunites on the left. The two limbs of the aorta completely encircle the trachea and esophagus, forming a ring. The anterior portion of the arch is usually smaller than the posterior part. When the aorta descends on the left (in about 75% of cases), the posterior arch is higher than the anterior arch; the reverse pattern is seen if the aorta descends on the right.

On plain chest radiographs, the two aortic limbs can appear as bulges on either side of the superior mediastinum, the right usually being larger and higher than the left. On barium swallow, a double aortic arch produces a characteristic reverse S-shaped indentation on the esophagus (Fig. 3-6). The upper curve of the S is produced by the larger posterior arch; the lower curve is related to the smaller anterior arch. Infrequently, a patient with a double aortic arch can have anterior and posterior esophageal indentations directly across from each other rather than in an S-shaped configuration.

The reverse S-shaped indentation of the esophagus is typical of all true vascular rings. For example, the vascular ring formed by an ascending right aortic arch, a left subclavian artery passing posteriorly to the esophagus, and a persistent ductus or ligamentum arteriosus extending from the left subclavian artery to the pulmonary artery produces a double impression on the esophagus essentially identical to that seen with a double aortic arch.

Coarctation of the aorta can produce a characteristic "figure-3" sign on plain chest radiographs (Fig. 3-7A) and a reverse figure-3 or "figure-E" impression on the barium-filled esophagus (Fig. 3-7B). The more cephalad bulge represents dilatation of the proximal aorta and base of the left subclavian artery (prestenotic dilatation); the lower bulge reflects poststenotic aortic dilatation. Coarctation of the aorta usually occurs at or just distal to the level of the ductus arteriosus; much less frequently, the area of narrowing lies proximal to this point. In the latter type of coarctation, a ventricular septal defect and patent ductus arteriosus are always present so that blood can be delivered to the descending aorta from the pulmonary artery through the patent ductus.

Most patients with coarctation of the aorta do not develop symptoms until late childhood or early adulthood. Narrowing of the aorta causes systolic overloading and hypertrophy of the left ventricle. There is usually a substantial difference in blood pressure between the upper and lower extremities. The relative obstruction of aortic blood flow leads to the progressive development of collateral circulation, often seen radiographically as rib notching (usually involving the posterior fourth to eighth ribs), caused by pressure erosion by the dilated, pulsating collateral vessels (Fig. 3-7C). Dilatation of mammary artery collaterals can produce retrosternal notching.

AORTIC ANEURYSM / TORTUOSITY

Elongation and unfolding of the descending thoracic aorta is frequently accompanied by a concomitant impression on the thoracic esophagus. Tortuosity of the epiphrenic segment of the aorta usually causes a sicklelike deformity with characteristic displacement of the esophagus anteriorly (Fig. 3-8A) and to the left (Fig. 3-8B). Localized aneurysmal dilatation of a segment of the thoracic aorta can also indent an adjacent portion of the esophagus.

ABERRANT RIGHT SUBCLAVIAN ARTERY

The most common nonaortic vascular lesion producing an impression on the barium-filled thoracic esophagus is an aberrant right subclavian artery. This artery, the last major vessel of the aortic arch, arises just distal to the left subclavian artery. In order to reach the right upper extremity, the aberrant right subclavian artery must course across the mediastinum behind the esophagus, and this produces a posterior esophageal indentation (Fig. 3-9A). On the frontal view, the esophageal impression runs obliquely upward and to the right (Fig. 3-9B). This appearance is so characteristic that no further radiographic investigation is required. An aberrant right subclavian artery rarely produces symptoms (other than occasional dysphagia), is usually an incidental finding during an upper gastrointestinal examination performed for other purposes, and is not associated with congenital heart disease.

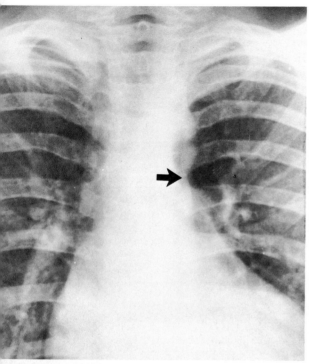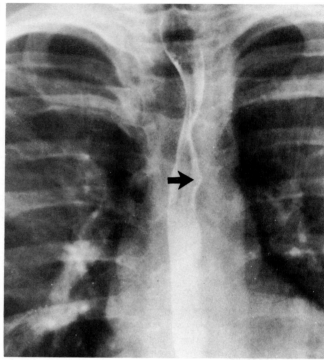

A B
C

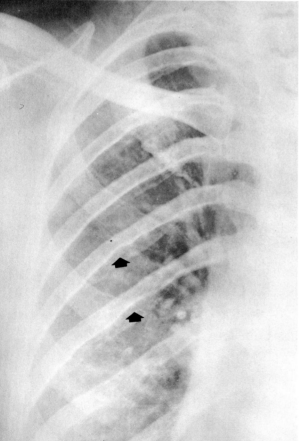

Fig. 3-7. Coarctation of the aorta. **(A)** Plain chest radiograph demonstrates the "figure-3" sign (the **arrow** points to the center of the 3). The upper bulge represents prestenotic dilatation, whereas the lower bulge represents poststenotic dilatation. **(B)** Barium swallow demonstrates the "reverse figure-3" sign (the **arrow** points to the center of the reverse figure-3). **(C)** Rib notching. There is notching of the posterior fourth through eighth ribs (the **arrows** point to two examples). (Swischuk LE: Plain Film Interpretation in Congenital Heart Disease. Baltimore, Williams & Wilkins, 1979)

ABERRANT LEFT PULMONARY ARTERY

Other nonaortic vascular impressions on the esophagus are rare. An aberrant left pulmonary artery arises from the right pulmonary artery and must cross the mediastinum to reach the left lung. As it courses between the trachea and esophagus, it produces a characteristic impression on the posterior aspect of the trachea just above the carina and a corresponding indentation on the anterior wall of the barium-filled esophagus (Fig. 3-10).

ANOMALOUS PULMONARY VENOUS RETURN

In patients with anomalous pulmonary venous return, blood from the lungs returns to the right side of the heart (right atrium, coronary sinus, or systemic vein) rather than emptying normally into the left atrium. In almost all cases, the anomalous pulmonary veins unite to form a single vessel posterior to the heart before entering a cardiac chamber or systemic vein. In the type-III anomaly, the anomalous pulmonary

Fig. 3-8. Tortuosity of the descending thoracic aorta producing characteristic displacement of the esophagus **(A)** anteriorly and **(B)** to the left. Note the retraction of the upper esophagus to the right. This is caused by chronic inflammatory disease, which simulates an extrinsic mass arising from the opposite side.

A B

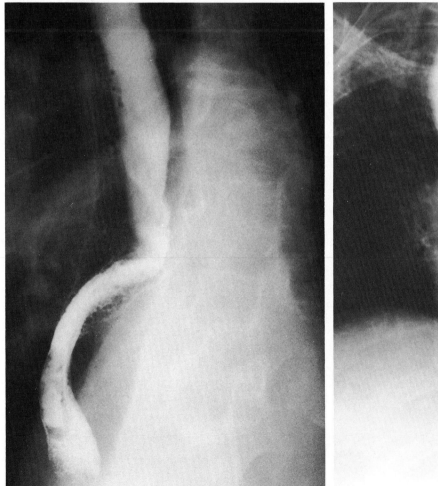
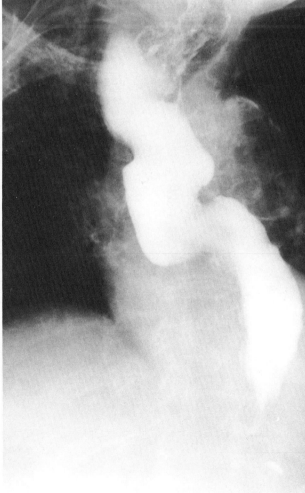

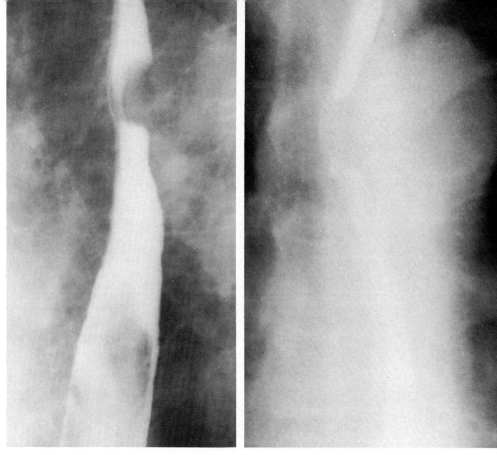

A B

Fig. 3-9. Aberrant right subclavian artery. **(A)** Posterior esophageal indentation on lateral view. **(B)** Esophageal impression running obliquely upward and to the right on frontal view.

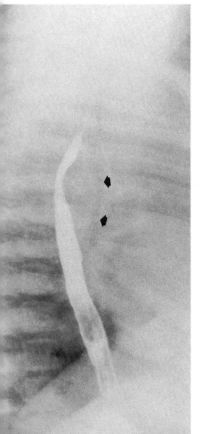

vein travels with the esophagus through the diaphragm and inserts into a systemic vein or, more commonly, into the portal vein, usually producing an anterior indentation on the lower portion of the barium-filled esophagus (Fig. 3-11). It is important to note that this indentation occurs above the diaphragm but slightly below the expected site of left atrial indentation.

PERSISTENT TRUNCUS ARTERIOSUS

Persistent truncus arteriosus is a relatively uncommon anomaly that is due to the failure of the common truncus arteriosus to divide normally into the aorta and pulmonary artery. This results in a single vessel draining both ventricles and supplying the systemic, pulmonary, and coronary circulations. In one form of persistent truncus arteriosus, the pulmonary artery is absent and the lungs are supplied by collateral bronchial arteries. These dilated bronchial vessels, which can be quite large, produce discrete indentations on the posterior wall of the esophagus (Fig. 3-12) that are somewhat lower than those usually seen with aberrant left subclavian arteries.

Fig. 3-10. Aberrant left pulmonary artery. The vessel crosses the mediastinum between the trachea **(arrows)** and the esophagus, producing impressions on the anterior aspect of the esophagus and the posterior margin of the trachea.

Fig. 3-11. Anomalous pulmonary venous return (type III). There is an anterior indentation on the lower border of the barium-filled esophagus **(arrow),** slightly below the expected site of the left atrium.

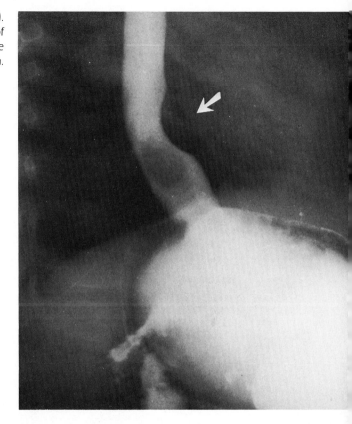

Fig. 3-12. Persistent truncus arteriosus. **(A)** Characteristic indentation on the posterior wall of the esophagus, which is somewhat lower than usually seen with an aberrant left subclavian artery. **(B)** Frontal view demonstrating a right-sided impression on the esophagus.

A B

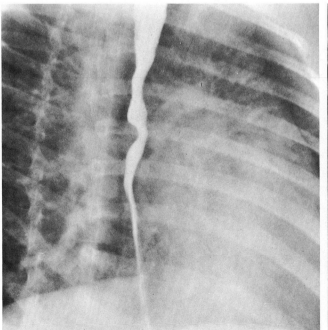
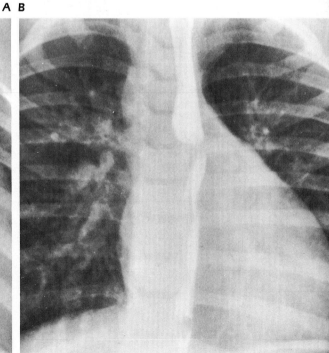

LEFT ATRIUM

The left atrium is in direct contact with the anterior aspect of the esophagus. Enlargement of the left atrium, whether secondary to congenital heart disease, as in ventricular septal defect, patent ductus arteriosus, or double outlet right ventricle (Fig. 3-13), acquired mitral valve disease (Fig. 3-14), or left atrial tumor (Fig. 3-15), produces a characteristic anterior impression and posterior displacement of the esophagus beginning about 2 cm below the carina. The impression of an enlarged left atrium on the barium-filled esophagus is best seen in the lateral and right anterior oblique projections. On the posteroanterior view, enlargement of the left atrium produces some displacement of the esophagus to the right. Even minimal left atrial enlargement can be detected on barium swallow; however, it must be remembered that slight esophageal indentation at this level may also be seen in some normal persons. Therefore, this finding must be correlated with clinical history and other radiographic signs of left atrial enlargement (*e.g.*, posterior displacement of the left main stem bronchus, widening of the carina, bulging in the region of the left atrial appendage, "double density" on the frontal view).

Fig. 3-13. Enlargement of the left atrium due to a double outlet right ventricle.

A B

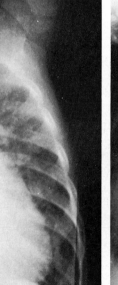
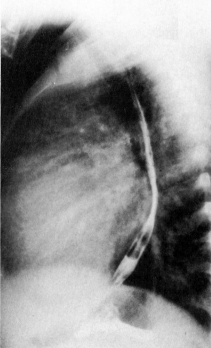

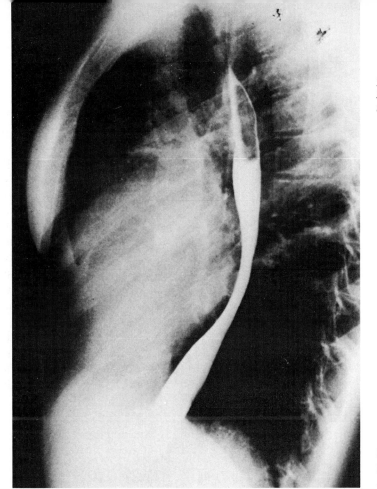

Fig. 3-14. Enlargement of the left atrium secondary to acquired mitral valve disease.

Fig. 3-15. Enlargement of the left atrium caused by a calcified left atrial tumor **(arrow).**

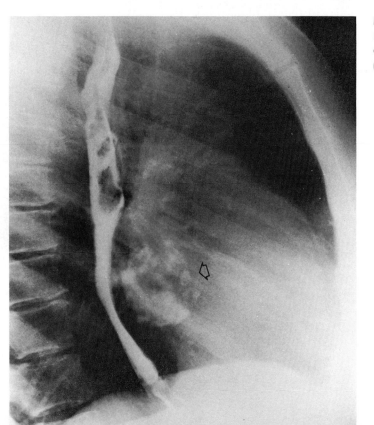

LEFT VENTRICLE

Enlargement of the left ventricle also produces anterior indentation and posterior displacement of the esophagus (Fig. 3-16). Whether secondary to aortic valvular disease or to cardiac failure, the enlarged left ventricle causes an esophageal impression that is best appreciated on the lateral view. The indentation is situated at a level somewhat inferior to the impression caused by an enlarged left atrium.

OTHER CAUSES

PERICARDIAL LESIONS

Just as enlargement of specific heart chambers results in esophageal indentation, so can a lesion of the pericardium. Pericardial tumors and cysts can cause localized impressions on the anterior aspect of the barium-filled esophagus; pericardial effusions tend to produce broader impressions on the esophagus.

INTRATHORACIC MASSES

Any mass lesion adjacent to the esophagus that arises within the mediastinum (Fig. 3-17), lung (Fig. 3-18), trachea, or lymph nodes can impress the barium-filled esophagus. Depending on the size and position of the mass, there can be a focal (Fig. 3-19) or broad (Fig. 3-20) impression on the esophagus and displacement of the esophagus in any direction. The most common entities producing esophageal impressions by this mechanism are inflammatory and metastatic lesions involving lymph nodes in the carinal and subcarinal regions.

PARAESOPHAGEAL HERNIA

The supradiaphragmatic portion of the stomach in a patient with a paraesophageal hernia can cause an impression on the distal esophagus as it courses toward the esophagogastric junction, which remains normally positioned below the diaphragm (Fig. 3-21). In this condition, the distal esophagus is usually displaced posteriorly and to the right, the extent of the impression depending on the amount of herniated stomach above the diaphragm.

APICAL PLEUROPULMONARY FIBROSIS

A "pseudoimpression" on the upper thoracic esophagus can be caused by apical pleuropulmonary fibrosis. This complication of chronic inflammatory disease, most commonly tuberculosis, produces retraction of the esophagus toward the side of the lesion, which can simulate the radiographic appearance of an extrinsic mass arising from the opposite side (see Fig. 3-8B). The margin of the esophagus on which the traction is exerted assumes an asymmetric pseudodiverticular appearance.

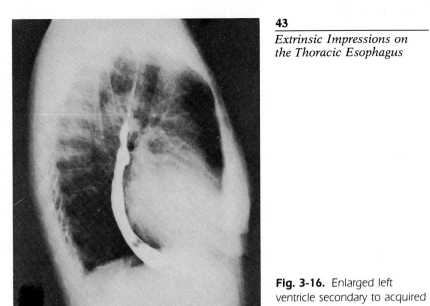

Fig. 3-16. Enlarged left ventricle secondary to acquired aortic stenosis.

Fig. 3-17. Enlargement of a substernal thyroid causing an impression on the upper thoracic esophagus.

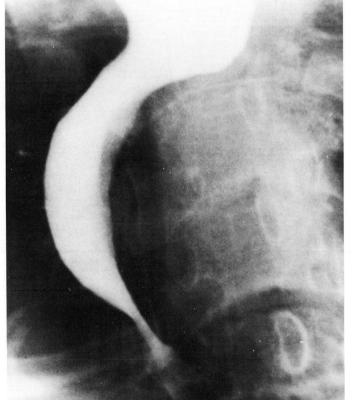

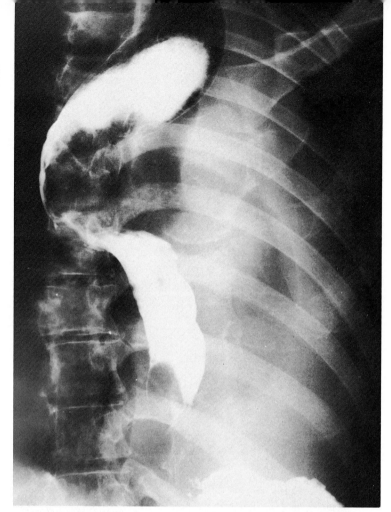

Fig. 3-18. Squamous carcinoma of the lung impressing and invading the midthoracic esophagus.

Fig. 3-19. Calcified mediastinal lymph nodes at the carinal level **(arrow)** causing a focal impression and displacement of the esophagus.

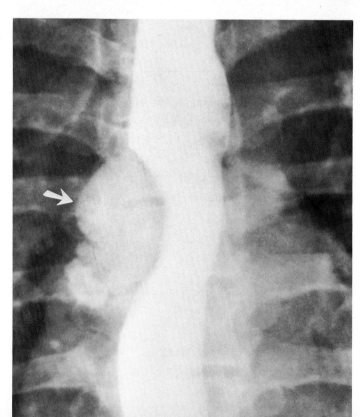

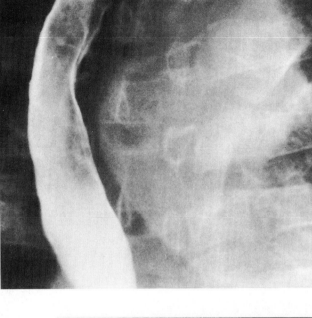

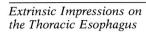

Fig. 3-20. Squamous
carcinoma of the lung
producing a broad impression
on the upper thoracic
esophagus.

Fig. 3-21. Paraesophageal
hernia impressing the distal
esophagus.

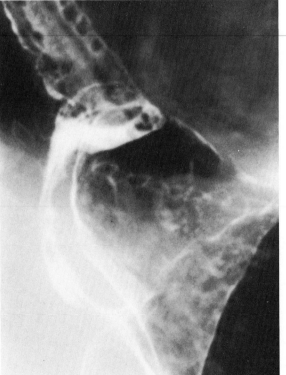

Esophagus

Margulis AR, Burhenne HJ: Alimentary Tract Roentgenology. St. Louis, C.V. Mosby, 1973

Shuford WH, Sybers RG, Milledge RD et al: The cervical aortic arch. AJR 116:519–527, 1972

Swischuk LE: Plain Film Interpretation in Congenital Heart Disease. Baltimore, Williams & Wilkins, 1979

Yeh HC, Wolf BS: A pulmonary venous indentation on the esophagus: A normal variant. Radiology 116:229–303, 1975

4

ESOPHAGEAL ULCERATION

Disease Entities

Reflux esophagitis
   Hiatal hernia
   Vomiting secondary to intra-abdominal disease
   Chalasia of infancy
   Pregnancy
   Scleroderma
   Medication
   Surgery
Barrett's esophagus
Infectious/granulomatous disorders
   Candidiasis
   Herpes simplex
   Tuberculosis
   Syphilis
   Histoplasmosis
   Crohn's disease
   Eosinophilic esophagitis
Malignant lesions
   Carcinoma
   Lymphoma
Corrosive esophagitis
Radiation injury
Drug-induced esophagitis
   Potassium chloride tablets
   Tetracycline
   Emepronium bromide
   Quinidine
   Ascorbic acid
Intramural pseudodiverticulosis

47

REFLUX ESOPHAGITIS

The most common cause of esophageal ulceration is esophagitis due to reflux of gastric or duodenal contents into the esophagus (Fig. 4-1). In most cases, a combination of gastric acid and pepsin causes mucosal irritation of the esophagus. Reflux esophagitis can occur even in the absence of stomach acid because of regurgitation of alkaline bile and pancreatic juice, which act as corrosive irritants to the esophageal mucosa.

PREDISPOSING CONDITIONS

Reflux esophagitis occurs when the lower esophageal sphincter fails to act as an effective barrier to stomach contents entering the distal esophagus. Rather than a simple mechanical barrier, the lower esophageal sphincter is a complex, dynamic structure that responds to a variety of physical, humoral, and neural stimuli to prevent reflux. Functional or structural changes at the gastroesophageal junction can disrupt the effectiveness of the barrier mechanism, thereby increasing the likelihood of reflux and the development of esophagitis and ulceration.

Fig. 4-1. Reflux esophagitis. Two dense lines of barium representing ulcers are surrounded by lucent rings of edema. The two views reveal distal mucosal irregularity, ulceration, and fold thickening.

A B

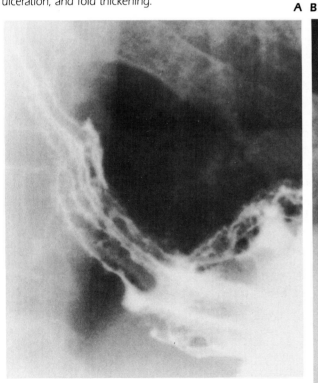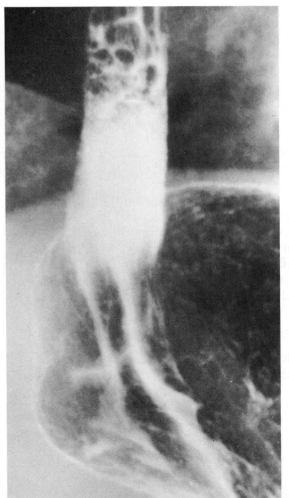

There is a higher than normal likelihood of gastroesophageal reflux in patients with sliding hiatal hernias. However, it must be emphasized that the competence of the lower esophageal sphincter is not dependent on its being situated above the diaphragm. In one endoscopic study, reflux esophagitis was observed in only 26% of patients with sliding hiatal hernias. Conversely, esophagitis is often encountered in patients in whom no hiatal hernia can be demonstrated. Reflux of acidic gastric contents into the esophagus can be caused by prolonged or repeated vomiting secondary to peptic ulcer, biliary colic, intestinal obstruction, acute alcoholic gastritis, pancreatitis, or migraine, or by vomiting following surgery or during pregnancy. Prolonged nasogastric intubation can decrease the competence of the lower esophageal sphincter and facilitate gastroesophageal reflux and subsequent esophagitis.

Chalasia is a functional disturbance in which the lower esophageal sphincter fails to remain normally closed between swallows, thereby permitting regurgitation of large amounts of gastric contents through it. Found during the immediate postnatal period, chalasia is a cause of vomiting in infants. However, as an infant matures, the development of neuromuscular control increases the competency of the lower esophageal sphincter, and free gastroesophageal reflux gradually disappears. Persistence of vomiting and reflux after several months suggests an abnormal sphincter or sliding hiatal hernia. Regurgitation and vomiting beginning after infancy are also abnormal and can result in nocturnal emesis, aspiration of gastric contents, and pulmonary complications.

Up to half of pregnant women experience heartburn, usually during the third trimester. These women demonstrate a reduction in lower esophageal sphincter pressure that returns to normal levels after delivery. This reversible incompetence of the lower esophageal sphincter is probably of hormonal origin and appears to reflect a generalized smooth muscle response to female hormones.

A patulous lower esophageal sphincter predisposing to reflux esophagitis is characteristically seen in patients with scleroderma (Fig. 4-2). Incompetence of the lower esophageal sphincter can also be related to drugs, such as anticholinergics, nitrites, beta-adrenergic agents, and some tranquilizers.

Surgical procedures in the region of the gastroesophageal junction can impair the normal function of the lower esophageal sphincter. Severing of the oblique muscles of the distal esophagus (Heller procedure for achalasia), total gastrectomy, and esophagocardiectomy can lead to reflux esophagitis. The disorder is particularly severe after vagotomy if the resulting stasis of gastric contents has not been relieved by a suitable drainage procedure.

CLINICAL SYMPTOMS

The symptoms of reflux esophagitis are due to gastric acid or alkaline bile and pancreatic juice irritating the distal esophageal mucosa. The

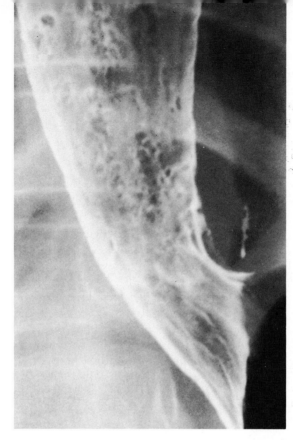

Fig. 4-2. Reflux esophagitis in scleroderma. Note the patulous esophagogastric junction.

most common symptom is heartburn, an uncomfortable burning sensation that starts below the sternum and tends to move up into the neck, waxing and waning in intensity. The retrosternal burning often occurs after eating and is aggravated by the ingestion of very hot or cold liquids, coffee, citrus juices, or alcoholic beverages. Reflux symptoms can be precipitated by any change in position that compresses the abdomen or increases intragastric pressure, such as bending or stooping, picking up objects from the floor, or lying flat after eating a large meal.

Regurgitation of gastric contents into the mouth is another classic symptom of reflux. This most frequently occurs during sleep and leads to the appearance of fluid on the pillow. The presence of gastric contents can cause a sour or metallic taste in the throat and mouth. Regurgitation implies severe reflux and often leads to aspiration and pulmonary complications.

Some patients with reflux have dysphagia. This does not reflect an organic stricture of the esophagus, since most patients with reflux esophagitis who have dysphagia have a normal intraluminal diameter. Hemorrhage related to esophagitis is usually a steady oozing of blood from the distal esophagus. Penetrating ulcers of the esophagus can cause brisk arterial bleeding.

A number of radiographic approaches have been suggested for demonstration of gastroesophageal reflux. One procedure is to increase intra-abdominal pressure by straight-leg raising or manual pressure on the abdomen with or without a Valsalva maneuver. Another approach is the water-siphon test, the significance of which is controversial. To perform this study, the physician pools barium in the cardia of the stomach (or in a hiatal hernia sac, if present) by turning the supine patient about 45° on his right side. The patient is then given several swallows of plain water. As the lower esophageal sphincter relaxes to allow passage of the water, barium may reflux from the stomach into the esophagus. Small amounts of reflux may be within normal limits. Reflux of barium of more than a few centimeters, however, is considered abnormal. At times, contrast can reflux as high as the aortic arch. Another method for demonstrating reflux is to have the patient change his position. As the patient turns from prone to supine or vice versa (either during fluoroscopy or for overhead views), reflux of barium from the stomach into the esophagus can often be detected.

It must be remembered that failure to demonstrate reflux radiographically does not exclude the possibility that a patient's esophagitis is related to reflux. As long as typical radiographic findings of reflux esophagitis are noted, there is little reason to persist in strenuous efforts to actually demonstrate retrograde flow of barium from the stomach into the esophagus. Conversely, demonstration of reflux in the absence of other radiographic findings in the distal esophagus does not permit the radiographic diagnosis of esophagitis. Whether or not reflux will lead to the development of esophagitis depends on such factors as the frequency with which the reflux occurs, the efficiency of secondary peristalsis in removing refluxed contents from the esophagus, and the acidity of the gastric contents. The presence or absence of a sliding hiatal hernia is of little practical significance, since reflux is not directly related to the presence of a hernia but rather is due to incompetence of the lower esophageal sphincter.

A new radionuclide technique for demonstrating and measuring gastroesophageal reflux is to scan the lower esophagus and stomach after the oral administration of ^{99m}Tc DTPA (Fig. 4-3). If no spontaneous reflux of radionuclide from the stomach into the distal esophagus is observed, an abdominal binder is used to raise intragastric pressure. This radionuclide technique has been reported to have an accuracy rate of about 90% in demonstrating gastroesophageal reflux.

RADIOGRAPHIC FINDINGS

Compared with direct esophagoscopy, the barium swallow has been considered a relatively insensitive procedure for demonstrating early esophageal changes consistent with reflux esophagitis. As the severity

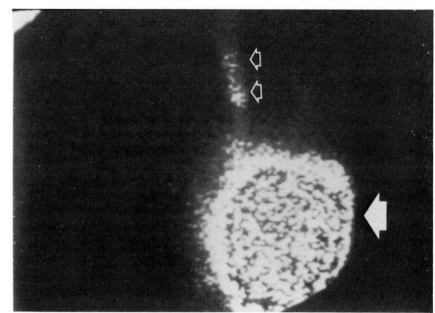

Fig. 4-3. Gastroesophageal reflux. Note the reflux of radionuclide into the esophagus **(small, open arrows)** from the stomach **(large, solid arrow)** following the oral administration of ^{99m}Tc DTPA.

Fig. 4-4. Reflux esophagitis. Superficial ulcerations or erosions appear as streaks or dots of contrast superimposed on the flat mucosa of the distal esophagus.

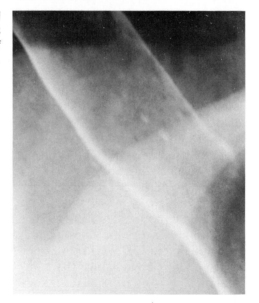

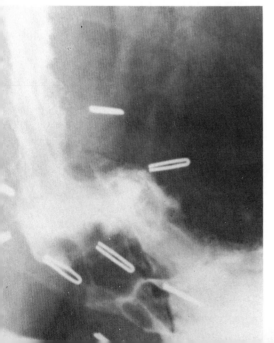

Fig. 4-5. Esophagitis following a failed Nissen procedure for a hiatal hernia and gastroesophageal reflux. The margins of the distal esophagus appear hazy and serrated.

of esophageal inflammation increases, the sensitivity and accuracy of the barium swallow improve.

The earliest radiographic findings in reflux esophagitis are detectable on double-contrast studies. They consist of superficial ulcerations or erosions that appear as streaks or dots of barium superimposed on the flat mucosa of the distal esophagus (Fig. 4-4). These ulcers often have a linear configuration and may be associated with fine radiating folds and slight retraction of the esophageal wall. In single-contrast studies of patients with esophagitis, the outer borders of the barium-filled esophagus are not sharply seen, but rather have a hazy, serrated appearance with shallow, irregular protrusions that are indicative of erosions of varying length and depth (Fig. 4-5). This marginal serration must be distinguished from the fine, regular transverse folds (feline esophagus, so named because it is characteristic of the distal third of the esophagus of the cat) that are found in normal patients, especially with the double-contrast technique (Fig. 4-6). These folds are transient in nature, are often seen on only one of a number of spot films during a given examination, and are probably caused by contraction of the muscularis mucosae. Instead of the normal, fine, sharply demarcated longitudinal folds of the collapsed esophagus, in esophagitis there is a

Fig. 4-6. Normal transverse esophageal folds (feline esophagus). (Gohel VK, Edell SL, Laufer I et al: Transverse folds in the human esophagus. Radiology 128:303–308, 1978)

A B

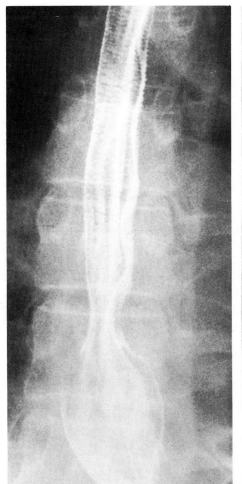
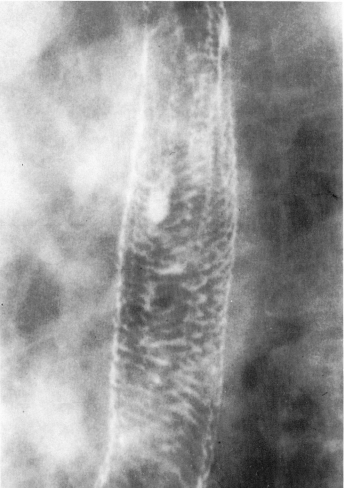

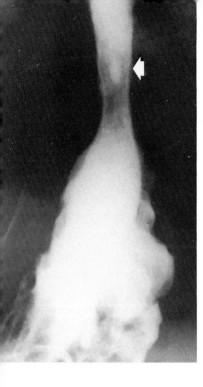

Fig. 4-7. Large, penetrating ulcer **(arrow)** in reflux esophagitis.

smudgy, irregular pattern of residual barium. In more severe disease, obvious erosions can be seen extending even into the midesophagus. Widening and coarsening of edematous longitudinal folds can simulate filling defects.

In addition to diffuse erosion, reflux esophagitis can result in large penetrating ulcers (marginal ulcers) in the region of the junction between the esophagus and stomach or hiatal hernia sac (Fig. 4-7), or in the hiatal hernia sac itself (Fig. 4-8). In about 15% of patients, a marginal ulcer penetrates through the wall of the esophagus into adjacent vital structures. Free perforation, though uncommon, is associated with such complications as peritonitis, subphrenic abscess, mediastinitis, pericarditis, and empyema. Marginal ulcers have a radiographic appearance similar to gastric ulcers due to chronic peptic disease. A nichelike projection is surrounded by intramural inflammation (ulcer collar), often with much local esophageal spasm and narrowing. Healing of a large or penetrating esophageal ulcer can result in stricture formation (Fig. 4-9).

Fig. 4-8. Two examples of ulcers **(arrows)** in large hiatal hernia sacs.

A B

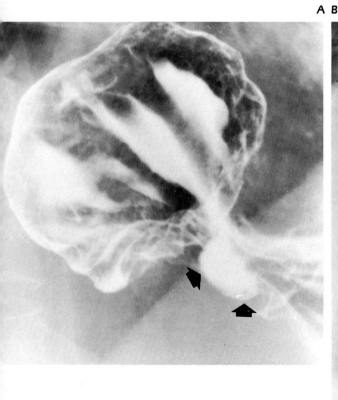
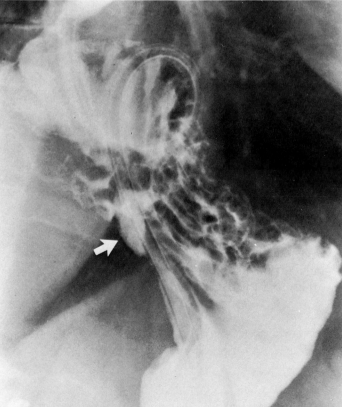

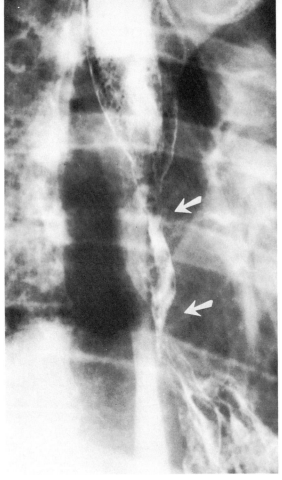

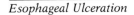

Fig. 4-9. Stricture **(arrows)** following healing of reflux esophagitis.

Fig. 4-10. Barrett's esophagus. Ulcerations **(arrow)** have developed at a distance from the esophagogastric junction.

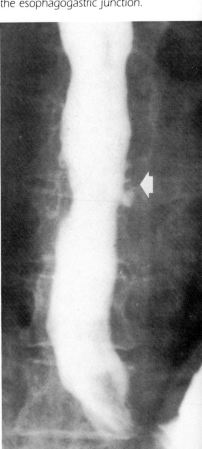

BARRETT'S ESOPHAGUS

Barrett's esophagus is a condition in which the normal stratified squamous lining of the lower esophagus is replaced by columnar epithelium similar to that of the stomach. This process is presumed to occur as a complication of reflux esophagitis, especially in view of the frequency with which the syndrome is associated with a sliding hiatal hernia and demonstrable gastroesophageal reflux.

RADIOGRAPHIC FINDINGS

Esophageal ulceration in Barrett's esophagus can occur anywhere along the columnar epithelium and tends to develop at a distance from the cardia, even as high as the aortic arch (Fig. 4-10). Unlike the shallow ulceration usually caused by reflux esophagitis in the squamous epithelium, the Barrett's ulcer tends to be deep and penetrating and identical to peptic gastric ulceration (Fig. 4-11). Stricture formation usually accompanies the ulceration. Not infrequently, no ulceration is evident, and only a smooth, tapered stricture is seen.

A sliding hiatal hernia with gastroesophageal reflux is commonly demonstrated in patients with Barrett's esophagus. In most cases, however, the Barrett's ulcer is separated from the hiatal hernia by a variable length of normal-appearing esophagus (Fig. 4-12), in contrast to reflux esophagitis, in which the distal esophagus is abnormal down to the level of the hernia.

Radionuclide examination with intravenous pertechnetate can be used to demonstrate a Barrett's esophagus. Because this radionuclide is actively taken up by the gastric type of mucosa, continuous concentration of the isotope in the distal esophagus to a level that corresponds approximately to that of the ulcer or stricture is indicative of a Barrett's esophagus and may obviate the need for mucosal biopsy (Fig. 4-13).

In addition to postinflammatory stricture, Barrett's esophagus has an unusually high propensity for developing malignancy in the columnar-lined portion (Fig. 4-14). In one series, adenocarcinoma, which is usually very rare in the esophagus, developed in 10% of patients with Barrett's esophagus.

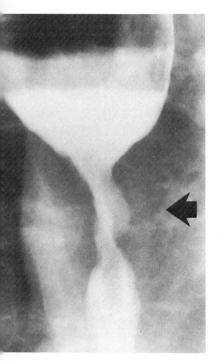

Fig. 4-11. Barrett's esophagus. Note the deep ulcer **(arrow)** with stricture formation.

Fig. 4-12. Barrett's esophagus. Several centimeters of relatively normal-appearing, nondilated esophagus separate the Barrett's ulcer **(arrow)** from the hiatal hernia sac.

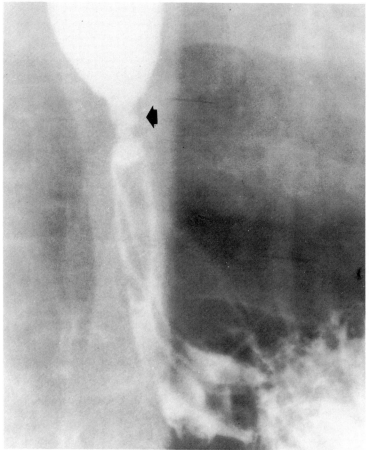

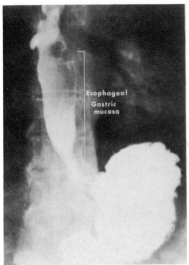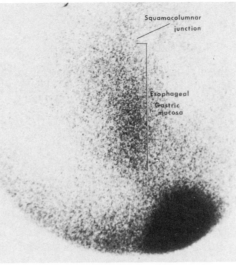

A B

Fig. 4-13. Barrett's esophagus. (A) Barium swallow. (B) ^{99m}Tc pertechnetate scintigram. The uptake of isotope extends above the esophagogastric junction to a level comparable to the esophageal stricture and ulcer on the radiograph. (Berquist TH, Nolan NG, Stephens DH et al: Radioisotope scintigraphy in diagnosis of Barrett's esophagus. AJR 123:401–411, 1975. Copyright 1975. Reproduced by permission)

CANDIDA ESOPHAGITIS

The most common infectious disease of the esophagus is candidiasis, caused by the usually harmless fungus *Candida albicans. Candida* is found in the mouth, throat, sputum, and feces of many normal children and adults. Acute infection by *Candida* develops when there is an immunologic imbalance between the host and the normal body flora. Esophageal candidiasis occurs most frequently in patients with leukemia or lymphoma and in patients receiving radiation therapy, chemotherapy, corticosteroids, or other immunosuppressive agents. Chronic debilitating diseases predisposing to the development of esophageal candidiasis include diabetes mellitus, systemic lupus erythematosus, multiple myeloma, primary hypoparathyroidism, and renal failure. Esophageal candidiasis can be found in otherwise healthy adults who have received antibiotics (especially tetracycline) for upper respiratory infection. It has been suggested that the fungi overgrow in this case because they do not have to compete for nutritive substances with the normal bacterial flora that have been destroyed by the antibiotics. Esophageal candidiasis has been reported as a complication of stasis secondary to functional or mechanical obstruction. On rare occasions, candidal infection may occur in patients who are in apparently good health and have no predisposing disease.

The symptoms of esophageal candidiasis can be acute or insidious. In acute disease, adynophagia (pain associated with swallowing) is usually intense and is localized to the upper retrosternal area, often radiating into the back. Chest pain may precede dysphagia and be so severe that a myocardial infarction is suggested. It is important to remember that esophageal candidiasis can occur with minimal or absent oral involvement (thrush). If it is promptly treated, complete recovery can be rapid. If the organism enters the circulation through ruptured esophageal vessels, systemic invasion can lead to the dissemination of *Candida* to other organs and often to a fatal outcome.

Fig. 4-14. Adenocarcinoma developing in Barrett's esophagus. Fungating filling defects in the lower third of the esophagus (**black arrows**) are associated with a small, sliding hiatal hernia. The **white arrow** points to the squamocolumnar junction. (Cho KJ, Hunter TB, Whitehouse WM: The columnar epithelial-lined lower esophagus and its association with adenocarcinoma of the esophagus. Radiology 115:563–568, 1975)

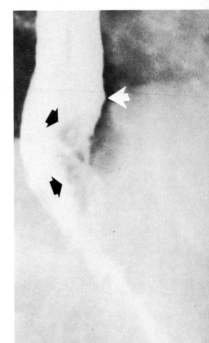

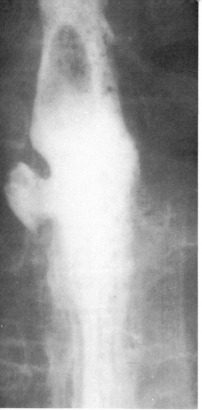

Fig. 4-15

Fig. 4-16

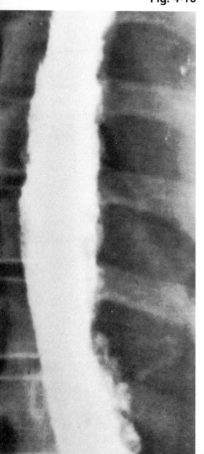

RADIOGRAPHIC FINDINGS

The radiographic changes in candidiasis frequently involve the entire thoracic esophagus, though the upper half is often relatively spared. Early in the course of disease, an esophagram generally shows only abnormal motility and a slightly dilated, virtually atonic esophagus. The earliest morphologic changes are small, marginal filling defects (simulating tiny air bubbles) with fine serrations along the outer border. As the disease progresses, an irregular cobblestone pattern is produced that reflects either submucosal edema in combination with ulceration or small pseudomembranous plaques composed of fungi and debris that cover the ulcerated esophageal mucosa (Fig. 4-15). The nodular appearance of the esophageal surface can also be due to the direct seeding of *Candida* colonies on the mucosa. The classic radiographic appearance of esophageal candidiasis is a shaggy marginal contour caused by deep ulcerations and sloughing of the mucosa (Fig. 4-16). Ulcerations are multiple and of varying size (Fig. 4-17); the intervening esophageal contour is nodular, with irregular round and oval defects that can resemble varices. The overlying pseudomembrane occasionally partially separates from the esophageal wall, permitting barium to penetrate under it and form a double track paralleling the esophageal lumen.

In patients with a hematologic malignancy or chronic debilitating disease, or in patients who have recently undergone a course of antibiotic or chemotherapy, the development of dysphagia and retrosternal pain should strongly suggest the diagnosis of esophageal candidiasis. A barium swallow usually confirms the diagnosis; only if the radiographic findings are not diagnostic is esophagoscopy indicated.

HERPETIC ESOPHAGITIS

A clinical and radiographic pattern indistinguishable from *Candida* esophagitis can be caused by herpes simplex infestation (Fig. 4-18). Herpetic esophagitis predominantly affects patients with disseminated malignancy or abnormal immune systems. Although the radiographic appearance of ulcers and plaquelike defects closely resembles candidiasis (Fig. 4-19), the presence of discrete ulcers on an otherwise normal background mucosa has been reported as strongly suggestive of herpetic esophagitis. Because the viral inflammation is usually self-limited, a

---

Fig. 4-15. Candidiasis. A nodular cobblestone pattern is seen in combination with large, discrete ulceration.

Fig. 4-16. Candidiasis. The shaggy marginal contour is caused by deep ulcerations and sloughing of the mucosa.

Fig. 4-17. *Candidiasis. Diffuse transverse ulcerations are evident with irregular esophageal narrowing. (Ott DJ, Gelfand DW: Esophageal stricture secondary to candidiasis. Gastrointest Radiol 2:323–325, 1978)*

Fig. 4-18. *Herpetic esophagitis. The diffuse irregularity and ulceration are indistinguishable from* Candida *esophagitis.*

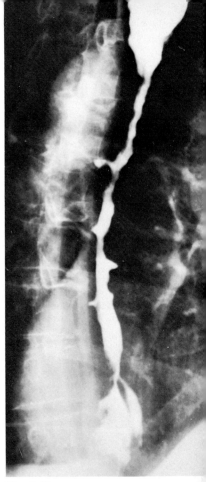

Fig. 4-17

Fig. 4-18

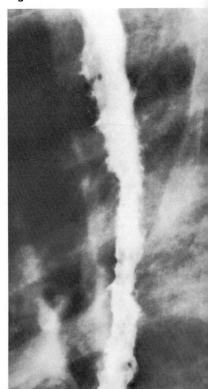

response to antifungal therapy cannot be considered proof that the characteristic radiographic changes are the result of *Candida* infection. For the diagnosis of herpetic esophagitis to be made, esophagoscopy with biopsy and cytology is required.

TUBERCULOUS ESOPHAGITIS

Tuberculosis of the esophagus is rare and almost invariably secondary to terminal disease in the lungs. Tuberculous involvement of the esophagus can result from the swallowing of infected sputum, direct extension from laryngeal or pharyngeal lesions, or contiguous extension from caseous hilar lymph nodes or infected vertebrae; it also can be part of generalized, disseminated miliary disease.

The most common manifestation of tuberculosis of the esophagus is single or multiple ulcers (Fig. 4-20). An intense fibrotic response often causes narrowing of the esophageal lumen. Numerous miliary granulomas in the mucosal layer occasionally give the appearance of multiple nodules. Sinuses and fistulous tracts are common; their presence in a patient with severe pulmonary tuberculosis who has a midesophageal ulcer or stricture in the region of the tracheal bifurcation should suggest a tuberculous etiology.

OTHER INFECTIOUS / GRANULOMATOUS CAUSES OF ESOPHAGITIS

One of the many appearances of syphilis involving the esophagus is fine mucosal irregularity or frank esophageal ulceration. An ulcerated midesophageal mass due to lymph node erosion can be seen in patients with mediastinal histoplasmosis. On rare occasions, diffuse or discrete esophageal ulceration can be demonstrated in patients with Crohn's disease of the esophagus. In patients with Crohn's disease elsewhere, the presence of esophageal ulceration, especially if it is associated with intramural fistulous tracts, should suggest the possibility of the same disease involving the esophagus (Fig. 4-21). Findings of mild esophagitis can progress to a cobblestone appearance of the mucosa and the development of intramural sinus tracts, esophagorespiratory fistula, or esophageal stenosis. Nodularity and fine superficial ulcerations have

Fig. 4-19. Herpetic esophagitis. Fine ulcerations are superimposed on a pattern of thickened folds and plaquelike defects.

Fig. 4-20. Tuberculosis. A large, midesophageal ulcer **(arrow)** with surrounding inflammatory edema mimics carcinoma. Note the generalized irregularity which represents diffuse ulcerative disease.

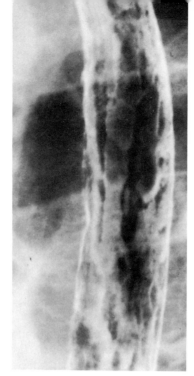

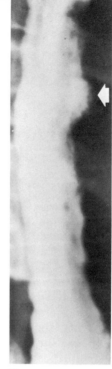

Fig. 4-19

Fig. 4-20

Fig. 4-22. Eosinophilic esophagitis. Fine, superficial ulcerations are visible with diffuse nodularity. (Picus D, Frank PH: Eosinophilic esophagitis. AJR 136:1001–1003, 1981. Copyright 1981. Reproduced by permission)

Fig. 4-23. Squamous carcinoma of the esophagus. Note the eccentric, ulcerated mass **(arrows)**.

Fig. 4-21. Crohn's disease. Long, intramural sinus tract **(arrow)**.

Fig. 4-22

Fig. 4-23

Fig. 4-21

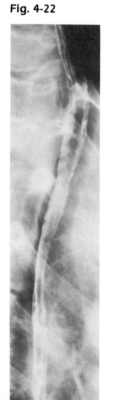

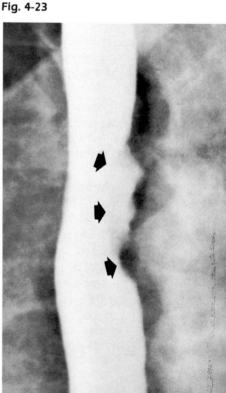

been described in a single case of esophagitis with peripheral and submucosal eosinophilia resembling eosinophilic gastroenteritis (Fig. 4-22).

CARCINOMA OF THE ESOPHAGUS

Carcinoma of the esophagus (95% squamous cell) is frequently associated with some degree of mucosal ulceration (Fig. 4-23). An ulcerating carcinoma typically appears as a crater surrounded by a bulging mass projecting into the esophageal lumen (Fig. 4-24). When examined in profile, the underside of the oval ulcer niche is often found to be bordered by a clear ridge extending from its upper to its lower limits, an excellent sign of malignancy. The ulcerated surface is rigid and remains unchanged by the passage of barium or primary peristaltic waves (Fig. 4-25). The wall opposite the niche may be normal but often demonstrates irregularity and lack of pliability, indicating mucosal destruction from an infiltrating tumor. In the relatively uncommon primary ulcerative esophageal carcinoma, ulceration of virtually all of an eccentric, flat mass produces a meniscoid appearance analogous to the Carman sign seen with gastric malignancy (Fig. 4-26, 4-27). Ulceration in a polypoid mass or an area of irregular narrowing is an infrequent manifestation of lymphoma of the esophagus.

CORROSIVE ESOPHAGITIS

The ingestion of corrosive agents causes acute and chronic inflammatory changes that are most commonly seen in the lower two-thirds of the esophagus (Fig. 4-28A). The most severe corrosive injuries are caused by alkali (lye, dishwasher detergents, washing soda) that penetrate the layers of the esophagus and cause a severe liquefying necrosis. Ingestion of acids (sulfuric, nitric, hydrochloric) is less likely to produce severe damage because of coagulation of the superficial layers, which forms a firm eschar limiting penetration to the deeper layers. The harmful effect of ingested acid is also partially neutralized by the alkaline pH of the esophagus.

Mucosal ulceration always occurs following the ingestion of corrosive materials. Superficial penetration of the toxic agent results in only minimal ulceration with mild erythema or mucosal edema. Deeper penetration into the submucosal and muscular layers causes sloughing of destroyed tissue and deep ulceration. In such cases, the resultant granulation tissue with numerous fibroblasts leads to the deposition of collagen, fibrous scarring, and gradual narrowing of the esophagus (Fig. 4-28B).

RADIATION INJURY

Esophagitis can be an undesirable side-effect of mediastinal radiation therapy, especially if combined with chemotherapy. Doses of radiation

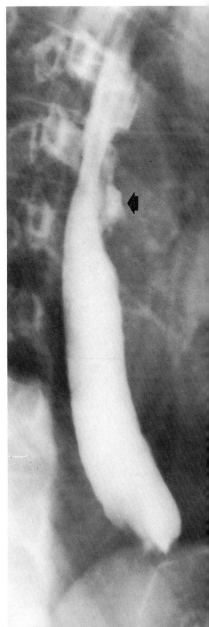

Fig. 4-24. Squamous carcinoma of the esophagus. On profile view, the lesion appears as an ulcer crater **(arrow)** surrounded by a bulging mass projecting into the esophageal lumen.

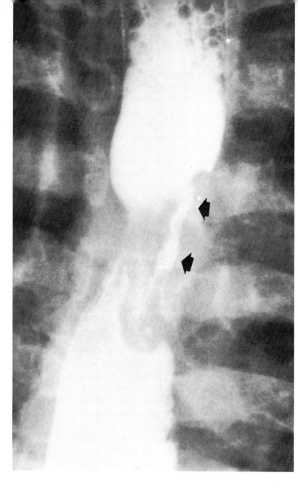

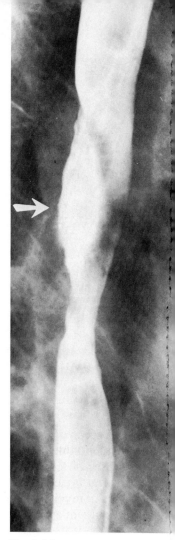

Fig. 4-25. Squamous carcinoma of the esophagus. Note the long ulceration **(arrows)** in the large, rigid lesion.

Fig. 4-26. Primary ulcerative carcinoma. An esophagram demonstrates a typical meniscoid ulcer **(arrow)** surrounded by a rim of neoplastic tissue. (Gloyna RE, Zornoza J, Goldstein HM: Primary ulcerative carcinoma of the esophagus. AJR 129:599–600, 1977. Copyright 1977. Reproduced by permission)

A B

Fig. 4-26

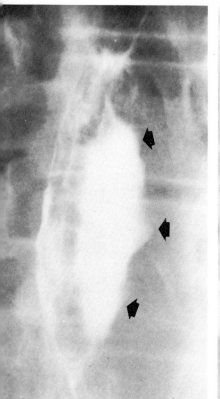

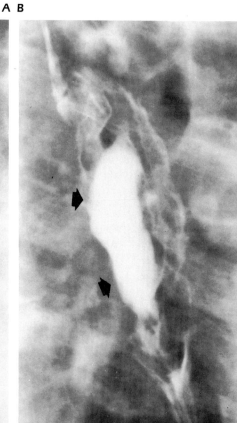

Fig. 4-27. Primary ulcerative carcinoma. Characteristic meniscoid ulceration **(arrows)** surrounded by a tumor mass is seen in **(A)** frontal and **(B)** lateral projections.

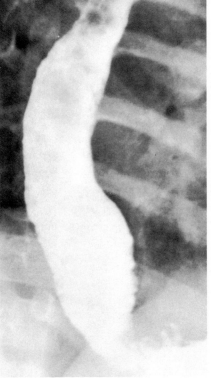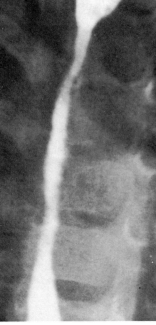

Fig. 4-28. Caustic esophagitis. **(A)** Dilated, boggy esophagus with ulceration 8 days after the ingestion of a corrosive agent. **(B)** Stricture formation is evident on an esophagram performed 3 months after the caustic injury.

A B

of greater than 4500 rad frequently lead to severe esophagitis with irreversible stricture formation. Similar complications can occur with doses of less than 2000 rads of mediastinal radiation in patients who simultaneously or sequentially receive Adriamycin (doxorubicin) or actinomycin D (Fig. 4-29). With each course of chemotherapy, there are recurrent episodes of esophagitis (recall phenomenon). The radiographic appearance of esophagitis in these patients is indistinguishable from that of *Candida* esophagitis, a far more common condition in patients undergoing chemotherapy and radiation therapy for malignant disease. The correct diagnosis should be suggested whenever a patient who develops esophagitis after radiation therapy and administration of Adriamycin (doxorubicin) has no clinical evidence of oral or pharyngeal candidiasis and does not respond to treatment with appropriate anti-fungal agents.

DRUG-INDUCED ESOPHAGITIS

Drug-induced ulceration of the esophagus may occur in patients who have delayed esophageal transit time, which permits prolonged mucosal contact with the ingested substance. In one study in which barium-sulfate tablets identical in size and shape to aspirin tablets were given to patients undergoing routine upper gastrointestinal series, more than half of the tablets remained in the esophagus longer than 5 minutes. Delay in passage of the tablets was particularly frequent in patients who were supine and in patients with a hiatal hernia and reflux or abnormal peristalsis. A relative obstruction, such as an esophageal

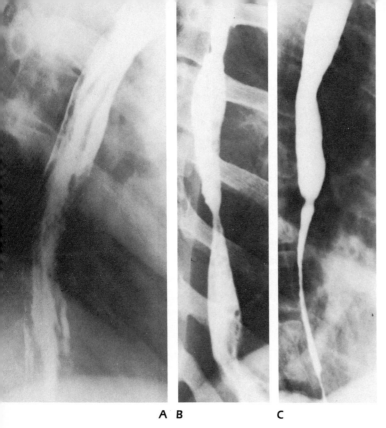

A B   C

Fig. 4-30. Intramural esophageal pseudodiverticulosis. Innumerable outpouchings representing dilated esophageal glands simulate the appearance of multiple esophageal ulcerations.

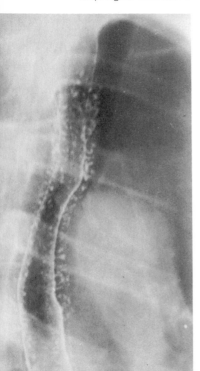

stricture or marked left atrial enlargement, may also lead to a drug remaining in prolonged contact with the mucosal surface of the esophagus.

The most common drug causing esophageal ulceration is potassium chloride in tablet form. Other medications implicated as causes of esophageal ulceration include tablets of tetracycline, emepronium bromide (an anticholinergic agent commonly used in the treatment of urinary frequency and nocturia), quinidine, and ascorbic acid. All of these drugs are apparently weak caustic agents that are innocuous when they pass rapidly through the esophagus.

INTRAMURAL ESOPHAGEAL PSEUDODIVERTICULOSIS

Intramural esophageal pseudodiverticulosis can simulate multiple esophageal ulcers (Fig. 4-30). Patients with this disease typically present with mild or moderate dysphagia that is intermittent or slowly progressive and usually of long duration. A proximal esophageal stricture is frequently seen. Radiographically, innumerable pinhead-sized outpouchings project from the lumen and end at the same level. The pseudodiverticula represent dilated esophageal glands that are radiographically similar to the Rokitansky–Aschoff sinuses in the gallbladder (Fig. 4-31) and probably result from a diffuse inflammatory process in the esophagus. Although *Candida albicans* is often cultured from the esophagus in patients with intramural pseudodiverticulosis, the presence of the fungus appears to be a secondary phenomenon rather than an etiologic factor.

Berquist HT, Nolan NG, Stephens DH et al: Radioisotope scintigraphy in the diagnosis of Barrett esophagus. AJR 123:401–411, 1975

Boal DKB, Newburger PE, Teel RL: Esophagitis induced by combined radiation and adriamycin. AJR 132:567–570, 1979

Castillo S, Aburashed A, Kimmelman J et al: Diffuse intramural esophageal pseudodiverticulosis: New cases and review. Gastroenterology 71:541–545, 1977

Cho KG, Hunter TB, Whitehouse WM: The columnar epithelial-lined lower esophagus and its association with adenocarcinoma of the esophagus. Radiology 115:563–568, 1975

Crowson TD, Head LH, Ferrante WA: Esophageal ulcers associated with tetracylcine therapy. JAMA 325:2747–2748, 1976

Crummy AB: The water test in the evaluation of gastroesophagel reflux: Its correlation with pyrosis. Radiology 78:501–504, 1966

Cynn WS, Chon HK, Gureghian PA et al: Crohn's disease of the esophagus. AJR 125:359–364, 1975

Donner MW, Saba GP, Martinez CR: Diffuse diseases of the esophagus: A practical approach. Semin Roentgenol 16:198–213, 1981

Evans KT, Roberts GM: Where do all the tablets go? Lancet 2:1237–1239, 1976

Franken EA: Caustic damage of the gastrointestinal tract: Roentgen features. AJR 118:77–85, 1973

Gloyna RE, Zornoza J, Goldstein HM: Primary ulcerative carcinoma of the esophagus. AJR 129:599–600, 1977

Gohel VK, Edell SL, Laufer I et al: Transverse folds in the human esophagus. Radiology 303–308, 1978

Ito J, Kobayashi S, Kasugai P: Tuberculosis of the esophagus. Am J Gastroenterol 65:454–456, 1976

Jenkins DW, Fisk DE, Byrd RB: Mediastinal histoplasmosis with esophageal abscess. Gastroenterology 70:190–211, 1976

Kavin H: Oesophageal ulceration due to emepronium bromide. Lancet 1:424–425, 1977

Levine MS, Laufer I, Kressel HY et al: Herpes esophagitis. AJR 136:863–866, 1981

Lewicki AM, Moore JP: Esophageal moniliasis: A review of common and less frequent characteristics. AJR 125:218–225, 1975

Margulis AR, Burhenne HJ: Alimentary Tract Roentgenology. St. Louis, C.V. Mosby, 1973

Meyers C, Durkin MG, Love L: Radiographic findings in herpetic esophagitis. Radiology 119:21–22, 1976

Muhletaler CA, Gerlock AJ, de Soto L et al: Acid corrosive esophagitis: Radiographic findings. AJR 134:1137–1140, 1980

Robbins AH, Hermos JA, Schimmel EM et al: The columnar-lined esophagus: Analysis of 26 cases. Radiology 123:1–7, 1977

Stone J, Friedberg SA: Obstructive syphilitic esophagitis. JAMA 177:711, 1961

Teplick JG, Teplick SK, Ominsky SH et al: Esophagitis caused by oral medication. Radiology 134:23–25, 1980

Walta DC, Giddens JD, Johnson LF et al: Localized proximal esophagitis secondary to ascorbic acid ingestion and esophageal motor disorder. Gastroenterology 70:766–769, 1976

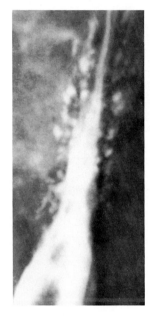

Fig. 4-31. Intramural esophageal pseudodiverticulosis. The multiple outpouchings mimic the pattern of Rokitansky–Aschoff sinuses in the gallbladder.

5

ESOPHAGEAL NARROWING

Disease Entities

Congenital conditions
    Esophageal web
    Lower esophageal ring (Schatzki ring)
    Cartilagenous esophageal ring
    Congenital stricture
Neoplastic lesions
    Carcinoma of the esophagus
    Carcinoma of the stomach
    Direct spread from adjacent malignancy
    Hematogenous/lymphangitic metastases
    Lymphoma
    Benign tumors
Reflux esophagitis
Corrosive esophagitis
Barrett's esophagus
Postsurgical stricture (*e.g.*, after hiatal hernia repair, gastric
    surgery)
Post-nasogastric intubation strictures
Infectious/inflammatory esophagitis
    Candidiasis
    Tuberculosis
    Syphilis
    Histoplasmosis
    Crohn's disease
    Eosinophilic esophagitis
Radiation injury
Motility disorders
    Achalasia pattern
    Esophageal spasm
Intramural esophageal pseudodiverticulosis
Mallory–Weiss syndrome

ESOPHAGEAL WEB

Congenital esophageal webs are smooth, thin, delicate membranes covered with normal-appearing mucosa (Fig. 5-1). Most congenital esophageal webs are situated in the cervical esophagus within 2 cm of the pharyngoesophageal junction. The typical transverse web arises from the anterior wall of the esophagus (never from the posterior wall) and is best seen in the lateral projection. It forms a right angle with the wall of the esophagus and protrudes into the esophageal lumen. A rarer circumferential type of web appears as a symmetric annular radiolucent band that concentrically narrows the barium-filled esophagus (Fig. 5-2). Webs are occasionally found in the distal esophagus (Fig. 5-3A); there may be multiple webs anywhere in the esophagus (Fig. 5-3B). Esophageal webs can usually be seen only when the barium-filled esophagus is maximally distended. Because rapid peristalsis permits cervical esophageal webs to be visible for only a fraction of a second, cinefluorography is often required for radiographic demonstration.

An esophageal web is usually an incidental finding of no clinical importance. Because it is not associated with any lack of distensibility, a transverse web only rarely occludes enough of the esophageal lumen to cause dysphagia. In contrast, circumferential webs can cause intermittent dysphagia because of constriction of the esophageal lumen. At times, the web itself is not visible, but a liquid bolus of barium can be demonstrated to squirt in a jet through the opening in the web (Fig. 5-4). The width of the jet immediately below the level of the web indicates the size of the orifice. This jet phenomenon occasionally simulates a long, smooth stenotic lesion.

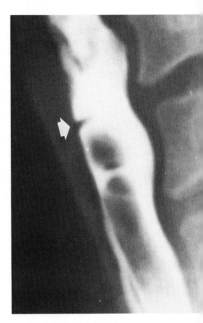

Fig. 5-1. Esophageal web. A smooth, thin membrane covered with normal-appearing mucosa protrudes into the esophageal lumen **(arrow)**.

DISORDERS ASSOCIATED WITH ESOPHAGEAL WEBS

Many diseases have been associated with esophageal webs. In most cases, the association appears to be coincidental. In certain skin diseases, such as epidermolysis bullosa and benign mucous membrane pemphigoid, a causal relationship seems likely. Epidermolysis bullosa is a rare hereditary disorder in which the skin blisters spontaneously or with injury. Subepidermal blisters characteristically affect the mucous membranes, giving rise to buccal contractures and feeding difficulties in infancy and childhood. Similar lesions in the esophagus can progress to the radiographic appearance of a stenotic web (Fig. 5-5). Benign mucous membrane pemphigoid, in contrast to other forms of pemphigus, particularly involves the mucous membranes of the mouth and conjunctiva, runs a chronic course, and tends to produce scarring. When the pharynx and esophagus are affected, postinflammatory scarring leads to adhesions that radiographically simulate esophageal webs (Fig. 5-6).

The Plummer–Vinson syndrome is a controversial entity in which esophageal webs have been reported in combination with dysphagia,

Fig. 5-2. Circumferential esophageal web **(arrows)**.

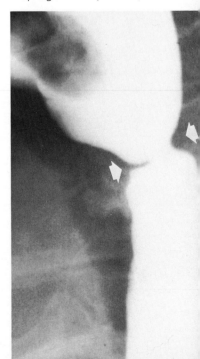

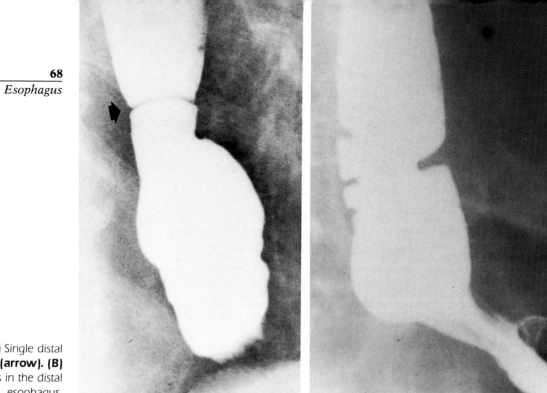

A B

Fig. 5-3. (A) Single distal esophageal web **(arrow)**. **(B)** Multiple webs in the distal esophagus.

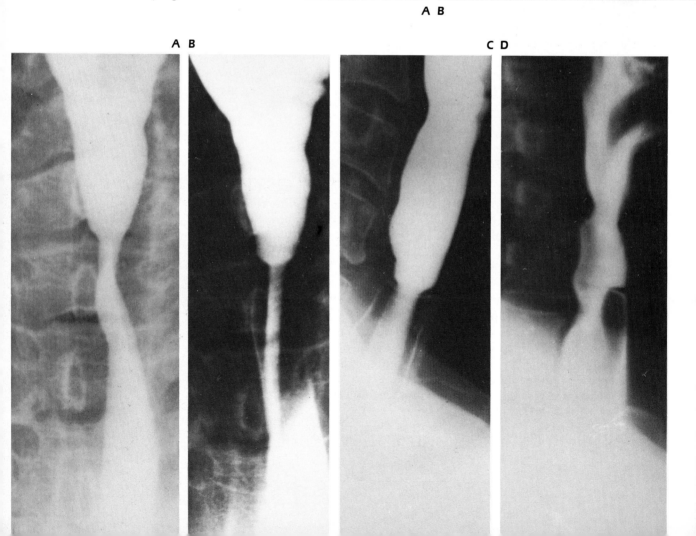

A B   C D

iron deficiency anemia, and mucosal lesions of the mouth, pharynx, and esophagus. The condition has been associated with a disturbance in iron metabolism, predominantly in middle-aged women. A correlation between the Plummer–Vinson syndrome and cancer has been suggested. In recent years, the validity of the Plummer–Vinson syndrome has been challenged because of the relative infrequency with which many of the component signs and symptoms have occurred together. Some authors consider that the discovery of an esophageal web in this "syndrome" merely represents a coincidental scar or adhesion from one of the variety of disease processes with which esophageal webs have occasionally been associated.

Fig. 5-5. Epidermolysis bullosa. A stenotic web **(arrow)** results from the healing of subepidermal blisters involving the mucous membranes.

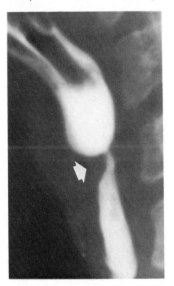

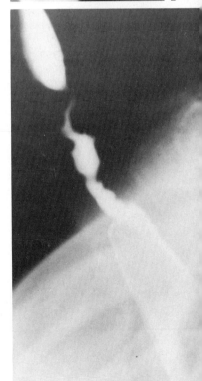

A
B

Fig. 5-6. Benign mucous membrane pemphigoid. Postinflammatory scarring causes a long, irregular area of narrowing suggestive of a malignant process.

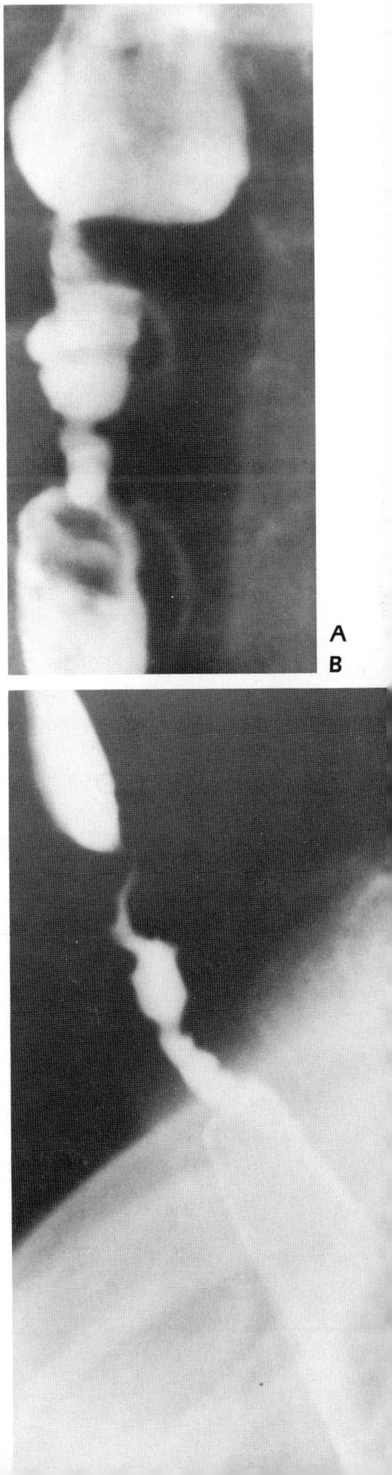

◀ **Fig. 5-4.** Jet phenomenon of esophageal web. **(A)** A frontal projection demonstrates an abruptly narrowed barium column simulating a long stenosing lesion in the upper esophagus. **(B)** The double-contrast effect below the web indicates the width of the jet and the normal caliber of the esophagus below the web. **(C)** The lateral projection better illustrates the annular constriction of the esophagus produced by the web. **(D)** Further opacification of the esophagus more graphically delineates the web. (Shauffer IA, Phillips HE, Sequeira J: The jet phenomenon: a manifestation of esophageal web. AJR 129:747–748, 1977. Copyright 1977. Reproduced by permission)

The lower esophageal ring (Schatzki ring) is a smooth, concentric narrowing several centimeters above the diaphragm that marks the junction between the esophageal and gastric mucosae (Fig. 5-7). The ring is present constantly and does not change in position. However, it is only visible when the esophagus above and below is filled sufficiently to dilate to a width greater than that of the ring (Fig. 5-8). If the luminal opening in the Schatzki ring is greater than 12 or 13 mm, symptoms of obstruction are unlikely. Rings with a narrowed luminal opening are prone to cause long-standing symptoms of intermittent dysphagia, particularly when large chunks of solid material are ingested. These symptoms can occasionally be reproduced if the patient swallows a barium capsule, radiopaque tablet, or marshmallow, any of which may temporarily become lodged in the esophagus just above the lower esophageal ring. Sudden, total esophageal obstruction can sometimes be caused by impaction of a large piece of meat.

CARTILAGENOUS RING (TRACHEOBRONCHIAL REST)

A cartilagenous ring consisting of tracheobronchial rests is an unusual cause of distal esophageal obstruction (Fig. 5-9). This anomaly probably results from sequestration of tracheal cartilage in the primitive esophagus before the two tubes have completely separated from each other. Because the cartilage is usually found in the distal esophagus, it is presumed that these cells were carried down the esophagus during the normal process of growth. Most cases of cartilagenous rings appear in infancy or early childhood with recurrent vomiting, failure to thrive, and aspiration pneumonia. Several adults, all of whom had long histories of dysphagia or other esophageal symptoms, have been described with this disorder. Characteristic radiographic findings are linear tracks of barium, representing ducts of tracheobronchial glands, that extend from the area of narrowing.

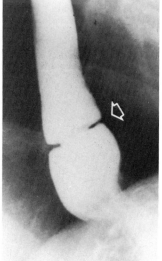

Fig. 5-7. Lower esophageal ring (Schatzki ring) **(arrow).** Smooth, concentric narrowing of the distal esophagus marks the junction between the esophageal and gastric mucosae.

Fig. 5-8. Lower esophageal ring. **(A)** Typical appearance in the filled esophagus. **(B)** The ring is not visible in the partially collapsed esophagus.

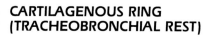

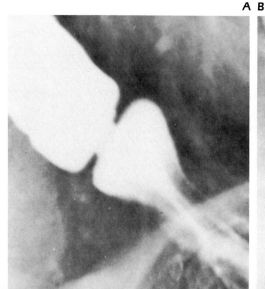

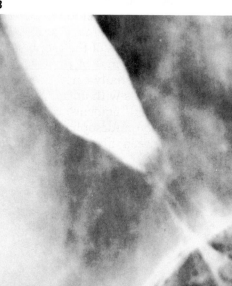

CONGENITAL STRICTURE

A congenital stricture of the esophagus is an uncommon lesion that represents an incomplete occlusion. It appears as a smooth fusiform narrowing of the esophageal lumen and causes a variable degree of obstruction and proximal dilatation. In the newborn, such a stricture is almost invariably of congenital origin; in the older infant or child, it may be impossible to distinguish between a congenital stricture and one of acquired origin caused by the swallowing of caustic material.

CARCINOMA OF THE ESOPHAGUS

Infiltrating carcinoma of the esophagus can extend under the esophageal mucosa and narrow the esophagus even in the absence of luminal proliferation. Unfortunately, symptoms of esophageal carcinoma tend to appear late in the course of the disease, so that the tumor is often in an advanced stage when first detected radiographically. Most carcinomas of the esophagus are of the squamous cell type. Excluding tumors of the gastric cardia that spread upward to involve the distal esophagus, about half of all esophageal carcinomas occur in the middle third. Of the remainder, slightly more occur in the lower than in the upper third. The incidence of carcinoma of the esophagus is far higher in men than in women, and the disease is more prevalent in blacks than in whites.

ETIOLOGIC FACTORS

Numerous etiologic factors have been suggested in the development of carcinoma of the esophagus. In the United States, there is a definite association between excessive alcohol intake, smoking, and esophageal carcinoma. Heavy use of alcohol and tobacco also significantly increases the risk of developing squamous carcinoma of the head and neck. Indeed, awareness of the not infrequent coexistence of tumors in these two sites may permit detection of small and potentially curable cancers of the esophagus in patients with known carcinoma of the head and neck. In Iran, China, and Russia, countries in which hot tea is a major beverage, carcinoma of the esophagus is very common and may be due to tissue damage secondary to raised intraesophageal temperature. Carcinoma of the esophagus occurs with significantly higher incidence than normal in patients with lye strictures, frequently developing at an unusually early age. The long-term stasis of esophageal contents in patients with untreated achalasia is also associated with a higher than normal incidence of carcinoma. Most of these lesions, however, occur in the midesophagus rather than in the distal portion. A relationship between hiatal hernia, reflux esophagitis, and carcinoma has been

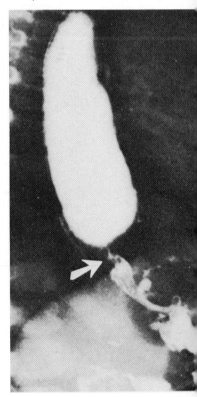

Fig. 5-9. Cartilaginous ring of tracheobronchial rests. Note the lower esophageal stricture **(arrow)** with proximal dilatation. (Rose JS, Kassner EG, Jurgens KH et al: Congenital oesophageal strictures due to cartilaginous rings. Br J Radiol 48:16–18, 1975)

Fig. 5-10. Adenocarcinoma arising in a patient with Barrett's esophagus. A constricting lesion may be seen in the midesophagus with a nodular margin and broad-based ulceration. The mucosal transition is just proximal to the constricting lesion. (Cho KJ, Hunter TB, Whitehouse WM: The columnar epithelial-lined esophagus and its association with adenocarcinoma of the esophagus. Radiology 115:563–568, 1975)

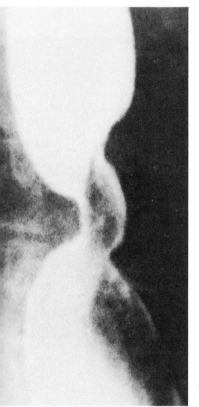

suggested. This is difficult to prove conclusively, since gastrointestinal reflux is so common in the general population. Patients with Barrett's esophagus have a definitely higher than normal risk of developing adenocarcinoma (up to a 10% incidence) (Fig. 5-10). Rare disorders that have been linked to the development of esophageal cancer include the Plummer–Vinson syndrome (sideropenic dysphagia) and tylosis, a genetically transmitted disease characterized by thickened skin of the hands and feet.

CLINICAL SYMPTOMS

Progressive dysphagia is the most common clinical presentation of carcinoma of the esophagus. In persons over 40 years of age, dysphagia must be assumed to be due to cancer until proven otherwise. Early in the disease, dysphagia is noted only with solid food; eventually, even fluids are regurgitated. Mild substernal pain or fullness may be an early sign of carcinoma of the esophagus. Persistent or severe discomfort, however, is usually due to extension of the tumor to the mediastinum and is therefore an unfavorable sign. Because the esophagus has no limiting serosa, direct extension of the tumor at the time of initial diagnosis is common and contributes to the dismal prognosis in this disease. Many patients with esophageal carcinoma have weight loss, which is closely related to the duration and severity of the esophageal obstruction. Hoarseness can occur if the recurrent laryngeal nerve is involved; anemia may be produced by slow, chronic blood loss. Pulmonary complications, such as aspiration pneumonia and esophago-respiratory fistula, are not infrequent (Fig. 5-11).

RADIOGRAPHIC FINDINGS

The earliest radiographic appearance of infiltrating carcinoma of the esophagus is a flat, plaquelike lesion, occasionally with central ulceration, that involves one wall of the esophagus (Fig. 5-12). At this stage, there is minimal reduction in the caliber of the lumen, and the lesion is seen to best advantage on double-contrast views of the distended esophagus. Unless the patient is carefully examined in various projections, this early form of esophageal carcinoma can be missed. As the infiltrating cancer progresses, luminal irregularities indicating mucosal destruction are noted (Fig. 5-13). Advanced lesions encircle the lumen completely, causing annular constrictions with overhanging margins, luminal narrowing, and, often, some degree of obstruction (Fig. 5-14). The lumen through the stenotic area is irregular, and mucosal folds are absent or severely ulcerated. Proximal dilatation of the esophagus is seen in obstructing carcinoma but is usually less pronounced than in achalasia. Because multiple synchronous foci of carcinoma of the

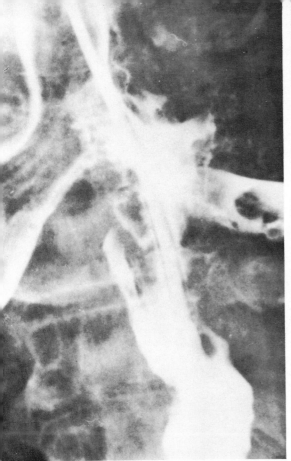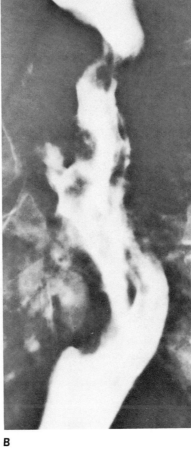

A B

Fig. 5-11. (A) Esophagorespiratory fistula as a complication of squamous carcinoma of the esophagus. **(B)** Esophagram showing the extensive malignant lesion.

Fig. 5-12. Early squamous carcinoma of the esophagus. A flat, plaquelike lesion **(arrows)** involves the posterior wall of the esophagus.

Fig. 5-13. Ulcerating squamous carcinoma of the esophagus.

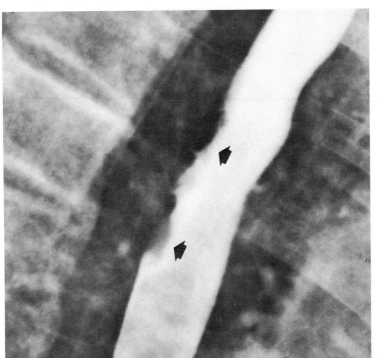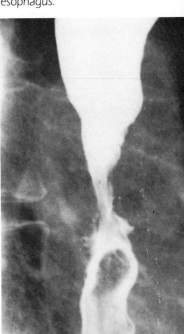

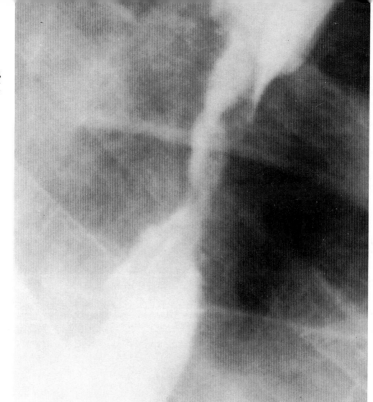

Fig. 5-14. Squamous carcinoma. An advanced lesion completely encircles the lumen, causing an annular constriction with overhanging margins.

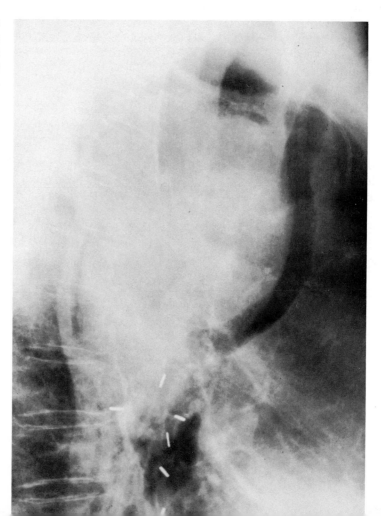

Fig. 5-15. Squamous carcinoma. Massive widening of the retrotracheal soft tissues causes anterior bowing of the tracheal air shadow.

esophagus sometimes occur, albeit rarely, a careful and complete examination of the remainder of the esophagus is essential, even when one obvious lesion has been demonstrated. High esophageal carcinoma usually causes difficulty in swallowing with frequent aspiration into the trachea. Carcinoma of the cervical portion of the esophagus can cause forward displacement of the tracheal air shadow on lateral view and the suggestion of a prevertebral mass. Upper thoracic lesions produce widening (> 3–4mm) of the retrotracheal soft-tissue stripe (Fig. 5-15).

TREATMENT AND PROGNOSIS

Because the nature of esophageal cancer brings the patient to medical attention relatively late in the course of the disease, the long-term survival rate is low. In some patients, a radical resection can be performed and reconstruction achieved with the stomach (Fig. 5-16), right or left colon, or jejunum pulled up through the intrathoracic, retrosternal, or antethoracic subcutaneous tissue. Unfortunately, tumor frequently recurs at the anastomotic site (Fig. 5-17). In many cases, only palliative treatment can be offered. The easiest method of restoring oral intake to these patients with esophageal cancer is by passing an indwelling tube through the lesion. A simple gastrostomy or jejunostomy can be performed to supply nutrition to the patient. Radiation therapy is often employed either in conjunction with a radical operation or as palliative therapy in patients in whom surgery cannot be performed. Squamous cell carcinoma of the esophagus responds to radiation therapy in a majority of patients; indeed, in up to 10% of cases, radiation therapy may be curative (Fig. 5-18).

CARCINOMA OF THE STOMACH

About 12% of adenocarcinomas of the stomach arising near the cardia invade the lower esophagus at an early stage and cause symptoms of esophageal obstruction. This process can produce an irregularly narrowed, sometimes ulcerated lesion simulating carcinoma of the distal esophagus (Fig. 5-19). A careful examination of the cardia is necessary to demonstrate the gastric origin of the tumor. Narrowing of the distal esophagus secondary to gastric carcinoma may be due not only to direct extension of tumor but also to destruction of cells in the myenteric plexus, which produces an achalasia-like pattern.

Fig. 5-16. Gastric pull-through following the radical resection of a large esophageal carcinoma. A surgical clip indicates the site of anastomosis with the remaining esophagus.

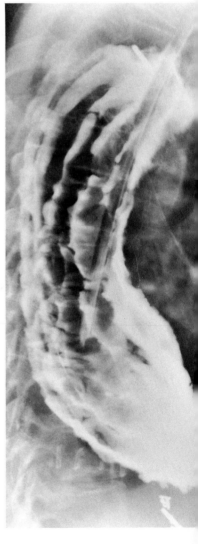

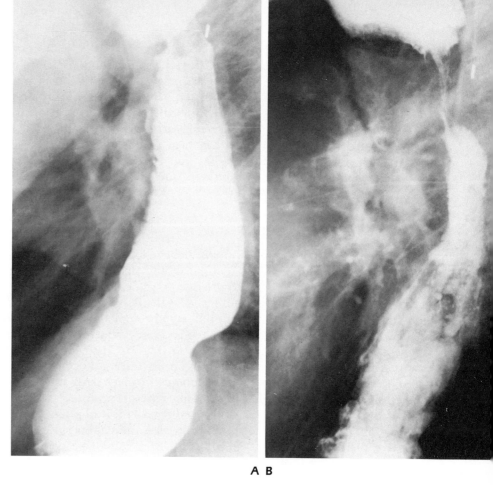

Fig. 5-17. Recurrent esophageal carcinoma at the anastomotic site. **(A)** Baseline barium swallow following surgical resection. There is mild narrowing, but the mucosal pattern at the anastomotic site (surgical clip) appears normal. **(B)** Ten months later, irregular, high-grade stenosis and the surrounding mass reflect tumor recurrence.

A B

A B

Fig. 5-18. Effect of radiation therapy on squamous carcinoma of the esophagus. **(A)** Original malignant lesion in the midthoracic esophagus. **(B)** Essentially normal esophagram in the same patient 9 years after radiation therapy.

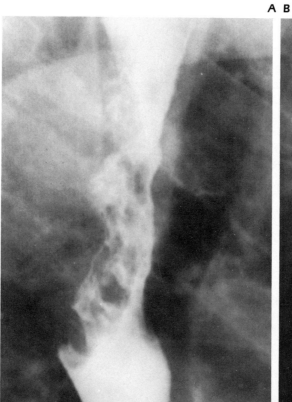

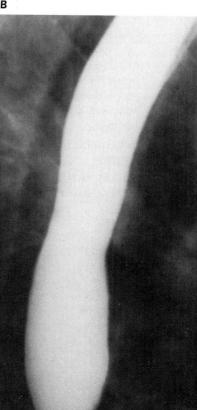

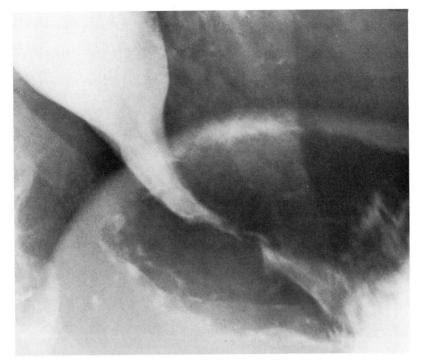

Fig. 5-19. Adenocarcinoma of the stomach invading the distal esophagus.

METASTATIC LESIONS

Other malignant lesions can spread to the esophagus and produce luminal narrowing. In the cervical region, direct extension from carcinoma of the larynx or thyroid can constrict the esophagus and cause relative obstruction (Fig. 5-20). Narrowing of the thoracic esophagus by tumor-containing lymph nodes or blood-borne metastases most commonly results from a primary site in either the breast or lung. This lesion typically appears radiographically as a symmetric stricture with smooth borders. Although concentric narrowing due to metastatic malignancy characteristically affects a short segment of the esophagus, long segmental stenosis occasionally occurs with metastatic carcinoma of the breast or diffuse mediastinal involvement by mesothelioma (Fig. 5-21). Irregular, ulcerated narrowing of the esophagus due to metastatic disease may also occur (Fig. 5-22).

LYMPHOMA

Transcardial extension of gastric lymphoma to involve the distal esophagus has been described in 2% to 10% of cases (Fig. 5-23). This typically presents as nodularity and nonobstructive narrowing and may be indistinguishable from distal esophageal involvement by gastric adenocarcinoma. Esophageal narrowing can also be caused by enlarged masses of lymphomatous nodes. Primary esophageal lymphoma is rare (Fig. 5-24).

Fig. 5-20. Metastatic carcinoma invading the esophagus. The direct extension of carcinoma of the thyroid causes constriction and relative obstruction of the lower cervical esophagus **(arrow).**

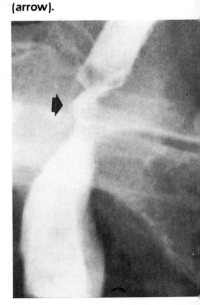

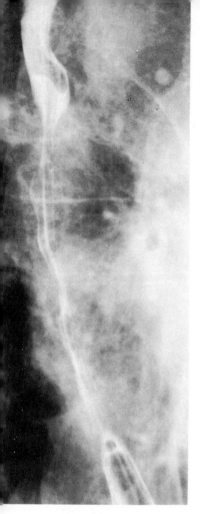

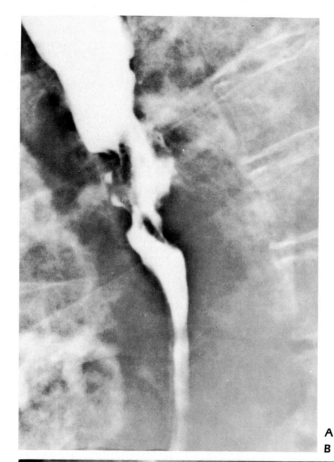

A
B

Fig. 5-21. Mesothelioma. Diffuse mediastinal involvement causes long, segmental stenosis of the esophagus.

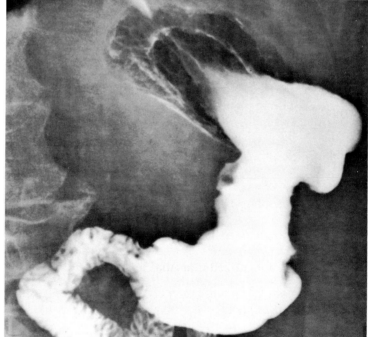

Fig. 5-22. Metastases to the esophagus from carcinoma of the stomach. **(A)** Irregular, ulcerated mass in the midesophagus. **(B)** Primary adenocarcinoma of the body of the stomach.

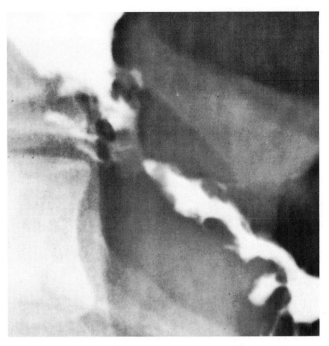

Fig. 5-23. Transcardial extension of gastric lymphoma to involve the distal esophagus.

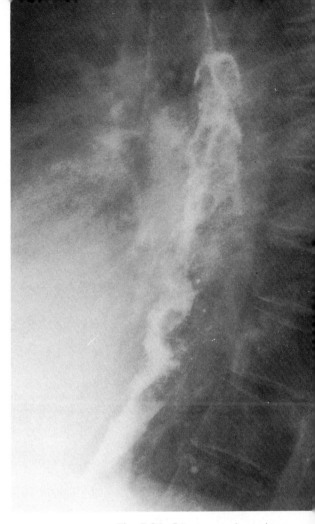

Fig. 5-24. Primary esophageal lymphoma. The diffuse, destructive process involves almost the entire thoracic esophagus.

BENIGN TUMORS

Benign tumors, primarily leiomyomas, are submucosal intramural masses that can appear to eccentrically narrow the esophageal lumen.

REFLUX ESOPHAGITIS

Distal esophageal narrowing is a severe complication of gastroesophageal reflux and peptic esophagitis (Fig. 5-25). The narrowing may be reversible if it is due to the intense spasm and inflammatory reaction that accompany a marginal ulcer at the gastroesophageal junction. A fixed, relatively obstructing stricture of the distal esophagus may be due to fibrotic healing of a localized marginal ulcer or to diffuse reflux esophagitis (Fig. 5-26). Strictures secondary to reflux esophagitis tend to be asymmetric, funnel-shaped, or broad-based, with no demonstrable mucosal pattern. An associated hiatal hernia is frequently detected (Fig. 5-27); however, the absence of a hernia in no way eliminates the possibility that a distal esophageal stricture is due to reflux esophagitis.

Fig. 5-25. Reflux stricture. Smooth narrowing of the distal esophagus extends to the level of the hiatal hernia.

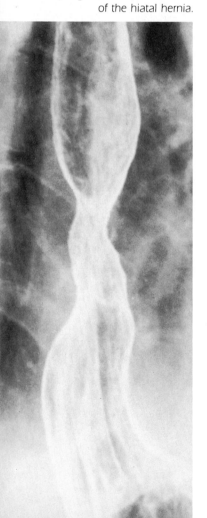

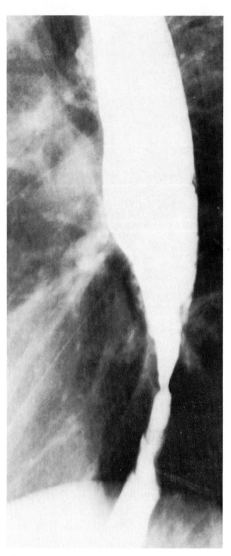

Fig. 5-26

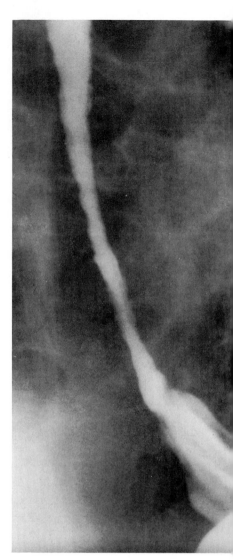

Fig. 5-27

Fig. 5-26. Esophageal stricture secondary to reflux esophagitis.

Fig. 5-27. Long esophageal stricture, due to reflux esophagitis, with an associated hiatal hernia.

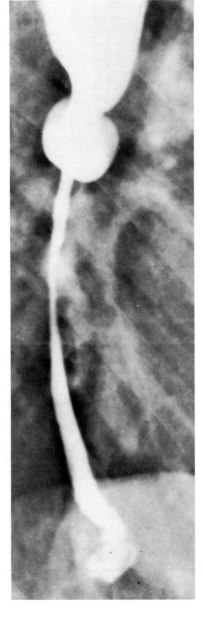

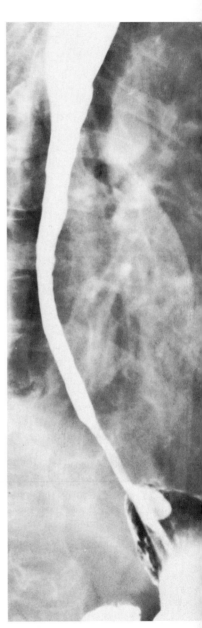

Fig. 5-28. Corrosive stricture resulting from the ingestion of lye.

CORROSIVE ESOPHAGITIS

A major complication of the ingestion of corrosive agents is the development of an esophageal stricture as the intense mucosal and intramural inflammation heals (Fig. 5-28). Strictures can appear as soon as 2 weeks after the ingestion of a caustic substance. Corrosive strictures tend to be long lesions involving large portions of the thoracic esophagus, sometimes extending the entire distance between the aortic knob and the diaphragm (Fig. 5-29).

Fig. 5-29. Extensive caustic stricture due to lye ingestion, involving almost the entire thoracic esophagus.

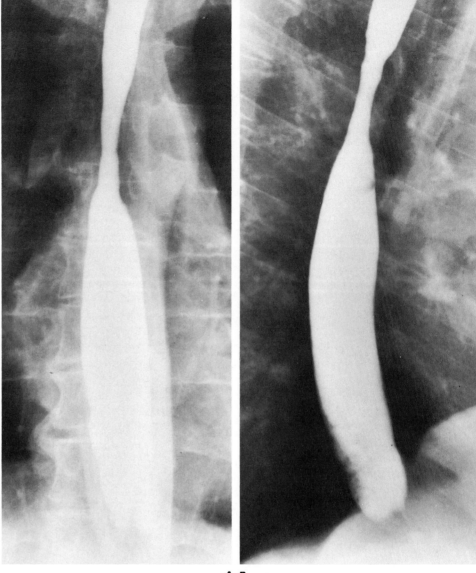

Fig. 5-30. Barrett's stricture. **(A)** Frontal and **(B)** lateral projections demonstrate a smooth upper thoracic esophageal stricture.

A B

Fig. 5-31. Postoperative esophageal stricture. There is severe narrowing near the esophagogastric junction and a large residual pouch, which developed 2 weeks after the surgical repair of a hiatal hernia.

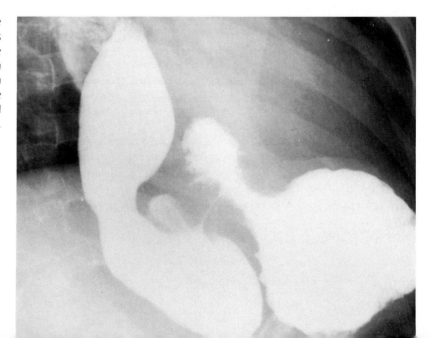

BARRETT'S ESOPHAGUS

Midesophageal strictures are commonly encountered in patients with a Barrett's esophagus (Fig. 5-30). In this condition, a variable length of the distal esophagus is lined by a gastric type of epithelium that is more susceptible to ulceration and inflammation with stricture formation than is the normal esophagus.

POSTSURGICAL / POSTINTUBATION STRICTURES

Strictures near the esophagogastric junction may occur postoperatively after surgical repair of a hiatal hernia (Fig. 5-31). Reflux of bile into the stomach after gastric surgery can cause severe esophagitis and stricture formation if gastroesophageal reflux permits bile to come in contact with the sensitive distal esophageal mucosa. Prolonged nasogastric intubation predisposes the patient to gastroesophageal reflux by preventing hiatal closure and by causing mucosal ischemia from compression of the esophageal mucosa. The resulting severe esophagitis can lead to the rapid development of a long stricture in the distal esophagus, often within several days of intubation (Fig. 5-32).

INFECTIOUS / GRANULOMATOUS ESOPHAGITIS

Strictures can develop during the healing phase of infectious and inflammatory processes involving the esophagus. In candidal infestation of the esophagus, compromise of luminal diameter can occur both from edema of the mucosa and from the presence of an overlying pseudomembrane. As the disease spreads through the esophageal wall, a long segment of the esophagus may become constricted (Fig. 5-33). The proximal and distal margins of the stricture are usually tapered, though there is occasionally asymmetry and an abrupt change in diameter simulating an infiltrating esophageal neoplasm.

Stricture formation is common during the healing phase of esophageal inflammation due to granulomatous diseases such as tuberculosis, syphilis, and histoplasmosis. Severe luminal narrowing also has been described in patients with Crohn's disease of the esophagus (Fig. 5-34), herpes simplex infestation (Fig. 5-35), and eosinophilic esophagitis (Fig. 5-36).

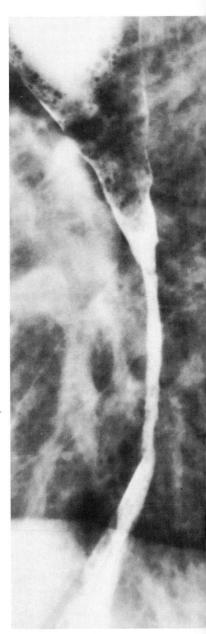

Fig. 5-32. Stricture due to prolonged nasogastric intubation. The severe esophagitis associated with the nasogastric intubation led to the development of a long stricture within 2 weeks.

Fig. 5-33. Candidiasis. There is irregular narrowing of the distal two-thirds of the esophagus with multiple transverse ulcerations. (Ott DJ, Gelfand DW: Esophageal strictures secondary to candidiasis. Gastrointest Radiol 2:323–325, 1978)

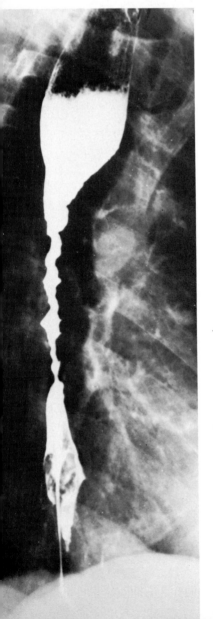

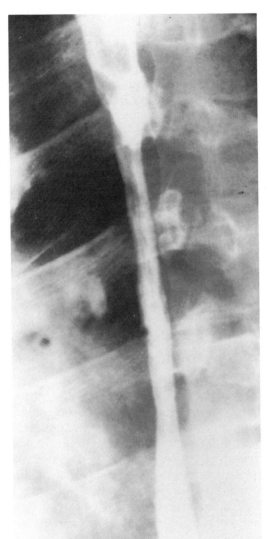

Fig. 5-34

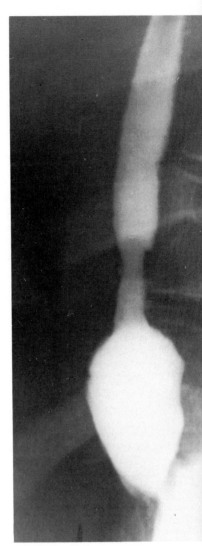

Fig. 5-35

Fig. 5-34. Crohn's disease. Note the long area of narrowing in the midesophagus.

Fig. 5-35. Herpes simplex. A short, smooth stricture is visible in the distal esophagus.

RADIATION INJURY

Esophageal stricture within the field of irradiation is a relatively infrequent long-term complication of mediastinal radiation therapy. Marked thickening of the submucosal and muscular layers due to edema and fibrosis can result in a stricture that has a benign appearance, with tapered margins and relatively smooth mucosal surfaces (Fig. 5-37). The narrowing may be due in part to radiation changes involving surrounding mediastinal structures.

MOTILITY DISORDERS

Severe narrowing of the distal esophagus with proximal dilatation is characteristic of the failure of relaxation of the lower esophageal sphincter in patients with achalasia (Fig. 5-38). In diffuse esophageal spasm, prolonged, strong contractions can cause marked narrowing of the esophageal lumen simulating the appearance of a fixed stricture.

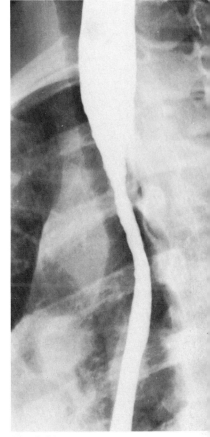

Fig. 5-36. Eosinophilic esophagitis. There is diffuse narrowing and surface irregularity of a 6-cm segment of the midthoracic esophagus. (Picus D, Frank PH: Eosinophilic esophagitis. AJR 136:1001–1003, 1981. Copyright 1981. Reproduced by permission)

Fig. 5-37. Radiation-induced stricture. The stricture, which developed after the administration of 6000 rad to the mediastinum for treatment of metastatic disease, has a benign appearance, with tapered margins and smooth mucosal surfaces.

Fig. 5-38. Achalasia. Failure of relaxation of the lower esophageal sphincter produces distal narrowing **(arrow)** and severe proximal dilatation.

Fig. 5-36

Fig. 5-37

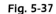

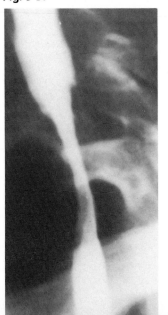

Fig. 5-38

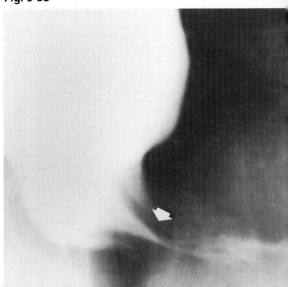

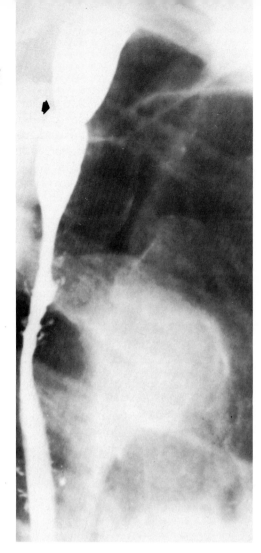

Fig. 5-39. Intramural esophageal pseudodiverticulosis. A stricture in the upper thoracic esophagus **(arrow)** is associated with diffuse filling of esophageal glands mimicking multiple ulcerations.

A B

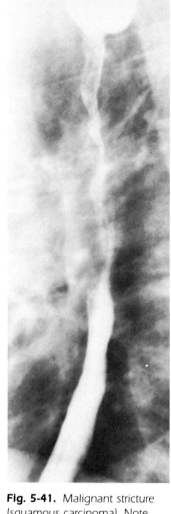

Fig. 5-41. Malignant stricture (squamous carcinoma). Note that the stricture is long, irregular, and eccentric.

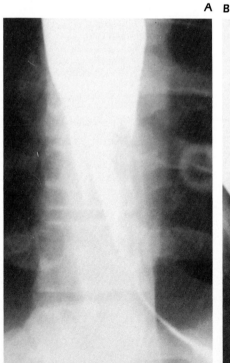

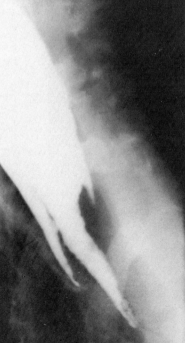

Fig. 5-40. Mallory–Weiss syndrome. Large mounds of adherent thrombus produce marked narrowing of the distal esophagus. (Curtin MJ, Milligan FD: Mallory–Weiss syndrome with esophageal obstruction secondary to adherent intraluminal thrombus. AJR 129:508–510, 1977. Copyright 1977. Reproduced by permission)

INTRAMURAL ESOPHAGEAL PSEUDODIVERTICULOSIS

A smooth stricture of the esophagus is found in about 90% of patients with intramural esophageal pseudodiverticulosis (Fig. 5-39). In about two-thirds of cases, it is located in the upper third of the esophagus. Dilatation of the stricture generally results in amelioration of symptoms of dysphagia. One case of conical narrowing of the esophagus has been described in association with the Mallory–Weiss syndrome (Fig. 5-40). In this patient, an intermediate degree of gastroesophageal mucosal injury and bleeding produced large mounds of adherent intraluminal thrombus, which caused esophageal obstruction.

DIFFERENTIATION BETWEEN BENIGN AND MALIGNANT CAUSES

In the patient with esophageal narrowing, the critical differential diagnosis is between carcinoma and a nonmalignant lesion. As a general rule, malignant neoplasms produce discrete, irregular, and fixed strictures, often with sharply demarcated filling defects with overhanging edges that bulge toward the lumen (Fig. 5-41). Associated ulceration is frequent and often has an irregular configuration. At times, however, esophageal narrowing due to malignancy can appear relatively smooth with tapering margins and closely simulate a benign lesion. Asymmetry or eccentricity of the stricture favors a malignant etiology (Fig. 5-42). Unless the clinical history and radiographic appearance is typical of a benign process and the patient improves on medical therapy, esophagoscopy and biopsy are necessary for an unequivocal diagnosis to be made.

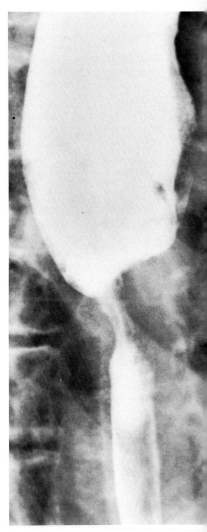

Fig. 5-42. Malignant stricture (squamous carcinoma). The marked asymmetry and eccentricity of the stricture favors a malignant etiology.

Esophagus

Benedict EB, Lever WF: Stenosis of the esophagus in benign mucus membrane pemphigus. Ann Otol Rhinol Laryngol 61:1121–1133, 1952

Burgess JN, Payne WS, Andersen HA et al: Barrett esophagus: The columnar-epithelial-lined lower esophagus. Mayo Clin Proc 46:728–734, 1971

Clements JL, Cox GW, Torres WE et al: Cervical esophageal webs—A roentgen-anatomic correlation. AJR 121:221–231, 1974

Curtin MJ, Milligan FD: Mallory–Weiss syndrome with esophageal obstruction secondary to adherent intraluminal thrombus. AJR 129:508–510, 1977

Cynn WS, Chon HK, Gurejhian PA et al: Crohn's disease of the esophagus. AJR 125:359–364, 1975

Donner MW, Saba GP, Martinez CR: Diffuse diseases of the esophagus: A practical approach. Semin Roentgenol 16:198–213, 1981

Fisher MS: Metastasis to the esophagus. Gastrointest Radiol 1:249–251, 1976

Franken EA: Caustic damage of the gastrointestinal tract: Roentgen features. AJR 118:77–85, 1973

Goldstein HM, Zornoza J: Association of squamous cell carcinoma of the head and neck with cancer of the esophagus. AJR 131:791–794, 1978

Goldstein HM, Zornoza J, Hopens T: Intrinsic diseases of the adult esophagus: Benign and malignant tumors. Semin Roentgenol 16:183–197, 1981

Han SY, Mihas AA: Circumferential web of the upper esophagus. Gastrointest Radiol 3:7–9, 1978

Hutton CF: Plummer–Vinson syndrome. Br J Radiol 29:81–85, 1956

Koehler RE, Moss AA, Margulis AR: Early radiographic manifestations of carcinoma of the esophagus. Radiology 119:1–5, 1976

Lansing PB, Ferrante WA, Ochsner JL: Carcinoma of the esophagus at the site of lye stricture. Am J Surg 118:108–111, 1973

Margulis AR, Burhenne HJ: Alimentary Tract Roentgenology. St. Louis, C.V. Mosby, 1973

Martel W: Radiologic features of esophagogastritis secondary to extremely caustic agents. Radiology 103:31–36, 1972

Nosher JL, Campbell WL, Seaman WB: The clinical significance of cervical esophageal and hypopharyngeal webs. Radiology 117:45–47, 1975

Ott DJ, Gelfand DW: Esophageal stricture secondary to candidiasis. Gastrointest Radiol 2:323–325, 1978

Parnell DD, Johnson SAM: Tylosis palmaris et plantaris: Its occurrence with internal malignancy. Arch Dermatol 100:7–9, 1969

Picus D, Frank PH: Eosinophilic esophagitis. AJR 136:1001–1003, 1981

Robbins AH, Hermos JA, Schimmel EM: The columnar-lined esophagus: Analysis of 26 cases. Radiology 123:1–7, 1977

Rose JS, Kassner EG, Jurgens KH et al: Congenital oesophageal strictures due to cartilaginous rings. Br J Radiol 48:16–18, 1975

Rosengren JE, Goldstein HM: Radiologic demonstration of multiple foci of malignancy in the esophagus. Gastrointest Radiol 3:11–13, 1978

Schatzki R, Gary JE: The lower esophageal ring. AJR 75:246–261, 1956

Seaman WB: The significance of webs in the hypopharynx and upper esophagus. Radiology 89:32–38, 1967

Shauffer IA, Phillips HE, Sequeira J: The jet phenomenon: A manifestation of esophageal web. AJR 129:747–748, 1977

ESOPHAGEAL
FILLING DEFECTS

6

Disease Entities

Neoplastic lesions
  Benign tumors
    Spindle cell tumor (*e.g.*, leiomyoma)
    Fibrovascular polyp
    Squamous papilloma
    Inflammatory esophagogastric polyp
    Adenomatous polyp
  Tumors of intermediate malignant potential
    Villous adenoma
  Malignant tumors
    Carcinoma of the esophagus
    Gastric carcinoma with upward extension
    Metastases
    Leiomyosarcoma
    Carcinosarcoma
    Pseudosarcoma
    Melanoma
    Lymphoma
    Verrucous squamous cell carcinoma
Lymph node enlargement (extrinsic lesions)
  Malignant lesion
  Granulomatous process
Candidiasis
Herpetic esophagitis
Varices
Duplication cyst
Foreign bodies/air bubbles
Prolapsed gastric folds

SPINDLE CELL TUMOR

Leiomyoma is the most common benign tumor of the esophagus (Fig. 6-1). Like the other benign spindle cell tumors of the esophagus, most leiomyomas are asymptomatic and are discovered during radiographic examination for nonesophageal complaints or incidentally at autopsy. In the few patients with symptoms, dysphagia and substernal pain are common complaints. Leiomyomas are most frequently found in the lower third of the esophagus. The vast majority are located intramurally and have little, if any, tendency to undergo malignant transformation. Unlike gastric leiomyomas, tumors of this cell type in the esophagus rarely ulcerate or bleed. Multiple tumors are occasionally present (Fig. 6-2).

When viewed in profile, an esophageal leiomyoma appears radiographically as a smooth, rounded intramural defect in the barium column (Fig. 6-3). The characteristic half-moon or crescent-shaped mass is sharply demarcated from adjacent portions of the esophageal wall. The superior and inferior margins of the tumor form a right or slightly obtuse angle with the wall of the esophagus. There is no evidence of infiltration, ulceration, or undercutting at the tumor margin. When examined *en face*, a leiomyoma appears as a round or lobulated filling defect sharply outlined by the barium flowing around each side.

Fig. 6-1. Leiomyoma. A smooth, rounded intramural defect is evident in the barium column **(arrows)**.

Fig. 6-2. Multiple esophageal leiomyomas. Several smoothly rounded filling defects in the barium column conform to the companion soft-tissue masses **(arrows)**. The masses move freely during swallowing, indicating a lack of adhesions or mediastinal infiltration. (Shaffer HA: Multiple leiomyomas of the esophagus. Radiology 118:29–34, 1976)

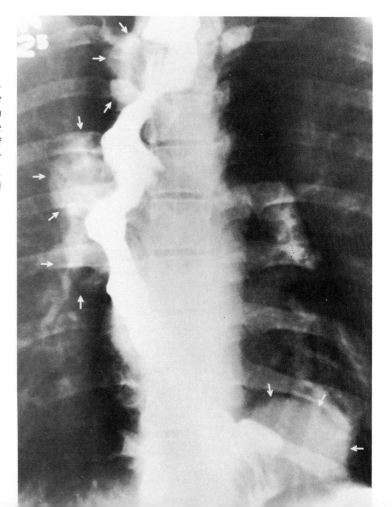

Esophageal motility is normal and dilatation above the tumor infrequent. An esophageal leiomyoma may have a large extramural component that is visible as it projects into the mediastinum and is outlined against adjacent lung. Rarely, leiomyomas of the distal esophagus contain enough calcium to be visible radiographically (Fig. 6-4). Because tumoral calcification has not been described in any other esophageal lesion, the presence of amorphous calcification in a retrocardiac esophageal mass is diagnostic of a leiomyoma.

Other benign spindle cell submucosal tumors are extremely rare. These include lipomas (Fig. 6-5), fibrolipomas (Fig. 6-6), myxofibromas, hemangiomas, lymphangiomas, schwannomas (Fig. 6-7), and granular cell myoblastomas (Fig. 6-8).

Fig. 6-3. Leiomyoma. Note the smooth, rounded intramural defect in the barium column **(arrows)**.

Fig. 6-4. Leiomyoma of the distal esophagus. Note the amorphous calcifications in the smoothly lobulated intramural tumor **(arrows)**. (Ghahremani GG, Meyers MA, Port RB: Calcified primary tumors of the gastrointestinal tract. Gastrointest Radiol 2:331–339, 1978)

Fig. 6-5. Lipoma. A sausage-shaped mass **(arrows)** is visible in the upper thoracic esophagus.

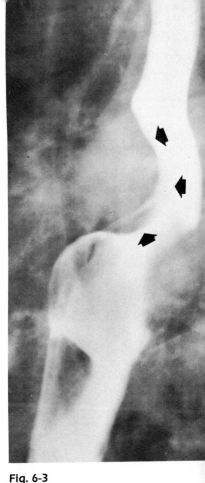

Fig. 6-3

Fig. 6-4

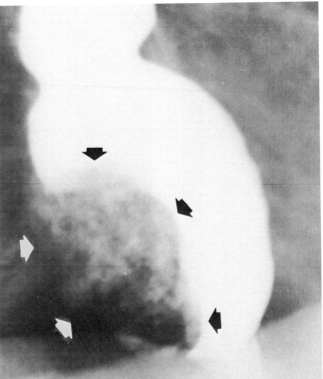

Fig. 6-5

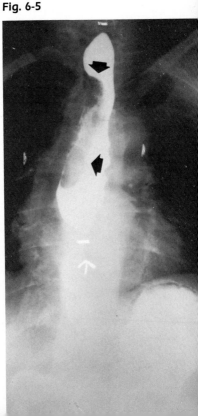

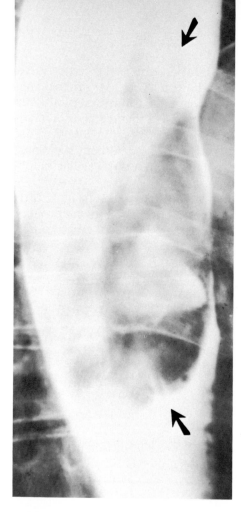

Fig. 6-6. Fibrolipoma
(arrows).

Fig. 6-7. Schwannoma
(arrow).

Fig. 6-8. Granular cell
myoblastoma **(arrows).**

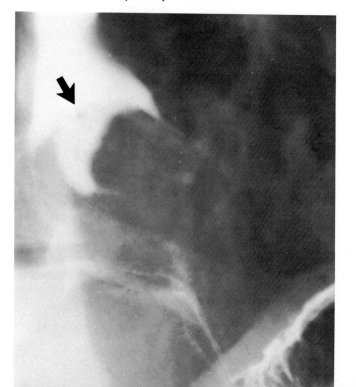

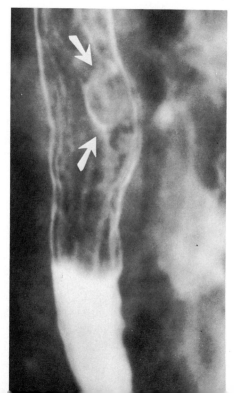

FIBROVASCULAR POLYP

Fibrovascular polyps, though rare, are the second most common type of solid benign tumor of the esophagus. They consist of varying amounts of fibrovascular tissue, adipose cells, and stroma that arise in the mucosa or submucosa and are covered by epidermoid epithelium, which can become secondarily eroded and bleed. Fibrovascular polyps can grow to a huge size without being suspected. Dysphagia is the most common symptom. Pain varies from severe epigastric distress to mild substernal and epigastric discomfort. Very large tumors can compress the trachea and cause respiratory distress. Occasionally, fibrovascular polyps present catastrophically by being regurgitated into the mouth, causing asphyxiation and death.

Fibrovascular polyps appear radiographically as large intraluminal filling defects (Fig. 6-9). They are oval-shaped or elongated, sausage-like masses with a smooth or mildly lobulated surface. At fluoroscopy, barium can be observed to flow around the intraluminal tumor and completely surround it. A large fibrovascular polyp can cause local widening of the esophagus but not the complete obstruction or wall rigidity that may be seen with an esophageal carcinoma.

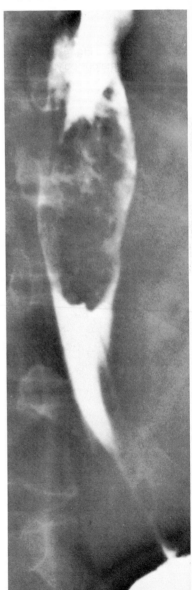

Fig. 6-9. Fibrovascular polyp. Note the bulky, sausage-shaped mass with a mildly lobulated surface.

OTHER BENIGN LESIONS

Squamous papillomas consist of a papillary structure lined with normal squamous epithelium. They are usually too small to be detected radiographically but occasionally present as large, movable, soft-appearing papillary intraluminal tumors (Fig. 6-10).

Fig. 6-10. Giant papilloma. There is a large, bubbly-appearing collection of tumor **(arrow)** in the distal esophagus. (Walker JH: Giant papilloma of the thoracic esophagus. AJR 131:519–520, 1978. Copyright 1978. Reproduced by permission)

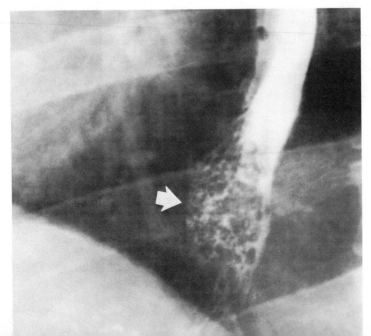

DUPLICATION CYST

A duplication cyst can produce an eccentric impression on the barium-filled esophagus simulating an intramural or mediastinal mass (Fig. 6-26). Duplications occur less commonly in the esophagus than in other portions of the gastrointestinal tract. These cystic structures are closely attached to the normal esophagus and are covered by muscle that is lined with gastric or enteric epithelium. As a duplication dilates with retained material, it may compress the esophagus and produce dysphagia. Cough, cyanosis, and respiratory distress may occur. Although contrast material infrequently fills a duplication (Fig. 6-27), in most cases there is no connection between the duplication and the esophageal lumen.

FOREIGN BODIES

A wide spectrum of foreign bodies can become impacted in the esophagus. Pieces of chicken bone (Fig. 6-28) or fishbones (Fig. 6-29) may be swallowed accidentally. If large enough, they will become impacted, predominantly in the cervical esophagus at or just above the level of the thoracic inlet. Metallic objects such as pins, coins (Fig. 6-30), and small toys (Fig. 6-31) are swallowed frequently by infants and young children. It is essential that a suspected foreign body be evaluated on two views in order for the physician to be certain that the dense object projected over the esophagus truly lies within it (Fig. 6-32). Most metals are very radiopaque and easily visualized on radiographs or during fluoroscopy. Objects made of aluminum and some light alloys may be impossible to detect radiographically, because the density of these metals is almost equal to that of soft tissue.

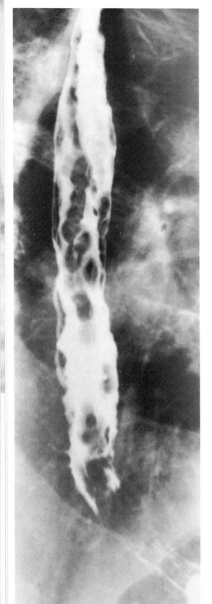

Fig. 6-25. Esophageal varices. Serpiginous submucosal masses represent dilated venous structures.

Fig. 6-26. Duplication cyst. Eccentric compression on the barium-filled esophagus simulates an intramural mass. ▶

Fig. 6-27. Esophageal duplication with postsurgical communication with the esophageal lumen. **Arrows** point to the duplication cyst. ▶

Fig. 6-28. Cornish game-hen bone **(arrow)** impacted in the lower cervical esophagus. ▶

Fig. 6-29. Fishbone impacted in the lower cervical esophagus. ▶

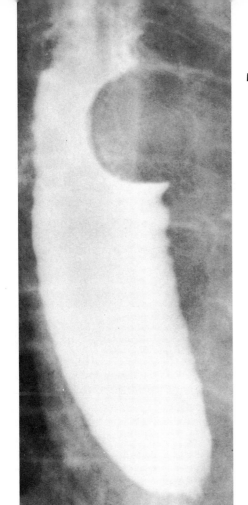

Fig. 6-26

Fig. 6-27

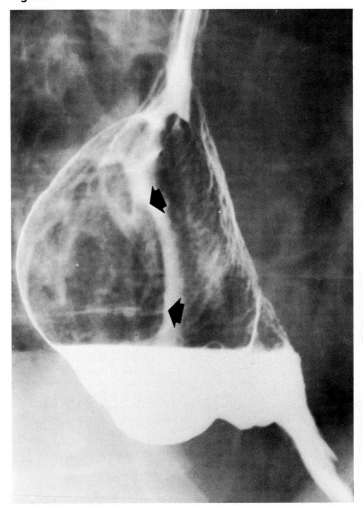

Fig. 6-28

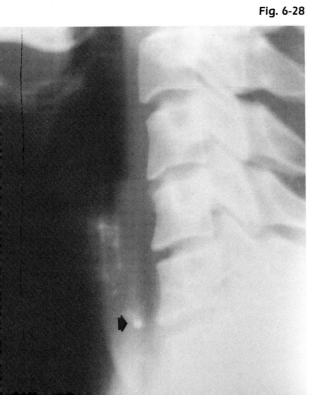

Fig. 6-29

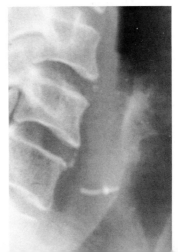

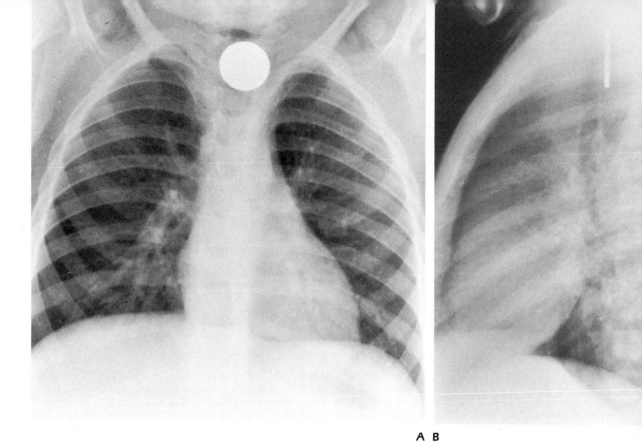

A B

Fig. 6-30. Metallic coin impacted in the esophagus. **(A)** Frontal and **(B)** lateral projections.

Fig. 6-31. Metallic jack impacted in the esophagus. **(A)** Frontal and **(B)** lateral projections.

A B

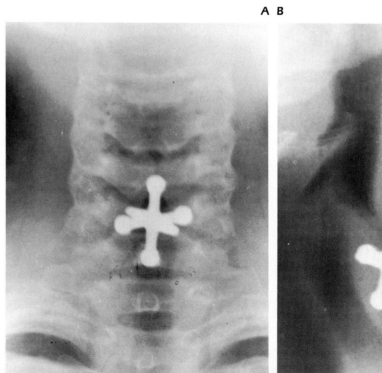

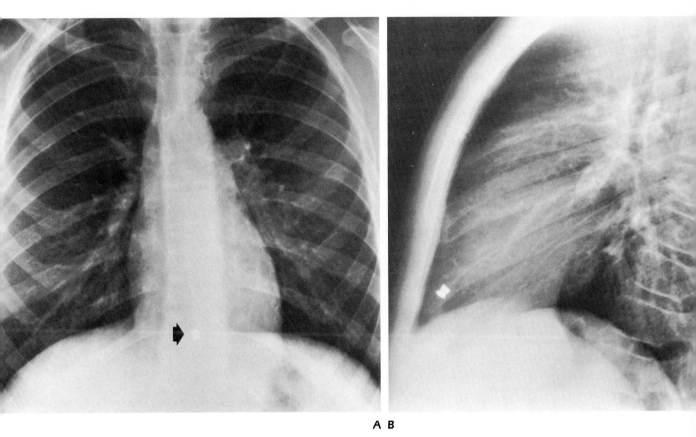

A B

Fig. 6-32. Bullet in the right atrium of a child simulating an esophageal foreign body. **(A)** The frontal view reveals the metallic density **(arrow)** to be situated at the level of the distal esophagus. **(B)** The lateral view clearly demonstrates the anterior, intracardiac location of the bullet. The child was shot in the neck, and the bullet travelled through the jugular vein and superior vena cava to the heart.

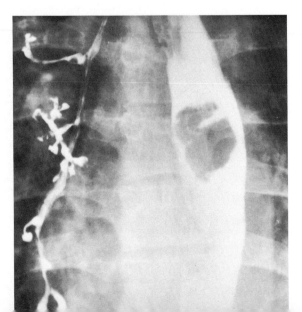

Fig. 6-33. Meat impaction. A large bolus of a hot dog is trapped in the midesophagus of a patient with quadriplegia. Barium in the bronchial tree is due to aspiration.

The presence of nonopaque foreign bodies in the esophagus, especially pieces of poorly chewed meat, can be demonstrated only after the ingestion of barium (Fig. 6-33). Such foreign bodies usually become impacted in the distal esophagus just above the level of the diaphragm and are often associated with a distal stricture (Fig. 6-34). These intraluminal filling defects usually have a nonhomogeneous surface that is either marbled or spotted and may resemble a completely obstructing carcinoma. Impactions may also be due to strictures in the cervical portion of the esophagus (Fig. 6-35).

Complications of ingested foreign bodies in the esophagus include penetration of the esophageal wall, which can lead to a periesophageal abscess or diffuse mediastinitis. In children, stridor or recurrent pneumonia can be caused by an esophageal foreign body not known to have been ingested.

PROLAPSED GASTRIC FOLDS

Prolapse of gastric mucosal folds can produce an irregular filling defect in the distal esophagus (Fig. 6-36*A*). Serial films demonstrate reduction of the prolapse, return of the gastric folds below the diaphragm, and a normal distal esophagus (Fig. 6-36*B*).

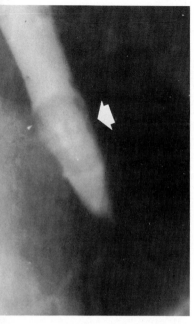

Fig. 6-34. Button **(arrow)** impacted in the distal esophagus just above the level of the diaphragm. The nonopaque plastic button appears as a filling defect in the barium column, with small amounts of contrast showing the four holes in it.

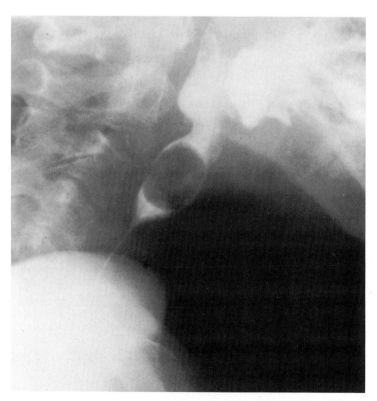

Fig. 6-35. Cherry pit impacted in the cervical esophagus proximal to a caustic stricture.

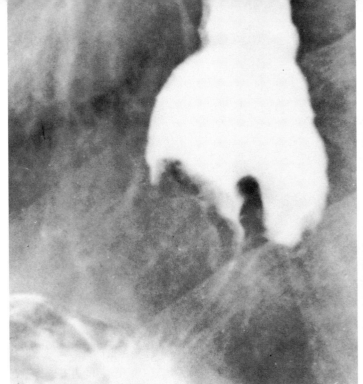
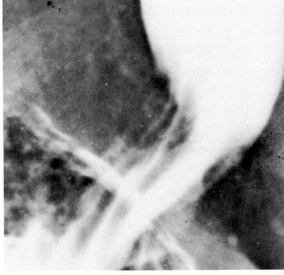

A B

Fig. 6-36. Prolapse of gastric mucosal folds. **(A)** Irregular filling defect in the distal esophagus. **(B)** After reduction of the prolapse, the distal esophagus appears normal.

BIBLIOGRAPHY

Anderson MF, Harell GS: Secondary esophageal tumors. AJR 135:1243–1246, 1980

Bleshman MH, Banner MP, Johnson RC et al: The inflammatory esophagogastric polyp and fold. Radiology 128:589–593, 1978

Carnovale RL, Goldstein HM, Zornoza J et al: Radiologic manifestations of esophageal lymphoma. AJR 128:751–754, 1977

Ghahremani GG, Meyers MA, Port RB: Calcified primary tumors of the gastrointestinal tract. Gastrointest Radiol 2:331–339, 1978

Goldstein HM, Zornoza J, Hopens T: Intrinsic diseases of the adult esophagus: Benign and malignant tumors. Semin Roentgenol 16:183–197, 1981

Jang GC, Clouse ME, Fleischner FG: Fibrovascular polyp: A benign intraluminal tumor of the esophagus. Radiology 92:1196–1200, 1969

Keshian JM, Alford PC: Granular cell myoblastoma of the esophagus. Am Surg 30:263–266, 1964

McCort JJ: Esophageal carcinosarcoma and pseudosarcoma. Radiology 102:519–524, 1972

Meyerowitz BR, Shea LT: The natural history of squamous verrucose carcinoma of the esophagus. J Thorac Cardiovasc Surg 61:646–649, 1970

Meyers C, Durkin MG, Love L: Radiographic findings in herpetic esophagitis. Radiology 119:21–22, 1976

Minielly JA, Harrison EG, Fontana RS et al: Verrucous squamous cell carcinoma of the esophagus. Cancer 20:2078–2087, 1967

Parnell S, Pepperom MA, Antoniola DA et al: Squamous cell papilloma of the esophagus. Gastroenterology 74:910–913, 1978

Schatzki R, Hawes LE: The roentgenologic appearance of extra-mucosal tumors of the esophagus. AJR 48:1–15, 1942

Shaffer HA: Multiple leiomyomas of the esophagus. Radiology 118:29–34, 1976

Smith PC, Swischuk LE, Fagan CJ: An elusive and often unsuspected cause of stridor or pneumonia (the esophageal foreign body). AJR 122:80–89, 1974

Walker JH: Giant papilloma of the thoracic esophagus. AJR 131:519–520, 1978

7

ESOPHAGEAL DIVERTICULA

Disease Entities

Cervical diverticula
    Zenker's (pharyngoesophageal)
    Traction (from surgery, infection)
Midesophageal diverticula
    Traction (interbronchial)
    Pulsion (interaorticobronchial)
Epiphrenic diverticula
Intramural esophageal pseudodiverticulosis

Esophageal diverticula are common lesions that are best divided according to the sites at which they occur. Their walls can contain all esophageal layers (traction) or be composed only of mucosa and submucosa herniating through the muscularis (pulsion). Almost all are acquired lesions.

ZENKER'S DIVERTICULA

A Zenker's diverticulum arises in the upper esophagus, its neck lying in the midline of the posterior wall at the pharyngoesophageal junction (approximately the C5-6 level). The development of a Zenker's diverticulum is apparently related to the premature contraction or other motor incoordination of the cricopharyngeus muscle, which produces increased intraluminal pressure and a pulsion diverticulum at a point of antomic weakness between the oblique and circular fibers of the muscle. Although many of these diverticula are asymptomatic, they may cause the insidious development of throat irritation with excessive mucus or the sensation during swallowing of the presence of a foreign body. A gurgling in the throat can be noted when liquids are swallowed.

As the diverticulum enlarges, dysphagia becomes more marked, and regurgitation of food and mucus may occur after meals and at night. Pulmonary complications secondary to aspiration pneumonia are not uncommon. A Zenker's diverticulum occasionally enlarges to such an extent that it compresses the esophagus at the level of the thoracic inlet and produces esophageal obstruction.

On plain radiographs of the neck, a Zenker's diverticulum may appear as a widening of the retrotracheal soft-tissue space, often with an air–fluid level (Fig. 7-1). Oral contrast is necessary to differentiate this appearance from a retrotracheal abscess. A Zenker's diverticulum presents as a saccular outpouching protruding from the esophageal lumen and connected to it by a relatively narrow neck (Fig. 7-2). Because the diverticulum arises from the posterior wall of the esophagus, it is best visualized at barium swallow in the lateral projection, though slight obliquity sometimes may be necessary. As the sac enlarges, it extends downward and posteriorly, displacing the cervical esophagus anteriorly and often causing marked narrowing of the adjacent esophageal lumen (Fig. 7-3). Barium and food may be retained in a Zenker's diverticulum for hours or even days after they have been ingested.

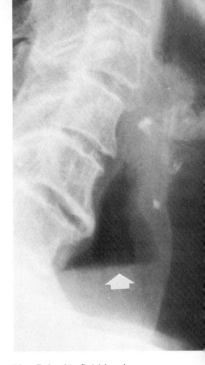

Fig. 7-1. Air–fluid level **(arrow)** in the retrotracheal soft-tissue space representing a Zenker's diverticulum.

CERVICAL TRACTION DIVERTICULA

Traction diverticula may also occur in the cervical esophagus. In this region, they can be the result of fibrous healing of an inflammatory process in the neck or be secondary to postsurgical changes (*e.g.*, laryngectomy; Fig. 7-4).

THORACIC DIVERTICULA

Diverticula of the thoracic portion of the esophagus are primarily found in the middle third opposite the bifurcation of the trachea in the region of the hilum of the lung. These interbronchial diverticula are almost invariably traction diverticula that develop in response to the pull of fibrous adhesions following infection of the mediastinal lymph nodes. Associated symptoms are rare, though mediastinal abscess or esophagorespiratory fistula may occur. Barium swallow demonstrates a diverticular collection of contrast that may have a funnel, cone, tent, or fusiform shape and is usually best visualized in the left anterior oblique projection (Fig. 7-5). Calcified mediastinal nodes from healed granulomatous disease (especially tuberculosis) are often seen adjacent to the diverticulum.

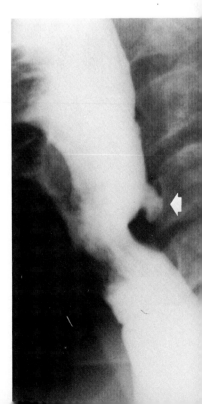

Fig. 7-2. Small Zenker's diverticulum. The saccular outpouching **(arrow)** arises just proximal to the posterior cricopharyngeus impression.

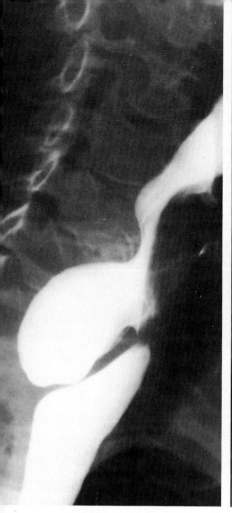
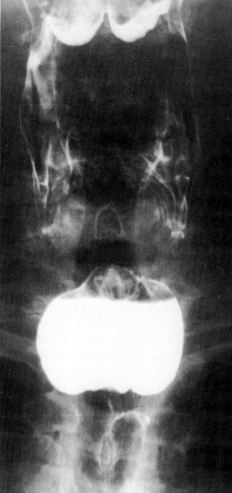

Fig. 7-3. (A) Oblique and **(B)** frontal views of a large Zenker's diverticulum almost occluding the esophageal lumen.

A B

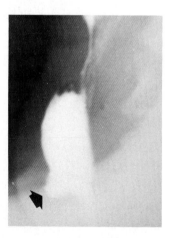
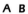

Fig. 7-4. Traction diverticulum **(arrow)** in the cervical esophagus caused by postoperative scarring following total laryngectomy.

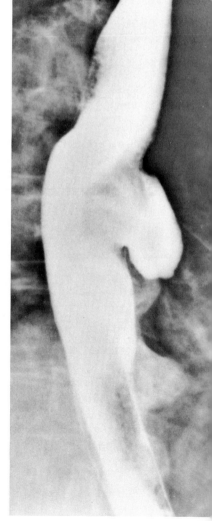

Fig. 7-5. Traction diverticulum of the midthoracic esophagus.

Much less frequently, midesophageal diverticula may be of the pulsion type. These interaorticobronchial diverticula arise in a relatively weak area on the left anterolateral wall of the esophagus between the inferior border of the aortic arch and the upper external margin of the left main bronchus. Because of its position, an interaorticobronchial diverticulum can be seen only in the right anterior oblique projection, in which it is separated from superimposition on the esophageal lumen.

EPIPHRENIC DIVERTICULA

Epiphrenic diverticula are usually of the pulsion type and occur in the distal 10 cm of the esophagus (Fig. 7-6). These diverticula appear to be associated with motor abnormalities of the esophagus and are probably related to incoordination of esophageal peristalsis and sphincter relaxation, resulting in the lower esophageal segment being subjected to increased intraluminal pressure. An epiphrenic diverticulum is rarely symptomatic, though it may produce symptoms because of its large size and the retention of food within it. Radiographically, an epiphrenic diverticulum tends to have a broad and short neck. If small, it can simulate an esophageal ulcer, though the normal appearance of the mucosal pattern of the adjacent esophagus usually permits differentiation between these two entities.

CARCINOMA DEVELOPING IN DIVERTICULA

Pulsion diverticula in the cervical or distal esophagus are usually smooth in contour. Irregularity of a diverticulum in either of these regions should suggest the possibility of infection or malignancy (Fig. 7-7). If prior radiographs are available for comparison, the interval development of an irregular margin in a previously smooth diverticulum is an ominous sign.

INTRAMURAL ESOPHAGEAL PSEUDODIVERTICULOSIS

Intramural esophageal pseudodiverticulosis can simulate diverticular involvement of the esophagus. In this extremely rare disorder, numerous small (1–3 mm), flask-shaped outpouchings represent dilated ducts coming from submucosal glands (Fig. 7-8). There is frequently a smooth stricture in the upper esophagus. Since these are not true diverticula of the muscular esophageal wall, the term pseudodiverticulosis is most correct. The radiographic appearance of multiple ulcerlike projections has been likened to a chain of beads and to the Rokitansky–Aschoff sinuses of the gallbladder. *Candida albicans* can be cultured from about half of patients with intramural pseudodiverticulosis, though there is no evidence to suggest the fungus as a causative agent.

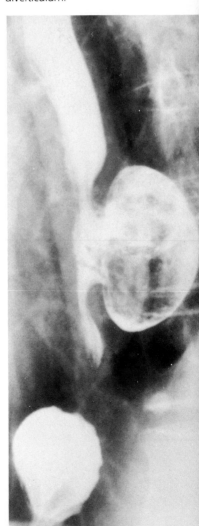

Fig. 7-6. Epiphrenic diverticulum.

Fig. 7-7. Carcinoma arising in an epiphrenic diverticulum. **(A)** The initial esophagram demonstrates a mild irregularity of the diverticulum that was not appreciated at the time of the examination. **(B)** Six months later, the large, ulcerating carcinoma of the esophagus is obvious.

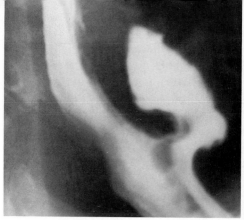
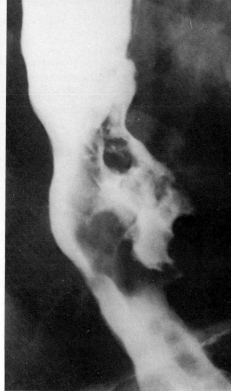

A

B

Fig. 7-8. Intramural esophageal pseudodiverticulosis. The numerous diverticular outpouchings represent dilated ducts coming from submucosal glands in the wall of the esophagus.

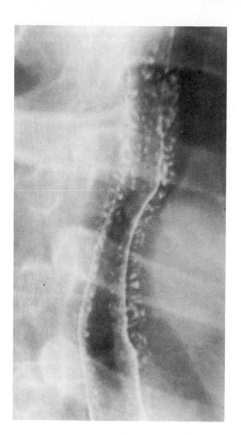

BIBLIOGRAPHY

Beauchamp JM, Nice CM, Belanger MA et al: Esophageal intramural pseudo-diverticulosis. Radiology 113:273–276, 1974

Bruggeman LL, Seaman WB: Epiphrenic diverticula: An analysis of 80 cases. AJR 119:266–276, 1973

Royd RM, Bogoch A, Greig JH et al: Esophageal intramural pseudodiverticulum. Radiology 113:267–270, 1974

Shirazi KK, Daffner RH, Gaede JT: Ulcer occurring in Zenker's diverticulum. Gastrointest Radiol 2:117–118, 1977

Wychulis RA, Gunnlaugsson HG, Clagett OT: Carcinoma occurring in pharyngoesophageal diverticulum. Surgery 66:976–979, 1969

ESOPHAGEAL VARICES

8

Disease Entities

Portal hypertension
   Hepatic cirrhosis
   Carcinoma of the pancreas
   Pancreatitis
   Retroperitoneal inflammatory disease
   High-viscosity–slow-flow states (*e.g.,* polycythemia)
Noncirrhotic liver disease
   Metastatic carcinoma
   Carcinoma of the liver
   Congestive heart failure
Superior vena cava obstruction
   Mediastinal tumors (*e.g.,* bronchogenic carcinoma)
   Chronic fibrosing mediastinitis
   Retrosternal goiter
   Thymoma

ETIOLOGY

Esophageal varices, dilated veins in the subepithelial connective tissue, are most commonly a result of portal hypertension (Fig. 8-1). Increased pressure in the portal venous system is usually secondary to cirrhosis of the liver. Other causes of portal hypertension include obstruction of the portal or splenic veins by carcinoma of the pancreas, pancreatitis, inflammatory diseases of the retroperitoneum, and high-viscosity–slow-flow states (*e.g.,* polycythemia), which predispose to intravascular thrombosis. In patients with portal hypertension, much of the portal blood cannot flow along its normal pathway through the liver to the inferior vena cava and then on to the heart. Instead, it must go by a circuitous collateral route through the coronary vein, across the eso-phagogastric hiatus, and into the periesophageal plexus before reaching **111**

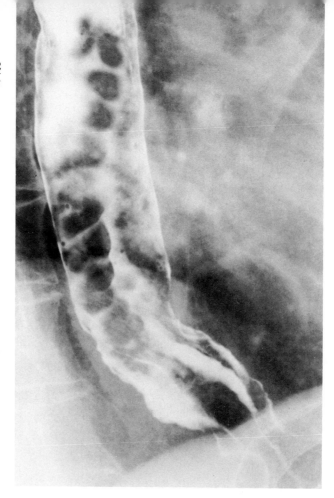

Fig. 8-1. Esophageal varices seen as a line of round filling defects representing dilated veins in the subepithelial connective tissue.

the azygos and hemiazygos systems, superior vena cava, and right atrium. The periesophageal plexus communicates with veins in the submucosa of the esophagus and gastric cardia. Increased blood flow through these veins causes the development of esophageal (and gastric) varices.

Esophageal varices are infrequently demonstrated in the absence of portal hypertension. They have been observed in patients with noncirrhotic liver disease such as metastatic carcinoma, carcinoma of the liver, and congestive heart failure. "Downhill" varices are produced when venous blood from the head and neck cannot reach the heart because of an obstruction of the superior vena cava (Fig. 8-2). This is usually secondary to progressive and prolonged compression of the superior vena cava by tumors or inflammatory disease in the mediastinum. In this situation, blood flows "downhill" through the azygos–hemiazygos system, the periesophageal plexus, and the coronary veins before eventually entering the portal vein, through which it flows to the inferior vena cava and right atrium. In patients with carcinomatous obstruction of the superior vena cava, the dilated submucosal veins tend to the confined to the upper esophagus. In patients with chronic venous obstruction due to mediastinal fibrosis, varices can involve the

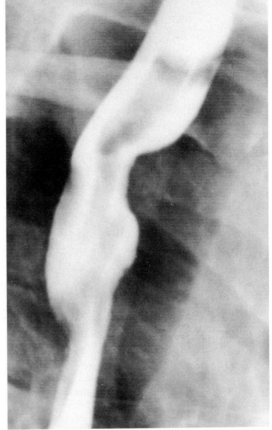

Fig. 8-2. "Downhill" varices in a patient with carcinomatous obstruction of the superior vena cava.

entire esophagus. Concomitant enlargement of intercostal vein collaterals occasionally causes rib notching.

CLINICAL SYMPTOMS

Bleeding, the major complication of esophageal varices, is nearly as likely to occur in small varices as in larger and more extensive lesions. Immediate death from exsanguination occurs in about 10% to 15% of patients with variceal bleeding. The diagnosis of esophageal varices in patients with cirrhotic liver disease implies significant portal venous hypertension and is an ominous sign. Up to 90% of the deaths from liver disease in patients with cirrhosis occur within 2 years of the diagnosis of varices.

RADIOGRAPHIC TECHNIQUES

The radiographic demonstration of esophageal varices requires precise technique. The object of the fluoroscopic examination is to line the esophageal mucosa with a very thin layer of barium so as to enhance the characteristic serpiginous appearance of the varices. Multiple radiographs must be taken during the resting stage following a swallow of barium. Complete filling of the esophagus with barium may obscure varices; powerful contractions of the esophagus may squeeze blood out of the varices and make them impossible to detect.

The examination for esophageal varices must include radiographs with the patient in a horizontal position. In this position, the transit of barium is slowed, mucosal coating is prolonged, and distention of varices is enhanced.

Varices related to portal hypertension are most commonly demonstrated in the lower third of the esophagus. When they are voluminous and extensive, varices can be seen in any projection. Early varices are generally situated on the right anterolateral wall of the distal segment of the esophagus and are therefore most easily identified in the left anterior oblique projection.

Numerous techniques have been suggested to enhance visualization of small esophageal varices. One maneuver is to obtain radiographs with the patient in deep, blocked inspiration. This lowers the position of the diaphragm and better demonstrates the distal esophagus. In addition, forced inspiration causes ballooning of the varices, making them easier to detect.

Pharmacologic agents have been used to better demonstrate small varices that cannot be identified on conventional studies. The use of 30 mg of Pro-Banthine (probantheline bromide) intramuscularly or intravenously several minutes before the administration of thick barium causes relaxation of the musculature of the distal esophagus and permits varices to fill better and remain dilated. However, the use of this anticholinergic drug is contraindicated in patients with a history of glaucoma, previous myocardial infarction, or urinary tract obstruction. Although some authors have employed glucagon to better demonstrate varices, the esophagus, unlike the rest of the gut, appears to be relatively insensitive to this drug.

RADIOGRAPHIC FINDINGS

The characteristic radiographic appearance of esophageal varices is serpiginous thickening of folds, which appear as round or oval filling defects resembling the beads of a rosary (Fig. 8-3). Initially, there is only mild thickening of folds and irregularity of the esophageal outline (Fig. 8-4). Distention with barium hides these thickened folds and causes the esophageal border to have an irregularly notched (worm-eaten) appearance (Fig. 8-5). Once the typical tortuous, ribbonlike defects are visible, the radiographic diagnosis of esophageal varices is usually easy to make (Fig. 8-6). In patients with severe portal hypertension, varices can be demonstrated throughout the entire thoracic esophagus (Fig. 8-7).

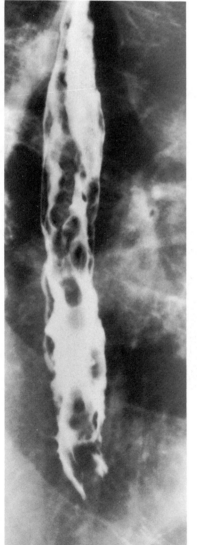

Fig. 8-3. Esophageal varices. Note the diffuse round and oval filling defects resembling the beads of a rosary.

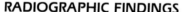

Fig. 8-4. Esophageal varices. There is moderate thickening of folds and irregularity of the esophageal outline. ▶

Fig. 8-5. Esophageal varices. Distention with barium obscures the thickened folds and causes an irregularly notched (worm-eaten) appearance. ▶

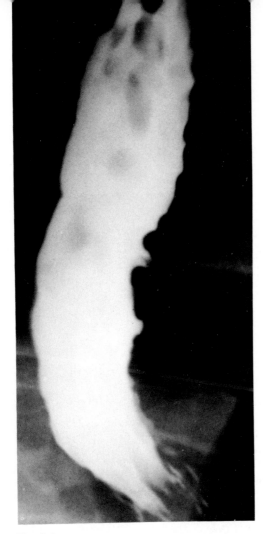

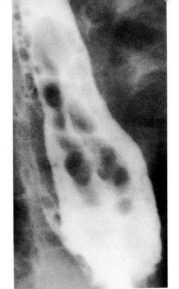

Fig. 8-6. Esophageal varices (Banti's syndrome).

Fig. 8-7. Esophageal varices. The varices extend to the level of the aortic arch in this patient with severe portal hypertension.

Fig. 8-4

Fig. 8-5

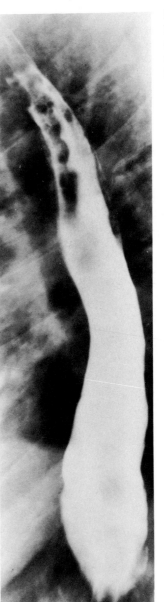

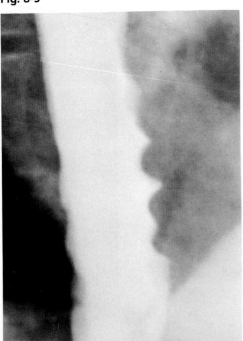

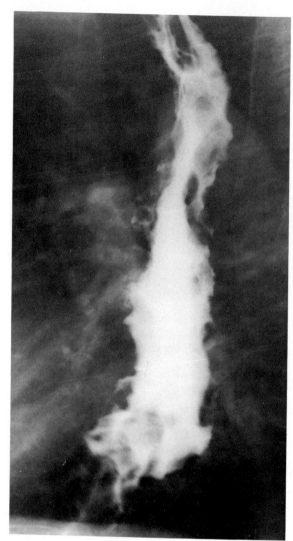

Fig. 8-8. Varicoid carcinoma.

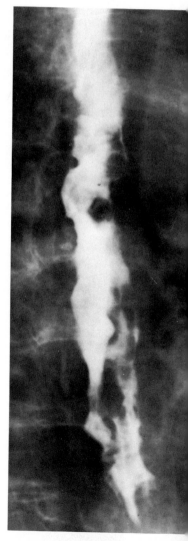

Fig. 8-9. Varicoid carcinoma.

DISORDERS SIMULATING VARICES

Several other disorders can simulate the radiographic appearance of esophageal varices. When varices are small, the thickening of mucosal folds and wall irregularity caused by them can be almost indistinguishable from mild chronic esophagitis. When varices are very large, irregular, and arrayed in a chaotic pattern, they may be confused with the varicoid form of esophageal carcinoma (Figs. 8-8, 8-9). Varices can be successfully differentiated from carcinoma in these cases by the demonstration of pliability of the walls of the esophagus, change in appearance when the esophagus is contracted and distended, and preservation of peristalsis. Rarely, lymphoma presents as a large intramural submucosal tumor with nodular folds closely resembling esophageal varices (Fig. 8-10).

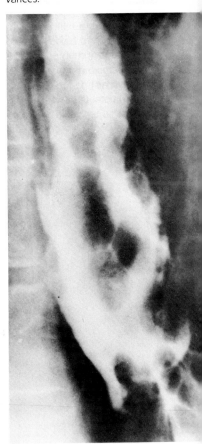

Fig. 8-10. Lymphoma presenting with thick, nodular folds that mimic esophageal varices.

BIBLIOGRAPHY

Cockerill EM, Miller RE, Chernish SM et al: Optimal visualization of esophageal varices. AJR 126:512–523, 1976

Felson B, Lessure AP: "Downhill" varices of esophagus. Dis Chest 46:740–746, 1964

Mikkelsen WJ: Varices of the upper esophagus in superior vena caval obstruction. Radiology 81:945–948, 1963

Nelson SW: The roentgenologic diagnosis of esophageal varices. AJR 77:599–611, 1957

Yates CW, LeVine MA, Jensen KM: Varicoid carcinoma of the esophagus. Radiology 122:605–608, 1977

the respiratory tract (Fig. 9-4). Fistulization is usually a late complication and often a terminal event. An esophagorespiratory fistula can also be a complication of erosion into the esophagus by carcinoma of the lung arising near or metastasizing to the middle mediastinum (Fig. 9-5) or by mediastinal metastases from other primary sites (Fig. 9-6). Regardless of therapy, the overall prognosis of malignant esophagorespiratory fistulas is dismal. About 80% of patients with this complication die within 3 months; only a few survive more than 1 year. The cause of death in these patients is either pulmonary infection due to repeated aspiration pneumonias, or uncontrollable hemorrhage.

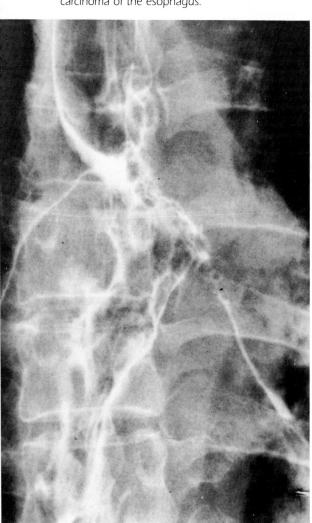

Fig. 9-4. Esophagorespiratory fistula due to squamous carcinoma of the esophagus.

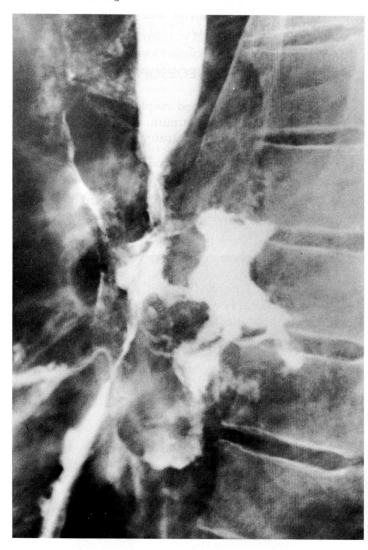

Fig. 9-5. Esophagorespiratory fistula secondary to squamous carcinoma of the lung.

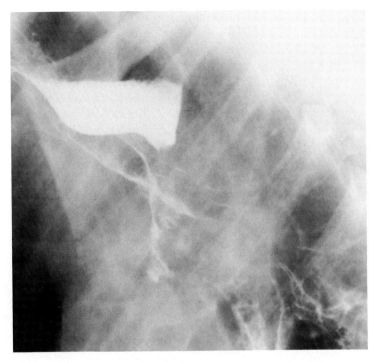

Fig. 9-6. Esophagorespiratory fistula caused by mediastinal metastases from adenocarcinoma of the cervix.

ESOPHAGEAL INSTRUMENTATION / VOMITING / TRAUMA

Fistulous communication between the esophagus and the trachea can be the result of esophageal instrumentation and perforation. This is most common after esophagoscopy but may also occur after dilatation of strictures by bouginage with direct vision, the use of weighted mercury nasogastric bougies (especially the Sengstaken–Blakemore tube for tamponade), pneumatic dilatation for the treatment of achalasia, or even insertion of a nasogastric tube (Fig. 9-7). The incidence of instrumental perforation depends to some extent on the underlying integrity of the esophagus; there is a higher than normal rate of postdilatation perforation in patients with caustic strictures, recent esophageal or periesophageal surgery, and malignant tumors (Fig. 9-8). Blunt or penetrating trauma to the chest, especially after crush injury, can result in esophageal perforation and fistulization. There is a relationship between the traumatic agent and the site of communication between the esophagus and the respiratory tract. Fistulas caused by instrumentation of esophageal strictures or ingested foreign bodies tend to communicate with either the right or the left main stem bronchus. Those caused by compression injury tend to communicate with the trachea.

Traumatic perforation of the thoracic esophagus leads to excruciating chest, back, or epigastric pain accompanied by dysphagia and respiratory distress. Chest radiographs demonstrate air dissecting within the mediastinum and soft tissues, often with pleural effusion or hydropneumothorax. The introduction of an oral contrast agent may demonstrate the site of perforation and the extent of fistulization.

Esophageal rupture caused by severe vomiting appears clinically as epigastric pain radiating to the shoulder-blades in a patient who appears gravely ill with pallor, sweatiness, tachycardia, and often shock. This disorder most frequently occurs in males and usually follows heavy drinking and a large meal (Boerhaave's syndrome) (Fig. 9-9). However, since this postemetic rupture usually occurs near the eso-phagogastric junction, it does not generally lead to development of an esophagorespiratory fistula.

Fig. 9-7. Esophagorespiratory fistula as a complication of nasogastric tube placement in a patient with squamous carcinoma of the esophagus.

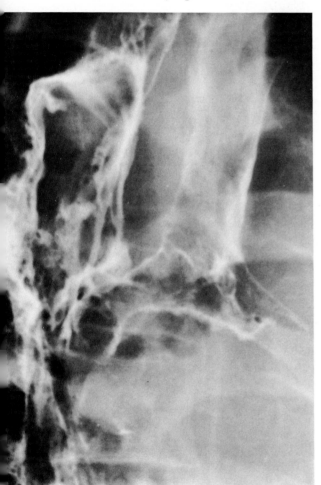

Fig. 9-8. Esophageal rupture following esophagoscopy in a patient with squamous carcinoma of the esophagus.

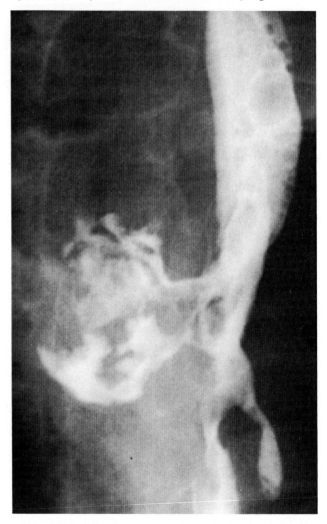

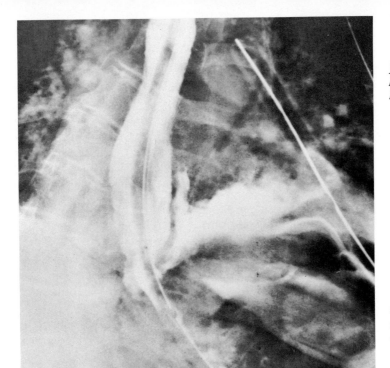

Fig. 9-9. Boerhaave's syndrome. Esophageal rupture occurred as a complication of severe vomiting in an elderly alcoholic.

CORROSIVE ESOPHAGITIS

Another form of traumatic insult to the esophagus is the ingestion of corrosive agents, especially alkali such as lye. Deep penetration of these toxic agents and necrosis through the entire wall of the esophagus can cause perforation, mediastinal inflammation, and fistulization, which may lead to a communication between the esophagus and respiratory tract (Fig. 9-10).

INFECTIOUS / GRANULOMATOUS ESOPHAGITIS

Fistulous communication between the esophagus and respiratory tract may be due to a variety of infectious processes. Mediastinal lymph nodes that undergo caseation or necrosis may rupture into the esophagus and tracheobronchial tree. In addition, any ulcerative lesion in the midesophagus or upper esophagus can extend through the wall and penetrate into the trachea or bronchus, causing an esophagorespiratory fistula.

In the early literature, tuberculosis and syphilis were reported as relatively common causes of esophagorespiratory fistulas. However, the esophagus is one of the organs least likely to be involved by tuberculosis. There is almost always evidence of the disease elsewhere, primarily in the lungs. In addition to its more common manifestations, such as ulceration and fibrotic narrowing, tuberculosis may result in sinuses or fistulous tracts.

Syphilis of the esophagus is a rare lesion. Inflammation of mediastinal lymph nodes in this disease may secondarily involve the esophagus.

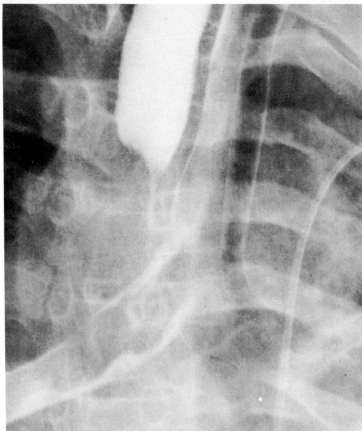

Fig. 9-10. Caustic esophagorespiratory fistula. The fistula developed in a patient who had ingested lye 1 month previously.

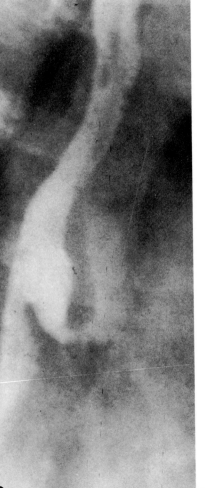

This process can cause extensive compression, resulting in esophageal obstruction, or necrosis and perforation, leading to a fistulous connection with the respiratory tract. The relentless pounding of a syphilitic aortic aneurysm can weaken the walls of the adjacent esophagus and trachea and lead to a communication between them.

Although histoplasmosis does not primarily affect the esophagus, the disease frequently causes a granulomatous inflammatory process involving mediastinal lymph nodes. Infrequently, this can lead to ulceration and fistulization between the esophagus and trachea.

Actinomycosis, though uncommonly involving the esophagus, can spread to that organ from adjacent foci by direct penetration or by hematogenous spread from a distant site. Radiographically, actinomycosis produces nonspecific ulceration, inflammation, and, not infrequently, an esophagorespiratory fistula. Fistulization between the esophagus and the respiratory tract is a rare complication of Crohn's disease involving the esophagus.

Fig. 9-11. Esophagorespiratory fistula secondary to ruptured traction diverticulum. There is a short, fistulous tract extending from the diverticulum to the left main stem bronchus. (Balthazar EJ: Esophagobronchial fistula secondary to ruptured traction diverticulum. Gastrointest Radiol 2:119–121, 1977)

OTHER CAUSES

Rarely, traction diverticula of the midesophagus perforate, causing the development of a mediastinal abscess or esophagorespiratory fistula (Fig. 9-11). These diverticula, which arise opposite the bifurcation of the trachea or near the left main stem bronchus, are generally related to fixation and traction exerted by the healing of inflamed lymph nodes (tuberculosis, histoplasmosis) adherent to the esophagus. On occasion, vertebral disease is the underlying factor.

Fistulization can occur between the esophagus and a pulmonary cyst or sequestered portion of the lung. Sequestration of the lung is a congenital pulmonary malformation in which a portion of pulmonary tissue is detached from the remainder of the normal lung and receives its blood supply from a systemic artery. Mediastinal cysts, especially if infected, can invade or erode the esophagus and trachea, causing esophagorespiratory fistulas similar to those secondary to mediastinal tumors.

On rare occasions, "spontaneous" fistulas occur between the esophagus and respiratory tract. In patients with this disorder, no evidence of pre-existing or concomitant disease can be demonstrated.

BIBLIOGRAPHY

Balthazar EJ: Esophagobronchial fistula secondary to ruptured traction diverticulum. Gastrointest Radiol 2:119–121, 1977

Caffey J: Pediatric X-ray Diagnosis, pp. 668–682. Chicago, Year Book Medical Publishers, 1978

Coleman FP: Acquired non-malignant esophagorespiratory fistula. Am J Surg 93:321–328, 1957

Martini N, Goodner JT, D'Angio GJ: Tracheoesophageal fistula due to cancer. J Thorac Cardiovasc Surg 59:319–324, 1970

Nelson RJ, Benfield JR: Benign esophagobronchial fistula. Arch Surg 100:685–688, 1970

10

DOUBLE-BARREL ESOPHAGUS

Disease Entities

Dissecting intramural hematoma
  Emetogenic injury
  Trauma
  Instrumentation
  Ingestion of a foreign body
  Spontaneous (bleeding diathesis)
Intramural abscess
Intraluminal diverticulum
Esophageal duplication

The term double-barrel esophagus refers to the radiographic appearance of an intramural dissecting channel opacified by barium that is separated by an intervening lucent line (mucosal stripe) from the normal esophageal lumen (Fig. 10-1). The radiographic pattern is strikingly similar to the typical findings in dissecting aneurysm of the aorta (Fig. 10-2), the esophageal mucosal stripe of the former being the equivalent of the undermined aortic intima of the latter.

INTRAMURAL HEMATOMA

EMETOGENIC INJURY

Vomiting consists of a complex series of movements controlled by the vagus nerve. The diaphragm descends to a deep inspiratory position as the expiratory muscles contract. As the glottis closes, the pyloric part of the stomach contracts while the body, cardia, and esophagus dilate. Compression of the flaccid stomach by raised intra-abdominal pressure due to the descent of the diaphragm and the contraction of abdominal

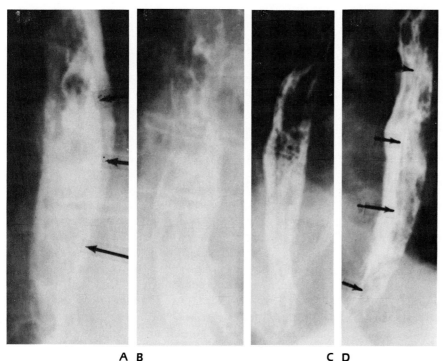

A B   C D

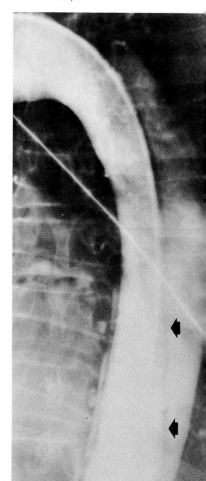

Fig. 10-2. Dissection of the aorta. Note the similarity of the undermined aortic intima **(arrows)** to the esophageal mucosal stripe.

Fig. 10-1. Intramural dissection of the esophagus (mucosal stripe sign.) **(A)** The sharply defined, lucent linear stripe **(arrows)** represents the dissected mucosa separating the two lumina. No extra-esophageal extravasation of barium is present. **(B)** After the barium has been washed out of the central lumen, the retained barium is contained in the outer cylinder. The mucosal stripe sign is now absent. **(C)** During the act of swallowing barium, the mucosal stripe sign persists. **(D) Arrows** outline the extent of the mucosal stripe sign. The rent in the mucosa was demonstrated by esophagoscopy. (Lowman RM, Goldman R, Stern H: The roentgen aspects of intramural dissection of the esophagus. Radiology 93:1329–1331, 1969)

wall muscles causes evacuation of stomach contents. Repeated vomiting at short intervals can impair neuromuscular coordination and produce muscular fatigue. If the cardia fails to open as the abdominal muscles vigorously contract, tears are likely to result.

The severity of emetogenic injury varies from a relatively minor mucosal laceration to complete rupture of the wall of the esophagus. Superficial mucosal lacerations result in little or no significant hemorrhage. In patients with severe vomiting, whether from dietary or alcoholic indiscretion or from any other cause, the sudden development of severe epigastric pain should suggest an esophageal perforation (Boerhaave's syndrome). In this condition, plain chest radiographs must be carefully examined for evidence of pneumomediastinum or cervical emphysema as well as for pleural changes at the left base. Contrast studies may demonstate extravasation through a transmural perforation (Fig. 10-3).

The Mallory–Weiss syndrome is characterized by upper gastrointestinal bleeding due to superficial mucosal lacerations or fissures near the esophagogastric junction that are caused by an increase in intraluminal and intramural pressure gradients. Most lacerations occur in the gastric mucosa or extend across the esophagogastric junction. In about 10% of cases, only the esophageal mucosa is involved (Fig. 10-4).

Mallory–Weiss tears usually occur in men over the age of 50 who have a history of alcohol excess. They present clinically with repeated vomiting followed by hematemesis. The syndrome occasionally develops without vomiting; coughing, defecation, and lifting of heavy loads have been implicated as causative factors.

Unlike the situation with complete esophageal perforation, radiographic findings are very rarely seen in patients with the Mallory–Weiss syndrome. An esophagram may sometimes demonstrate barium penetration into the wall of the esophagus (Fig. 10-5).

Between the two extremes, emetogenic injury infrequently causes an intermediate laceration with bleeding into the wall of the esophagus and dissection of the esophageal wall in the submucosal plane. Unless spontaneously decompressed into the lumen or externally by rupture, the ensuing hematoma within the esophagus may be extensive.

RADIOGRAPHIC FINDINGS

An intramural esophageal hematoma that is not connected to the lumen produces compression and displacement of the barium-filled esophagus. Its appearance is similar to that seen in arteriographic studies of dissecting aortic aneurysms. If the hematoma has decompressed into the lumen, barium examination reveals contrast filling the false intra-

Fig. 10-3. Boerhaave's syndrome. An esophagram demonstrates the extravasation of contrast **(arrows)** through a transmural perforation.

Fig. 10-4. Mallory–Weiss tear confined to the esophageal mucosa **(arrows).**

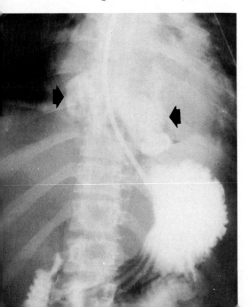

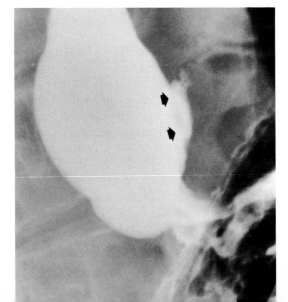

mural channel as well as the true lumen of the esophagus (Fig. 10-6). The close approximation of the intraluminal and intramural collections of barium and the relatively rapid emptying of the intramural channel should permit differentiation from complete rupture of the esophagus, in which contrast material enters the mediastinum and is retained in periesophageal tissues.

TRAUMA / INSTRUMENTATION

Intramural hematomas may occur following trauma or instrumentation. The incidence of esophageal perforation during esophagoscopy has been estimated at 0.25% with a mortality rate of 0.06%. The rate of perforation associated with esophageal dilatation using mercury bougies is about 0.5%; with pneumatic dilators, it is even higher. Perforation can be complete or be incomplete and confined to the mucosa. In the latter instance, a submucosal hematoma can produce dissection of the esophageal wall resulting in a double-barrel esophagus, with the true and false lumens separated by a radiolucent mucosal stripe.

Dissecting intramural hematomas of the esophagus can occur after the ingestion of sharp foreign bodies. Intramural hemorrhage related to a bleeding diathesis may also develop without trauma. This has been

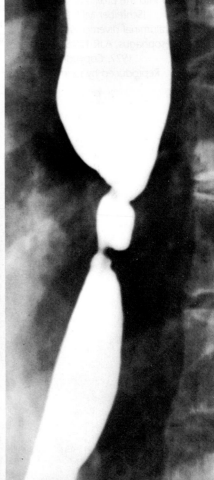

Fig. 10-5. Mallory–Weiss tear (arrows).

A B

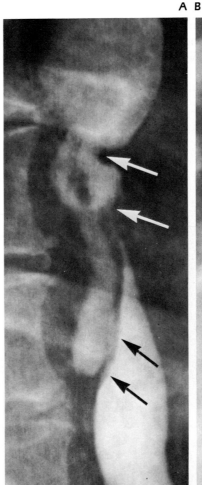

Fig. 10-6. Intramural esophageal hematoma. **(A)** An esophagram with gastrografin demonstrates two midesophageal strictures **(white arrows).** Distal to the lower stricture are two columns of contrast material separated by a radiolucent stripe **(black arrows).** The smaller, posterior column represents the intramural collection of contrast material. **(B)** A follow-up esophagram shows the complete resolution of the intramural hematoma. Only strictures are demonstrated. (Bradley JL, Han SY: Intramural hematoma (incomplete perforation) of the esophagus associated with esophageal dilatation. Radiology 130:59–62, 1979)

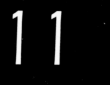

11

DIFFUSE FINELY NODULAR LESIONS OF THE ESOPHAGUS

Disease Entities

Leukoplakia
Superficial spreading esophageal carcinoma
Acanthosis nigricans
Candidiasis
Reflux esophagitis
Corrosive esophagitis
Tuberculosis

LEUKOPLAKIA

Leukoplakia refers to small round foci of epithelial hyperplasia that appear on esophagoscopy as tiny white patches. They can occasionally be seen radiographically as small, superficial nodular filling defects with somewhat poorly defined borders (Fig. 11-1). Peristalsis is not impaired. Prominent lesions of leukoplakia are most commonly located in the middle third of the esophagus.

SUPERFICIAL SPREADING ESOPHAGEAL CARCINOMA

Superficial spreading esophageal carcinoma, if its invasion is limited to the submucosal layer, may appear radiographically as a granular pattern (Fig. 11-2). Impaired distensibility of the wall of the esophagus in addition to multiple finely nodular filling defects suggest the diagnosis of superficial spreading esophageal carcinoma.

ACANTHOSIS NIGRICANS

Acanthosis nigricans is a premalignant skin disorder characterized by papillomatosis, pigmentation, and hyperkeratosis. When it involves the esophagus, multiple verrucous proliferations throughout the mucosa similar to the skin changes may produce the radiographic appearance of finely nodular filling defects (Fig. 11-3). Acanthosis nigricans has been associated with a higher than normal incidence of malignant tumors, usually in the stomach or elsewhere in the abdomen.

Fig. 11-1. Leukoplakia. Small, superficial nodular filling defects with somewhat poorly defined borders are visible. (Itai J, Kogure P, Okujama J et al: Diffuse finely nodular lesions of the esophagus. AJR 128:563–566, 1977. Copyright 1977. Reproduced by permission)

Fig. 11-2. Superficial spreading esophageal carcinoma with dense, granular lesions in the midesophagus. A nasogastric tube used for air insufflation is seen at the level of the aortic knob. (Itai, J, Kogure P, Okujama J et al: Diffuse finely nodular lesions of the esophagus. AJR 128:563–566, 1977. Copyright 1977. Reproduced by permission)

Fig. 11-3. Acanthosis nigricans. Innumerable elevations are seen without evidence of serration of the esophageal margins. (Itai J, Kogure P, Okujama J et al: Diffuse finely nodular lesions of the esophagus. AJR 128:563–566, 1977. Copyright 1977. Reproduced by permission)

Fig. 11-1   **Fig. 11-2**

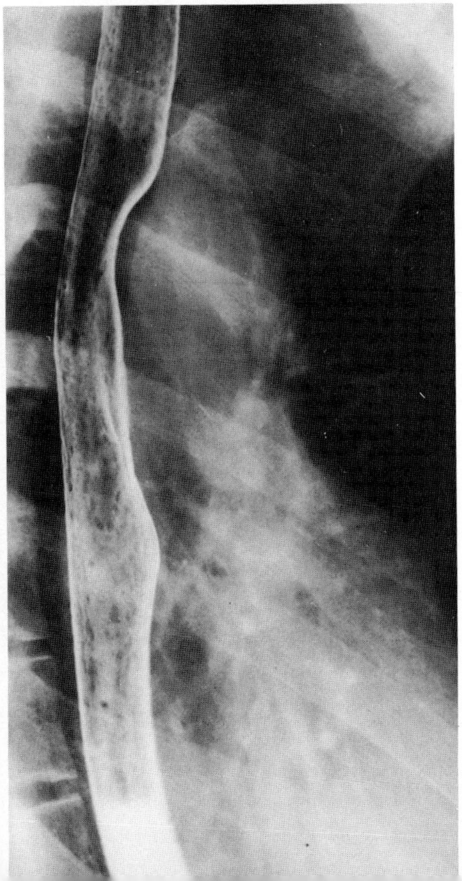

Fig. 11-3

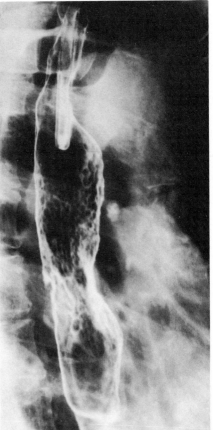
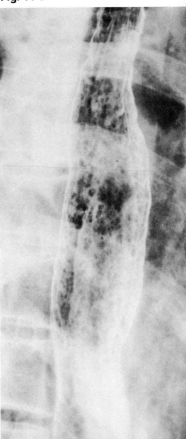

ESOPHAGITIS

In esophageal candidiasis, the earliest morphologic abnormalities consist of subtle marginal filling defects due to small pseudomembranous plaques that can be mistaken for tiny air bubbles (Fig. 11-4). Similarly, a diffuse granular pattern can be seen on double-contrast examination in an early stage of reflux (Fig. 11-5) or corrosive (Fig. 11-6) esophagitis. If the esophagus is involved with diffuse tuberculosis, numerous miliary granulomas may produce the radiographic appearance of multiple finely nodular lesions.

Fig. 11-4 Candidiasis. Filling defects representing small pseudomembranous plaques simulate tiny air bubbles.

Fig. 11-5. Reflux esophagitis. Note the diffuse granular appearance.

Fig. 11-6. Caustic esophagitis following lye ingestion.

Fig. 11-4   **Fig. 11-5**   **Fig. 11-6**

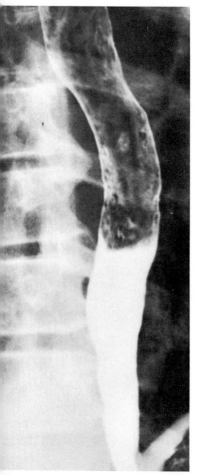
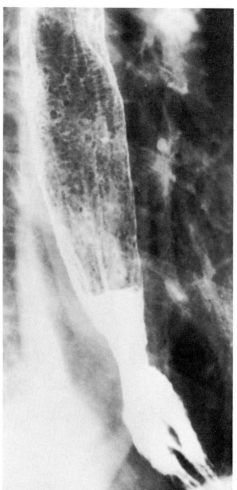
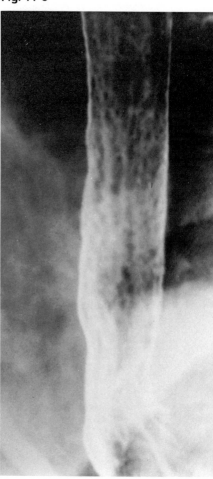

BIBLIOGRAPHY

Guyer PB, Brunton FJ, Rooke HWP: Candidiasis of the oesophagus. Br J Radiol 44:131–136, 1971

Itai Y, Kogure T, Okuyama Y et al: Diffuse fine nodular lesions of the esophagus. AJR 128:563–566, 1977

Itai Y, Kogure T, Okuyama Y et al: Radiological manifestations of esophageal involvement in acanthosis nigricans. Br J Radiol 49:592–593, 1976

Itai Y, Kogure T, Okuyama Y et al: Superficial esophageal carcinoma. Radiology 126:597–601, 1978

Koehler RE, Weyman PJ, Oakley HF: Single- and double-contrast techniques in esophagitis. AJR 135:15–19, 1980

Ott DJ, Gelfand DW, Wu WC: Reflux esophagitis: Radiographic and endoscopic correlation. Radiology 130:583–588, 1979

PART TWO

DIAPHRAGM

The diaphragm is a muscular structure separating the thoracic and abdominal cavities. It is attached to the xiphoid process and lower costal cartilages anteriorly, the ribs laterally, and the ribs and upper three lumbar vertebrae posteriorly. The diaphragm has a central membranous portion (central tendon) in which there is no muscle. The muscles of the diaphragm arch upward toward the central tendon to form a smooth, dome-shaped appearance on both sides.

The height of the diaphragm varies considerably with the phase of respiration. On full inspiration, the diaphragm is usually at about the level of the tenth posterior intercostal space. In expiration, it may appear 2 or 3 intercostal spaces higher. The position of the diaphragm in children and young adults is somewhat higher than in full-grown adults; in the aged, the diaphragm is usually lower in position. The level of the diaphragm rises as a patient moves from an upright to a supine position. The dome of the diaphragm tends to be about half an interspace higher on the right than on the left. However, in about 10% of patients, the hemidiaphragms are at the same height or the left is higher than the right.

EVENTRATION OF THE DIAPHRAGM

Eventration of the diaphragm is a congenital abnormality in which one hemidiaphragm (very rarely both) is hypoplastic, consisting of a thin, membranous sheet attached peripherally to normal muscle at points of origin from the rib cage. The peripheral musculature and phrenic innervation are intact. Because the thinned, weakened musculature is inadequate to restrain the abdominal viscera, the diaphragm rises to a more cephalad position than normal. Total eventration occurs almost exclusively on the left (Fig. 12-1). If only a portion of the diaphragm is weakened, a localized bulge may be seen. This usually involves the anteromedial portion of the right hemidiaphragm, through which a portion of the right lobe of the liver bulges (Fig. 12-2). Local eventration can also occur elsewhere, particularly posteriorly, where upward displacement of the kidney can produce a rounded mass simulating a neoplasm (Fig. 12-3A,B). In this situation, excretory urography clearly demonstrates the nature of the lesion (Fig. 12-3C).

Eventration of the diaphragm is usually asymptomatic and an incidental radiographic finding. Infrequently, nonspecific dyspepsia, epigastric discomfort or burning, and eructation can occur. Cardiopulmonary distress is uncommon in adults, though cardiovascular embarrassment can be a result of eventration of the diaphragm in neonates.

Radiographically, eventration appears as localized bulging or generalized elevation of the diaphragm (Fig. 12-4). At fluoroscopy, movement of the diaphragm may be normal or diminished; absent respiratory excursion on the affected side may be noted. The cardiomediastinal structures may be displaced toward the contralateral side. Paradoxical diaphragmatic motion is occasionally demonstrated, though it is much more commonly seen in patients with paralysis of the diaphragm. In

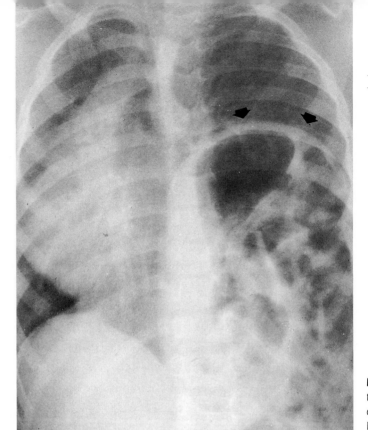

Fig. 12-1. Total eventration of the left hemidiaphragm of a child. The dome of the left hemidiaphragm is at the level of the sixth posterior rib **(arrow).**

Fig. 12-2. Partial eventration of the right hemidiaphragm **(arrow).**

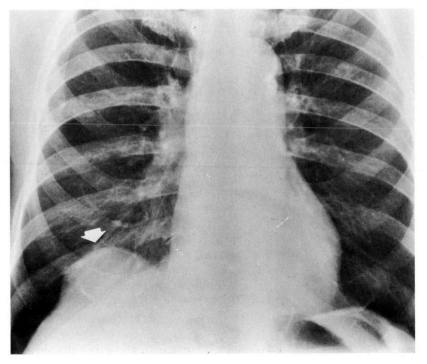

Fig. 12-3. (A) Frontal and **(B)** lateral radiographs of the chest demonstrate a rounded mass simulating a neoplasm posteriorly at the left base **(arrows). (C)** An excretory urogram clearly shows that the mass represents upward displacement of a normal kidney **(arrow)** in a patient with local eventration of the left hemidiphragm.

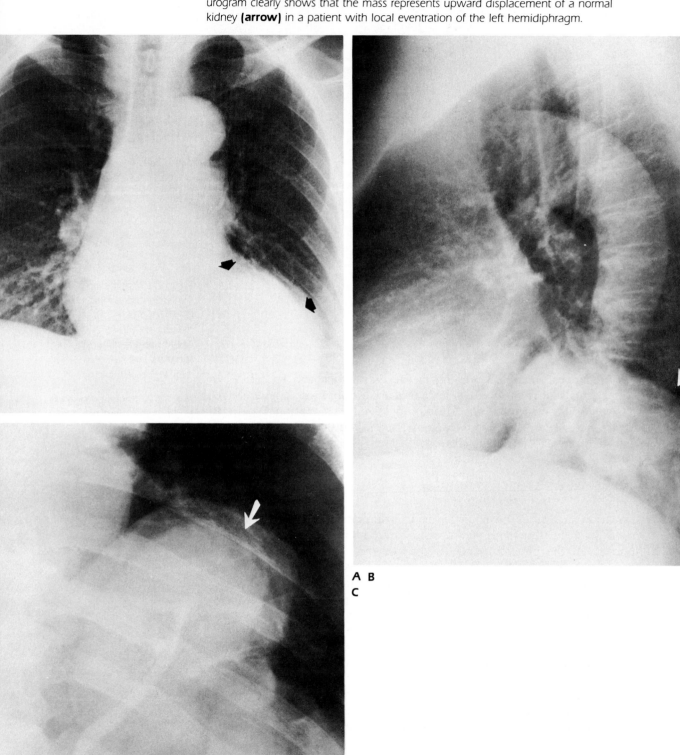

A   B
C

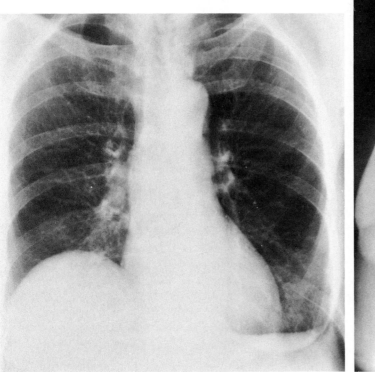 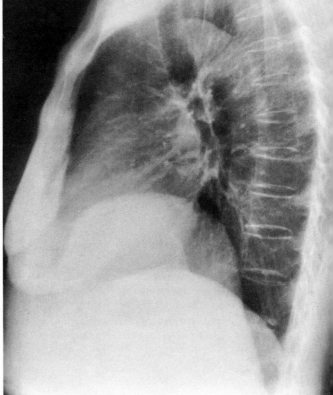

A B

Fig. 12-4. Eventration of the right hemidiaphragm viewed on **(A)** frontal and **(B)** lateral projections.

rare instances, localized bulging of the diaphragm can be caused by tumors, cysts, or inflammatory lesions of the diaphragm. Differentiation of these rare entities from simple localized eventration is usually impossible without a strongly suggestive clinical history or an interval change from prior radiographs.

PARALYSIS OF THE DIAPHRAGM

Elevation of one or both leaves of the diaphragm can be caused by paralysis resulting from any process that interferes with the normal function of the phrenic nerve. It may be due to inadvertent surgical transection of the phrenic nerve, involvement of the nerve by primary bronchogenic carcinoma (Fig. 12-5) or metastatic malignancy in the mediastinum, or a variety of intrinsic neurologic diseases. Diaphragmatic paralysis can be caused by injury to the phrenic nerve as a result of trauma to the thoracic cage or cervical spine or as a consequence of damage during brachial plexus block or forceps delivery, in which injury to the phrenic nerve may be accompanied by an associated brachial palsy or Erb's paralysis. Pressure on the phrenic nerve from a substernal thyroid or aortic aneurysm can cause diaphragmatic paralysis on a mechanical basis. Infectious processes involving the lung and mediastinum, such as tuberculosis and acute, nonnecrotizing, non-

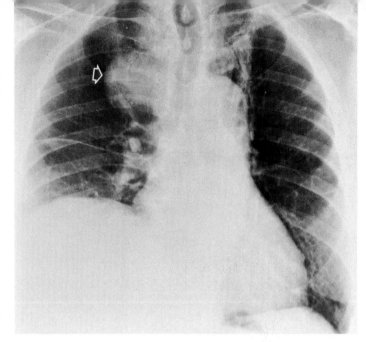

Fig. 12-5. Paralysis of the right hemidiaphragm due to involvement of the phrenic nerve by primary bronchogenic carcinoma **(arrow).**

organizing pneumonia, can result in temporary or permanent diaphragmatic paralysis. In some cases, there is no obvious cause for the loss of diaphragmatic motion, and the paralysis must be termed idiopathic.

A radiographic hallmark of diaphragmatic paralysis is paradoxical motion of the diaphragm in response to the "sniff" test. Under fluoroscopic observation of the diaphragm, the patient is instructed to close his mouth, relax his abdomen, and inhale rapidly. This rapid inspiration causes a quick, downward thrust of a normal leaf of the diaphragm. The paralyzed diaphragm, in contrast, tends to ascend with inspiration because of the increased intra-abdominal pressure. Although small amounts of unilateral paradoxical excursion of the diaphragm on sniffing are not infrequent, a marked degree of paradoxical motion is a valuable aid in discriminating between paralysis of the diaphragm and limited diaphragmatic motion secondary to intrathoracic or intra-abdominal inflammatory disease.

OTHER CAUSES OF ELEVATION OF THE DIAPHRAGM

Diffuse elevation of the diaphragm can be caused by ascites, obesity, pregnancy, or any other process in which the intra-abdominal volume is increased (Fig. 12-6). In these instances, intact innervation and musculature permits some diaphragmatic movement, albeit possibly decreased.

Intra-abdominal inflammatory diseases can lead to elevation of one or both leaves of the diaphragm, with severe limitation of diaphragmatic motion. This appearance is especially marked in patients with sub-

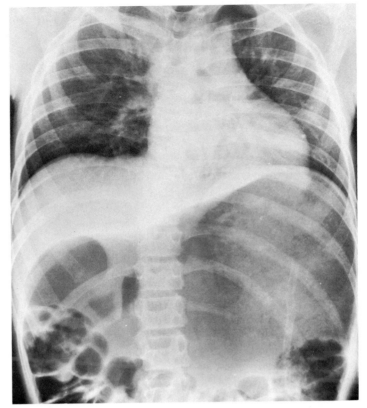

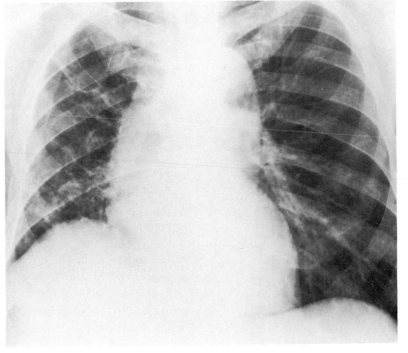

Fig. 12-6. Diffuse elevation of both leaves of the diaphragm caused by severe, acute gastric dilatation.

Fig. 12-7. Elevation of the right hemidiaphragm caused by a huge gumma of the liver.

phrenic abscesses, in whom there is associated blunting of the costo-phrenic angle and often subphrenic collections of gas. The limitation of diaphragmatic motion in patients with intra-abdominal inflammation is probably related to an attempt to avoid the pain associated with deep inspiration. The degree of limitation of movement is related to the severity of the disease process and its location in relation to the diaphragm. Thus, an abscess in the pelvis has far less effect on the position and motion of the diaphragm than does acute cholecystitis or a subphrenic abscess.

Intra-abdominal masses arising in the upper quadrants can also cause diaphragmatic elevation. Localized or generalized bulging of the diaphragm may be due to a cyst or tumor in the liver (Fig. 12-7), spleen, kidney, adrenal, or pancreas. One case of left hemidiaphragmatic elevation has been reported to be secondary to a large suprarenal abdominal aortic aneurysm (Fig. 12-8).

Acute intrathoracic processes can also cause elevation of the diaphragm due to splinting of the diaphragm secondary to chest wall injury, atelectasis, or pulmonary embolus. An infrapulmonic effusion can closely simulate an elevated diaphragm. Pleural effusions initially form inferior to the lung. With increasing amounts of fluid, spillover into the costophrenic sulci produces the classic radiographic sign of blunting of the costophrenic angles. For unclear reasons, fluid can continue to accumulate in an infrapulmonary location without spilling into the costophrenic sulci or extending up along the chest wall. This produces a radiographic pattern (pseudodiaphragmatic contour) that mimics diaphragmatic elevation on the erect film.

On the posteroanterior projection, the peak of the pseudodiaphragmatic contour is lateral to that of the normal hemidiaphragm (Fig.

Fig. 12-8. Elevation of the left hemidiaphragm due to an abdominal aortic aneurysm. **(A)** Frontal and **(B)** lateral projections reveal the opacified, saccular abdominal aortic aneurysm elevating the left hemidiaphragm. (Phillips G, Gordon D: Abdominal aortic aneurysm: Unusual cause for left hemidiaphragmatic elevation. AJR 136:1221–1223, 1981. Copyright 1981. Reproduced by permission)

A B

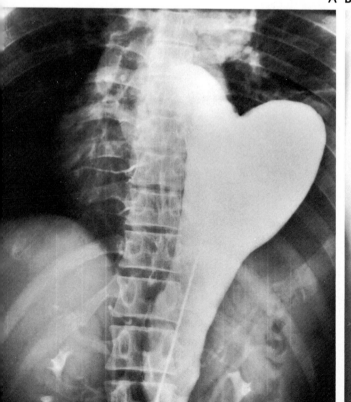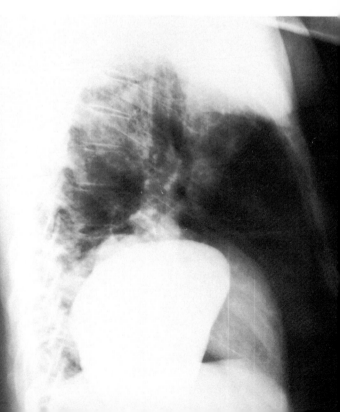

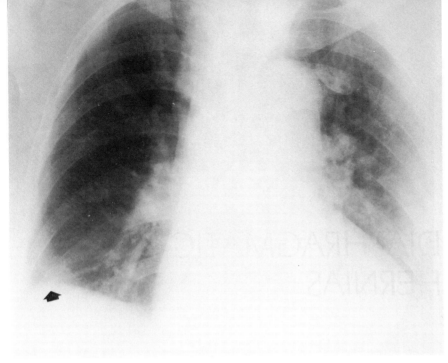

Fig. 12-9. Pseudodiaphragmatic contour (subpulmonic effusion). The peak of the right hemidiaphragm **(arrow)** is situated more laterally than normal.

12-9) and situated near the junction of the middle and lateral thirds, rather than near the center. In addition, the pseudodiaphragmatic contour slopes down rapidly toward the lateral costophrenic recess. On lateral projection, the ascending portion of the pseudodiaphragmatic contour rises abruptly in almost a straight line to the region of the major fissure, rather than assuming a normal, more rounded configuration. At fluoroscopy, the patient with an infrapulmonic effusion demonstrates no impairment of diaphragmatic excursion during respiration. Tilting the patient to one side causes fluid to spill over into the lateral costophrenic sulcus.

BIBLIOGRAPHY

Alexander C: Diaphragm movements and the diagnosis of diaphragmatic paralysis. Clin Radiol 17:79–83, 1966

Campbell JA: The diaphragm in roentgenology of the chest. Radiol Clin North Am 1:395–410, 1963

Laxdall OE, McDougall HA, Mellin GW: Congenital eventration of the diaphragm. N Engl J Med 250:401–408, 1954

Lundius B: Intrathoracic kidney. AJR 125:678–681, 1975

Lundstrom CH, Allen PR: Bilateral congenital eventration of the diaphragm. AJR 97:216–217, 1966

Phillips G, Gordon DG: Abdominal aortic aneurysm: Unusual cause for left hemidiaphragmatic elevation. AJR 136:1221–1223, 1981

Riley EA: Idiopathic diaphragmatic paralysis. Am J Med 32:404–415, 1962

Thomas T: Nonparalytic eventration of the diaphragm. J Thorac Cardiovasc Surg 55:586–593, 1968

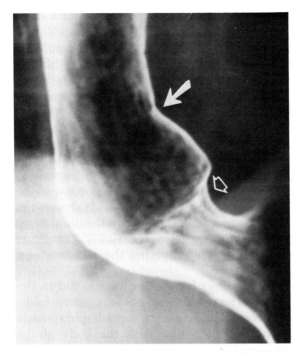

Fig. 13-10. "A" ring. An indentation **(solid arrow)** separates the tubular esophagus above from the dilated vestibule below. The **open arrow** marks the level of the junction between the esophageal and the gastric mucosae.

Fig. 13-11. "B" ring. The presence of a second indentation **(solid arrows)** below the "A" ring **(open arrows)** implies the existence of a hiatal hernia.

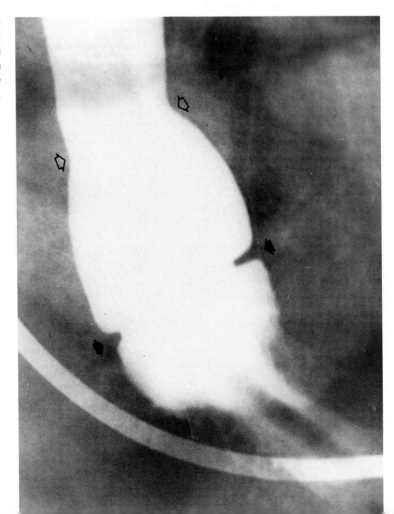

PARAESOPHAGEAL HERNIA

A paraesophageal hernia is progressive herniation of the stomach anterior to the esophagus, usually through a widened esophageal hiatus but occasionally through a separate adjacent gap in the diaphragm (Fig. 13-12). Unlike the situation with a hiatal hernia, the terminal esophagus in the patient with a paraesophageal hernia remains in its normal position, and the esophagogastric junction is situated below the diaphragm (Fig. 13-13). True paraesophageal hernias are uncommon, appearing in only 5% of all patients operated on for hiatal hernia. Initially, only the fundus of the stomach is situated above the diaphragm. As herniation progresses, increasing amounts of the greater curvature roll into the hernia sac, inverting the stomach so that the greater curvature lies uppermost. At times, spleen, omentum, transverse colon, or small bowel may accompany the herniated stomach into the thorax.

Infrequently, acquired paraesophageal hernias develop following hiatal hernia repair. Regardless of the type of surgical procedure done, the distal end of the esophagus and the cardia are firmly anchored below the diaphragm, whereas the free part of the fundus of the stomach lies against the old hiatus, which has been sutured closed. Re-expansion of the hiatus around the esophagus may permit the fundus to slide through the opening and become a paraesophageal hernia. Acquired paraesophageal hernias can even develop through a diaphragmatic opening created for admission of the surgeon's fingers (Fig. 13-14).

Fig. 13-13. Paraesophageal hernia. Note that the esophagogastric junction remains below the level of the left hemidiaphragm.

Fig. 13-12. Paraesophageal hernia.

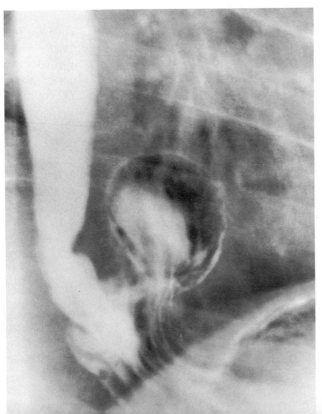

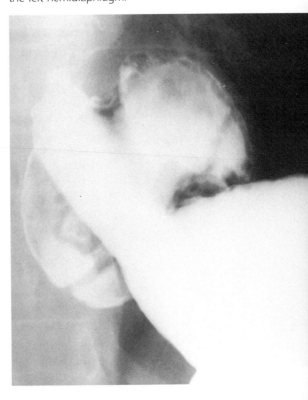

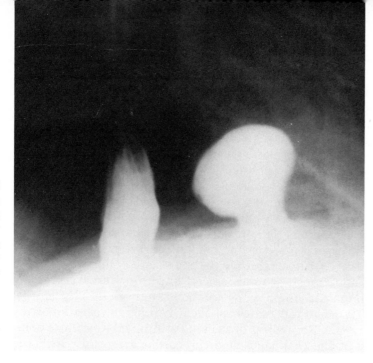

Fig. 13-14. Paraesophageal hernia through an opening in the left hemidiaphragm that had been created for admission of the surgeon's fingers during a previous hiatal hernia repair. (Hoyt T, Kyaw MM: Acquired paraesophageal and disparaesophageal hernias. AJR 121:248–251, 1974. Copyright 1974. Reproduced by permission)

Many patients with paraesophageal hernias are asymptomatic, even if the condition has progressed to herniation of the entire stomach into the thorax. Not infrequently, paraesophageal hernias are first identified on routine chest radiographs when an air–fluid level is detected behind the cardiac silhouette (Fig. 13-15). Patients can present with vague symptoms of postprandial indigestion, substernal fullness, nausea, occasional retching, and, if the hernia is large, dyspnea after meals. Unlike sliding hiatal hernias, paraesophageal hernias are associated with normal functioning of the gastroesophageal junction, and reflux esophagitis does not occur.

Although paraesophageal hernias usually have a relatively long, benign clinical course, they occasionally have serious complications. Asymptomatic anemia can be caused by blood loss from hemorrhagic gastritis of the herniated fundus; this complication is presumably related to enlarged rugal folds that are edematous because of venous and lymphatic obstruction and therefore prone to erosion. Patients with paraesophageal hernias frequently develop gastric ulcers at the point at which the herniated stomach crosses the crus of the diaphragm. The most serious complication of large paraesophageal hernias is gastric volvulus. If not promptly recognized and relieved by insertion of a nasogastric tube or by surgical repair, gastric volvulus can rapidly progress to incarceration and strangulation of the stomach. Because of the risk of serious complications and the ineffectiveness of medical treatment, paraesophageal hernias are frequently considered for surgical repair.

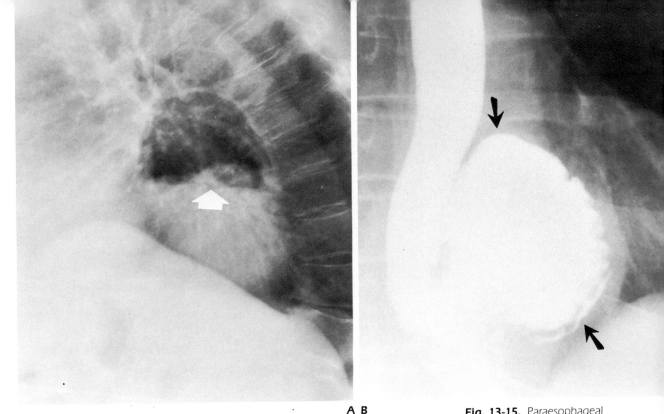

A B

Fig. 13-15. Paraesophageal hernia. **(A)** A lateral plain chest radiograph reveals an air–fluid level **(arrow)** behind the cardiac silhouette. **(B)** A barium swallow clearly shows the paraesophageal hernia **(arrows)**.

OTHER DIAPHRAGMATIC HERNIAS

Diaphragmatic hernias through orifices other than the esophageal hiatus are due to congenital abnormalities in the formation of the diaphragm. Many small diaphragmatic hernias contain only omentum. Larger lesions usually include parts of the stomach, transverse colon, and greater omentum. In most cases, these abdominal structures are not fixed within a diaphragmatic hernia and can be withdrawn with ease. Infrequently, the small bowel, cecum, liver, or pancreas can be found in a diaphragmatic hernia.

The symptoms caused by large diaphragmatic hernias depend on the size of the hernia, the viscera that have herniated, and whether the herniated structures are fixed or capable of sliding back and forth between the abdomen and the thorax. Because the stomach is usually situated within large diaphragmatic hernias, some degree of postprandial distress is common. Symptoms of intermittent partial bowel obstruction are frequent, and, if there is interference with the blood supply of the portion of intestine that is within the hernia sac, strangulation and gangrenous necrosis may result.

Large diaphragmatic hernias can produce pressure on the heart and a shift of mediastinal structures that result in intermittent episodes of syncope, vertigo, tachycardia, palpitations, and cyanosis, all aggravated by physical effort, eating, and change of position. The hernia can

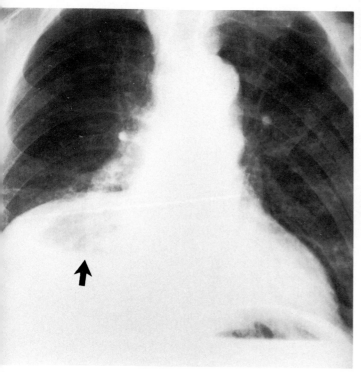

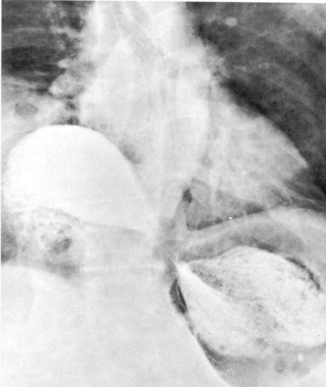

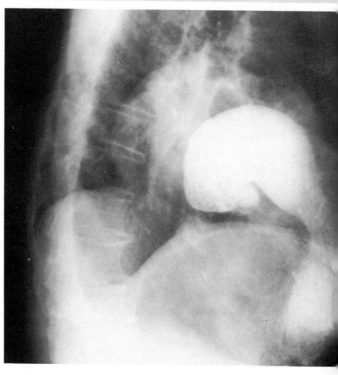

A B
C

Fig. 13-16. Herniation through the anteromedial foramen of Morgagni. **(A)** A chest radiograph demonstrates a soft-tissue mass in the right cardiophrenic angle. In this view, the gas within the mass **(arrow)** is in the inverted gastric antrum. The gas on the left is in the fundus. **(B)** Frontal and **(C)** lateral views with barium show typical herniation of the stomach through the right foramen of Morgagni with volvulus. The anterior position of the hernia is clearly visible on the lateral view. (Rennell CL: Foramen of Morgagni hernia with volvulus of the stomach. AJR 117:248–250, 1973. Copyright 1973. Reproduced by permission)

cause decreased aeration of the ipsilateral lung and lead to respiratory complaints, such as dyspnea, cyanosis, and irritating cough, that are most marked after exercise. Superimposed pneumonia often develops. Large hernias can even irritate the phrenic nerve, resulting in spasm of the diaphragm and severe left chest pain, which can be referred to the left shoulder and arm and be indistinguishable from angina pectoris.

FORAMEN OF MORGAGNI HERNIA

Herniations through the anteromedial foramina of Morgagni can occur on either side of the attachment of the diaphragm to the sternum. They are more common on the right, possibly because the pericardial attachment to the diaphragm is more extensive on the left. Herniation through the foramen of Morgagni typically presents radiographically as a large, smoothly marginated soft-tissue mass in the right cardiophrenic angle (Fig. 13-16A). On lateral view, the anterior position of the hernia is evident. When a loop of gas-filled bowel (especially transverse colon) is seen within the soft-tissue mass, the proper diagnosis is easy to make. However, if the hernia contains only omentum and no gas-filled bowel, it may be impossible on plain chest radiographs to distinguish a hernia through the foramen of Morgagni from a pericardial cyst (Fig. 13-17), pulmonary hamartoma (Fig. 13-18), or epicardial fat pad. In this situation, a contrast examination is required (Fig. 13-16B,C).

FORAMEN OF BOCHDALEK HERNIA

Herniations through the posterolateral foramina of Bochdalek more commonly occur on the left than on the right, presumably because of

Fig. 13-17. Pericardial cyst **(arrows)** mimicking herniation through the foramen of Morgagni. **(A)** Frontal and **(B)** oblique views.

A B

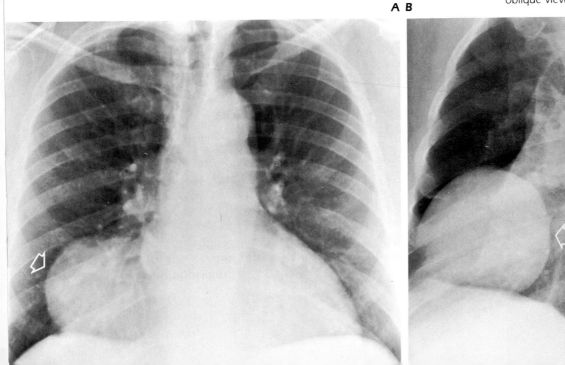

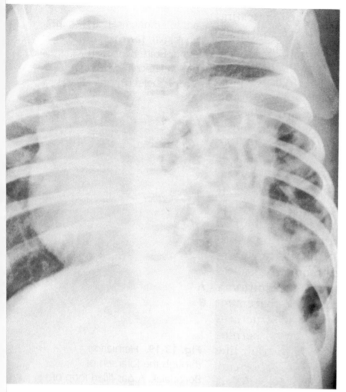

Fig. 13-20. Congenital diaphragmatic hernia. A plain chest radiograph demonstrates multiple radiolucencies in the chest due to gas-filled loops of bowel. Contrast examination is not required for diagnosis.

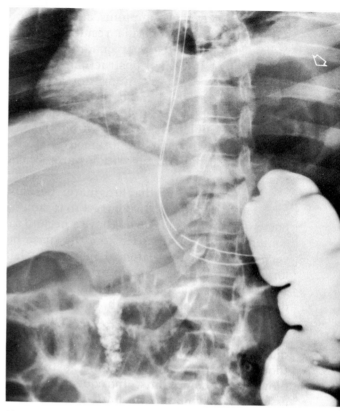

Fig. 13-21. Post-traumatic diaphragmatic hernia. Herniation of a portion of the splenic flexure **(arrow)** with obstruction to the retrograde flow of barium.

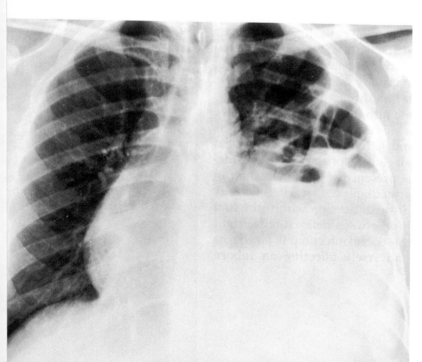

Fig. 13-22. Post-traumatic diaphragmatic hernia due to a motor vehicle accident. A plain frontal radiograph of the chest reveals herniated bowel contents above the expected level of the left hemidiaphragm.

TRAUMATIC DIAPHRAGMATIC HERNIA

Traumatic diaphragmatic hernias most commonly follow direct laceration by a knife, bullet, or other penetrating object (Fig. 13-21). They can also occur as a result of a marked increase in intra-abdominal pressure and should be suspected in any patient with a history of blunt abdominal trauma who develops vague upper abdominal symptoms. Traumatic hernias occur much more frequently (90%–95% of the time) on the left than on the right, both because of an embryologic point of weakness in the left hemidiaphragm and because of the protecting effect of the liver on the right. Stomach, colon, omentum, spleen, or small bowel can be found above the diaphragm. The early clinical course tends to be dominated by accompanying injuries, so that signs of visceral herniation are delayed. Symptoms of postprandial fullness, cramps, nausea, vomiting, chest pain, dyspnea, bowel obstruction, or strangulation may not develop until many years after the traumatic episode. In addition, the hernia may not arise immediately after injury but may follow an additional violent effort or blow that causes the previous scar to weaken. The association of an old traumatic diaphragmatic hernia with bleeding in the chest can result in the development of adhesions that cause fixation of abdominal viscera within the thorax. A potentially fatal complication is the spill of septic bowel contents or highly irritating gastric juice into the pleural cavity. This catastrophic event may be misdiagnosed as coronary occlusion or pulmonary embolism if no history of prior herniation is available.

Plain radiographs of the chest usually demonstrate herniated bowel contents above the expected level of the diaphragm (Fig. 13-22). Often, the diaphragm itself cannot be delineated. The radiographic appearance can simulate eventration or diaphragmatic paralysis, since the herniated viscera can parallel the diaphragm on both frontal and lateral projections (Fig. 13-23A). This apparent elevation tends to change in shape with altered patient position, strongly suggesting the presence of a hernia. Administration of barium by mouth or by rectum may be required to demonstrate the relationship of the gastrointestinal tract to the diaphragm (Fig. 13-23B). A major differential point is the constriction of the afferent and efferent loops of bowel as they traverse a laceration in the diaphragm, in contrast to the wide separation of loops that is typically seen with eventration or paralysis of the diaphragm.

INTRAPERICARDIAL HERNIA

Intrapericardial diaphragmatic hernias (peritoneal–pericardial) are extremely rare. They can be either congenital (Fig. 13-24) or post-traumatic (Fig. 13-25) and can contain (in decreasing order of frequency) omentum, colon, small bowel, liver, or stomach. Although patients with intrapericardial diaphragmatic hernias may be asymptomatic for long periods, most eventually present with either cardiorespiratory (angina, shortness of breath, cardiac tamponade) or gastrointestinal (cramping abdominal pain, constipation, abdominal distention) complaints. Radiographically, gas-filled loops of bowel can be seen lying alongside the heart (see Fig. 13-24). On multiple projections, including decubitus views, the herniated loops can be seen to remain in conformity with the heart border.

BIBLIOGRAPHY

Ahrend T, Thompson B: Hernia of the foramen of Bochdalek in the adult. Am J Surg 122:612–615, 1971

Bartley O, Wickbom I: Roentgenologic diagnosis of rupture of the diaphragm. Acta Radiol [Diagn] (Stockh) 53:33–41, 1960

Botha GSM: Radiological localization of the diaphragmatic hiatus. Lancet 1:662–664, 1957

Carter BN, Giuseffi J, Felson B: Traumatic diaphragmatic hernia. AJR 65:56–71, 1951

Fagan CJ, Schrieber MH, Amparo EG et al: Traumatic diaphragmatic hernia into the pericardium: Verification of diagnosis by computed tomography. J Comput Assist Tomogr 3:405–408, 1979

Hill LD: Incarcerated paraesophageal hernia: A surgical emergency. Am J Surg 126:286–291, 1973

Hood R: Traumatic diaphragmatic hernia. Ann Thorac Surg 12:311–324, 1971

Hoyt T, Kyaw MM: Acquired paraesophageal and disparaesophageal hernias: Complications of hiatal hernia repair. AJR 121:248–251, 1974

Linsman JF: Gastroesophageal reflux elicited while drinking water (water siphonage test): Its clinical correlation with pyrosis. AJR 94:325–332, 1965

McCarten KM, Rosenberg HK, Borden S et al: Delayed appearance of right diaphragmatic hernia associated with group B streptococcal infection in newborns. Radiology 139:385–389, 1981

Rennell CL: Foramen of Morgagni hernia with volvulus of the stomach. AJR 117:248–250, 1973

Stein GN, Finkelstein A: Hiatal hernia: Roentgen incidence and diagnosis. Am J Dig Dis 5:77–87, 1960

Vestby G, Aakhus T: Incidence of sliding hiatus hernia. Invest Radiol 1:379–385, 1966

Wallace DB: Intrapericardial diaphragmatic hernia. Radiology 122:596, 1977

Wolf BS, Brahms SA, Khilnani MT: The incidence of hiatal hernia in routine barium meal examinations. J Mount Sinai Hosp NY 26:598–600, 1959.

PART THREE

STOMACH

GASTRIC ULCERS

The detection of gastric ulcers and the decision as to whether these represent benign or malignant processes are major parts of the upper gastrointestinal examination. It is estimated that 90% to 95% of gastric ulcers can be revealed by expert radiographic study. This requires demonstration of the ulcer crater in both profile and *en face* views. The latter is particularly helpful in evaluating the surrounding gastric mucosa to differentiate between benign and malignant ulcers.

Certain technical factors preclude demonstration of a small percentage of gastric ulcers. The ulcer can be shallow or filled with residual mucus, blood, food, or necrotic tissue that prevents barium from filling it. Similarly, the margins of an ulcer can be so edematous that barium cannot enter it; a small ulcer can be obscured by large rugal folds. Scattered radiation in obese patients can impair image quality and detail, especially on lateral views. In contrast, false-positive ulcerlike patterns can be caused by barium trapped between gastric folds. These "non-ulcers" are most commonly noted along the greater curvature and the upper body and antrum of the lesser curvature. Careful technique with graded compression and distention of the stomach usually permits obliteration of these non-ulcers.

The classic appearance of a gastric ulcer on profile view is a conical or button-shaped projection from the gastric lumen (Fig. 14-1). On the *en face* view, the ulcer appears as a round or oval collection of barium that is denser than the barium or air–barium mixture covering the surrounding gastric mucosa (Fig. 14-2).

On double-contrast studies, an ulcer crater on the dependent wall can collect a pool of barium as on single-contrast studies. If the ulcer crater is very shallow, however, it can be coated by only a thin layer of barium, resulting in a ring shadow (Fig. 14-3A). Turning the patient may permit barium to flow across the surface of the ulcer and fill the crater (Fig. 14-3B). The walls of an ulcer crater on the nondependent wall of the stomach may remain coated with barium even after contrast has flowed out of the crater. The significance of the resulting ring shadow can be confirmed by demonstration of the ulcer in a profile view or by turning the patient so that the ulcer is in the dependent position and fills with barium.

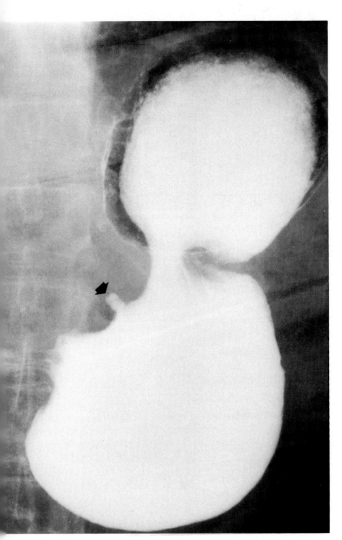

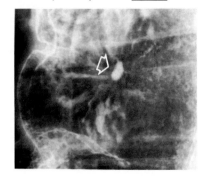

Fig. 14-1. Benign gastric ulcer **(arrow)** projecting from the lumen of the stomach.

Fig. 14-2. Benign gastric ulcer appearing as an oval collection of barium **(arrow)** on the <u>en face</u> view.

Fig. 14-3. Ring sign of gastric ulcer. **(A)** A thin layer of barium coats the margin of the ulcer crater **(arrows)**. **(B)** Turning the patient permits barium to flow across the surface of the ulcer and fill the crater **(arrows)**. Note the smooth mucosal folds radiating to the edge of this benign gastric ulcer.

A B

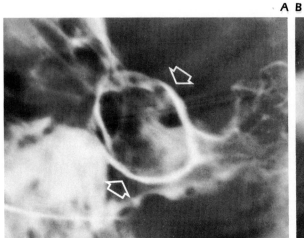

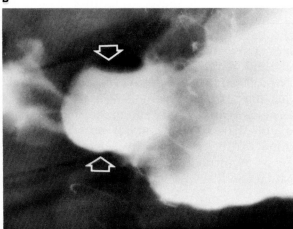

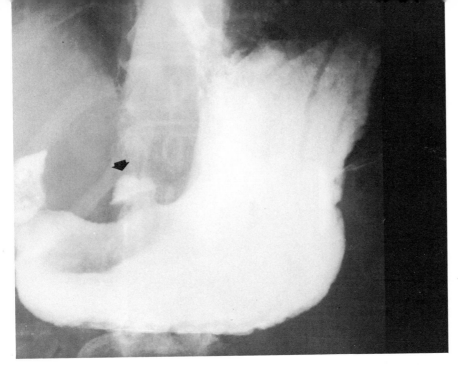

Fig. 14-4. Penetration of a benign gastric ulcer. The crater **(arrow)** clearly projects beyond the expected confines of the inner margin of the stomach.

SIGNS OF BENIGN GASTRIC ULCERS

The traditional sign of a benign gastric ulcer on profile view is penetration—the clear projection of the ulcer outside of the normal barium-filled gastric lumen due to the ulcer representing an excavation in the wall of the stomach (Fig. 14-4). Three other features seen on profile view are additional evidence for benignity of a gastric ulcer: the Hampton line, an ulcer collar, and an ulcer mound. These signs are related to undermining of the mucosa due to the relative resistance to peptic digestion of the mucosal layer compared to the submucosa. This results in the more resistant mucosa appearing to overhang the more rapidly destroyed submucosa. With minimal edema of the overhanging mucosa, a perfect profile view may demonstrate a thin, sharply demarcated lucent line (Hampton line) with parallel straight margins at the base of the crater (Fig. 14-5). An increased amount of mucosal edema due to inflammatory exudate results in a larger, lucent ulcer collar separating the ulcer from the gastric lumen (Fig. 14-6). If this collar is irregular or more prominent on one side than the other, malignancy must be suspected. An ulcer mound is produced by extensive mucosal edema and lack of distensibility of the gastric wall (Fig. 14-7). Unlike the Hampton line or ulcer collar, the ulcer mound can extend considerably beyond the limits of the ulcer itself. If the mound is large, the niche may not project beyond the contour of the stomach when viewed in profile. This appearance can simulate a neoplasm. The benignancy of this process is suggested by the central location of the ulcer within the mound; the smooth, sharply delineated, gently sloping, and symmetrically convex tissue around the ulcer; and the smooth,

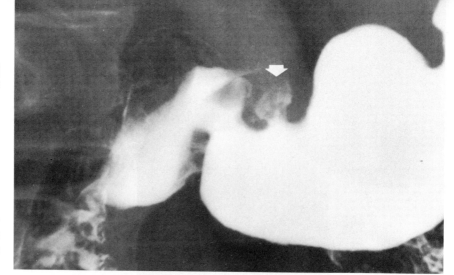

Fig. 14-10. Benign lesser curvature ulcer with an appearance mimicking a diverticulum **(arrow).**

Fig. 14-11. Two examples of radiation of mucosal folds to the edge of benign gastric ulcer craters **(arrows). (A)** Single-contrast and **(B)** double-contrast examinations.

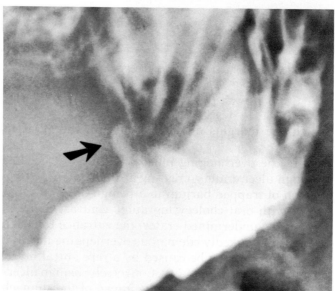

A

B

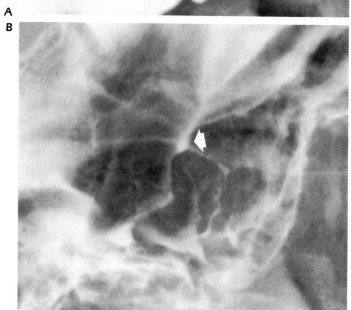

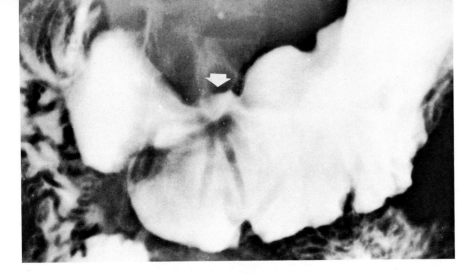

Fig. 14-12. Radiating folds in a benign gastric ulcer. The small, slender folds extending to the edge of the crater **(arrow)** indicate the benignancy of the ulcer.

Fig. 14-13. Malignant gastric ulcer. Thick folds radiate to an irregular mound of tissue around the ulcer **(arrow).**

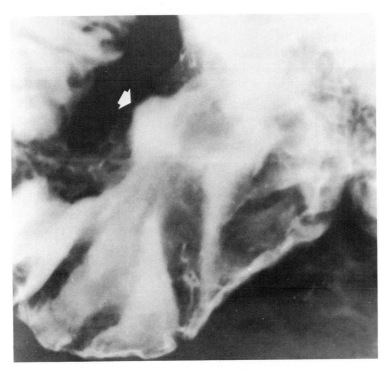

extensive edema about the ulcer, *en face* views demonstrate a wide, lucent band that symmetrically surrounds the ulcer (halo defect). Radiation of mucosal folds to the margin of the halo indicates benignancy. Even if there are no radiating folds, the smooth contour of the surrounding edematous tissue suggests a benign ulcer, as opposed to the nodularity associated with a malignant ulcer. The halo defect caused by benign edematous tissue has a somewhat hazy and indistinct border, in contrast to the sharp demarcation and abrupt transition of the junction between neoplastic tissue and the normal gastric wall.

The size, shape, number, and location of gastric ulcers have in the past been suggested as criteria for distinguishing between benign and malignant lesions. For the most part, however, these "signs" have proved to be of no practical value.

Gastric ulcers can be of any size. Although large gastric ulcers used to be considered malignant by virtue of their size alone, it is now generally accepted that the size of an ulcer bears no relationship to the presence of malignancy (Fig. 14-14). Similarly, the contour of the ulcer base is of little diagnostic value. Although a benign ulcer tends to have a smooth base, it can be irregular if blood, mucus, or necrotic or exogenous debris is lodged within it (Fig. 14-15). With the increasing use of double-contrast techniques, linear (Fig. 14-16), rod-shaped, rectangular, and flame-shaped ulcers have been described in addition to the classic appearance of an ulcer crater as a circular collection of barium.

Although multiplicity of gastric ulcers has been suggested as a sign of benignancy (Fig. 14-17), the demonstration of synchronous gastric ulcers is of little value in distinguishing benign from malignant ulcers. The frequency of multiple gastric ulcers on single-contrast barium studies has ranged up to 12.5%; an even higher incidence has been reported with double-contrast techniques. In one study, 20% of patients with multiple ulcers had a malignant lesion. Therefore, each gastric ulcer must be individually evaluated according to classic radiographic criteria for the possibility of malignancy.

Except for the gastric fundus above the level of the cardia, where essentially all ulcers are malignant, the location of an ulcer has no significance with respect to whether an ulcer is benign or malignant. Although benign gastric ulcers are most commonly found along the lesser curvature of the stomach or on its posterior wall, they can be found almost anywhere. In young patients, ulcers tend to occur in the distal part of the stomach; in older persons, ulcers are more frequently seen high on the lesser curvature.

BENIGN ULCERS ON THE GREATER CURVATURE

Benign greater curvature ulcers can cause diagnostic difficulty, since they sometimes do not demonstrate the same characteristic radiographic features of benignancy that are seen on profile views of lesser curvature ulcers. Indeed, a benign greater curvature ulcer typically demonstrates features that would suggest malignancy if the ulcer were situated on the lesser curvature. Benign ulcers on the greater curvature frequently have an apparent intraluminal location rather than clearly penetrating beyond the expected limit of the wall of the stomach (Fig. 14-18). Spasm of the circular muscles of the portion of the gastric wall surrounding the ulcer causes the more mobile greater curvature to be pulled toward the relatively fixed lesser curvature, producing an in-

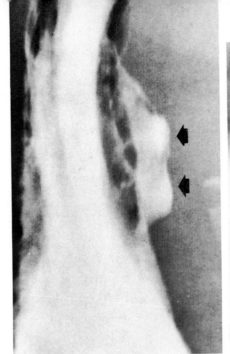
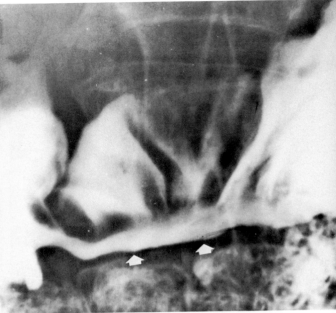

A B

Fig. 14-14. Long ulcers **(arrows)** of **(A)** the body and **(B)** the antrum. Both ulcers were histologically benign.

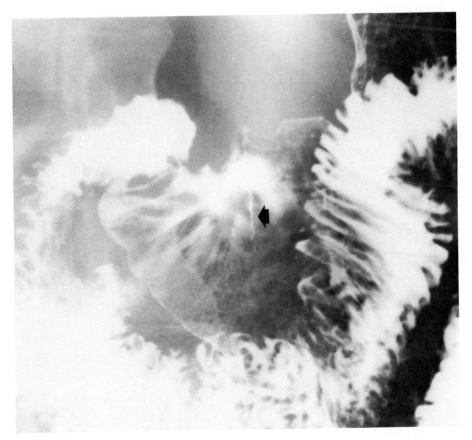

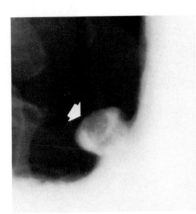

Fig. 14-15. Irregular filling defect (blood clot) in a benign ulcer **(arrow)** on the lesser curvature of the stomach.

Fig. 14-16. Linear ulcer **(arrow)** in the gastric antrum.

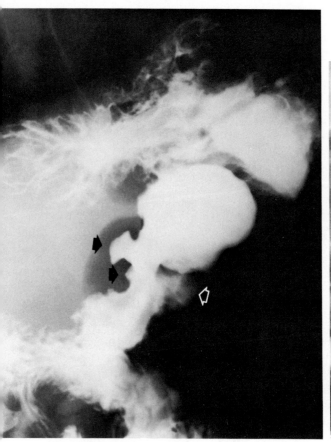

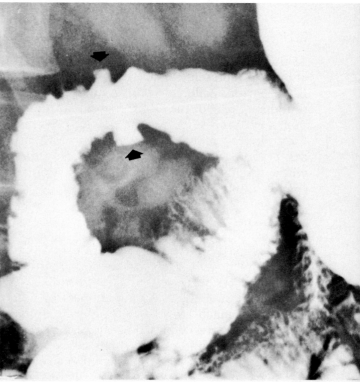

Fig. 14-17. Multiple benign gastric ulcers **(arrows)** in two patients.

A B

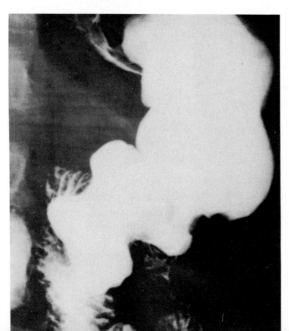

Fig. 14-18. Benign greater curvature ulcer. The ulcer has an apparent intraluminal location, shouldered edges, and a scalloped border proximal to it, all of which would suggest a malignant lesion if the ulcer were on the lesser curvature. (Zboralske FF, Stargardter FL, Harrell GS: Profile roentgenographic features of benign gastric curvature ulcers. Radiology 127:63–67, 1978)

dentation (incisura) along the greater curvature. Since the ulcer is at the base of the incisura, it projects into the gastric lumen and may simulate an ulcerated mass. In addition, a scalloped or nodular gastric contour suggesting a malignant lesion can be seen adjacent to a benign greater curvature ulcer, probably due to spasm of the surrounding circular muscles.

ELLIPSE SIGN

At times, it may be difficult to decide whether a persistent collection of barium represents an acute ulceration or a nonulcerating deformity. If the barium collection has an elliptic configuration, the orientation of the long axis of the ellipse can be an indicator of the nature of the pathologic process (ellipse sign). If the long axis is parallel to the lumen, the collection represents an acute ulceration (Fig. 14-19). If the long axis is perpendicular to the lumen, the collection represents a deformity without acute ulceration (Fig. 14-20). Both ulcer and deformity can coexist in the same area (Fig. 14-21).

HEALING

The vast majority of gastric ulcers (more than 95%) are benign and heal completely with medical therapy. Most benign ulcers diminish to one-half or less of their original size within 3 weeks and show complete healing within 6 weeks. Complete healing does not necessarily mean that the stomach returns to an absolutely normal radiographic appearance; bizarre deformities can result (Fig. 14-22). As healing proceeds, the surrounding ulcer mound subsides, and the ulcer crater decreases in size and depth. Retraction and stiffening of the wall of the stomach can lead to residual deformity or stenosis. On double-contrast studies, gastric ulcer scars characteristically appear as a collection of

Fig. 14-19. Ellipse sign. Two benign gastric ulcers are seen as persistent barium collections **(arrows)** running parallel to the lumen. (Eisenberg RL, Hedgcock MW: The ellipse sign: An aid in the diagnosis of acute ulcers. J Can Assoc Radiol 30:26–29, 1979)

A B

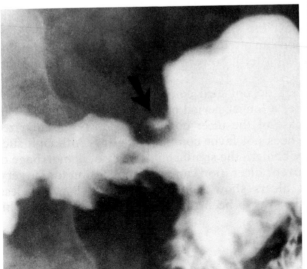

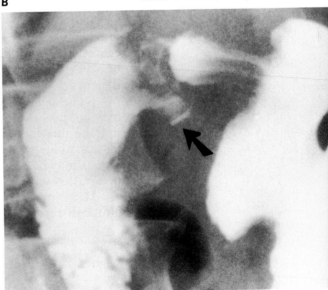

BENIGN CAUSES

The overwhelming majority of gastric ulcers are a manifestation of peptic ulcer disease (Fig. 14-27). However, gastric ulceration can also be a complication or primary manifestation of other benign disorders involving the stomach. Localized or diffuse nonmalignant ulcers can be the result of inflammatory disease, such as any form of gastritis (Fig. 14-28) or granulomatous infiltration of the stomach. Benign gastric tumors, especially leiomyomas, can present as ulcerated masses (Fig. 14-29). All of these disease entities are more extensively discussed in other sections.

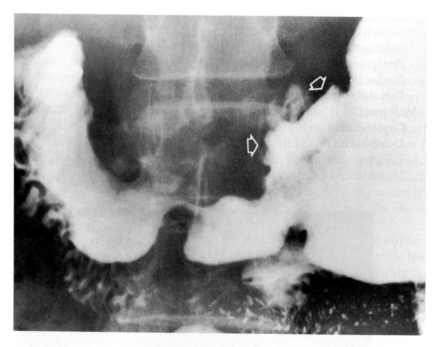

Fig. 14-26. Malignant gastric ulcer. There is an abrupt transition between the normal mucosa and the abnormal tissue surrounding the irregular gastric ulcer **(arrows).**

Fig. 14-27. Benign pyloric channel ulcer **(arrow).**

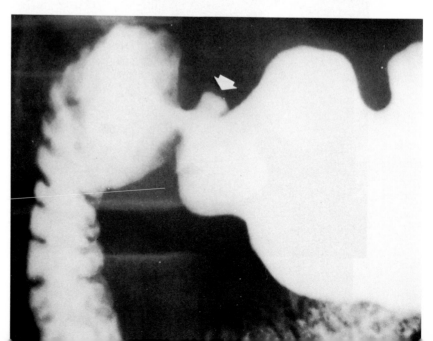

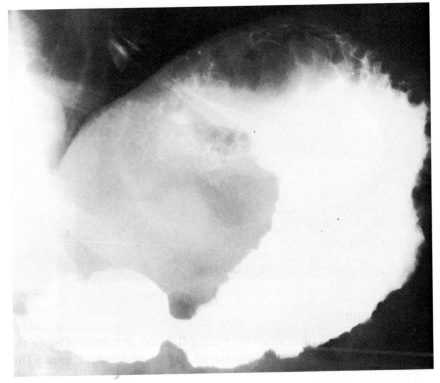

Fig. 14-28. Corrosive gastritis. Diffuse ulceration involving the body and antrum is due to the ingestion of hydrochloric acid.

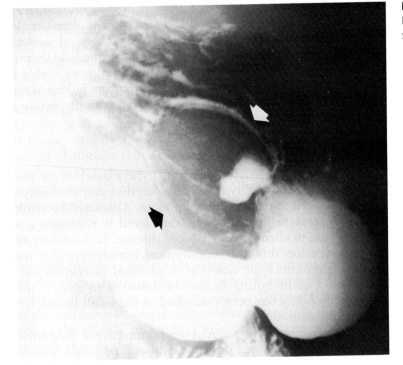

Fig. 14-29. Ulcerated leiomyoma of the body of the stomach **(arrows).**

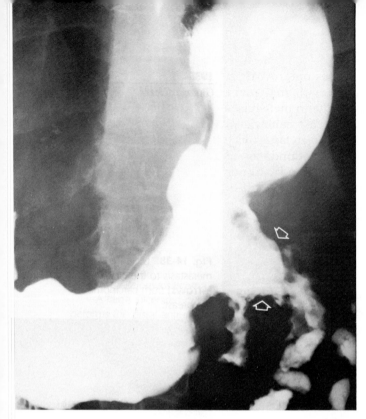

Fig. 14-39. Huge malignant ulcer (arrows) on the greater curvature representing direct invasion by carcinoma of the pancreas.

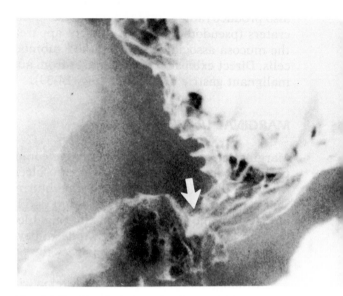

Fig. 14-40. Marginal ulceration (arrow) following Billroth-I anastomosis.

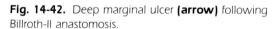

Fig. 14-41. Marginal ulceration (arrow) following gastrojejunostomy. The ulcer appears in the jejunum within the first few centimeters of the anastomosis.

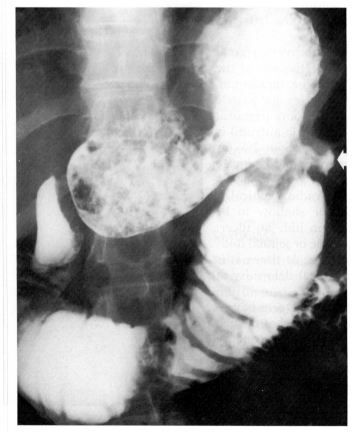

Fig. 14-42. Deep marginal ulcer (arrow) following Billroth-II anastomosis.

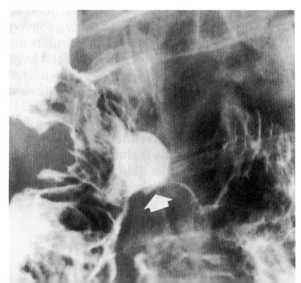

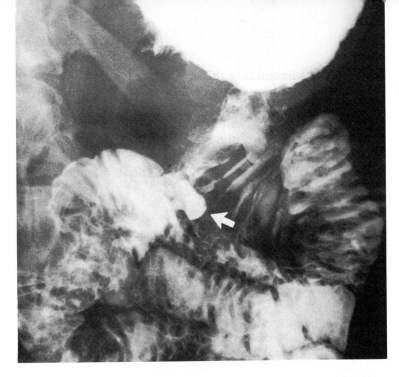

Fig. 14-43. Marginal ulcer with conical configuration **(arrow)** following Billroth-II anastomosis.

Fig. 14-44. Marginal ulcer **(arrow)** following Billroth-II anastomosis. Marked edema of jejunal folds at the anastomotic site suggests recurrent ulcer disease. There is also narrowing of the stoma with relative separation of the jejunal and gastric segments.

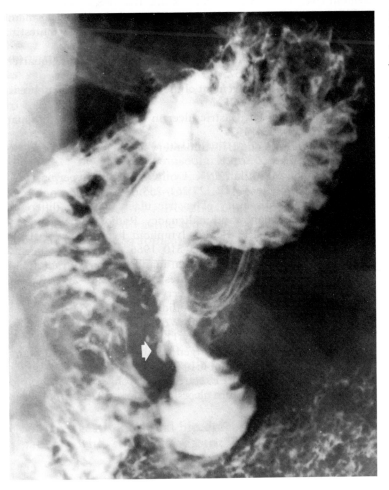

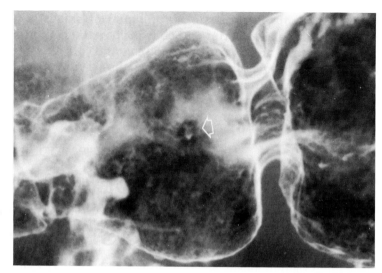

Fig. 15-1. Superficial gastric erosions in a patient with gastritis. The collection of barium represents a shallow erosion surrounded by a radiolucent halo **(arrow)**.

dyspepsia or epigastric pain often indistinguishable from peptic ulcer disease. The relationship of the erosions to the patient's symptoms is unclear.

RADIOGRAPHIC FINDINGS

Fig. 15-2. Superficial gastric erosion. A radiolucent halo of edema surrounds the small, barium-filled erosion **(arrow)**.

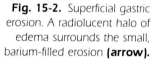

The classic radiographic appearance of a superficial gastric erosion is a tiny fleck of barium, which represents the erosion, surrounded by a radiolucent halo, which represents a mound of edematous mucosa (Fig. 15-2). The resultant target lesions are usually multiple, though a solitary erosion is occasionally demonstrated. The number of erosions is usually underestimated on radiographic examination, probably because of difficulty in performing a double-contrast study of the anterior wall of the stomach. Superficial gastric erosions can also appear as flat epithelial defects without surrounding reaction that coat with barium and are represented by reproducible linear streaks or dots of contrast. These incomplete erosions are more difficult to demonstrate radiographically, since they require optimal gastric distention and mucosal coating.

ETIOLOGY

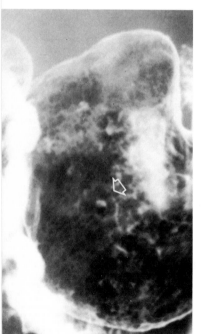

Superficial gastric erosions in many patients have no known predisposing cause. Specific etiologic factors include alcohol, anti-inflammatory agents (aspirin, steroids, phenylbutazone, indomethacin), analgesics, and emotional stress. Aphthoid ulcers in the stomach in patients with Crohn's disease are indistinguishable radiographically from su-

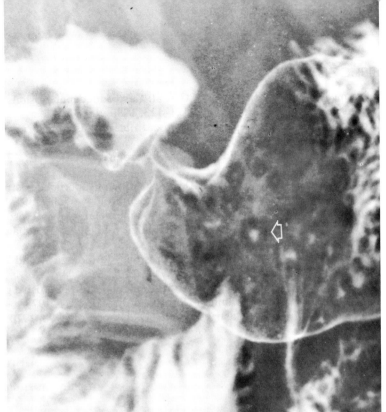

Fig. 15-3. Aphthoid ulcer in Crohn's disease **(arrow)**. The radiographic appearance is indistinguishable from that of other types of superficial gastric erosions.

perficial gastric erosions (Fig. 15-3) and are similar to the erosions seen in the colon in the early stages of Crohn's disease. They probably represent early, asymptomatic Crohn's disease in the stomach, which can progress to deeper ulcers, scarring, and stenosis. Biopsies of the aphthoid gastric ulcers of Crohn's disease reveal them to be noncaseating granulomas, unlike mucosal biopsies of superficial gastric erosions which usually show only a nonspecific chronic inflammatory reaction. Similar aphthoid erosions have been described as the earliest radiographically detectable changes in patients with gastric candidiasis, (Fig. 15-4).

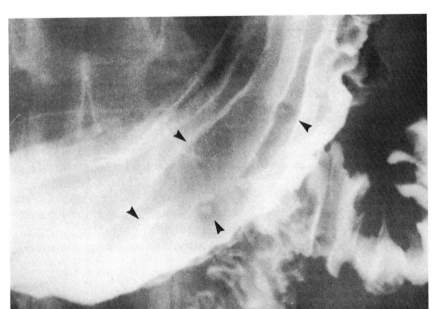

Fig. 15-4. Aphthoid ulcerations in gastric candidiasis. Coned view demonstrates numerous aphthoid ulcers **(arrowheads)**. The black ring represents the slightly raised, inflammatory edge surrounding the shallow, barium-filled depression. (Cronan J, Burrell M, Trepeta R: Aphthoid ulcerations in gastric candidiasis. Radiology 134:607–611, 1980)

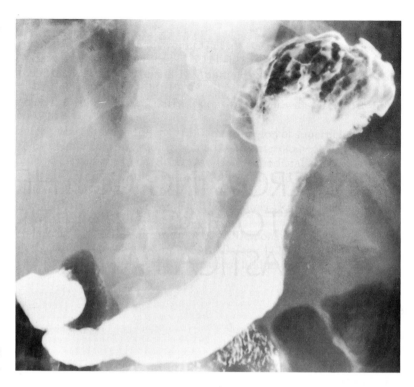

Fig. 16-1. Scirrhous carcinoma of the stomach.

CARCINOMA

Linitis plastica (leather bottle stomach) refers to any condition in which marked thickening of the gastric wall causes the stomach to appear as a narrowed, rigid tube. By far the most common cause of this radiographic pattern is scirrhous carcinoma of the stomach (Fig. 16-1). Tumor invasion of the gastric wall stimulates a desmoplastic response, which produces diffuse thickening and fixation of the stomach wall (Fig. 16-2). The involved stomach is contracted into a tubular structure without normal pliability. At fluoroscopy, peristalsis does not pass through the tumor site. Extension of tumor growth into the mucosa can produce nodular or irregular mucosal folds. Although scirrhous carcinoma can arise anywhere in the stomach, it usually begins near the pylorus and progresses slowly upward, the fundus being the area least involved (Fig. 16-3). The infiltration does not end abruptly but merges gradually into normal tissue. The duodenal bulb is often dilated and tends to remain filled because of rapid emptying of the rigid, pipelike stomach.

Another major manifestation of gastric carcinoma is narrowing of a segment of the stomach. At an early stage, gastric malignancy can appear as a plaquelike infiltrative lesion along one curvature (Fig. 16-4). Advanced carcinoma can encircle a segment of stomach and cause a constricting lesion similar to that produced by annular carcinoma of the colon (Fig. 16-5).

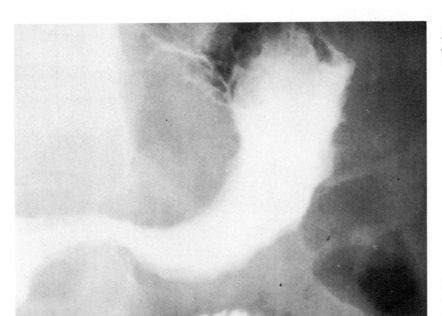

Fig. 16-2. Scirrhous carcinoma of the stomach. An intense desmoplastic reaction causes nodular thickening and fixation of the gastric wall.

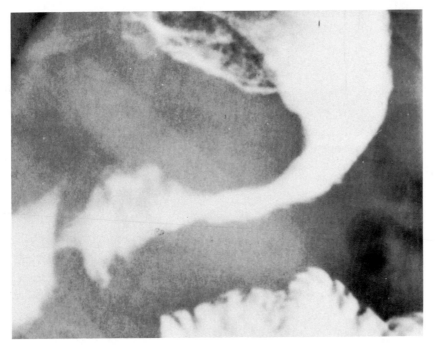

Fig. 16-3. Scirrhous carcinoma of the stomach. Generalized luminal narrowing tends to spare the fundus.

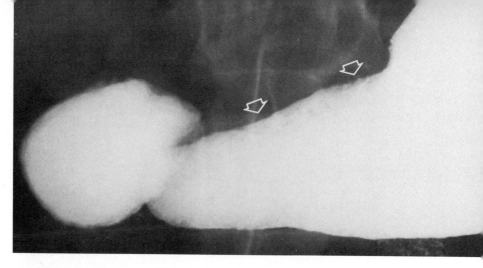

Fig. 16-4. Early adenocarcinoma of the stomach. A plaquelike lesion infiltrates the lesser curvature of the antrum **(arrows).**

Fig. 16-5. Two patients with constricting adenocarcinomas of the antrum of the stomach.

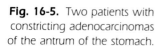

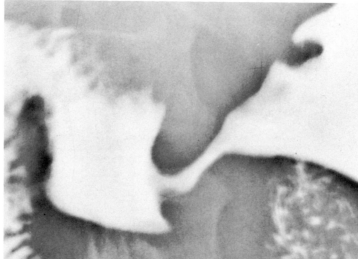

A

B

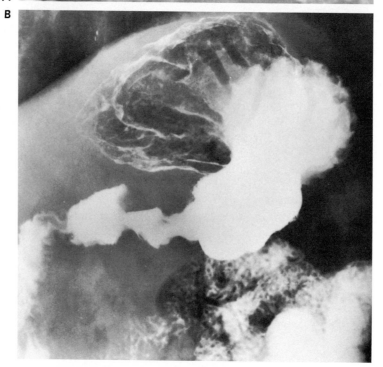

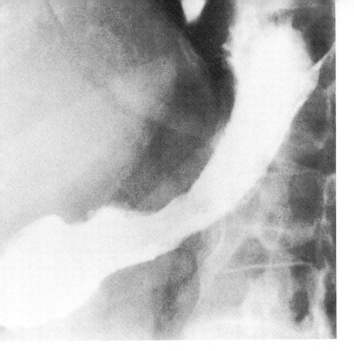 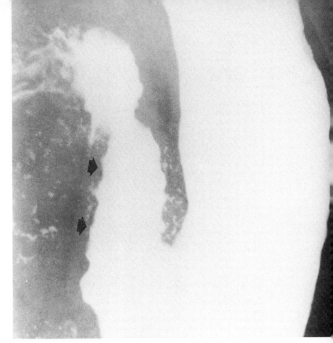

Fig. 16-6. Gastric lymphoma. A severe desmoplastic reaction produces a radiographic pattern that mimics scirrhous carcinoma.

Fig. 16-7. Gastric lymphoma. Infiltrative Hodgkin's disease causes irregular narrowing of the distal antrum **(arrows).**

LYMPHOMA

Invasion of the gastric wall by an infiltrative type of lymphoma (especially the Hodgkin's type) can cause a severe desmoplastic reaction and a radiographic appearance that mimics scirrhous carcinoma (Fig. 16-6). Thickening of the gastric wall narrows the lumen, especially in the antral region (Fig. 16-7). The overlying mucosal pattern is often effaced and indistinct, though without discrete ulceration. Unlike the rigidity and fixation of scirrhous carcinoma, residual peristalsis and flexibility of the stomach wall are often preserved in Hodgkin's disease.

METASTATIC LESIONS

Carcinoma of the pancreas is the major extragastric malignancy that produces a linitis plastica pattern. Circumferential narrowing of the stomach due to direct extension of tumor (Fig. 16-8) or metastases to perigastric nodes (Fig. 16-9) can result in an appearance indistinguishable from primary gastric carcinoma. A similar pattern can be caused by carcinoma of the transverse colon spreading to the stomach by way of the gastrocolic ligament. Hematogenous metastases, primarily from poorly differentiated carcinoma of the breast, can diffusely infiltrate the wall of the stomach with highly cellular deposits and produce a linitis plastica appearance (Fig. 16-10). The changes may involve the

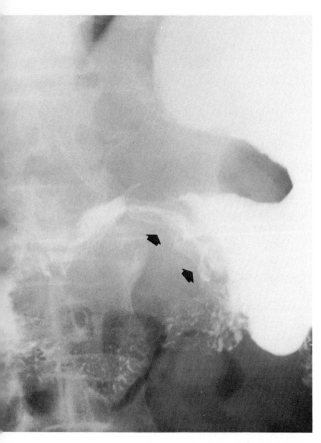

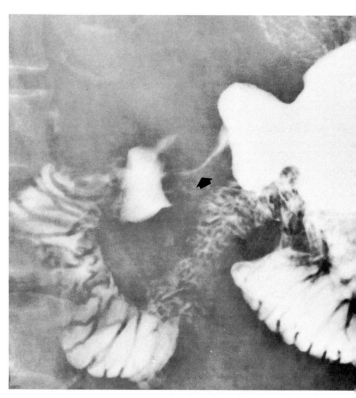

Fig. 16-9. Circumferential narrowing of the distal stomach **(arrow)** secondary to pancreatic carcinoma metastatic to perigastric lymph nodes.

Fig. 16-8. Direct extension of carcinoma of the pancreas causing severe narrowing of the distal antrum **(arrows)**.

Fig. 16-10. Scirrhous metastatic carcinoma of the breast infiltrating the wall of the stomach and narrowing the gastric lumen.

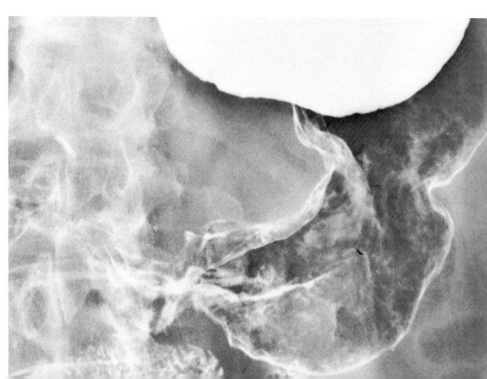

entire stomach or be more limited. At an early stage, the mucosa is often intact; a spiculated or nodular mucosal pattern can develop. Because the linitis plastica pattern in patients with metastatic lesions rarely occurs in the absence of far-advanced carcinoma with multiple sites of metastatic disease, the proper diagnosis is usually evident.

BENIGN CAUSES

GASTRIC ULCER DISEASE

Although the contracted, rigid pattern of linitis plastica of the stomach is almost always the result of malignant disease, benign processes can produce a radiographically indistinguishable appearance. Antral narrowing and rigidity can be caused by the intense spasm associated with a distal gastric ulcer (Fig. 16-11). Indeed, the ulcer sometimes cannot even be seen because of the lack of antral distensibility. In contrast to the linitis plastica pattern produced by malignant lesions, peptic-induced rigidity should not persist in the case of benign ulcers, most of which heal with adequate antacid therapy. An unusual cause of narrowing of a short segment of the stomach is the "geriatric" ulcer. Whereas gastric ulcers in young patients are relatively infrequent in the proximal half of the stomach, ulcers in elderly patients are particularly prone to arise high on the posterior wall of the stomach. As fibrous healing progresses, a typical "hourglass" deformity may result.

CROHN'S DISEASE

Crohn's disease involving the stomach can result in a smooth, tubular antrum that is poorly distensible and exhibits sluggish peristalsis. The

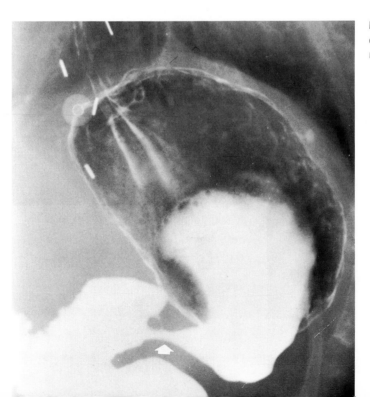

Fig. 16-11. Peptic ulcer disease causing antral narrowing and rigidity.

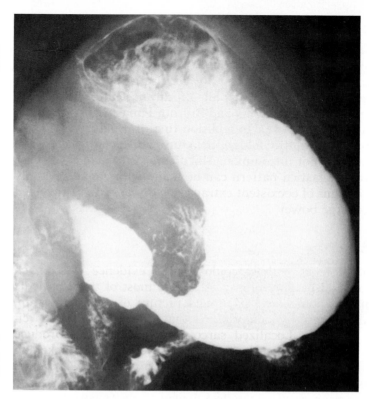

Fig. 16-15. Tuberculosis of the stomach. Fibrotic healing produces narrowing and rigidity of the distal antrum.

TUBERCULOSIS

Primary tuberculosis of the stomach is unusual; involvement of the stomach secondary to tuberculosis elsewhere is exceedingly rare. The most common symptoms are ulcerlike epigastric distress, vomiting suggesting pyloric obstruction, loss of weight and strength, fever, and hemorrhage. Diffuse inflammation or fibrotic healing causes rigidity of the distal stomach and a linitis plastica pattern (Fig. 16-15). Ulcerations and fistulas between the antrum and small bowel can simulate the radiographic appearance of gastric involvement by Crohn's disease. In extremely rare instances, histoplasmosis and actinomycosis also infiltrate the wall of the stomach.

EOSINOPHILIC GASTRITIS AND POLYARTERITIS NODOSA

Thickening of the muscle layer of the wall of the stomach due to edema and a diffuse infiltrate of predominantly mature eosinophils can produce the linitis plastica pattern in persons with eosinophilic gastritis (Fig. 16-16). Extensive disease can irregularly narrow the distal antrum and cause some degree of gastric outlet obstruction. If the subserosal layer of the stomach is also involved, eosinophilic ascites or pleural effusion can occur. Although eosinophilic gastritis can simulate a more aggressive process, it is essentially a benign condition that is self-limited, and it often completely returns to normal after steroid therapy. In the patient with the linitis plastica pattern, associated peripheral eosino-philia and a history of abdominal distress following the ingestion of specific foods should suggest the diagnosis of eosinophilic gastritis, especially if there is also relatively long contiguous spread of disease into the small bowel (eosinophilic gastroenteritis).

A radiographic appearance identical to eosinophilic gastroenteritis may be due to polyarteritis nodosa (Fig. 16-17). In this condition, irregular narrowing of the antrum secondary to ischemia and inflammation can coexist with thickening of folds in the small bowel.

INFECTION

Phlegmonous gastritis is an extremely rare condition in which bacterial invasion causes thickening of the wall of the stomach associated with discolored mucosa and an edematous submucosa. Bacteria can be seen enmeshed in a fibrinopurulent exudate on histologic sections of the stomach wall. Most cases of phlegmonous gastritis are due to alpha-hemolytic streptococci, though pneumococci, staphylococci, *Escherichia coli*, and, rarely, *Proteus vulgaris* and *Clostridium welchii* can also be the causative organisms. Although the exact mechanism is unclear, infections of the gastric wall appear to arise from direct invasion of the gastric mucosa, hematogenous spread from a septic focus (*e.g.*, endo-carditis), or lymphatic spread from a contiguous process (*e.g.*, chole-cystitis). The duodenum and esophagus are usually spared.

Clinically, the patient with phlegmonous gastritis is usually a woman over the age of 40 who presents with symptoms of acute abdominal catastrophe (abrupt onset of midepigastric pain, nausea, and vomiting). Purulent emesis, an extremely rare occurrence, is pathognomonic of phlegmonous gastritis. Many patients with this condition have signs of peritoneal irritation (muscle guarding, rebound tenderness on palpation) as well as fever, chills, severe prostration, and hiccups (due to diaphragmatic irritation). The abdominal pain may disappear if the patient assumes a sitting position (Dienenger's sign), a finding that has been suggested as specific for diffuse phlegmonous gastritis. Immediate surgery with vigorous antimicrobial therapy has somewhat reduced the previous 100% mortality rate following medical treatment of the disease.

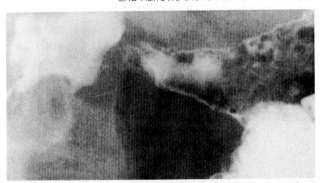

Fig. 16-16. Eosinophilic gastritis. Diffuse infiltration of predominantly mature eosinophils thickens the muscular layer and narrows the lumen of the stomach.

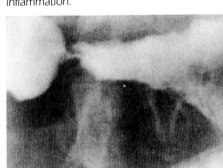

Fig. 16-17. Polyarteritis nodosa. Moderately irregular narrowing of the antrum is due to ischemia and inflammation.

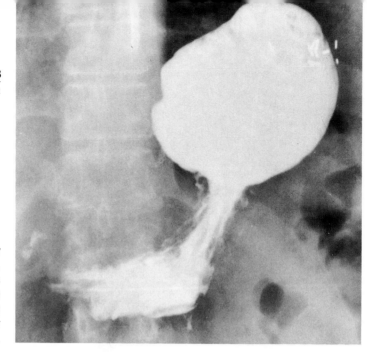

Fig. 16-26. Gastroplasty surgery for weight reduction. The presence of surgical clips and sutures in combination with distal gastric narrowing should suggest the proper diagnosis.

BIBLIOGRAPHY

Du Plessis DJ: Primary hypertrophic stenosis in the adult. Br J Surg 53:485–492, 1966

Franken EA: Caustic damage of the gastrointestinal tract: Roentgen features. AJR 118:77–85, 1973

Ghahremani GG: Nonobstructive mucosal diaphragms or rings of the gastric antrum in adults. AJR 121:236–247, 1974

Goldstein HM, Rogers LF, Fletcher GH et al: Radiological manifestations of radiation-induced injury to the normal upper gastrointestinal tract. Radiology 117:135–140, 1975

Gonzalez G, Kennedy T: Crohn's disease of the stomach. Radiology 113:27–29, 1974

Hall DA, Clouse ME, Gramm HF: Gastroduodenal ulceration after hepatic arterial infusion chemotherapy. AJR 136:1216–1218, 1981

Joffe N: Metastatic involvement of the stomach secondary to breast carcinoma. AJR 123:512–521, 1975

Margulis AR, Burhenne HJ: Alimentary Tract Roentgenology. St. Louis, C.V. Mosby, 1973

Martel W, Abell MR, Allan TNK: Lymphoreticular hyperplasia of the stomach (pseudolymphoma). AJR 127:261–265, 1976

McLaughlin JS, Van Eck W, Thayer W et al: Gastric sarcoidosis. Ann Surg 153:283–288, 1961

Messinger NH, Bobroff LM, Beneventano T: Lymphosarcoma of the colon. AJR 117:281–286, 1973

Nicks AJ, Hughes F: Polyarteritis nodosa "mimicking" eosinophilic gastroenteritis. Radiology 116:53–54, 1975

Turner MA, Beachley MC, Stanley D: Phlegmonous gastritis. AJR 133:527–528, 1979

Vuthibhagdee A, Harris NF: Antral stricture as a delayed complication of iron intoxication. Radiology 103:163–164, 1972

Wehnut WD, Olmsted WW, Neiman HL et al: Eosinophilic gastritis. Radiology 120:85–89, 1976

Fi(

g

narro

dis

with

folds al

and ma

alor

(T

ga

Rep

THICKENING OF GASTRIC FOLDS

17

Disease Entities

Normal variant
Gastritis
  Alcoholic
  Hypertrophic
  Antral
  Corrosive
  Infectious
  Postradiation
  Postfreezing
Peptic ulcer disease
Zollinger–Ellison syndrome
Menetrier's disease
Lymphoma
Pseudolymphoma
Carcinoma
Varices
Infiltrative processes
  Eosinophilic gastritis
  Crohn's disease
  Sarcoidosis
  Tuberculosis
  Syphilis
  Amyloidosis
Adjacent pancreatic disease
  Acute pancreatitis
  Extension of carcinoma of the pancreas

219

The gastric mucosa is normally thrown into numerous longitudinal folds or rugae that run predominantly in the direction of the long axis of the stomach. Folds in the vicinity of the lesser curvature run lengthwise in parallel fashion and form the magenstrasse that permits the rapid transport of fluid toward the duodenum. Gastric folds are not only composed of epithelium but also contain the lamina propria, the muscularis mucosae, and varying amounts of the submucosa. Therefore, edema of the mucosa or submucosa, as well as infiltration by neoplastic or inflammatory cells or vascular engorgement, can result in the radiographic pattern of thickened gastric folds.

There is much variability in the normal radiographic appearance of gastric folds. Folds in the fundus tend to be thicker and more tortuous than those in the distal part of the stomach. Antral folds measuring more than 5 mm in width are generally considered abnormal; folds of the same size in the fundus would probably be within normal limits. When the stomach is filled, the mucosa may be stretched evenly and smoothly and appear thinned. Conversely, when the stomach is partially empty or partially contracted, the gastric rugae are more prominent. Thus, in many patients, apparent thickening of the mucosal folds, especially in the fundus and proximal body to the stomach, merely represents a normal variant rather than a true pathologic process.

GASTRITIS

ALCOHOLIC

Many inflammatory diseases involving the stomach can result in the radiographic appearance of thickened rugal folds. Overindulgence in alcoholic beverages is the most common cause of acute exogenous gastritis. The radiographic appearance of thickened gastric folds (Fig. 17-1) parallels the pathologic observation of hyperemic engorged rugae, which usually subside completely after withdrawal of alcohol. Bizarre rugal thickening occasionally mimics malignant disease (Fig. 17-2). In patients with long drinking histories, chronic gastritis and a relative absence of folds is fequently seen (Fig. 17-3), though this can be related to such factors as cirrhosis, age, malnutrition, medication, and other systemic disease in addition to the alcohol itself.

HYPERTROPHIC

Hypertrophic gastritis is thickening of the mucosa due to localized or diffuse hyperplasia of surface epithelial cells (Fig. 17-4). This is a controversial entity that appears to be related to chronic inflammation of the gastric mucosa in which there is thickening, without destruction, of glandular elements. The pathogenesis is not clear, though many investigators have considered hypertrophic gastritis to be a functional lesion possibly related to transient edema, neuromuscular disturbances, or high acid output.

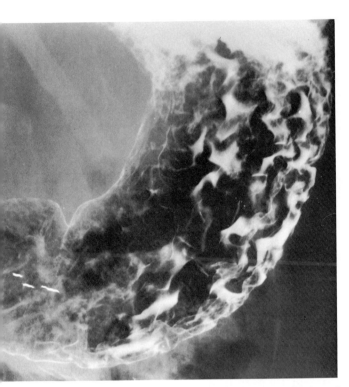

Fig. 17-1. Alcoholic gastritis. Diffuse thickening of gastric rugal folds.

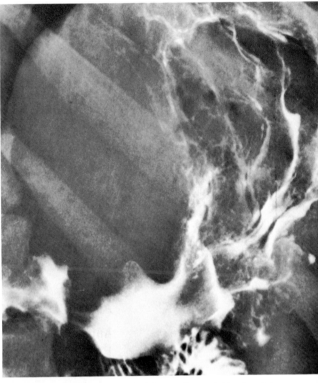

Fig. 17-2. Alcoholic gastritis. Bizarre, large folds simulate a malignant process.

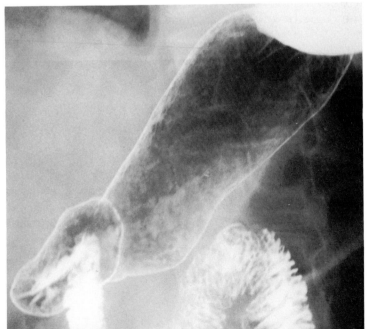

Fig. 17-3. Chronic atrophic gastritis with relative absence of folds in a patient with a long drinking history.

or irregularly corrugated appearance of the antrum) and antral spasm (Fig. 17-8). Patients with antral gastritis usually have epigastric pain, frequently of long duration, that has little relation to eating and is not completely relieved by antacids. The radiographic findings of antral gastritis may persist even when the patient is clinically well and tend to increase when symptoms recur.

CORROSIVE

The ingestion of corrosive agents results in a severe form of acute gastritis characterized by intense mucosal edema and inflammation. Radiographically, thickened gastric folds are associated with mucosal ulcerations, atony, and rigidity (Fig. 17-9). A fixed, open pylorus is usually seen, probably due to extensive damage to the muscular layer. The presence of gas in the wall of the stomach after the ingestion of corrosive agents is an ominous sign; free gastric perforation may occur.

Caustic ingestion occurs primarily in children and young adults. Most cases in children are accidental; those in young adults are usually associated with suicide attempts. Accidental ingestion of caustic materials in adults most often occurs in alcholics and psychotics.

Strong corrosives descend down the lesser curvature along the magenstrasse and accumulate in the antrum. Once a caustic agent reaches the distal antrum, it produces a tetanic contraction of the pylorus that prevents the noxious substance from passing further down the gastrointestinal tract. Because the bulk of the corrosive agent is thus concentrated in the lower part of the gastric body and antrum of the stomach, the resultant injury is most severe in these areas.

Acids generally produce more severe gastric damage than do ingested alkali. This is presumably due to partial neutralization of alkaline agents by the gastric acidity. Highly concentrated alkali, however, especially in liquid form, are also capable of causing severe damage to the wall of the stomach.

Fig. 17-8. Two patients with antral gastritis, which is seen as the flattening of the prepyloric shoulder of the lesser curvature with the corrugated appearance of mucosal crenulation **(arrows)**.

A B

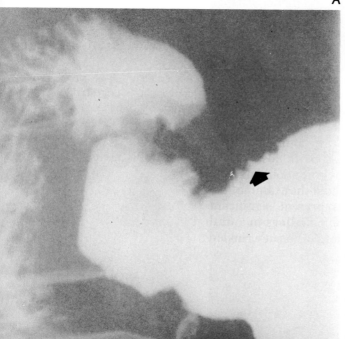 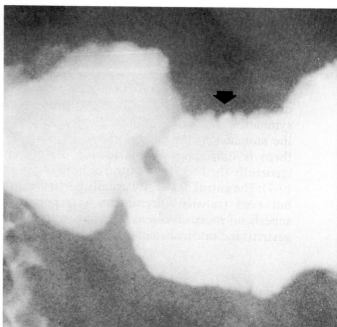

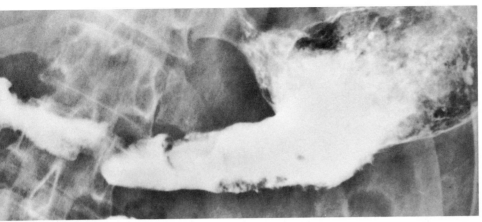

Fig. 17-9. Caustic gastritis following the ingestion of hydrochloric acid. Thickened folds along the greater curvature are associated with ulceration and rigidity.

INFECTIOUS

In infectious gastritis, bacterial invasion of the stomach wall or bacterial toxins (*e.g.,* botulism, diphtheria, dysentery, typhoid fever) result in hyperemia of the mucosa, edema, exudation, and a layering of fibrinous material on the mucosa that produces the radiographic appearance of thickened gastric folds. Involvement by gas-forming organisms can produce the characteristic pattern of gas within the wall of the stomach.

An unusual infestation of the stomach is acute anisakiasis, a form of visceral larva migrans acquired by the ingestion of raw or poorly cooked fish containing *Anisakis* larvae. This ascaris-like nematode spends its larval stage within tiny crustaceans that are eaten by such salt-water fish as herring, cod, and mackerel. Marine mammals, such as the whale and dolphin, are its final hosts. When humans break the natural chain and consume infected fish, the *Anisakis* worms penetrate the mucosa of the gastrointestinal tract and cause symptoms of acute, cramping abdominal pain within 4 hr to 6 hr of ingestion. The disease is self-limited, because the worms cannot grow in humans and die within a few weeks.

In the appropriate clinical setting, the presence of localized or generalized coarse, broad gastric folds due to mucosal edema is suggestive of, though not specific for, the diagnosis of anisakiasis (Fig. 17-10*A*). A definitive radiologic diagnosis requires the demonstration of a threadlike filling defect about 30 mm in length that represents the larva itself (Fig. 17-10*B*). The worms can appear serpiginous, circular, or ringlike and can change their shape during the examination.

POSTRADIATION / POSTFREEZING

Thickening of gastric folds can be seen after radiation or freezing therapy for gastric ulcer disease. Although a decrease in gastric secretion can be achieved by these techniques, they are rarely performed since less hazardous medical therapy has become available.

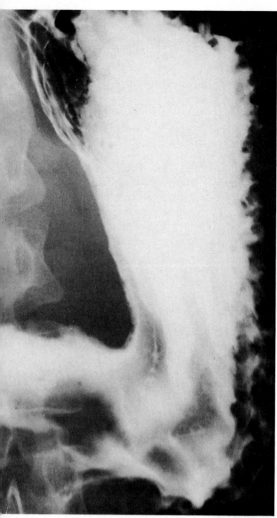

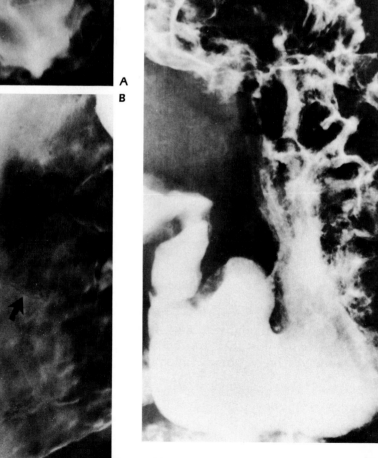

Fig. 17-10. Anisakiasis. **(A)** Generalized fold thickening representing mucosal edema in a patient who developed abdominal pain and nausea 8 hr after eating raw mackerel. **(B)** A double-contrast study shows a small collection of barium at the site at which the parasite penetrated the gastric mucosa **(arrowhead)** and reveals the thin outline of the larva itself **(arrow)**. (Nakata H, Takeda K, Nakayama T: Radiological diagnosis of acute gastric anisakiasis. Radiology 135:49–53, 1980)

Fig. 17-11. Zollinger–Ellison syndrome. There is diffuse thickening of gastric folds in this patient with hypersecretion of acid and peptic ulcer disease.

A
B

Hypersecretion of acid in patients with peptic ulcer disease or the Zollinger–Ellison syndrome is one of the most common causes of diffuse thickening of gastric folds (Fig. 17-11). In the body and fundus of the stomach (not the antrum), there appears to be a close correlation between the degree of enlargement of gastric folds and the level of acid secretions. In the Zollinger–Ellison syndrome, great glandular length and encroachment of fundal-type mucosa into the antrum produce characteristic increased rugosity and gastric secretions. Localized thickening of mucosal folds due to inflammatory edema can be seen surrounding an acute ulcer crater. The presence of thickened gastric folds radiating toward the crater is a traditional radiographic sign of a benign gastric ulcer (Fig. 17-12).

Hypersecretory states result in large amounts of retained gastric fluid despite fasting and lack of any organic obstruction. This is especially prominent in the Zollinger–Ellison syndrome, in which the gastric mucosa responds maximally to the stimulus of the gastrinlike hormone produced by the ulcerogenic tumor or its metastases.

MENETRIER'S DISEASE

Menetrier's disease (giant hypertrophic gastritis) is an uncommon disorder that is characterized by massive enlargement of rugal folds due to hyperplasia and hypertrophy of the gastric glands. There is usually hyposecretion of acid and excessive secretion of gastric mucus that can be associated with protein loss into the lumen of the stomach. The thickened gastric rugae become contorted and folded on each other

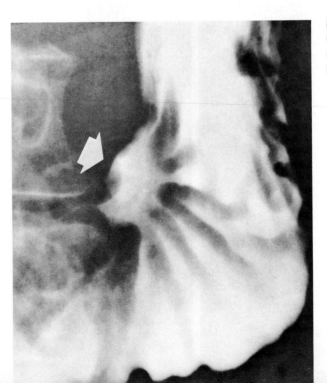

Fig. 17-12. Benign gastric ulcer. Thickened gastric folds radiate toward the crater **(arrow)**.

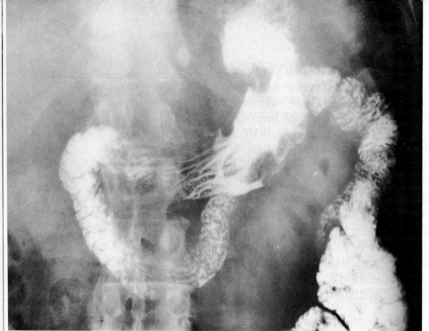
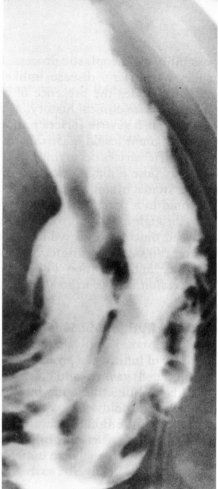

A B

Fig. 17-23. Nonfundic gastric varices. **(A)** Giant "folds" in the body of the stomach, particularly along the greater curvature, produce lobulated filling defects. There is no evidence of fundic varices or splenomegaly. **(B)** Fluoroscopic pressure spot-film reveals discrete varices as the cause of the enlarged rugae. (Sos T, Meyers MA, Baltaxe HA: Nonfundic gastric varices. Radiology 105:579–580, 1972)

associated increase in the eosinophil count in the peripheral blood and intolerance to specific foods.

Granulomatous processes, such as Crohn's disease, sarcoidosis, tuberculosis, and syphilis, can produce a pattern of rugal enlargement before the more characteristic antral narrowing and rigidity develop. Infiltration of the stomach wall by amyloid can also result in thickening of the gastric rugal folds (Fig. 17-25).

ADJACENT PANCREATIC DISEASE

Thickened gastric folds are a manifestation of adjacent pancreatitis, often with pseudocyst formation (Fig. 17-26). Selective prominence of nodular, serpentine mucosal folds on the posterior wall and lesser curvature of the stomach has been reported as a frequent and reliable sign of acute pancreatitis (Fig. 17-27). The rugal folds in the fundus and body along the greater curvature are normally more prominent than those on the lesser curvature and posterior wall of the barium-filled stomach. Selective enlargement of folds along the lesser curvature and posterior wall in patients with acute pancreatitis is presumably due either to activated enzymes producing mural irritation with spasm of the muscular layer or to a severe perigastric inflammatory response

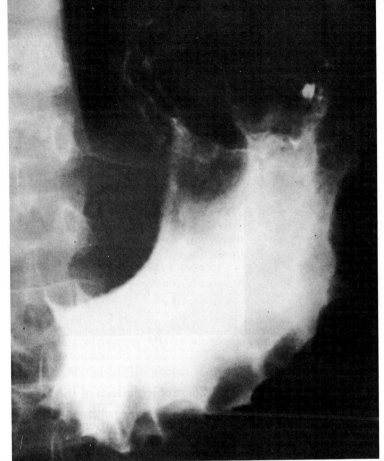

Fig. 17-24. Eosinophilic gastritis. Marked enlargement of rugal folds is caused by diffuse infiltration of eosinophilic leukocytes.

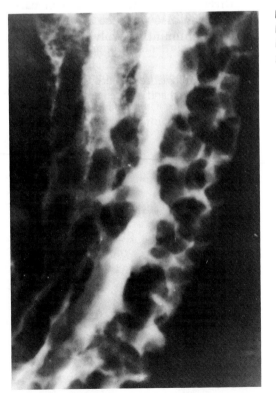

Fig. 17-25. Amyloidosis. Huge, nodular folds are caused by diffuse infiltration of the stomach by amyloid.

pattern include nonspecific inflammation, intestinal metaplasia, and benign lymphoid hyperplasia.

BENIGN TUMORS

With the increased use of the double-contrast technique, gastric polyps are being detected more frequently. In one series, polyps were demonstrated in 1.6% of upper gastrointestinal examinations. Although most gastric polyps are asymptomatic and discovered as incidental findings, some can bleed and produce hematemesis or melena. On rare occasions, a gastric polyp may prolapse through the pylorus and cause gastric outlet obstruction. The vast majority of epithelial polyps of the stomach can be divided into two groups: hyperplastic (regenerative) polyps and adenomas. Although there is some overlap, these two types of polyp can usually be distinguished by their radiographic appearance.

HYPERPLASTIC POLYP

Hyperplastic polyps are the most common causes of discrete filling defects in the stomach. These polyps are not true neoplasms but the result of excessive regenerative hyperplasia in an area of chronic gastritis. They are typically asymptomatic, small and smooth-surfaced, often multiple, and randomly distributed throughout the stomach. The polyps are composed of hyperplastic glands that are often cystic and are lined by a single layer of mature mucus cells with abundant cytoplasm and small, basally located nuclei. Mitoses are rare, except in areas of surface inflammation. The stroma shows varying degrees of inflammation and granulation tissue. Although malignant transformation virtually never occurs, hyperplastic polyps can be associated with an independent, coexisting carcinoma elsewhere in the stomach.

ADENOMATOUS POLYP

Adenomas are true neoplasms that are composed of dysplastic glands and are capable of continued growth. They have a definite tendency toward malignant transformation, and the reported incidence of this complication increases with the size of the polyp (average, about 40%). Most adenomas are relatively large with an irregular, lobulated surface and deep fissures extending down to the base. They can be sessile or pedunculated. The majority are single lesions situated in the antrum. Histologically, adenomas have a papillary configuration with frequent mitoses in pseudostratified and poorly differentiated component cells. Inflammatory changes are not a prominent feature.

Radiographic Findings of Hyperplastic and Adenomatous Polyps

The radiographic appearances of hyperplastic and adenomatous polyps reflect their pathologic characteristics. The hyperplastic polyp is seen

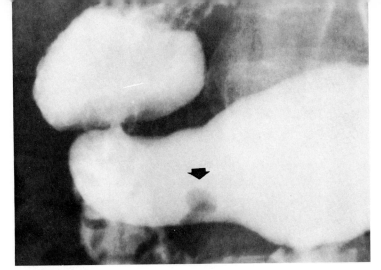

Fig. 18-3. Hyperplastic polyp. Note the small, sharply defined filling defect with a smooth contour **(arrow)**. A short stalk connects the head of the polyp to the stomach wall.

as a small (average, 1 cm), sharply defined filling defect with a smooth contour and no evidence of contrast in it (Fig. 18-3). When hyperplastic polyps are multiple, as is frequently the case, they all tend to be of about the same size (Fig. 18-4).

The adenomatous polyp is usually a large (greater than 2 cm) sessile lesion with an irregular surface (Fig. 18-5). Contrast material entering deep fissures and furrows in the polyp tends to produce a papillary or villous appearance. Adenomatous polyps are usually single and are most commonly found in the antrum.

Active peristalsis in the stomach may permit a gastric polyp to develop a fairly long pedicle. This appears as a narrow, stalklike defect extending from the head of the polyp to the stomach wall (Fig. 18-6).

Unfortunately, simple hyperplastic polyps can present any or all of the radiographic criteria (large size, lobulated or irregular contour) suggestive of gastric adenomas or even frank malignancy. On rare occasions, a hyperplastic polyp demonstrates substantial growth within a relatively short time. Therefore, if a gastric polyp is 1 cm or larger, endoscopy and biopsy are recommended. If there is no histologic

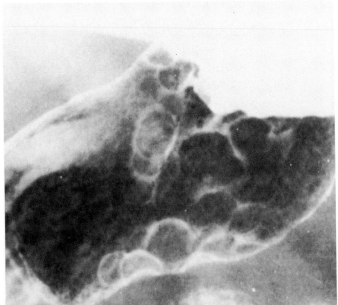
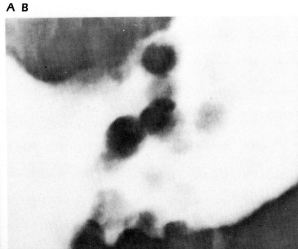

Fig. 18-4. Hyperplastic polyps. Multiple smooth filling defects of similar size are seen on **(A)** double-contrast and **(B)** filled views.

A B

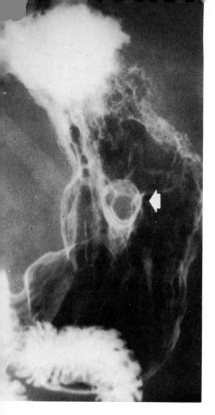

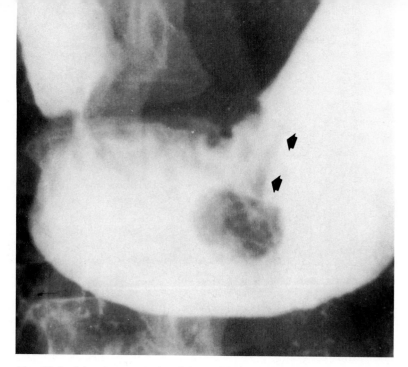

Fig. 18-6. Adenomatous polyp. A long, thin pedicle **(arrows)** extends from the head of the polyp to the stomach wall.

Fig. 18-5. Adenomatous polyp **(arrow)**.

Fig. 18-7. Gastric polyposis associated with familial polyposis of the colon. (Denzler TB, Harned RK, Pergram CJ: Gastric polyps in familial polyposis coli. Radiology 130:63–66, 1979)

A B

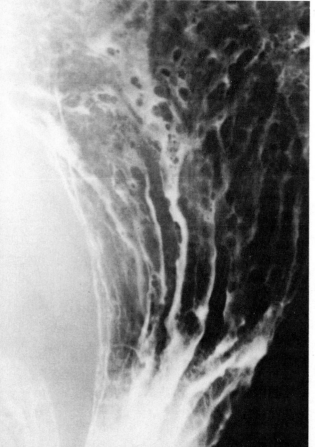

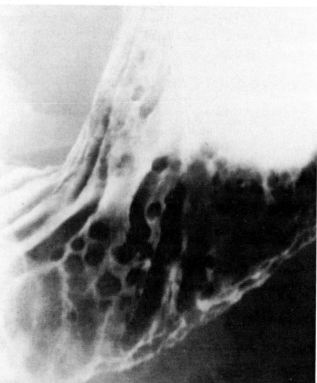

evidence of neoplasia, no additional investigation or treatment is necessary.

Both hyperplastic and adenomatous polyps tend to develop in patients with chronic atrophic gastritis, a condition known to be associated with a high incidence of carcinoma. Thus, even though a gastric polyp is proved to be benign, the entire stomach must be carefully examined for the possibility of a coexisting carcinoma.

There is a higher than normal incidence of adenomatous and hyperplastic gastric polyps in patients with familial polyposis of the colon (Fig. 18-7). Gastric polyposis also occurs in the Cronkhite–Canada syndrome (colon polyposis, nail and hair changes), in which enlarged rugal folds and whiskering (multiple tiny projections due to barium trapped between nodular excrescences of rugae) have also been described.

HAMARTOMAS

Multiple gastric polyps can develop in patients with the Peutz–Jeghers syndrome (Fig. 18-8). The polyps, which are hamartomas with essentially no malignant potential, are composed of normal constituents of the mucosa arranged in a different manner. The true nature of the gastric filling defects in this condition is usually evident when other manifestations of the Peutz–Jeghers syndrome (small bowel polyps, mucocutaneous pigmentation) are present. In Cowden's disease (multiple hamartoma syndrome), hamartomas in the stomach and other parts of the gastrointestinal tract can be associated with the characteristic circumoral papillomatosis and nodular gingival hyperplasia (Fig. 18-9).

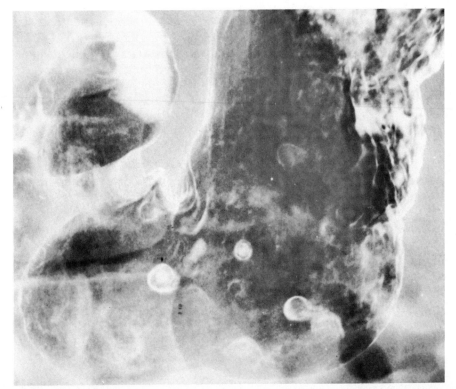

Fig. 18-8. Peutz–Jeghers syndrome. Note the multiple hamartomas of the stomach. The patient had small bowel polyps and mucocutaneous pigmentation.

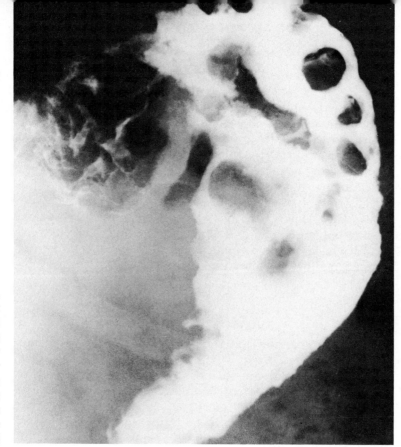

Fig. 18-9. Cowden's disease.
Note the multiple gastric
hamartomas. The patient had
characteristic circumoral
papillomatosis and nodular
gingival hyperplasia. (Hauser
H, Ody B, Plojoux O et al:
Radiological findings in
multiple hamartoma syndrome
(Cowden disease). Radiology
137:317–323, 1980)

SPINDLE CELL TUMOR

Spindle cell tumors constitute the overwhelming majority of benign submucosal gastric neoplasms. These lesions vary in size from tiny nodules (Fig. 18-10), often discovered incidentally at laparotomy or autopsy, to bulky tumors with large intraluminal components that can be associated with hemorrhage, obstruction, or perforation (Fig. 18-11). Some spindle cell tumors have extensive exogastric components that can mimic extrinsic compression of the stomach by normal or enlarged liver, spleen, pancreas, or kidney. It is therefore essential that an apparent mass be identified on several projections with the patient in various positions so that the physician may be certain that the mass represents a true lesion and not merely extrinsic compression by a contiguous structure (Fig. 18-12). It may be extremely difficult to distinguish radiographically between benign spindle cell tumors and their malignant counterparts. Although large, markedly irregular filling defects with prominent ulcerations suggest malignancy, a radiographically benign tumor can be histologically malignant.

Leiomyoma is the most common spindle cell tumor of the stomach. Usually single rather than multiple, leiomyomas are composed of well-differentiated smooth muscle cells forming criss-crossing bundles that separate a richly vascularized collagen tissue. Small intramural tumor nodules cause circumscribed, rounded filling defects that closely resemble sessile gastric polyps. Leiomyomas can be extremely large and

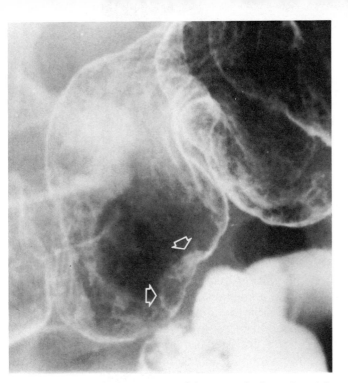

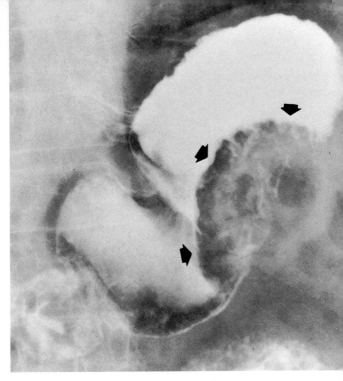

Fig. 18-10. Leiomyoma of the stomach. A small nodule **(arrows)** is seen on double-contrast examination.

Fig. 18-11. Large leiomyoma involving the greater curvature of the stomach **(arrows).**

Fig. 18-12. Pseudomass **(arrows). (A)** On the filled, supine film, the large "mass" simulates a spindle cell tumor on the greater curvature. **(B)** On the double-contrast view with the patient in a different position, the "mass" has disappeared. It therefore clearly represented a transient, extrinsic compression by a contiguous structure.

A B

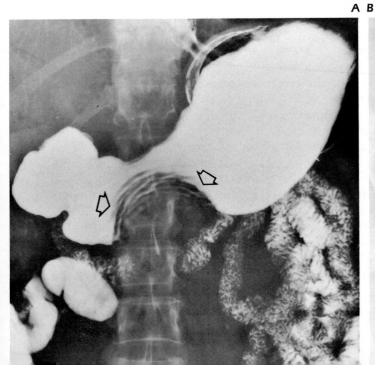

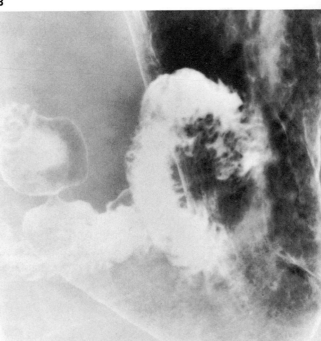

predominantly located in intraluminal (Fig. 18-13), intramural (Fig. 18-14), or extramural (Fig. 18-15) locations. Because of their tendency toward central necrosis and ulceration, bleeding is common as the tumor grows. Hematemesis or melena are frequent symptoms. Up to 5% of gastric leiomyomas demonstrate coarse calcification simulating uterine fibroids. Multiplicity of tumors suggests malignancy, though evidence of metastases is often the only radiographic indication that the lesion is not benign.

Lipomas, fibromas, hemangiomas, and neurogenic tumors, all of which can be radiographically indistinguishable from leiomyomas, are far less common submucosal gastric neoplasms. Lipomas are usually single and of moderate size (Fig. 18-16). They occur primarily in the antrum and tend to develop toward the lumen of the stomach and become pedunculated. Deep ulceration frequently occurs. As with the very rare hemangiomas, gastric lipomas change shape in response to peristalsis and produce compressible nodular defects. Fibromas are firm, elastic tumors consisting of fibroblasts grouped together in dense, intricate bundles. These very slow-growing tumors are usually found in the antrum. Neurogenic tumors include neurolemmomas (Fig. 18-17) and neurofibromas and are sometimes a manifestation of von Recklinghausen's disease.

VILLOUS ADENOMA

Villous adenomas of the stomach are rare lesions that histologically and radiographically resemble colon tumors of the same type. Retention of contrast material among the villous projections results in a fine lacework of radiodense particles interspersed throughout the sessile mucosal lesion, producing a soap-bubble or frondlike appearance (Fig. 18-18). Often multiple, villous adenomas of the stomach are soft, pliable, and nonobstructing. As with this type of tumor in the colon, villous adenomas of the stomach have a substantial incidence of malignancy. In one large series of 16 villous adenomas of the stomach, all had evidence of *in situ* or invasive carcinoma.

Fig. 18-13. Leiomyoma presenting as an intraluminal gastric mass **(arrows).**

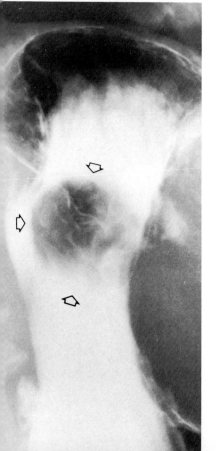

Fig. 18-14. Leiomyoma presenting as an intramural gastric mass **(arrows).**

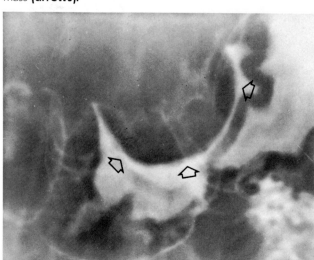

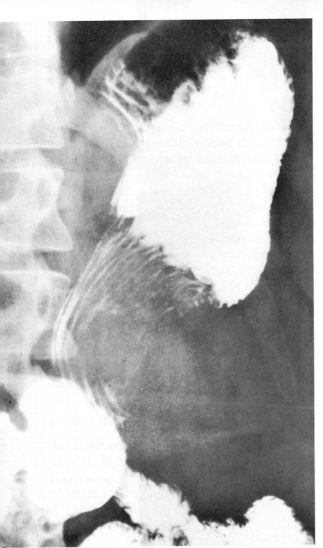

Fig. 18-15. Leiomyoma with a large exophytic component simulating an extrinsic mass.

Fig. 18-16. Lipoma. A smooth, polypoid mass may be seen in the body of the stomach **(arrow).**

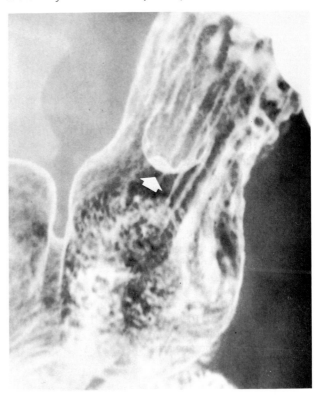

Fig. 18-17. Neurolemmoma. The antral mass is large and smooth with central ulceration.

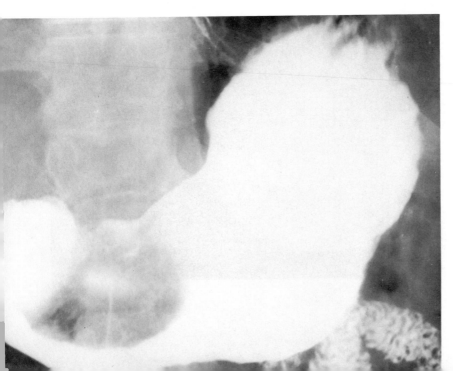

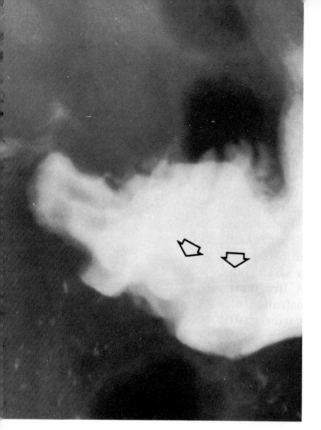

Fig. 18-21. Lymphoma. Multiple ulcerated, polypoid gastric masses are visible **(arrows).**

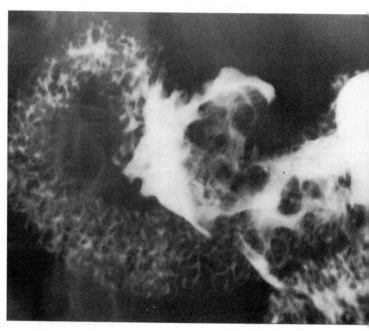

Fig. 18-22. Lymphoma. Multiple polypoid filling defects with generalized thickening of folds involve the antrum and duodenal bulb.

lymphoma) (Fig. 18-22) or separated by a normal-appearing mucosal pattern, unlike the atrophic mucosal background that is seen with multiple carcinomatous polyps in patients with pernicious anemia. Filling defects in the stomach are unusual manifestations of Burkitt's lymphoma (Fig. 18-23).

METASTASES

Hematogenous metastases infrequently involve the stomach and produce single or multiple gastric filling defects (Fig. 18-24). Abdominal symptoms tend to be relatively nonspecific or entirely absent. Anorexia, nausea, vomiting, and epigastric distress are the most common complaints, but these symptoms are frequently attributed to other gastric disorders or to the side-effects of chemotherapeutic drugs. On rare occasions, gastric hemorrhage or outlet obstruction develops.

Metastatic melanoma is the most common hematogenous metastasis to cause single or multiple filling defects in the barium-filled stomach. These lesions are usually ulcerated or umbilicated and have a bull's-eye appearance (Fig. 18-25). Gastric metastases from malignant

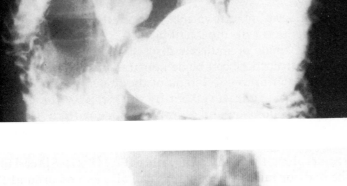

Fig. 18-23. Burkitt's
lymphoma. A solitary mass
(arrow) is evident in the body
of the stomach.

Fig. 18-24. Undifferentiated
carcinoma metastatic to the
stomach. Note the ulcerated
filling defect **(arrow)**.

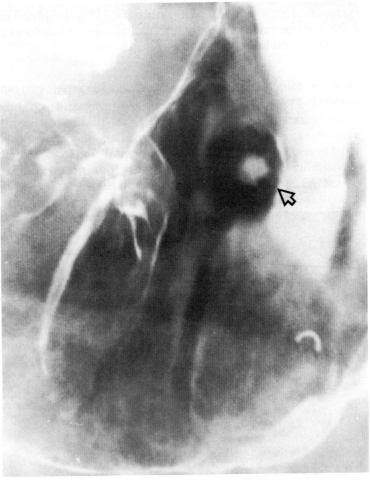

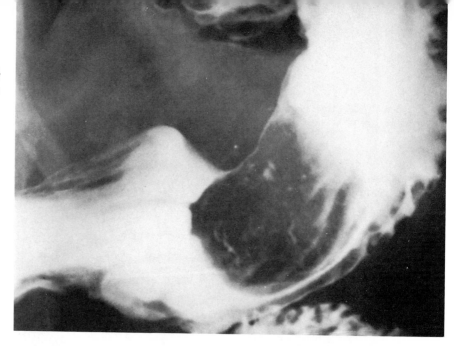

Fig. 18-29. Leiomyosarcoma. The bulky tumor, which arises in the body of the stomach, contains some central ulceration.

Fig. 18-30. Leiomyosarcoma. **(A)** Full and **(B)** coned-down views demonstrate the large exogastric component of the lesion. The liver is enormously enlarged. **(C)** The <u>en face</u> view demonstrates the intramural portion of the mass, suggesting a tumor of the spindle cell type.

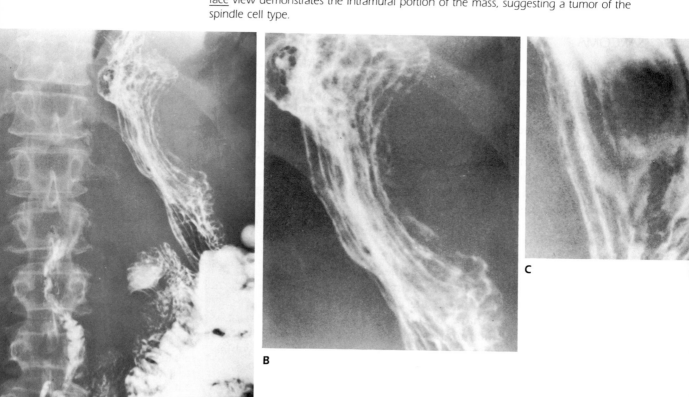

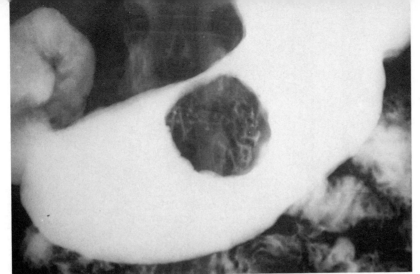

Fig. 18-31. Liposarcoma. The
mildly irregular antral filling
defect is extremely radiolucent,
probably reflecting its fatty
composition.

Fig. 18-32. Leiomyoblastoma.
The antral mass is huge and
irregular.

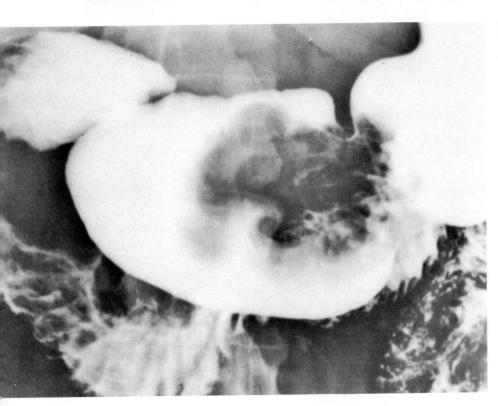

EXTRINSIC CYSTIC OR INFLAMMATORY MASSES

Cystic and inflammatory masses arising outside the stomach can cause
extrinsic impressions mimicking intramural or intraluminal gastric
lesions. Cysts of the liver (Fig. 18-33), spleen, kidney, or adrenal and
upper abdominal abscesses (Fig. 18-34) can produce this radiographic
appearance.

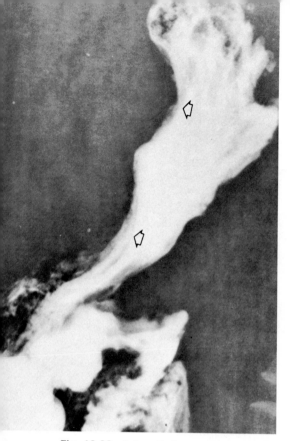

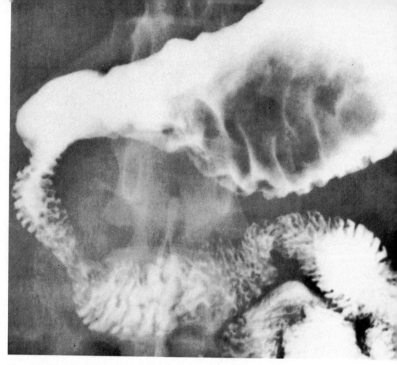

Fig. 18-34. Pancreatic abscess. The large retrogastric inflammatory process causes edema and effacement of rugal folds. Radiographically, the abscess appears as a discrete mass in the body and antrum of the stomach.

Fig. 18-33. Polycystic liver. The two large, extrinsic impressions **(arrows)** on the anterior aspect of the stomach mimic intramural lesions.

ECTOPIC PANCREAS

Aberrant pancreatic tissue (ectopic pancreas) can be found in many areas of the gastrointestinal tract but is most common on the distal greater curvature of the gastric antrum within 3 cm to 6 cm of the pylorus (Fig. 18-35). About half of patients with ectopic pancreas are symptomatic and complain of vague abdominal pain, nausea, and occasional vomiting. Bleeding can occur if the overlying mucosa becomes ulcerated. Radiographically, ectopic pancreas appears as a smooth submucosal mass, rarely more than 2 cm in diameter, that often has a central dimple or umbilication representing the orifice of the duct associated with the aberrant pancreatic tissue.

ENLARGED GASTRIC FOLDS

Enlarged gastric folds, when viewed on end, can produce a radiographic pattern of multiple nodular filling defects suggesting polyps (Fig. 18-36). This appearance can be seen in patients with Menetrier's disease (Fig. 18-37) or gastric varices (Fig. 18-38), as well as in persons with thickened rugal folds due to granulomatous infiltration (Crohn's disease, sarcoidosis, tuberculosis) or eosinophilic gastritis.

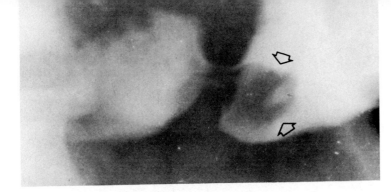

Fig. 18-35. Ectopic pancreas. There is a filling defect in the distal antrum **(arrows)** with a central collection of barium.

Fig. 18-36. Multiple nodular filling defects suggesting polyps. The filling defects are due to enlarged gastric folds, which are viewed on end in this patient with alcoholic gastritis.

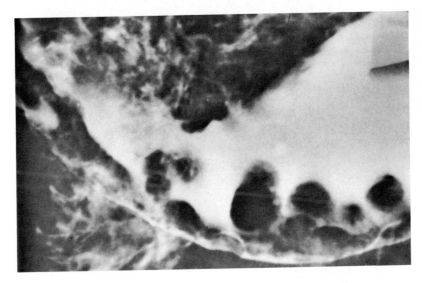

Fig. 18-37. Menetrier's disease. Diffuse thickening of rugal folds simulates the appearance of multiple polypoid filling defects.

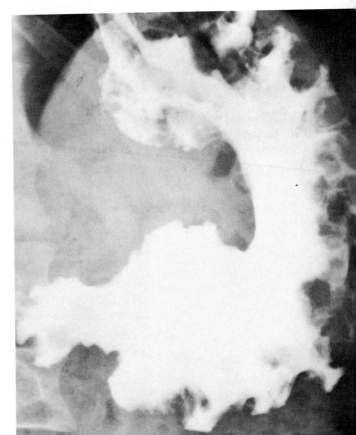

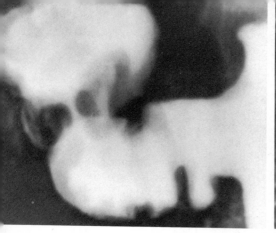
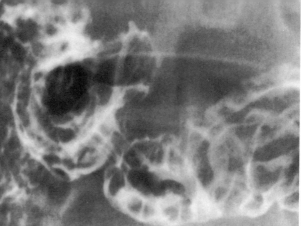

A B

Fig. 18-38. Antral varices. Dilated venous structures in **(A)** single- and **(B)** double-contrast views simulate multiple polypoid filling defects.

BEZOAR

A bezoar is an intragastric mass composed of accumulated ingested material (Fig. 18-39). Phytobezoars, which are composed of undigested vegetable material, have classically been associated with the eating of unripe persimmons, a fruit containing substances that coagulate on contact with gastric acid to produce a stickly gelatinous material, which then traps seeds, skin, and other foodstuffs. Numerous other substances that can apparently form bezoars include glue (especially in persons making model airplanes), tar, paraffin, shellac, asphalt, bismuth carbonate, magnesium carbonate, laundry starch, and wood fibers.

Trichobezoars (hairballs) occur predominantly in females, especially those with schizophrenia or other mental instability. The accumulated matted mass of hair can enlarge to occupy the entire volume of the stomach, often assuming the shape of the organ. A small percentage of bezoars are composed of both hair and vegetable matter and are termed trichophytobezoars.

Symptoms of gastric bezoars result from the mechanical presence of the foreign body. They include cramplike epigastric pain and a sense of dragging, fullness, lump, or heaviness in the upper abdomen. The

Fig. 18-39. Bezoar. The large intragastric filling defect is composed of accumulated ingested material.

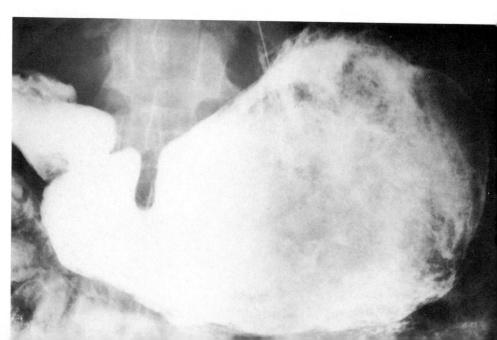

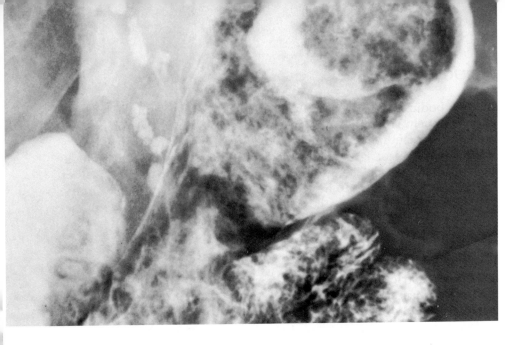

Fig. 18-40. Bezoar. Infiltration of contrast into the interstices of the mass results in a characteristic mottled appearance.

incidence of associated peptic ulcers is high, especially with the more abrasive phytobezoars. When bezoars are large, symptoms of pyloric obstruction can clinically simulate symptoms of a gastric carcinoma.

Plain abdominal radiographs often show the bezoar as a soft-tissue mass floating in the stomach at the air–fluid interface. On barium studies, contrast coating of the mass and infiltration into the interstices result in a characteristic mottled or streaked appearance (Fig. 18-40). The filling defect is occasionally completely smooth, simulating an enormous gas bubble that is freely movable within the stomach (Fig. 18-41).

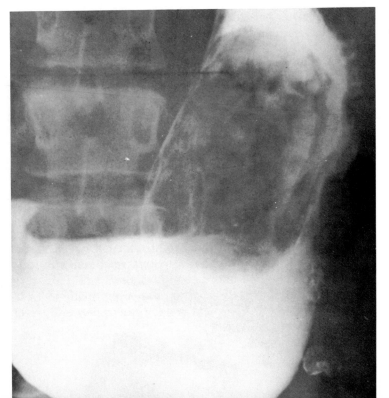

Fig. 18-41. Glue bezoar in a young model-airplane builder. The smooth mass simulates an enormous gas bubble.

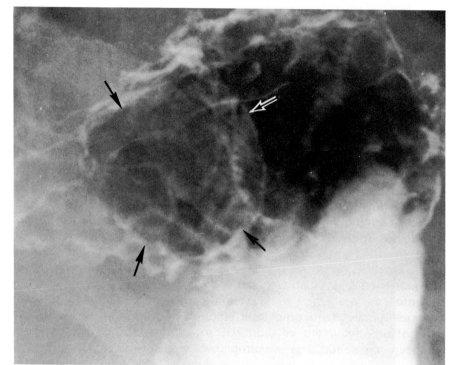

Fig. 18-48. Tumefactive extramedullary hematopoiesis. There is a sharply marginated smooth-walled gastric mass adjacent to the esophagogastric junction. (Gomes AS, Harell GS: Tumefactive extramedullary hematopoiesis of the stomach. Gastrointest Radiol 1:163–165, 1976)

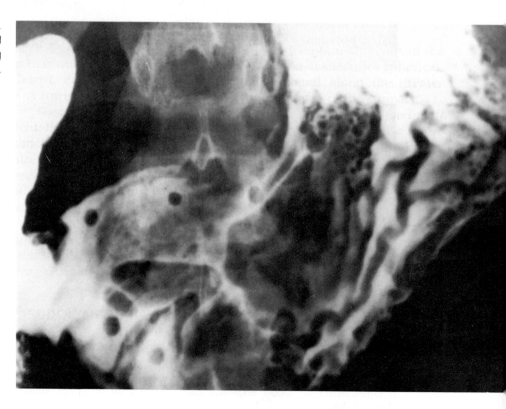

Fig. 18-49. Amyloidosis. Submucosal masses of amyloid appear as multiple lucent filling defects simulating air bubbles.

INTRAGASTRIC GALLSTONE

An extremely rare cause of filling defects in the stomach is intragastric gallstones. A gallstone may pass from the duodenum into the stomach either by retrograde flow from the duodenum following cholecysto-duodenal fistula or directly through a cholecystogastric fistula. Like other foreign bodies in the stomach, intragastric gallstones can cause mucosal irritation leading to ulceration, bleeding, perforation, and even gastric outlet obstruction.

TUMEFACTIVE EXTRAMEDULLARY HEMATOPOIESIS

Tumefactive extramedullary hematopoiesis of the stomach very rarely produces a submucosal gastric mass (Fig. 18-48). Extramedullary hematopoiesis develops when normal blood-forming sites cannot maintain a rate of red-blood-cell formation sufficient for body demand, as in patients with leukemia, myelofibrosis, severe anemia, polycythemia, Hodgkin's disease, and chronic poisoning with marrow-toxic substances. Extramedullary hematopoietic collections, usually microscopic, are most commonly found in the liver, spleen, and lymph nodes. Infrequently, extramedullary hematopoiesis can form significant tumor masses involving multiple organs, including the upper gastrointestinal tract. In patients with chronic myelogenous leukemia, tumefactive extramedullary hematopoiesis of the stomach may be indistinguishable from a gastric polypoid mass secondary to leukemic infiltrate.

AMYLOIDOSIS

A gastric filling defect, often with ulceration, can be produced by localized deposition of amyloid within the wall of the stomach. Although amyloidosis is usually associated with diffuse involvement of the gastrointestinal tract, isolated amyloidomas of the stomach can occur (Fig. 18-49).

CANDIDIASIS

Candidal infection in an immunosuppressed patient has been reported to cause multiple scattered, nodular filling defects in the stomach. Central ulcerations or depressions in the lesions tend to produce a bull's-eye appearance.

BIBLIOGRAPHY

Allman RM, Cavanagh RC, Helwig EB et al: Inflammatory fibroid polyp. Radiology 127:69–73, 1978

Athey PA, Goldstein HM, Dodd GD: Radiologic spectrum of opportunistic infections of the upper gastrointestinal tract. AJR 129:419–424, 1977

Bahk YW, Ahn JS, Choi HJ: Lymphoid hyperplasia of the stomach presenting as umbilicated polypoid lesions: Report of two cases. Radiology 100:277–280, 1971

Braxton M, Jacobson G: Intragastric gallstone. AJR 78:631–632, 1957

Burgess JN, Dockerty MB, ReMine WH: Sarcomatous lesions of the stomach. Ann Surg 173:758–766, 1971

Chiles JT, Platz CE: The radiographic manifestations of pseudolymphoma of the stomach. Radiology 116:551–556, 1975

Dastur KJ, Ward JF: Amyloidoma of the stomach. Gastrointest Radiol 5:17–20, 1980

Dunnick NR, Harell GS, Parker BR: Multiple "bull's-eye" lesions in gastric lymphoma. AJR 126:965–969, 1976

Faegenburg D, Farman J, Dallemand S et al: Leiomyoblastoma of the stomach: Report of nine cases. Radiology 117:297–300, 1975

Gomes AS, Harell GS: Tumefactive extramedullary hematopoiesis of the stomach. Gastrointest Radiol 1:163–165, 1976

Gordon R, Laufer I, Kressel HY: Gastric polyps found on routine double-contrast examination of the stomach. Radiology 134:27–30, 1980

Hegedus V, Poulsen PE, Reichardt J: The natural history of the double pylorus. Radiology 126:29–34, 1978

Jamshidnejad J, Koehler RE, Narayan D: Double channel pylorus. AJR 130:1047–1050, 1978

Joffe N: Metastatic involvement of the stomach secondary to breast carcinoma. AJR 123:512–521, 1975

Kavlie H, White TT: Leiomyomas of the upper gastrointestinal tract. Surgery 71:842–848, 1972

Kilcheski T, Kressel HY, Laufer I et al: The radiographic appearance of the stomach in Cronkhite–Canada syndrome. Radiology 141:57–60, 1981

Margulis AR, Burhenne HJ: Alimentary Tract Roentgenology. St. Louis, C.V. Mosby, 1973

Meltzer AD, Ostrum BJ, Isard HJ: Villous tumors of the stomach and duodenum: Report of three cases. Radiology 78:511–513, 1966

Meyers MA, McSweeny J: Secondary neoplasms of the bowel. Radiology 105:1–11, 1972

Ming SC: Malignant potential of gastric polyps. Gastrointest Radiol 1:121–125, 1976

Op den Orth JO, Dekker W: Gastric adenomas. Radiology 141:289–293, 1981

Perez CA, Dorfman RF: Benign lymphoid hyperplasia of the stomach and duodenum. Radiology 87:505–510, 1966

Pomerantz H, Margolin HN: Metastases to the gastrointestinal tract from malignant melanoma. AJR 88:712–717, 1962

Privett JTJ, Davies ER, Roylance J: The radiological features of gastric lymphoma. Clin Radiol 28:457–463, 1977

Rappaport AS: Gastroduodenal fistulae and double pyloric canal. Gastrointest Radiol 2:341–346, 1978

Sherrick DW, Hodgson JR, Dockerty MB: The roentgenologic diagnosis of primary gastric lymphoma. Radiology 84:925–932, 1965

Thoeni RF, Gedgaudas RK: Ectopic pancreas: Usual and unusual features. Gastrointest Radiol 5:37–42, 1980

Tim LO, Banks S, Marks IN et al: Benign lymphoid hyperplasia of the gastric antrum: Another cause of "*état mammelonné*." Br J Radiol 50:29–31, 1977

Tsukamoto Y, Nishitani H, Oshiumi Y et al: Spontaneous disappearance of gastric polyps: Report of four cases. AJR 129:893–897, 1977

Wright FW, Matthews JM: Hemophilic pseudotumor of the stomach. Radiology 98:547–549, 1971

FILLING DEFECTS IN THE GASTRIC REMNANT

Disease Entities

Surgical deformity
Suture granuloma
Bezoar
Carcinoma
  Gastric stump carcinoma
  Recurrent carcinoma
Hyperplastic polyps and bile (alkaline) reflux gastritis
Jejunogastric intussusception

Partial resection of the stomach is most commonly performed for peptic ulcer disease. Although the 1.5% mortality rate that is associated with partial gastric resection and vagotomy is somewhat higher than that for vagotomy with a drainage procedure alone, the rate of recurrent ulcers of less than 2% after vagotomy and hemigastrectomy is far less than the rate of 6% to 8% after vagotomy and a drainage procedure. Resection of a portion of the stomach can also be performed as surgical therapy for gastric malignancy.

SURGICAL DEFORMITY

Anastomosis after partial gastrectomy can be either a gastroduodenostomy (Billroth I) or gastrojejunostomy (Billroth II). In both of these procedures, the cut end of the stomach is usually partially oversewn to minimize problems associated with a large gastric stoma. The oversewn area produces a typical deformity or plication defect on subsequent contrast examinations. One example is the characteristic plication defect associated with the Hofmeister type of anastomosis, a procedure developed to minimize the problems associated with a large gastric stoma (Fig. 19-1). With this technique, the open end of the gastric stump is closed, with a line of sutures extending from the lesser curvature for one-half to two-thirds of the distance to the greater curvature, and the anastomosis then performed. The resulting filling defect corresponds to the closure line of the invaginated cut surface of the stomach. It is frequently apparent on initial postoperative studies and can decrease in size or disappear on subsequent examinations.

Surgical deformities, especially in patients undergoing partial gastric resection for malignancy, can closely simulate neoplastic processes. Therefore, it is essential that a baseline upper gastrointestinal series be obtained soon after partial gastric resection. Filling defects and extrinsic impressions demonstrated within the first few months of surgery clearly represent surgical deformities rather than discrete lesions. In contrast, subsequent development of a new filling defect or distortion of the region of the anastomosis should be viewed with concern and be considered an indication for gastroscopy.

Another surgery-induced filling defect in the gastric remnant is a suture granuloma (Fig. 19-2). This lesion appears as a well-defined, rounded filling defect at the level of the surgical anastomosis. Although asymptomatic and merely an incidental finding, the radiographic appearance can mimic a gastric neoplasm and lead to unnecessary reoperation. Because suture granulomas occur only after gastric surgery with nonabsorbable suture material, the use of completely absorbable sutures should eliminate them as well as other complications related to nonabsorbable sutures, such as suture-line ulcers, abscesses, and adhesions.

Fig. 19-1. Surgical deformity (Hofmeister defect). **(A)** Large defect on the lesser curvature and posterior aspect of the gastric remnant **(arrow)** several weeks after surgery. **(B)** Smaller defect **(arrow)** 4 years later. (Fisher MS: The Hofmeister defect: A normal change in the postoperative stomach. AJR 84:1082–1086, 1960. Copyright 1960. Reproduced by permission)

BEZOAR

Bezoars in the gastric remnant are a not infrequent complication following partial gastric resection with Billroth-I or -II anastomoses.

A   B

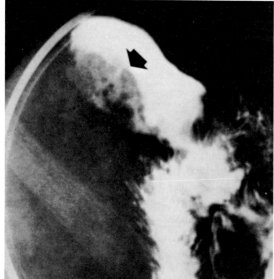
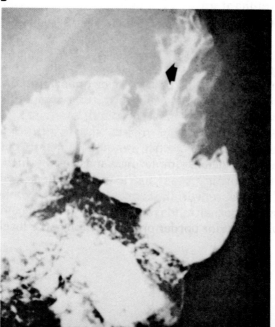

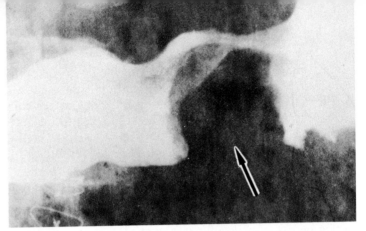

Fig. 19-2. Suture granuloma. A large mass at the greater curvature side of the antrum **(arrow)** projects as a smooth tumor into the gastric lumen. (Gueller HA, Shapiro HA, Nelson JA et al: Suture granulomas simulating tumors: A preventable postgastrectomy complication. Dig Dis 21:223–228, 1976)

The chief constituent of postgastrectomy bezoars is the fibrous, pithy component of fruits (especially citrus) and vegetables. These congeal to form masses that entrap varying amounts of stems, seeds, fruit skins, and fat globules. The resulting conglomerate mass of fiber becomes coated by gastric mucus secretions. Masses containing yeast organisms have also been reported in the gastric remnant, but these bezoars usually disappear without any therapy.

Both acid–pepsin secretion and the mixing and agitation of gastric contents are essential for the digestion of fibrous foods, especially oranges. After vagotomy, hydrochloric acid secretion is markedly reduced, if not eliminated. Resection of the pylorus and antral portion of the stomach results in loss of the normal gastric churning action. Inadequate chewing of food related to impaired dentition is also a contributing factor in the development of postgastrectomy bezoars. Stenosis of the anastomosis does not appear to predispose to bezoar formation in the gastric remnant, since, in most cases, the size of the stoma is adequate for the passage of food of up to 4 cm in diameter.

Bezoars in the gastric remnant vary in size, consistency, and number. They can be large enough to fill and distend the entire gastric remnant or small and easily overlooked. Their consistency varies from rubbery and firm to mushy and soft. Although most bezoars in the gastric remnant are single, several separate masses can be formed.

Many small bezoars in the gastric remnant are entirely asymptomatic. If there is substantial reduction in gastric volume due to encroachment upon the lumen or retardation of gastric emptying by obstruction of the stoma, a sensation of fullness, early satiety, nausea, vomiting, or epigastric or left upper quadrant pain can result. A ball–valve mechanism can cause intermittent symptoms. Although bezoars can erode the gastric mucosa, blood loss (either acute or chronic) is rarely encountered and, if present, should suggest another diagnosis.

A bezoar in the gastric remnant appears radiographically as a mottled filling defect simulating a mass of retained food particles (Fig. 19-3). It conforms to the gastric outline and tends to trap barium in spongelike fashion within its matrix. When the patient is in the upright position, the bezoar tends to float in the barium column like an iceberg, its convex superior border projecting above the level of the barium into

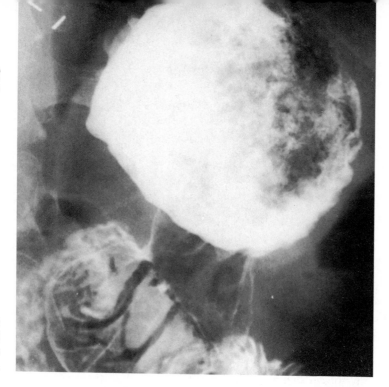

Fig. 19-3. Bezoar in the gastric remnant. A mottled filling defect simulates a mass of retained food particles.

the gastric air bubble. Bezoars are usually freely movable with change in the patient's position, unlike neoplasms, which are fixed to the gastric wall.

In addition to causing gastric outlet obstruction, a bezoar arising in the gastric remnant can pass into and obstruct the small bowel, usually in the relatively narrow terminal ileum.

To prevent the development of bezoars in the gastric remnant, postgastrectomy patients must be counseled with regard to both the foods they can safely eat and how to chew them properly. All fibrous foods, especially citrus fruits, should be avoided or else minced prior to ingestion. It has been suggested that about 90% of all bezoars in the gastric remnant could be prevented by the elimination of oranges from the diets of postgastrectomy patients.

GASTRIC STUMP CARCINOMA

Gastric stump carcinoma refers to a malignancy occurring in the gastric remnant after resection for peptic ulcer or other benign disease (Fig. 19-4). The development of recurrent symptoms after a long period of relatively good health following partial gastrectomy should suggest the possibility of gastric stump carcinoma. A neoplasm at the anastomotic site can ulcerate and clinically mimic a benign ulcer. However, simple stomal ulceration rarely occurs after many years of freedom from symptoms. For the possibility to be excluded that the carcinoma was undetected at the time of the original resection, most authors stipulate that at least 5 years must have elapsed since the initial gastric surgery.

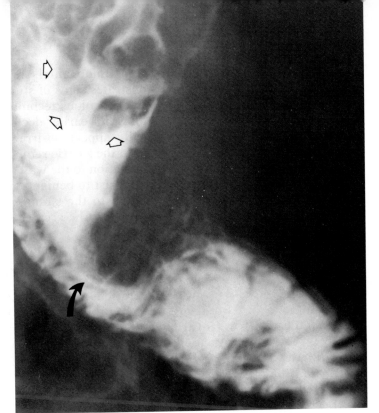

Fig. 19-4. Gastric stump carcinoma. A large, irregular polypoid mass is visible in the proximal portion of the gastric remnant **(open arrows).** The smooth filling defect at the anastomosis **(curved, solid arrow)** represents a benign leiomyoma.

Fig. 19-5. Gastric stump carcinoma. A large, irregular polypoid mass **(arrows)** arises near the anastomosis and fills much of the distal gastric remnant.

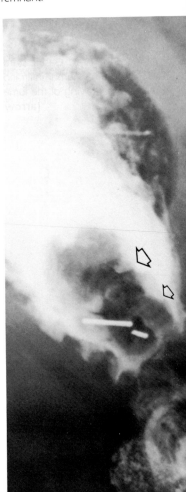

The incidence of carcinoma in the gastric remnant is 2 to 6 times higher than in the intact stomach. This complication is especially high in Europe, where gastric stump carcinoma has been reported to occur in about 15% of patients within 10 years of initial surgery and in about 20% after 20 years. In view of these statistics, some authors advise that gastric resection for benign disease should be avoided whenever possible, especially in young patients. If partial resection of the stomach is performed, an annual endoscopic examination beginning 10 years after the intial surgery is recommended.

The increased incidence of carcinoma in the gastric remnant is probably related to the chronic reflux of bile and pancreatic juice into the gastric remnant after partial gastrectomy. When gastric mucosa is subjected to a constant flow of bile and pancreatic juice, chronic and atrophic gastritis, intestinal metaplasia, adenomatous transformation of gastric mucosa, and submucosal ectopic glandular hyperplasia can occur. These changes may be seen singly or in combination and can vary in degree. The predilection for malignant transformation to occur in the perianastomotic region may well reflect these probably premalignant dysplastic changes in the gastric mucosa.

RADIOGRAPHIC FINDINGS

The rate of detection of gastric stump carcinoma by means of barium swallow has been poor. In most series, a majority of carcinomas have

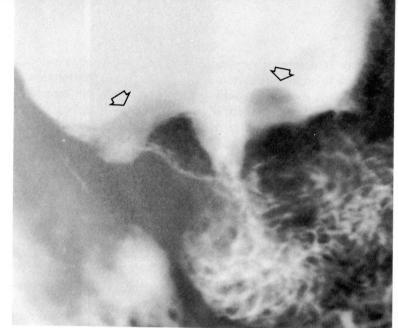

Fig. 19-8. Recurrent adenocarcinoma of the stomach. There is symmetric narrowing of the stoma with nodular masses **(arrows)** on the gastric side of the anastomosis.

Fig. 19-9. Bile reflux gastritis. There is thickening of rugal folds in the gastric remnant.

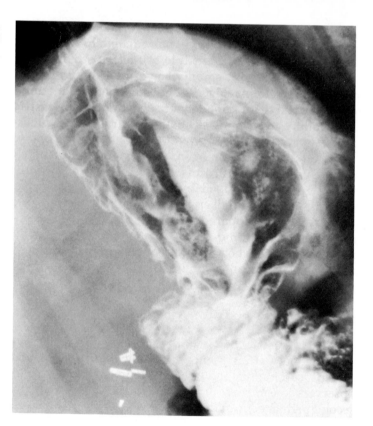

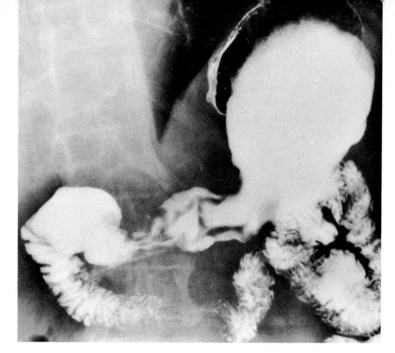

Fig. 19-10. Bile reflux gastritis. The patient had undergone gastroenterostomy for previous peptic disease. Because the patient could produce no gastric acid even on stimulation tests, the thickened antral folds and ulceration were attributed to bile reflux gastritis.

HYPERPLASTIC POLYPS / BILE (ALKALINE) REFLUX GASTRITIS

Hyperplastic polyps in the gastric remnant probably represent a reactive response to reflux of bile and pancreatic juices from the jejunum into the stomach. These highly alkaline digestive secretions are normally prevented from entering the stomach by an intact pylorus. When the pyloric mechanism is destroyed or circumvented by partial gastric resection, free reflux can produce severe gastritis and ulceration. Damage to the stomach mucosa is often multifocal or diffuse, resulting in the development of hyperplastic gastric polyps in multiple areas.

Fig. 19-11. Marginal (stomal) ulceration. The large ulcer **(arrow)** has arisen on the jejunal side of the anastomosis.

Bile reflux gastritis appears radiographically as thickened folds in the gastric remnant (Fig. 19-9). The most servere changes tend to occur near the anastomosis. Extensive swelling of gastric rugae can produce a discrete mass effect. Ulcerations due to bile reflux gastritis occur on the gastric side of the remnant (Fig. 19-10). True stomal ulceration due to the residual action of acid and pepsin on the sensitive intestinal mucosa occurs on the jejunal side of the anastomosis (Fig. 19-11).

Typical symptoms of alkaline reflux gastritis include postprandial pain, bilious vomiting, and weight loss. Gastric analysis demonstrates achlorhydria. If the symptoms of alkaline reflux gastritis cannot be managed effectively by conservative measures (diet, antispasmodics, cholestyramine), a surgical procedure is needed to divert bile and other duodenal contents from the gastric remnant.

Discrete polypoid lesions developing in the gastric remnant within a few years of surgery are more likely to be hyperplastic polyps than

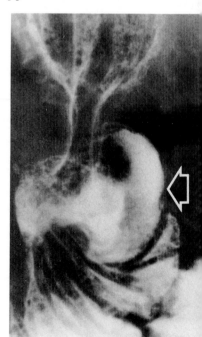

carcinoma. Nevertheless, endoscopy and biopsy are essential for confirmation of the diagnosis. Most postgastrectomy hyperplastic polyps produce few, if any, symptoms. Progressive increase in the size and number of these polyps, however, can lead to the formation of large conglomerate masses in the gastric remnant immediately proximal to the stoma. Surgical or endoscopic removal of these polyps may be required if they produce symptoms of intermittent gastric outlet obstruction, epigastric pain, vomiting, or gastrointestinal hemorrhage.

JEJUNOGASTRIC INTUSSUSCEPTION

Jejunogastric intussusception is a rare but potentially lethal complication of partial gastrectomy with Billroth-II anastomosis. In this condition, a portion of the full thickness of the jejunum invaginates back into the stomach. The efferent loop alone accounts for about 75% of jejunogastric intussusceptions; the afferent loop alone or in combination with the efferent loop constitutes the remaining cases.

The precise etiology of jejunogastric intussusception is unclear. Widely patent gastroenteric anastomoses may favor jejunogastric intussusception by permitting the loose mucosa at the anastomotic site to prolapse into the gastric pouch during normal peristalsis. Hyperperistalsis in the small bowel after gastric surgery, as well as excessive mobility of the jejunum (especially with antecolic anastomoses), are also contributing factors.

Jejunal intussusception can be either acute or chronic recurrent. Acute but delayed jejunogastric intussusception can occur months or years after gastric surgery. The patient with this condition presents as an acute surgical emergency, with sudden, severe colicky abdominal pain, intractable vomiting, and hematemesis. These symptoms reflect incarceration of the intussusceptum, and mortality rises sharply with delay in surgical decompression of the upper intestinal obstruction.

Chronic jejunogastric intussusception often produces only vague symptoms of recurrent abdominal pain relieved by vomiting. Because chronic recurrent intussusception is intermittent, gastroscopy or laparotomy may fail to demonstrate the lesion.

Retrograde jejunogastric intussusception appears radiographically as a clearly defined spherical or ovoid intraluminal filling defect in the gastric remnant (Fig. 19-12). Contrast material may be seen outlining the jejunal folds and surrounding the intussusceptum. These folds are stretched or enlarged, because of pressure edema, and appear as thin, curvilinear, concentric parallel stripes or striations (coiled-spring appearance).

Recent reports have demonstrated that some jejunogastric intussusceptions can be reduced at fluoroscopy because of the favorable direction of the pressure exerted by the barium. Glucagon-induced hypotonia can also promote reduction of the intussucception.

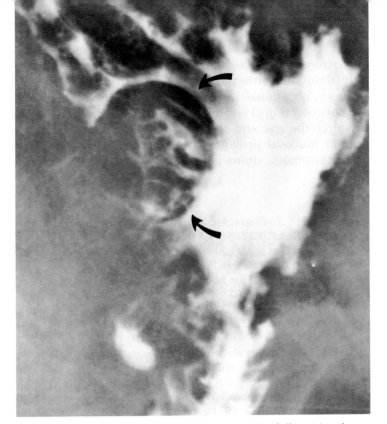

Fig. 19-12. Retrograde jejunogastric intussusception (afferent loop) producing a large, sharply defined filling defect **(arrows)**.

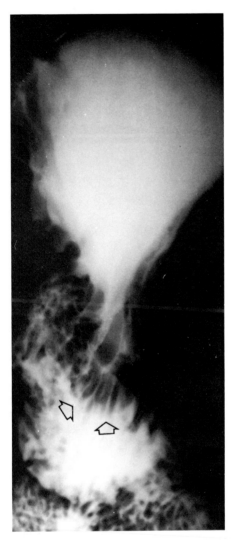

Fig. 19-13. Gastrojejunal mucosal prolapse. There is a sharply marginated, smooth mass in the efferent loop **(arrows)**.

Fig. 19-14. Antegrade gastrojejunal mucosal prolapse producing a large, partially obstructing mass in the efferent loop **(arrows)**.

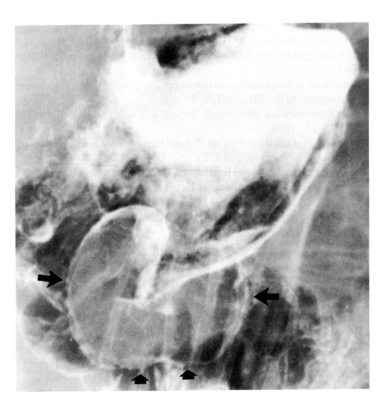

Fig. 20-1. Gastric outlet obstruction caused by peptic ulcer disease.

Fig. 20-2. Gastric outlet obstruction due to a giant duodenal ulcer. **(A)** The mottled density of nonopaque material represents excessive overnight gastric residual. **(B)** A delayed film shows the giant duodenal ulcer **(arrow).** (Eisenberg RL, Margulis AR, Moss AA: Giant duodenal ulcers. Gastrointest Radiol 2:347–353, 1978)

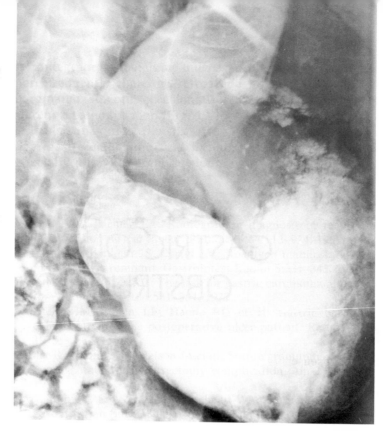

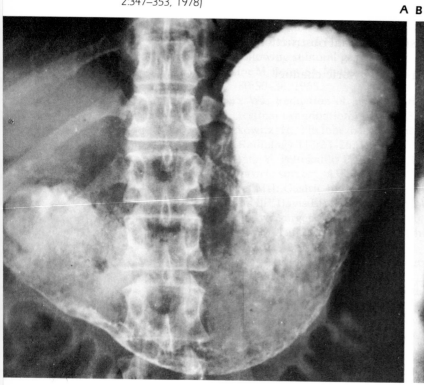
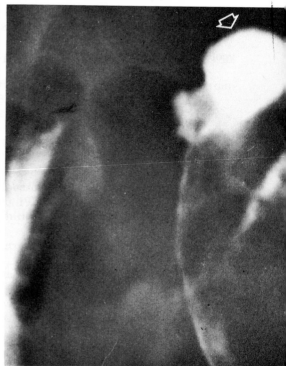

A B

PEPTIC ULCER DISEASE

In adults, peptic ulcer disease is by far the most common cause of gastric outlet obstruction (about 60%–65% of cases) (Fig. 20-1). The obstructing lesion in peptic ulcer disease is usually in the duodenum, occasionally in the pyloric channel or prepyloric gastric antrum, and rarely in the body of the stomach. Narrowing of the lumen due to peptic ulcer disease can result from spasm, acute inflammation and edema, muscular hypertrophy, or contraction of scar tissue. In most patients, several of these factors combine to produce gastric outlet obstruction.

Most patients with peptic disease causing pyloric obstruction have a long history of ulcer symptoms. Indeed, gastric outlet obstruction as the initial manifestation of peptic ulcer disease is very unusual and should raise the suspicion of gastric malignancy. Vomiting is a characteristic clinical symptom. Although the constant presence of large amounts of bile in the retained secretions suggests that the descending duodenum is included in the obstructed segment, bile-stained gastric aspirate is not inconsistent with pyloric stenosis. Vomiting secondary to obstruction is usually delayed for several hours after meals, unlike that which occurs rapidly in response to an irritant in the stomach. In patients with peptic disease who develop gastric outlet obstruction, ulcer pain tends to be constant, and vomiting becomes a major means of pain relief.

RADIOGRAPHIC FINDINGS

Plain abdominal radiographs often demonstrate the shadowy outline of a distended stomach in patients with gastric outlet obstruction. On upright films, there is frequently a fuzzy air–fluid level distinct from the sharp, even air–fluid levels seen elsewhere in the bowel. On barium examination, a mottled density of nonopaque material represents excessive overnight gastric residual (Fig. 20-2A). There is a marked delay in gastric emptying, with barium often retained in the stomach for 24 hr or longer. The stomach may become huge and, with the patient in the upright position, hang down into the lower abdomen or pelvis. The critical differential diagnosis is between a benign (primarily peptic ulcer disease) and malignant cause of gastric outlet obstruction. The presence of a persistent fleck of barium in a narrowed pyloric channel suggests peptic disease. However, a discrete filling defect suggests malignancy, as does nodularity or irregularity of the mucosa proximal to the constricted area. It is essential that every effort be made to express barium into the duodenal bulb. The finding of distortion and scarring of the bulb with formation of pseudodiverticula makes peptic ulcer disease the most likely etiology (Fig. 20-2B). Conversely, a radiographically normal duodenal bulb increases the likelihood of underlying malignant disease. In many patients, unfortunately, it is impossible to differentiate confidently on barium studies between a benign and a malignant cause of gastric outlet obstruction. In these cases, endoscopy or surgical exploration is required to exclude the possibility of a malignant lesion.

An annular constricting lesion near the pylorus (Fig. 20-3), representing carcinoma of the antrum, is the second leading cause of gastric outlet obstruction (about 30–35% of cases). Other infiltrative primary malignant tumors or metastatic lesions obliterating the lumen of the distal stomach and proximal duodenum can also produce the radiographic pattern of gastric outlet obstruction.

Unlike patients with gastric outlet obstruction caused by peptic disease, who typically have a long history of ulcer pain, about one-third of patients with obstruction due to malignancy have no pain. A large majority have a history of pain of less than 1 year's duration. Vomiting and weight loss are prominent clinical symptoms.

Primary scirrhous carcinoma of the pyloric channel is a cause of gastric outlet obstruction that can be indistinguishable radiographically from benign stricture. The tumor originates in the pyloric channel and grows circumferentially. It has a definite tendency for submucosal, muscular, and serosal invasion with preservation of the mucosal lining. Although the pyloric lesion associated with this tumor appears radiographically to be relatively benign, early development of metastases is the rule. Distal antral involvement can be seen in advanced cases, but the duodenum is usually spared.

The cellular neoplastic and nonspecific inflammatory infiltrate, as well as a secondary desmoplastic reaction, contributes to the formation of a short, concentric stricture without peristalsis. The pylorus is elongated, symmetrically smooth, and rigid, often with gradual tapering of the proximal margin. The major differential point between pyloric narrowing due to primary scirrhous carcinoma and that due to a healed ulcer is the frequent presence of acute ulceration (gastric, antral, pyloric, duodenal) and duodenal deformity in patients with peptic disease.

Fig. 20-3. Gastric outlet obstruction caused by annular constricting carcinoma of the stomach **(arrow)**.

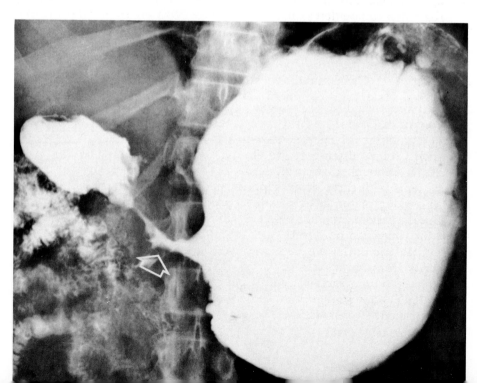

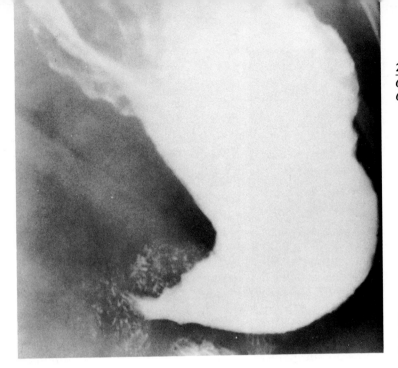

Fig. 20-4. Gastric outlet obstruction caused by Crohn's disease involving the stomach.

BENIGN TUMORS

PROLAPSED ANTRAL POLYP

Rarely, prolapse of a benign antral polyp into the duodenum produces intermittent gastric outlet obstruction. As the gastric polyp is propelled by peristalsis through the pylorus into the duodenum, it pulls a segment of stomach with it. Radiographically, the prolapsed polyp appears as an intraluminal filling defect in the duodenal bulb (see Fig. 30-32). Shortening of the gastric antrum with convergence of distal gastric folds can sometimes be identified. At fluoroscopy, the defect caused by the polyp can be demonstrated to change position, sometimes being in the pyloric antrum and then prolapsing into the duodenal bulb.

INFLAMMATORY DISORDERS

Inflammatory disease involving the distal stomach and proximal duodenum can cause infiltration or spasm resulting in clinical and radiographic signs of gastric outlet obstruction. Up to two-thirds of patients with Crohn's disease of the stomach develop this complication (Fig. 20-4). Although rare, granulomatous involvement of the stomach in patients with sarcoidosis, syphilis, or tuberculosis can cause sufficient thickening of the gastric wall to produce an obstructive appearance. Severe pancreatitis and cholecystitis can incite inflammatory spasm, which leads to obliteration of the lumen of the proximal duodenum and gastric outlet obstruction (Fig. 20-5). Stricture of the antrum can result from fibrous healing after the ingestion of corrosive substances (Fig. 20-6). On rare occasions, deposition of amyloid in the stomach wall can be so pronounced as to produce severe luminal narrowing and gastric outlet obstruction.

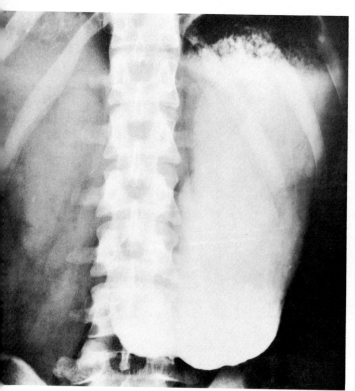

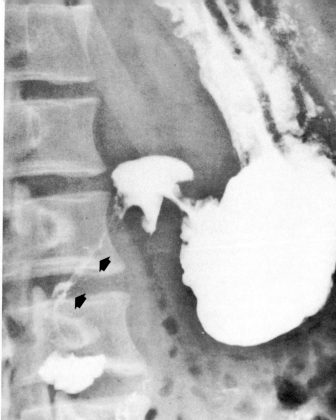

Fig. 20-5. Acute pancreatitis. **(A)** Complete gastric outlet obstruction. **(B)** As the acute inflammatory process subsides, some barium is seen to pass through the severely spastic and narrowed second portion of the duodenum **(arrows)**.

Fig. 20-6. Gastric outlet obstruction. The obstruction was caused by a caustic stricture that developed within 1 month of the ingestion of hydrochloric acid.

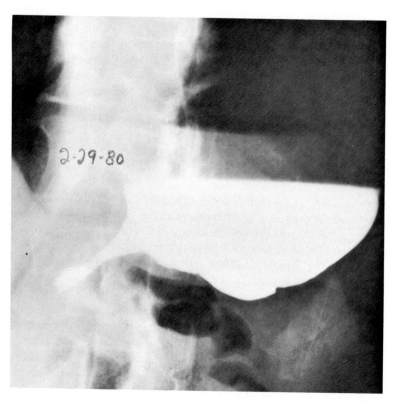

ANTRAL MUCOSAL DIAPHRAGM

Antral mucosal diaphragms are thin membranous septa that are usually situated within 3 cm of the pyloric canal and run perpendicular to the long axis of the stomach. They can be seen in infants and children and are probably congenital anomalies resulting from failure of the embryonic foregut to recanalize. Because a large percentage of proved cases have been in patients with peptic ulcer disease, it has been suggested that an antral mucosal diaphragm may result from healing of a circumferential gastric ulcer. However, this inflammatory origin is doubtful, since the diaphragm histologically is composed of a layer of mucosa on each side of a common submucosa and muscularis, with no evidence of inflammation or fibrosis.

Clinical symptoms of partial gastric outlet obstruction (upper epigastric pain, fullness, and vomiting, particularly after a heavy meal) correlate with the size of the central aperture of the antral mucosal diaphragm. Symptoms of obstruction do not occur if the diameter of the diaphragm is more than 1 cm. Even with minute central orifices as small as 2 mm, no obstructive symptoms may be produced until adult life. Infrequently, infants with mucosal diaphragms present with projectile vomiting in the neonatal period. In severe obstruction, gastric emptying is greatly delayed, and barium can be seen to pass in a thin stream (jet effect) from the center of the obstruction.

The nonobstructing antral mucosal diaphragm appears radiographically as a persistent, sharply defined, 2-cm- to 3-cm-wide bandlike defect in the barium column that arises at right angles to the gastric wall (Fig. 20-7). Although this appearance can be simulated by a prominent transverse mucosal fold that is often found in the antrum, this fold does not extend across the gastric lumen, nor is it generally perfectly straight. The antral mucosal diaphragm is best seen when the stomach proximal and distal to it are distended. The portion of the antrum proximal to the pylorus and distal to the mucosal diaphragm can mimic a second duodenal bulb (Fig. 20-8). The distal antrum can sometimes even be confused with a gastric diverticulum or ulcer, though, on close inspection, it clearly lies within the line of the stomach and changes size and shape during the examination.

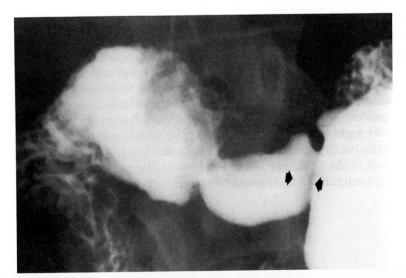

Fig. 20-7. Antral mucosal diaphragm. The bandlike defect **(arrows)** arises at right angles to the gastric wall.

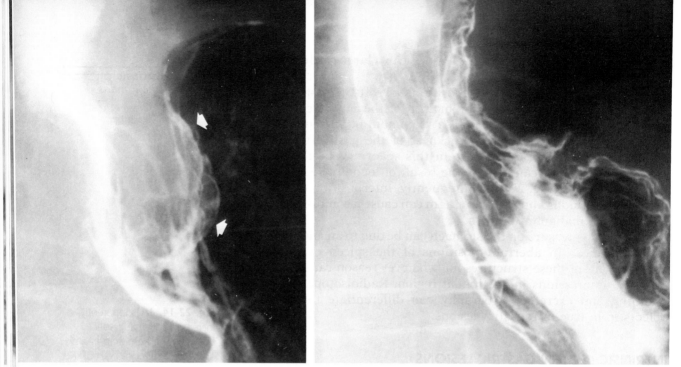

A B

Fig. 22-15. **(A)** Fundal pseudotumor **(arrows)** caused by a reduced hiatal hernia. **(B)** The pseudotumor disappears when the hiatal hernia is fully distended and situated above the diaphragm.

Fig. 22-16. Gastric varix. A single fundal mass **(arrows)** in the region of the esophagogastric junction simulates a neoplastic process.

Fig. 22-17. Gastric varices. Irregular filling defects in the fundus **(black arrows)** are associated with serpiginous varices in the esophagus **(white arrow).**

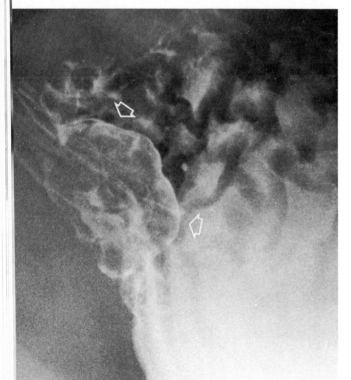

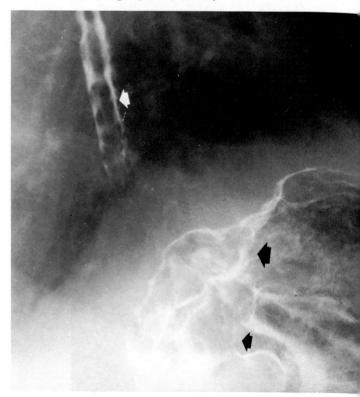

portion often leads to gastric bleeding. Redundancy of soft tissue associated with a reduced hiatal hernia can produce a discrete mass in the fundus (Fig. 22-15A). In some patients, a notchlike defect is seen. This form of fundal pseudotumor disappears when the hiatal hernia is fully distended and is located above the diaphragm (Fig. 22-15B).

Gastric varices can be difficult to distinguish from a primary fundal tumor (Fig. 22-16), especially without esophageal varices, splenomegaly, or a history of cirrhosis. The thick, tortuous mucosal folds or lobulated polypoid mass caused by varices frequently demonstrate alteration in size and shape when the patient changes position and phase of respiration (Fig. 22-17).

Thickened gastric rugae in the fundus may be caused by a true pathologic process or may merely be due to poor distention. When prominent fundal folds reflect a clinically significant entity, there are usually similar changes elsewhere in the stomach that offer a clue to the diagnosis. If thickened mucosal folds are localized to the fundus and cannot be effaced by overdistention of the stomach, gastroscopy is required to exclude the possibility of malignancy.

Postoperative distortion of normal anatomic relationships can cause extrinsic masses in the fundus. A typical example is the pseudotumor secondary to a Nissen fundoplication. This method of hiatal hernia repair involves wrapping the gastric fundus around the lower esophagus to create an intra-abdominal esophageal segment with a natural valve mechanism at the esophagogastric junction. The surgical procedure characteristically results in a prominent filling defect at the esophagogastric junction (Fig. 22-18) that is generally smoothly marginated and symmetric on both sides of the distal esophagus. An irregular outline may be present if part of the stomach is incompletely filled with barium or air. The distal esophagus appears to pass through the center of the concave mass (pseudotumor), which impresses the superomedial aspect of the fundus. If an adequate clinical history has not been obtained, the pseudotumor may be confused with a neoplasm in this area. Demonstration of a preserved esophageal lumen and mucosal pattern, as well as good delineation of the gastroesophageal junction, should permit exclusion of the possibility of a neoplastic process.

A left subphrenic abscess can displace the fundus of the stomach caudad, abnormally widening the distance between it and the diaphragm (Fig. 22-19). Concomitant findings of splinting of the left hemidiaphragm, irritative phenomena at the base of the left lung, or the presence of gas within the abscess can clarify the diagnosis. This pattern can be simulated by a large infrapulmonary effusion that appears to widen the distance between the left hemidiaphragm and fundus in the absence of a true abdominal process. Abscesses can also extrinsically impress the fundus without widening the space between it and the left hemidiaphragm (Fig. 22-20).

Fig. 22-18. Fundal mass caused by Nissen fundoplasty **(arrows).** The distal esophagus appears to pass through the center of the concave mass.

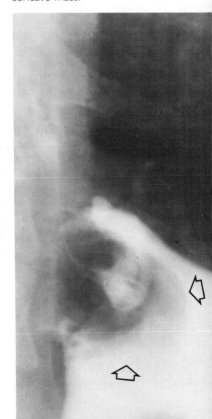

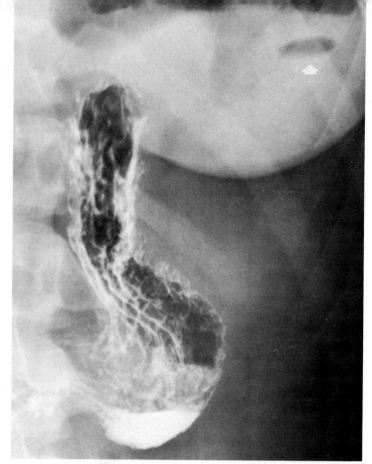

Fig. 22-19. Left subphrenic abscess. The mass narrows the fundus and displaces it from the hemidiaphragm. Note the collection of gas **(arrow)** in the abscess.

Fig. 22-20. Post-traumatic abscess extrinsically impressing the fundus **(arrows)** without widening the space between the fundus and the left hemidiaphragm. The patient sustained a gunshot wound in which the bullet penetrated the pancreas and left kidney.

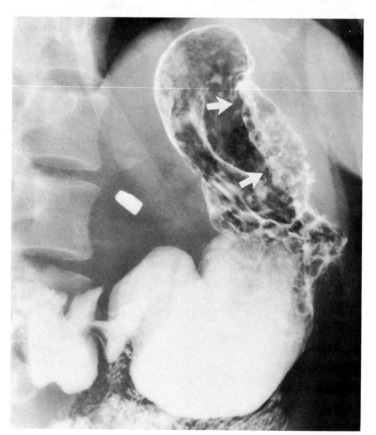

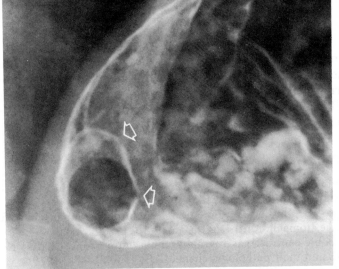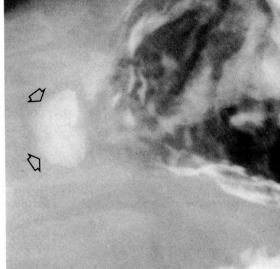

A B

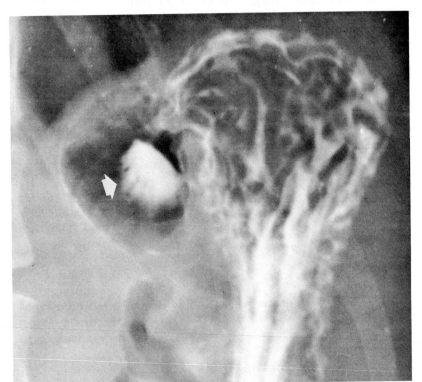

Fig. 22-21. (A) Gas-filled gastric diverticulum mimicking a discrete fundal mass **(arrows)**. (B) On repeat examination, barium within the diverticulum **(arrows)** is clearly separated from the fundus, revealing the true nature of the process.

Fig. 22-22. Gastric diverticulum. Pooling of barium **(arrow)** simulates an acute ulceration.

An apparent filling defect in the posterior portion of the fundus can be due to a large gastric diverticulum that fails to fill with gas or barium and mimics a smooth-bordered, submucosal mass (Fig. 22-21A). On repeat examination, barium can usually be demonstrated to enter the diverticulum, thereby establishing the diagnosis (Fig. 22-21B). At times, a collection of barium may pool in a gastric diverticulum and mimic an acute ulceration (Fig. 22-22). Inflammatory or neoplastic enlargement

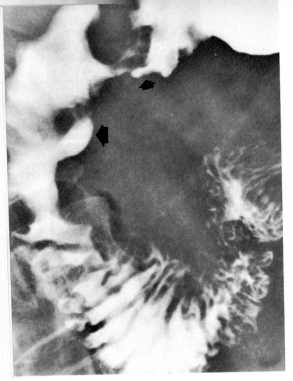

Fig. 27-3. Zollinger–Ellison syndrome. There is diffuse thickening of folds in the proximal duodenal sweep with bulbar and postbulbar ulceration **(arrows)**.

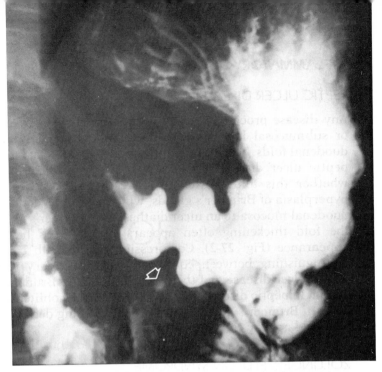

Fig. 27-4. Zollinger–Ellison syndrome. Note the ulcer **(arrow)** in the fourth portion of the duodenum. There is diffuse thickening of folds in the duodenal sweep.

PANCREATITIS / CHOLECYSTITIS

Acute pancreatitis is the other major cause of thickening of duodenal folds (Fig. 27-5). Severe inflammatory spasm secondary to pancreatitis can make the duodenal sweep so irritable that it does not completely fill with barium (Fig. 27-6). The radiographic appearance of edematous, thickened folds in the periampullary region and proximal second portion of the duodenum, especially if associated with elevation of serum amylase and a mass impression on the duodenum from the swollen head of the pancreas, should suggest the diagnosis of acute pancreatitis. Thickening of duodenal folds, often with narrowing of the lumen, can also be associated with other types of adjacent periduodenal inflammation, such as acute cholecystitis (Fig. 27-7).

UREMIA (CHRONIC DIALYSIS)

Gastrointestinal complaints such as nausea and vomiting are not infrequent long-term complications in uremic patients undergoing chronic dialysis. Prominence of the mucosal pattern can be seen with irregular, swollen, and stiffened folds in the duodenal bulb and second portion of the duodenum. Although an increase in the incidence of peptic ulceration has been reported in patients on chronic dialysis, the nodular thickening of duodenal folds is apparently not related to hyperacidity or peptic ulcer disease. Indeed, the thickening of duodenal

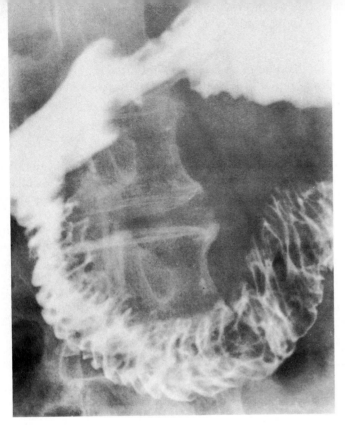

Fig. 27-5. Acute pancreatitis causing thickening of duodenal folds. Note the widening of the duodenal sweep, the double-contour effect, and sharp spiculations.

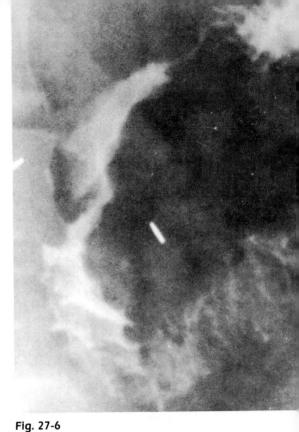

Fig. 27-6

Fig. 27-7

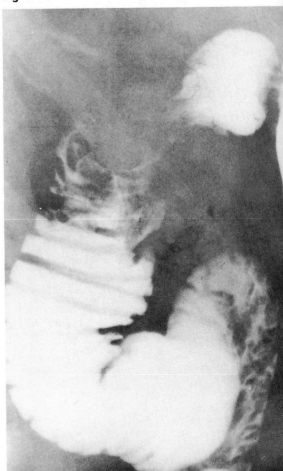

Fig. 27-6. Acute hemorrhagic pancreatitis following pancreatic biopsy. There is diffuse thickening of duodenal folds, although the severe inflammatory spasm makes the duodenal sweep so irritable that it does not completely fill with barium.

Fig. 27-7. Acute cholecystitis. An adjacent inflammatory process produces fold thickening, luminal narrowing, and a mass effect involving the proximal second portion of the duodenum.

folds in patients on chronic dialysis often simulates the appearance of pancreatitis, a disease that frequently complicates prolonged uremia and may be responsible for producing the radiographic pattern.

CROHN'S DISEASE / TUBERCULOSIS

Chronic inflammatory disorders can also cause thickening of duodenal folds. Crohn's disease can affect the duodenum and produce a spectrum of radiographic appearances, including mucosal thickening, ulceration, and stenosis (Fig. 27-8). Although duodenal involvement is occasionally an isolated process in Crohn's disease, concomitant disease in the terminal ileum can usually be detected. Tuberculosis of the duodenum, although rare even in patients with pulmonary or gastrointestinal disease, can produce a pattern of nodular, hyperplastic fold thickening, diffuse ulceration, and luminal narrowing identical to that seen in Crohn's disease (Fig. 27-9). When tuberculosis involves the duodenum, associated antral and pyloric disease is almost always present.

OTHER INFLAMMATORY DISORDERS

Nodular thickening of duodenal folds can be seen with parasitic infestations such as giardiasis and strongyloidiasis (Fig. 27-10). In

Fig. 27-8. Crohn's disease of the duodenum. There is thickening of mucosal folds in a narrowed second portion of the duodenum.

Fig. 27-9. Tuberculosis of the duodenum. There is diffuse fold thickening, spasm, and ulceration of the proximal duodenum.

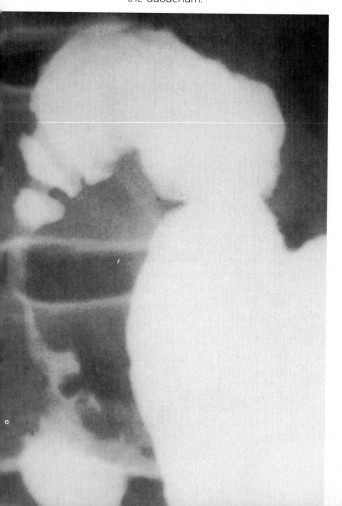

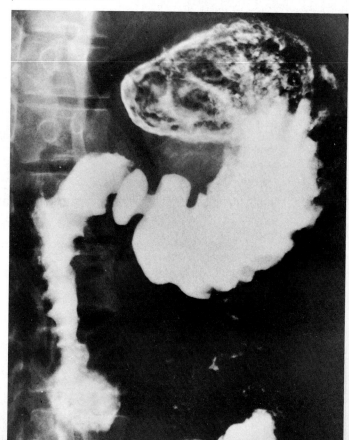

giardiasis, hyperperistalsis and increased secretions produce a blurred, thickened, edematous mucosal fold pattern involving the duodenum and jejunum. Strongyloides infestation of the duodenum causes diffuse thickening of folds, ulceration, and luminal stenosis that can closely simulate Crohn's disease. A bizarre pattern of nodular fold thickening in the duodenum has also been described in early stages of nontropical sprue.

NEOPLASTIC DISORDERS

Lymphoma occasionally involves the duodenal bulb and sweep and produces a radiographic pattern of coarse, nodular, irregular folds (Fig. 27-11). Metastases to peripancreatic lymph nodes can result in localized impressions on the duodenum simulating thickened folds (Fig. 27-12). Fold thickening can also be secondary to impaired lymphatic drainage due to malignant replacement of normal lymph node architecture (Fig. 27-13).

INFILTRATIVE DISORDERS

Diffuse small bowel infiltrative diseases can also affect the duodenum, though duodenal involvement as an isolated finding has not been reported. In Whipple's disease, periodic acid-Schiff (PAS)-positive mac-

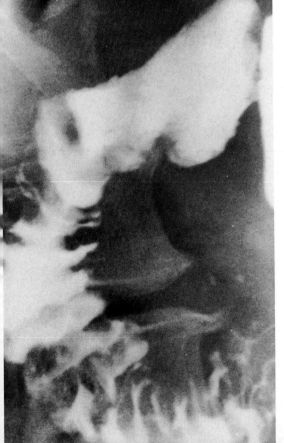

Fig. 27-10. Strongyloidiasis. Irregular, at times nodular, thickening of folds throughout the duodenal sweep.

Fig. 27-11. Lymphoma. There is localized luminal narrowing of the proximal second portion of the duodenum with a pattern of coarse, nodular, irregular folds.

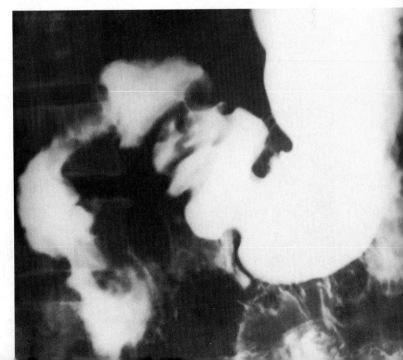

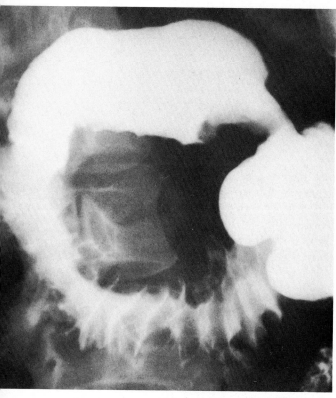

Fig. 27-12. Metastases to peripancreatic lymph nodes causing localized impressions on the duodenum. The impressions simulate thickened folds.

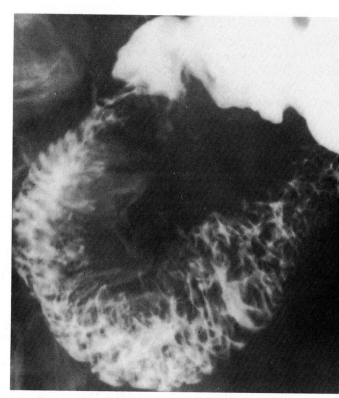

Fig. 27-13. Metastases to peripancreatic lymph nodes. Impaired lymphatic drainage, which is due to tumor replacement of normal lymph nodes, causes a pattern of diffuse fold thickening in the duodenal sweep.

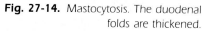

Fig. 27-14. Mastocytosis. The duodenal folds are thickened.

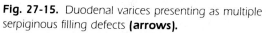

Fig. 27-15. Duodenal varices presenting as multiple serpiginous filling defects **(arrows).**

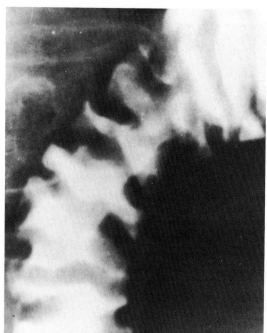

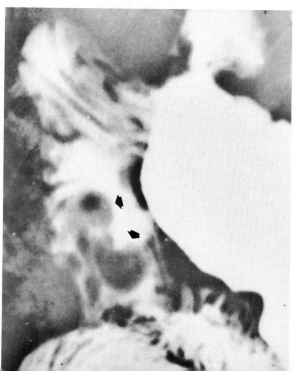

rophages can infiltrate the duodenal submucosa and produce diffuse thickening of folds. A similar pattern can be caused by infiltration of the duodenal wall in amyloidosis, mastocytosis (Fig. 27-14), and eosinophilic enteritis. The gross dilatation of lymphatics seen in patients with intestinal lymphangiectasia can also present the radiographic appearance of thickening of duodenal folds.

VASCULAR DISORDERS

DUODENAL VARICES

Duodenal varices are collateral vessels that can result from extrahepatic obstruction of the portal or splenic veins as well as from intrahepatic portal hypertension. Esophageal varices are almost always also present. Duodenal varices have four major radiographic appearances. First, collateral flow in a dilated superior pancreaticoduodenal vein can cause a vertical compression defect on the duodenal bulb about 1 cm distal to the pylorus. Second, small varices produce a diffuse polypoid mucosal pattern in the duodenum that can be difficult to distinguish from inflammatory fold thickening due to Brunner's gland hyperplasia. Third, larger, dilated submucosal veins can project into the lumen and cause serpiginous filling defects similar to the typical appearance of esophageal varices (Fig. 27-15). Finally, an isolated duodenal varix occasionally presents as a discrete filling defect on the medial aspect of the descending duodenum. In patients with known portal hypertension, unusual polypoid, mural, or extrinsic defects in the duodenum should suggest the possibility of duodenal varices.

MESENTERIC ARTERIAL COLLATERALS

Arteriosclerotic occlusive disease of the mesenteric vessels primarily involves the origins of the celiac axis and superior mesenteric artery. Occlusion of either of these arterial trunks causes enlargement and tortuosity of the collateral pathways between them. The initial loops of the pancreaticoduodenal arcade lie roughly parallel and in close proximity to the descending duodenum. The gastroduodenal artery also lies adjacent and parallel to the descending duodenum for a variable distance. When these arteries serve as enlarged collaterals, they can appear as serpiginous, nodular filling defects simulating thickened duodenal folds (Fig. 27-16). In addition, enlarged arterial collaterals can produce discrete filling defects on the medial aspect of the duodenum with widening of the sweep. Tortuous enlargement of an aberrant right hepatic artery arising from the superior mesenteric artery instead of from the celiac axis can cause a sharply marginated extrinsic defect on the superior aspect of the duodenal bulb.

INTRAMURAL HEMORRHAGE / DUODENAL CONGESTION

Hemorrhage into the duodenal wall can produce the radiographic pattern of mucosal fold thickening (stacked-coins appearance). Duodenal intramural hemorrhage can be caused by anticoagulant therapy or a bleeding diathesis or can be a complication of trauma to the upper abdomen. Chronic congestion of the duodenum secondary to portal hypertension (cirrhosis) or congestive heart failure can also give rise to peptic symptoms and thickening of duodenal mucosal folds.

CYSTIC FIBROSIS

A thickened, coarse fold pattern in the duodenum is commonly demonstrated in patients with cystic fibrosis of the pancreas (mucoviscidosis) (Fig. 27-17). Associated findings include nodular indentations along the duodenal wall, smudging or poor definition of the mucosal fold pattern, and redundancy, distortion, and kinking of the duodenal contour. These changes are usually confined to the first and second portions of the duodenum, though the thickened fold pattern occasionally extends into the proximal jejunum. The cause of duodenal fold thickening in cystic fibrosis is obscure. It is postulated that the lack of pancreatic bicarbonate in patients with cystic fibrosis results in inadequate buffering of normal amounts of gastric acid, causing mucosal irritation and muscular contractions that produce the thickened mucosal folds.

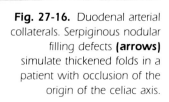

Fig. 27-16. Duodenal arterial collaterals. Serpiginous nodular filling defects **(arrows)** simulate thickened folds in a patient with occlusion of the origin of the celiac axis.

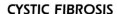

Fig. 27-17. Cystic fibrosis of the pancreas (mucoviscidosis). The duodenal folds have a thick, coarse pattern.

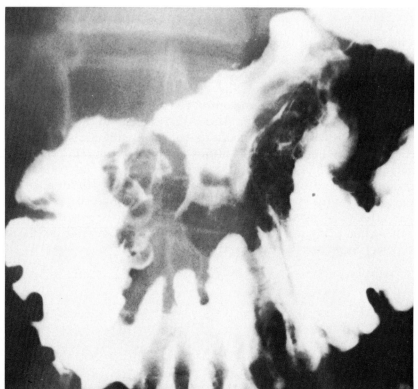

BIBLIOGRAPHY

Bateson EM: Duodenal and antral varices. Br J Radiol 42:744–747, 1969

Baum S, Stein GN, Baue A: Extrinsic pressure defects on the duodenal loop in mesenteric occlusive disease. Radiology 85:866–874, 1965

Dodds WJ, Spitzer RM, Friedland GW: Gastrointestinal roentgenographic manifestations of hemophilia. AJR 110:413–416, 1970

Eaton SB, Benedict KT, Ferrucci JT et al: Hypotonic duodenography. Radiol Clin North Am 8:125–137, 1970

Eaton SB, Ferrucci JT: Radiology of the Pancreas and Duodenum. Philadelphia, WB Saunders, 1973

Fleming RJ, Seaman WB: Roentgenographic demonstration of unusual extra-esophageal varices. AJR 103:281–290, 1968

Fraser GM, Pitman RG, Lawrie JH et al: The significance of the radiological finding of coarse mucosal folds in the duodenum. Lancet 2:979–982, 1964

Govoni AF: Benign lymphoid hyperplasia of the duodenal bulb. Gastrointest Radiol 1:267–269, 1976

Itzchak Y, Glickman MG: Duodenal varices in extrahepatic portal obstruction. Radiology 124:619–624, 1977

Legge DA, Carlson HC, Judd ES: Roentgenologic features of regional enteritis of the upper gastrointestinal tract. AJR 110:355–360, 1970

Perez CA, Dorfman RF: Benign lymphoid hyperplasia of the stomach and duodenum. Radiology 87:505–510, 1966

Schulman A: The cobblestone appearance of the duodenal cap, duodenitis and hyperplasia of Brunner's glands. Br J Radiol 43:787–795, 1970

Shimkin PM, Pearson KD: Unusual arterial impressions upon the duodenum. Radiology 103:295–297, 1972

Taussig LM, Saldino RM, di Sant'Agnese PA: Radiographic abnormalities of the duodenum and small bowel in cystic fibrosis of the pancreas (mucoviscidosis). Radiology 106:369–376, 1973

Wiener SN, Vertes V, Shapiro H: The upper gastrointestinal tract in patients undergoing chronic dialysis. Radiology 92:110–114, 1969

28

WIDENING OF THE DUODENAL SWEEP

Disease Entities

Normal variant
Pancreatic lesions
  Pancreatitis
  Pancreatic pseudocyst
  Pancreatic cancer
  Metastatic replacement of the pancreas
  Cystadenoma/cystadenocarcinoma
Lymph node enlargement
  Metastases
  Lymphoma
  Inflammation
Cystic lymphangioma of the mesentery
Mesenteric arterial collaterals
Retroperitoneal masses (tumors, cysts)
Aortic aneurysm
Choledochal cyst

Widening of the duodenal sweep is often considered evidence suggestive of malignancy or inflammation in the head of the pancreas. However, this finding frequently does not represent pancreatic pathology and thus must be interpreted with great caution. There is great variation in the configuration of the doudenal sweep among normal patients, and slight degrees of enlargement are difficult to recognize with confidence. In heavy patients, the combination of a high transverse stomach and long vertical course of the descending duodenum can create the illusion of a large sweep, which is actually within normal limits. In addition, widening of the sweep can be related to upward pressure on the

Fig. 28-1. Acute pancreatitis. Severe inflammation causes widening of the sweep and a high-grade duodenal obstruction. ▶

duodenal bulb or downward pressure on the third portion of the duodenum rather than to an impression by the head of the pancreas on the medial aspect of the second portion of the duodenum.

Enlargement of the duodenal sweep can reflect benign pancreatic disease (pancreatitis or pseudocyst) or pancreatic malignancy. Although there are numerous radiographic criteria for distinguishing between benign and malignant pancreatic disease, a precise diagnosis is often extremely difficult to make.

ACUTE PANCREATITIS

Most patients with acute pancreatitis have a history of alcohol abuse. Abdominal pain is almost universal; radiation of pain to the back occurs in about half of patients. Nausea, vomiting, and a feeling of prostration are common, as are fever and epigastric tenderness.

In acute pancreatitis, the gland may enlarge to 3 times its normal size. Involvement of the head of the pancreas may produce a smooth mass indenting the inner border of the duodenal sweep (Fig. 28-1). Duodenal paresis and edema of duodenal folds is common, as is edema of the papilla of Vater (Fig. 28-2). Gastric atony and dilatation, as well as edema of folds in the proximal jejunum, can be seen. Swelling of the pancreas can also cause an extrinsic impression on the posterior surface or greater curvature of the stomach.

RADIOGRAPHIC FINDINGS

Abnormalities on chest or plain abdominal radiographs can suggest the diagnosis of acute pancreatitis. Hemidiaphragmatic elevation, plate-like subsegmental atelectasis, consolidation (pneumonia or segmental

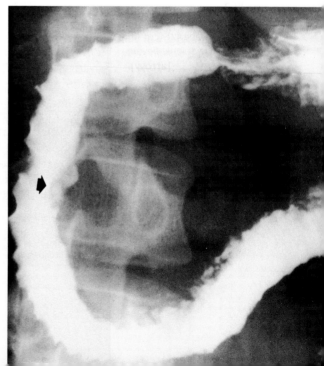

Fig. 28-2. Hemorrhagic pancreatitis with severe inflammatory changes involving the duodenal sweep (thickened folds and mucosal ulcerations) and probably edematous enlargement of the papilla of Vater **(arrow)**.

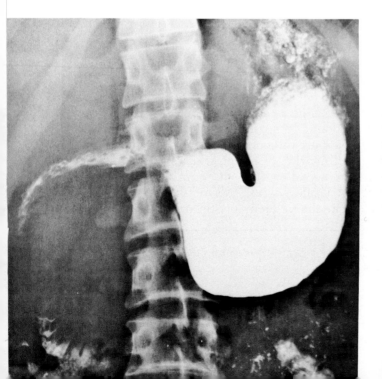

and spiculation of the mucosa (Fig. 28-5), as well as enlargement of the papilla, can be seen, though identical findings can be demonstrated in patients with pancreatic carcinoma and impacted ampullary gallstones, respectively. Unusual appearances in chronic pancreatitis include thumbprintlike indentations on the duodenal bulb and nodular, bulbar filling defects with central ulceration.

PANCREATIC PSEUDOCYST

Pancreatic pseudocysts are encapsulated collections of fluid with a high concentration of pancreatic enzymes. They are so named because they do not possess the epithelial lining that is characteristic of true cysts. A pseudocyst can develop following a severe episode of acute pancreatitis (especially if secondary to alcohol abuse) in which pancreatic juices exuding from the surface of the gland or from ductal disruption are walled off by adjacent serosal, mesenteric, and peritoneal surfaces. Because of the high protein content, osmotic pressure draws fluid into the pseudocyst and increases its size. If the fluid within the cyst is not resorbed, the inflamed membranes become a thickened and fibrotic cyst wall. The true incidence of pseudocysts complicating pancreatitis is not known. With the advent of ultrasound, pseudocysts can now be demonstrated in more than half of patients with pancreatitis.

Pseudocysts can develop after injury to the pancreas. Although most commonly the result of blunt abdominal trauma, pseudocysts can also be secondary to iatrogenic damage from previous abdominal surgery. Up to 20% of pseudocysts arise in the absence of any known predisposing pancreatic disorder.

Fig. 28-5. Chronic pancreatitis. There is mucosal spiculation along the inner border of the descending duodenum. Note the mass impression on the duodenal sweep by the markedly enlarged head of the pancreas.

Fig. 28-6. Pancreatic pseudocyst. There is huge enlargement of the duodenal sweep.

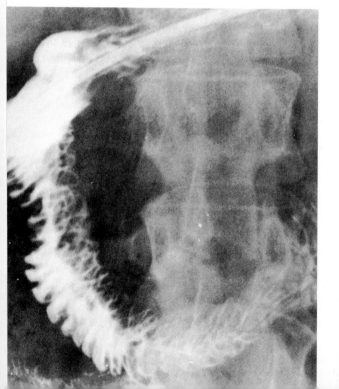

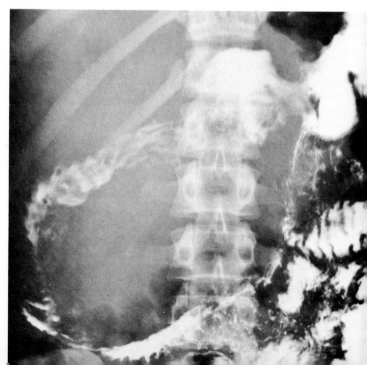

About 70% of pseudocysts arise from the body and tail of the pancreas. Those arising from the head of the gland cause widening and compression of the duodenal sweep. Pancreatic pseudocysts can appear to migrate and have been demonstrated in the mediastinum, chest, and even the neck. The great majority, however, develop between the pancreas and the stomach, though they can become large enough to fill the entire abdomen.

Small pancreatic pseudocysts are often asymptomatic. Like patients with chronic pancreatitis, patients with large pseudocysts complain of abdominal pain frequently radiating to the back. An upper abdominal mass can sometimes be palpated. Although jaundice is uncommon, it can be caused by compression of the bile duct due to a pseudocyst in the head of the pancreas. Jaundice can also be due to underlying hepatocellular disease in the absence of any extrahepatic biliary obstruction.

RADIOGRAPHIC FINDINGS

Plain abdominal radiographs often demonstrate pancreatic calcification consistent with chronic alcoholic pancreatitis. Rarely, calcification occurs in the wall of the pseudocyst itself. On barium examination, pseudocysts tend to produce large mass impressions on the inner border of the second portion of the duodenum or on the inferior or posterior wall of the stomach (Fig. 28-6). These impressions are usually smooth, without any evidence of invasion (pad effect) (Fig. 28-7). At times, however, the adjacent stomach or duodenal wall appears irregular or ragged (Fig. 28-8), implying invasion of the pseudocyst into adjacent viscera due to enzymatic action, pressure necrosis, or intense inflammation. In these instances, it can be extremely difficult to differentiate radiographically between a pseudocyst and a pancreatic malignancy.

COMPLICATIONS

Infection, rupture, and hemorrhage can complicate pancreatic pseudocysts. Infection by organisms from the adjacent stomach and bowel produces a high fever, chills, and leukocytosis. Sudden perforation of a pseudocyst into the peritoneal cavity results in a severe chemical peritonitis with boardlike abdominal rigidity, intense pain, and an often fatal outcome. Hemorrhage from a pancreatic pseudocyst can be caused by enzymatic digestion of small vessels lining the cyst wall, erosion into nearby major vessels (*e.g.*, gastroduodenal, splenic), or perforation into an adjacent viscus. Like cyst rupture, hemorrhage from a pancreatic pseudocyst is associated with a high mortality rate.

CARCINOMA OF THE PANCREAS

In patients with a malignancy in the head of the pancreas, significant widening of the duodenal sweep generally indicates advanced disease. Because diffuse widening of the duodenal sweep is such a late sign of carcinoma of the pancreas, subtle changes in the duodenum produced by enlargement of the head of the pancreas must be carefully evaluated. These include flattening and indentation of the medial wall, formation of double contours, deformity and displacement of diverticula, and alteration of the height, width, and direction of mucosal folds on the medial aspect of the duodenum. The extent of radiographic abnormalities does not necessarily reflect the size of the pancreatic lesion. Small, strategically located tumors close to the duodenum or stomach produce radiographic abnormalities at a much earlier stage than large lesions arising at points relatively removed from these organs.

RADIOGRAPHIC FINDINGS

Fig. 28-7. Pancreatic pseudocyst. There is a pad effect (impression without invasion) on the inner aspect of the duodenal sweep.

Fig. 28-8. Pancreatic pseudocyst. The irregular, ragged appearance of the inner margin of the duodenal sweep reflects intense adjacent inflammation.

Masses in the head of the pancreas typically cause impressions on either the stomach or the duodenal sweep (Fig. 28-9). Indentation on the greater curvature of the antrum results in the "antral pad" sign (Fig. 28-10). More commonly, mass impressions on the inner aspect of the duodenum create a double-contour effect (Fig. 28-11). This appearance results from differential filling of the duodenum, with the interfold spaces along the inner aspect of the sweep containing less barium than the corresponding spaces along the outer aspect. Localized impressions on the sweep can cause nodular indentations. Malignant disease infiltrating the wall of the duodenum can produce an "inverted-3" (Frostberg) sign (Fig. 28-12), though this nonspecific sign, which is seen in

Fig. 28-7   **Fig. 28-8**

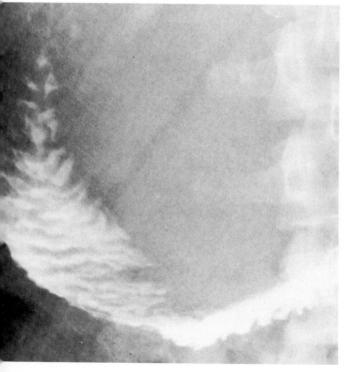

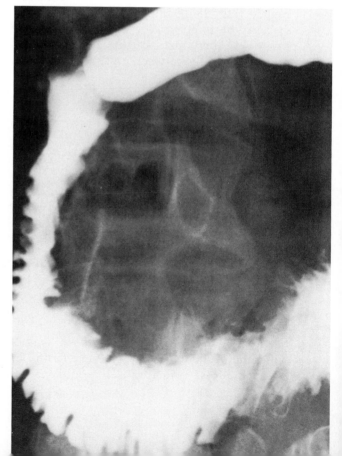

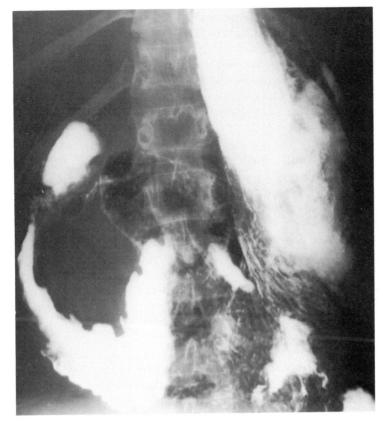

Fig. 28-9. Gastrin-secreting islet cell carcinoma of the pancreas causing widening of the duodenal sweep. Pronounced irregularity of the duodenal margin indicates neoplastic invasion.

Fig. 28-11. Double-contour effect along the medial aspect of the duodenal sweep caused by carcinoma of the pancreas.

Fig. 28-10. Antral pad sign **(arrow)** caused by adenocarcinoma of the pancreas.

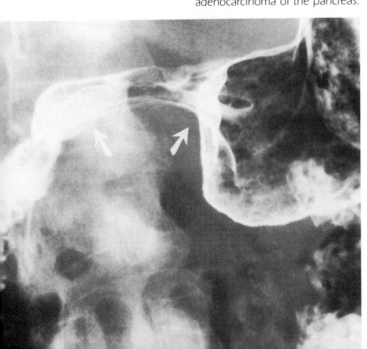

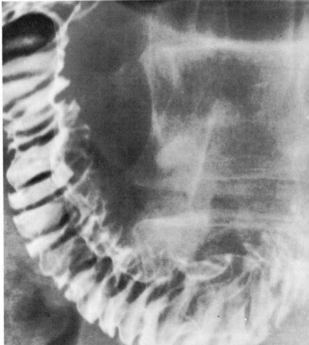

less than 10% of patients with pancreatic carcinoma, is probably more common in inflammatory disorders such as acute pancreatitis (Fig. 28-13) and postbulbar ulcer disease (Fig. 28-14). The central limb of the "3" represents the point of fixation of the duodenal wall where the pancreatic and common bile ducts insert into the papilla. The impressions above and below this point reflect either edema of the minor and major papillae or smooth muscle spasm and edema in the duodenal wall.

Distortion of a duodenal diverticulum is an infrequent but highly suggestive indication of an enlarging mass in the pancreas (Fig. 28-15). This finding is not pathognomonic but merely indicates an expanding process in the head of the pancreas or peripancreatic area. Flattening, indentation, or any other contour distortion of a duodenal diverticulum is more suggestive of malignancy than is mere displacement.

Fine or coarse sharpening and elongation of barium-filled crevices between duodenal plical folds (spiculation) is secondary to mucosal edema and neuromuscular irritation. This appearance can be seen in patients with pancreatitis (Fig. 28-16) or pancreatic carcinoma (Fig. 28-17). Displacement or frank splaying of the spikes suggests tumor infiltration of the wall causing traction and fixation of folds.

Irregular nodularity along the medial aspect of the second portion of the duodenum is more suggestive of malignancy than inflammation. This finding is of importance primarily in the duodenum distal to the papilla, since postbulbar peptic disease can also produce nodular filling defects in the proximal duodenum.

Fig. 28-12. Frostberg's inverted-3 sign **(arrow)** in a patient with carcinoma of the head of the pancreas.

Fig. 28-13. Frostberg's inverted-3 sign **(arrow)** in a patient with acute pancreatitis and no evidence of malignancy.

Fig. 28-12   **Fig. 28-13**

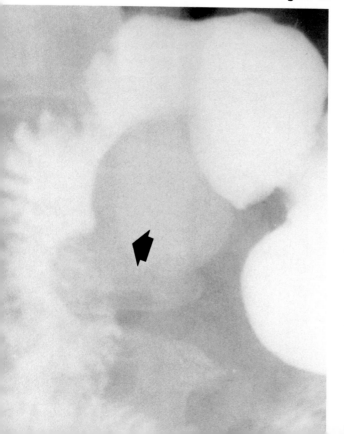

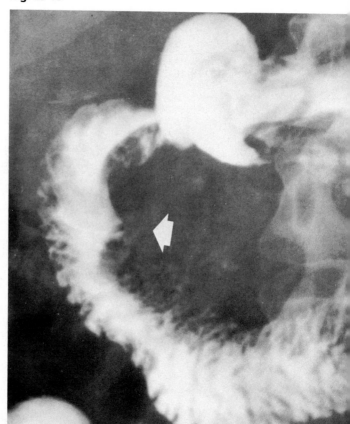

Although mucosal flattening with fold effacement and a slight reduction in luminal caliber can be seen in patients with pancreatic carcinoma, this appearance is more consistent with chronic pancreatitis. Severe tumor involvement can cause ulceration and frank duodenal obstruction.

METASTATIC LESIONS

Widening of the duodenal sweep can be caused by metastatic replacement of the head of the pancreas. Secondary malignant involvement of the pancreas is usually due to direct extension of a cancer arising in an adjacent organ (stomach, colon, kidney). True hematogenous metastases to the pancreas are rare.

CYSTADENOMA / CYSTADENOCARCINOMA

Although most cystadenomas and cystadenocarcinomas occur in the body or tail of the pancreas, tumors arising in the head of the pancreas can widen the duodenal sweep. These uncommon lesions have certain clinical features that can permit their differentiation from solid neoplasms. They occur in younger persons than pancreatic carcinoma and have a heavy predominance in women. Symptoms are infrequent; the presenting complaint is usually a poorly defined upper abdominal mass that is not tender. The incidence of concomitant metabolic and endocrine

Fig. 28-14. Frostberg's inverted-3 sign in a patient with a large postbulbar ulcer **(arrow)** and no evidence of malignancy.

Fig. 28-15. Distorted duodenal diverticulum **(arrow)** in a patient with carcinoma of the pancreas. Note the double contour (mass effect) and spiculations.

Fig. 28-14

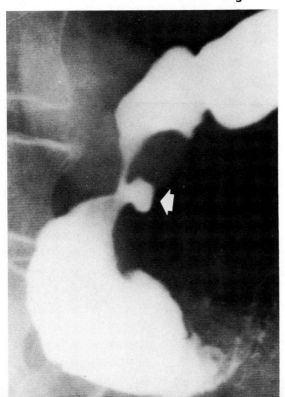

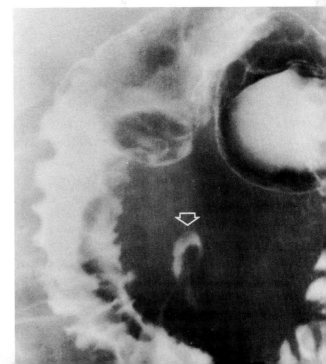

abnormalities (diabetes, obesity, sterility, infertility, thyroid dysfunction, hypertension) is high. Cystadenocarcinomas of the pancreas have a much better prognosis than solid adenocarcinomas. Many of the tumors are surgically resectable, and complete excision is associated with a high cure rate.

LYMPH NODE ENLARGEMENT

Enlargement of lymph nodes near the head of the pancreas can widen the duodenal sweep. The subpyloric lymph nodes lie below the flexure that forms the junction between the first and second portions of the duodenum. The pancreaticoduodenal nodes lie medial to the head of the pancreas in the groove between it and the duodenum. Any enlargement of these peripancreatic lymph nodes (due to lymphoma, metastases to lymph nodes, or inflammatory disease) can produce the radiographic pattern of widening of the duodenal sweep (Fig. 28-18).

OTHER CAUSES

Cystic lymphangiomas of the mesentery can also widen the duodenal sweep (Fig. 28-19). These benign, unilocular or multilocular cystic structures contain serous or chylous fluid. They can be the result of

Fig. 28-16. Spiculation of duodenal folds in acute pancreatitis **(arrow).**

Fig. 28-17. Spiculation of duodenal folds in carcinoma of the pancreas **(arrows).** Note the mass effect on the medial wall of the descending duodenum.

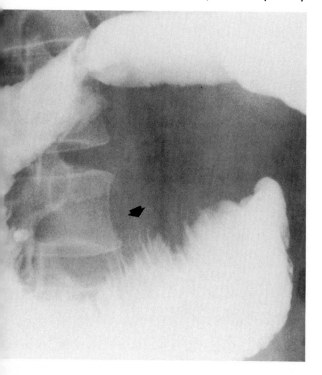

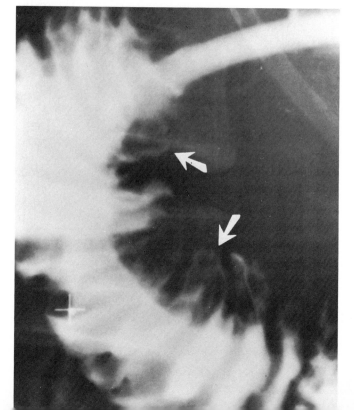

congenital or developmental misplacement and obliteration of draining lymphatics or be secondary to acquired lymphatic obstruction (*e.g.*, trauma). Similar to the findings in lymphangiectasia, associated protein-losing enteropathy and hypoproteinemic edema have been reported in cystic lymphangiomas.

Dilated pancreaticoduodenal collateral vessels in patients with occlusion of the celiac axis or superior mesenteric artery infrequently produce a smooth, concave impression on the medial aspect of the descending duodenum. This double-contour effect can simulate a mass in the head of the pancreas.

Retroperitoneal masses (primary or metastatic neoplasms, cysts) can widen the duodenal sweep (Fig. 28-20). Downward displacement of the third portion of the duodenum by an aortic aneurysm can produce a similar radiographic appearance. Choledochal cysts (localized dilatations of the common bile duct) occurring near the ampulla of Vater can result in generalized widening of the duodenal sweep (Fig. 28-21) or a localized impression near the papilla.

Fig. 28-18. Lymphoma involving the peripancreatic lymph nodes and causing widening of the duodenal sweep. Note the spiculations and double-contour effect simulating primary pancreatic carcinoma.

Fig. 28-19. Cystic lymphangioma of the mesentery. Note the scattered clumps of calcification in the lesion.

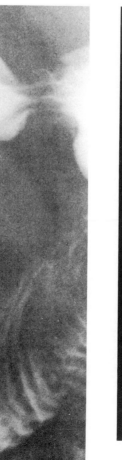

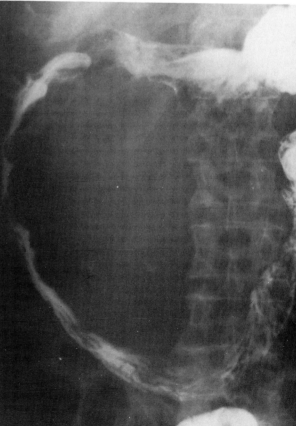

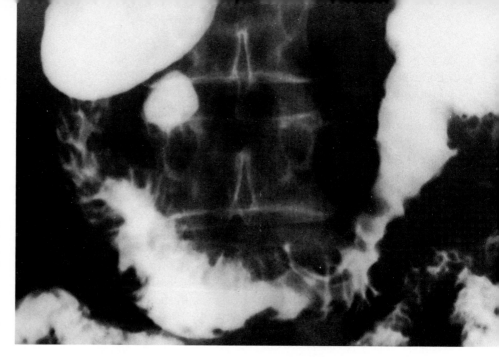

Fig. 28-20. Squamous carcinoma of the lung metastatic to the retroperitoneum. Widening of the duodenal sweep with multiple nodular indentations and spiculation simulates the appearance of primary pancreatic carcinoma.

Fig. 28-21. Huge choledochal cyst causing generalized widening of the duodenal sweep.

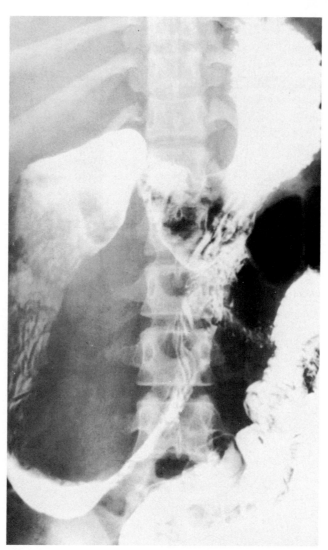

Bellon EM, George CR, Schreiber H: Pancreatic pseudocysts of the duodenum. AJR 133:827–831, 1979

Benedict KT, Ferrucci JT, Eaton SB: Hypotonic duodenography: Current concepts in technique, interpretation, and clinical usefulness. CRC Crit Rev Radiol Sci 1:567–578, 1970

Beranbaum SL: Carcinoma of the pancreas: A bidirectional roentgen approach. AJR 96:447–467, 1966

Bilbao MK, Rosch J, Frische LH et al: Hypotonic duodenography in the diagnosis of pancreatic disease. Semin Roentgenol 3:280–287, 1968

Eaton SB, Benedict KT, Ferrucci JT et al: Hypotonic duodenography. Radiol Clin North Am 8:125–137, 1970

Eaton SB, Rerrucci JT: Radiology of the Pancreas and Duodenum. Philadelphia, WB Saunders, 1973

Eaton SB, Ferrucci JT, Margulis AR et al: Unusual roentgen findings in pancreatic disease. AJR 116:396–405, 1972

Eyler WR, Clark MD, Rian RL: An evaluation of the roentgen signs of pancreatic enlargement. JAMA 181:967–971, 1962

Ferrucci JT, Benedict JT, Page DL et al: Radiographic features of the normal hypotonic duodenogram. Radiology 96:401–408, 1970

Frostberg N: Characteristic duodenal deformity in cases of different kinds of perivaterial enlargement of the pancreas. Acta Radiol 19:164–173, 1938

Hodes PJ, Pendergrass EP, Winston NJ: Pancreatic, ductal and vaterian neoplasms: Their roentgen manifestations. Radiology 62:1–15, 1954

Jacquemet P, Liotta D, Mallet-Guy P: The Early Radiological Diagnosis of Diseases of the Pancreas and Ampulla of Vater: Elective Exploration of the Ampulla of Vater and the Head of the Pancreas by Hypotonic Duodenography. Springfield, IL, Charles C Thomas, 1965

Leonidas JC, Kopel FB, Danese CA: Mesenteric cyst associated with protein loss in the gastrointestinal tract. AJR 112:150–154, 1971

Renert WA, Hecht HL: Lymphangiographic demonstration of impression upon the duodenum by retroperitoneal lymph nodes. Br J Radiol 44:189–194, 1971

Renert WA, Pitt MJ, Capp MP: Acute pancreatitis. Semin Roentgenol 8:405–414, 1973

Rubinstein ZS, Bank S, Marks IN et al: Hypotonic duodenography in chronic pancreatitis. Br J Radiol 44:142–149, 1971

Schultz EH: Aids to diagnosis of acute pancreatitis by roentgen study. AJR 89:825–836, 1963

Shockman AT, Marasco JA: Pseudocysts of the pancreas. AJR 101:628–638, 1967

Thomford NR, Jesseph JE: Pseudocyst of the pancreas: A review of 50 cases. Am J Surg 118:86–94, 1969

29 EXTRINSIC PRESSURE ON THE DUODENUM

Disease Entities

Bile ducts
  Normal impression
  Enlargement
  Choledochal cyst
Gallbladder
  Normal impression
  Enlargement
    Hydrops
    Courvoisier phenomenon
  Carcinoma
  Pericholecystic abscess
Liver
  Generalized hepatomegaly (especially enlargement of the caudate lobe)
  Cyst
  Tumor
  Lymphadenopathy in the periportal region
Right kidney
  Enlargement due to bifid collecting system/hydronephrosis

Multiple cysts/polycystic disease
Hypernephroma
  Mass effect
  Direct invasion of duodenum
Right adrenal
  Enlargement (Addison's disease)
  Carcinoma
Pancreas
  Annular pancreas
  Carcinoma (wrapped around the duodenum)
Postbulbar ulcer (lateral incisura appearance)
Colon
  Duodenocolic apposition
  Carcinoma of the hepatic flexure
Vascular structures
  Duodenal varices
  Mesenteric arterial collaterals
  Aortic aneurysm
  Intramural or mesenteric hematoma

The duodenal bulb and sweep are intimately related anatomically to other structures in the right upper quadrant. The liver and gallbladder are in immediate contact with the anterior–superior aspect of the first portion of the duodenum. The transverse colon normally crosses the second portion of the duodenum anteriorly. A mesenteric bridge attaches the hepatic flexure of the colon to the lower portion of the descending duodenum. Posteriorly, the duodenum is extraperitoneal and has a variable relationship to the medial portion of the anterior aspect of the right kidney in the neighborhood of the hilus. As the superior mesenteric artery and vein emerge from the root of the mesentery, they cross the transverse portion of the duodenum near the midline. Thus, any disease state involving an organ within the right upper quadrant can cause displacement of or extrinsic pressure on the duodenal bulb and sweep.

BILE DUCTS

Even when normal, the common bile duct can produce a linear or small, rounded impression on the duodenal bulb. A dilated common bile duct tends to cause a large tubular impression on the duodenal bulb or the postbulbar area (Fig. 29-1). This broad radiolucent defect arises superiorly and to the right of the barium-filled duodenum.

A choledochal cyst is a segmental dilatation of the common bile duct that can also involve the adjacent cystic and common hepatic ducts. Much more common in females than in males, about 60% occur in children under the age of 10. The classic clinical triad of jaundice, right upper quadrant abdominal mass, and abdominal pain is found in less than 40% of cases. Depending on the size of the cyst and the portion of the bile duct involved, various patterns of impression and displacement of the duodenal bulb and sweep can be seen. A choledochal cyst can become so large that it widens and stretches the duodenal loop; it can even displace the stomach upward.

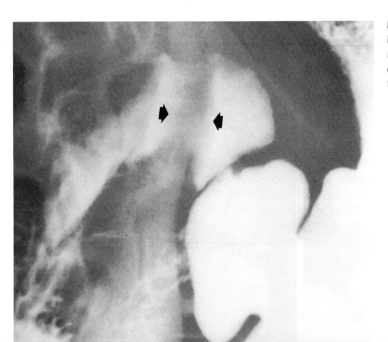

Fig. 29-1. Dilated common bile duct producing a tubular impression **(arrows)** on the duodenum near the apex of the bulb.

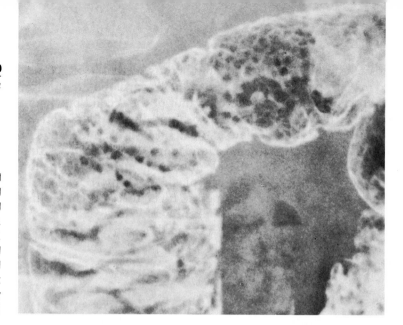

Fig. 30-13. Benign lymphoid hyperplasia. Multiple round elevations are evenly spread over the duodenal surface. (Langkamper R, Hoek AC, Dekker W et al: Elevated lesions in the duodenal bulb caused by heterotopic gastric mucosa. Radiology 137:621–624, 1980)

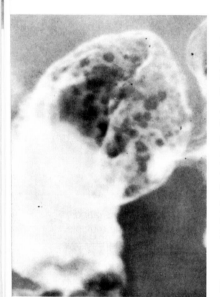

Fig. 30-14. Heterotopic gastric mucosa in the duodenal bulb producing a diffuse, finely nodular pattern.

HETEROTOPIC GASTRIC MUCOSA

Heterotopic gastric mucosa in the duodenal bulb can present as multiple elevated lesions. These abruptly marginated, angular filling defects range from 1 mm to 6 mm in diameter and are scattered over the surface of the bulb in one or more clusters, predominantly in the juxtapyloric region (Fig. 30-14). They are best visualized on double-contrast views of an optimally distended bulb. The irregular clusters of elevated lesions caused by heterotopic gastric mucosa must be differentiated from other causes of multiple filling defects in the bulb. In benign lymphoid hyperplasia, the smoothly demarcated, round elevations are similar in size and are evenly scattered on the duodenal surface rather than being restricted to the bulb. In Brunner's gland hyperplasia, the elevations tend to be larger and more uniform in size, rather round, and often less numerous.

PAPILLA OF VATER

In patients with filling defects in the second portion of the duodenum, it is essential that it be determined whether the mass represents the duodenal papilla, an elevated mound of tissue projecting into the duodenal lumen. The duodenal papilla can usually be precisely localized on hypotonic studies by identification of the promontory, straight segment, and longitudinal fold (Fig. 30-15). The papilla generally sits on or immediately below the promontory, a localized bulging along the medial contour of the mid-descending duodenum that results in slight widening of the lumen. The straight segment is the flat, smooth portion of the medial wall of the duodenum that extends 2 cm to 3 cm inferior to the promontory. Contrary to the appearance on the lateral wall at this level, regular interfold indentations are not visible within the straight segment. The longitudinal fold is a vertically oriented ridge

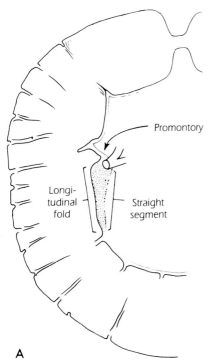

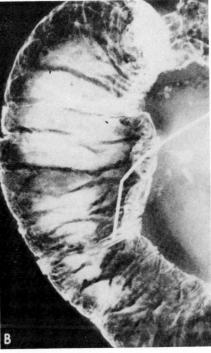

Fig. 30-15. Normal duodenal anatomy on hypotonic study. **(A)** Schematic representation of the descending duodenum showing the typical arrangement of the promontory, papilla, straight segment, and longitudinal fold. **(B)** Radiograph of a specimen demonstrating the characteristic appearance of the inner duodenal profile. Note the relationship of the papilla to the promontory and the position of the longitudinal fold along the straight segment. (Eaton SB, Ferrucci JT: Radiology of the Pancreas and Duodenum. Philadelphia, WB Saunders, 1973)

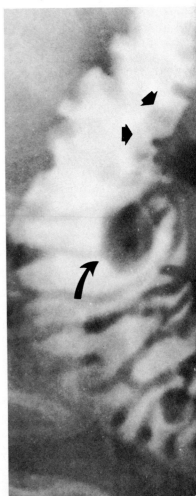

Fig. 30-16. Benign polyp in the duodenal sweep. The large polyp **(curved arrow)** is clearly separate from the duodenal papilla **(straight arrows)**.

of mucosa and submucosa that arises as a mucosal hood above the papilla and extends distally for 2 cm to 3 cm parallel to the straight segment. This fold runs perpendicular to the typical transverse plical folds of the duodenum. Any filling defects situated within the triangle bordered by these three structures is most likely related to the papilla. Lesions outside this area should suggest another pathologic process (Fig. 30-16).

Enlargement of the papilla (greater than 1.5 cm in length) can be due to papillary edema or neoplasm of the ampulla of Vater (the slightly dilated segment of bile duct within the papilla). Differential diagnosis of enlargement of the papilla is discussed in Chapter 64.

CHOLEDOCHOCELE

A choledochocele is a cystic dilatation of the intraduodenal portion of the common bile duct in the region of the ampulla of Vater. On barium studies of the upper gastrointestinal tract, a choledochocele causes a well-defined, smooth filling defect projecting into the lumen on the medial wall of the descending duodenum (Fig. 30-17A). At cholangiography, the bulbous terminal portion of the common bile duct is evident (Fig. 30-17B).

DUPLICATION CYST

Duodenal duplication cysts can appear as intramural filling defects and are usually detected early in life (Fig. 30-18). Communication with the duodenal lumen has been reported to occur in about 10% to 20% of these rare congenital lesions. Duodenal duplication cysts most commonly present as abdominal masses, often with nausea and vomiting. They are occasionally so large as to cause duodenal obstruction.

Two radiographic patterns of duodenal duplication cysts have been described. The first is a well-defined oval filling defect. The second and more characteristic pattern is a sharply defined intramural defect, usually situated in the concavity of the first and second portions of the duodenum. Because the cysts are filled with fluid, they often change shape with compression and on serial films.

PANCREATIC PSEUDOCYST

Rarely, pancreatic pseudocysts extend into the wall of the duodenum and produce an intramural filling defect (Fig. 30-19). If a pseudocyst is tensely distended, the bulging mucosa or muscularis can compromise the lumen and cause varying degrees of duodenal obstruction.

Fig. 30-17. Choledochocele. **(A)** On barium study, the lesion appears as a smooth filling defect **(arrows)** projecting into the lumen on the medial wall of the descending duodenum. **(B)** At cholangiography, the bulbous terminal portion of the common bile duct is evident **(arrow)**.

A B

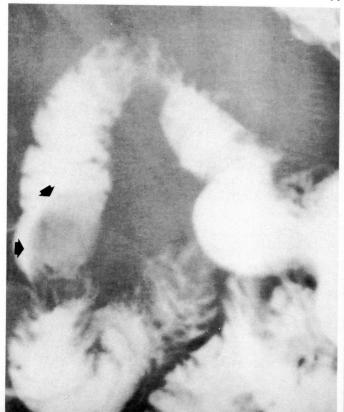
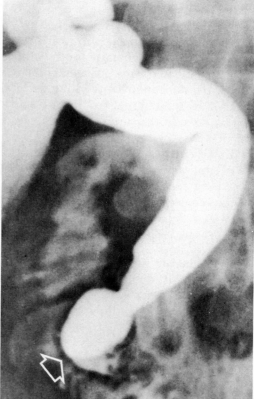

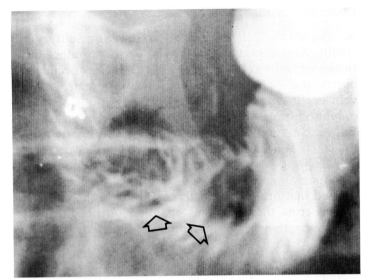

Fig. 30-18. Duodenal duplication cyst. A lobulated filling defect **(arrows)** may be seen in the region of the junction of the second and third portions of the duodenum.

Fig. 30-19. Pancreatic pseudocyst extending into the wall of the duodenum and producing a large intramural filling defect **(arrows)**.

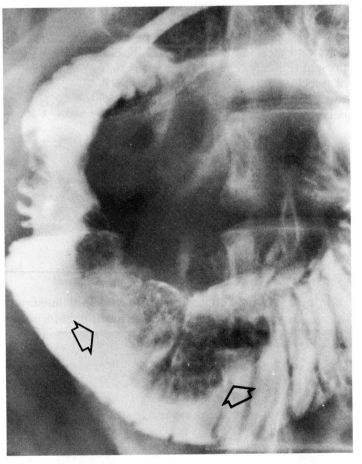

Pedunculated polyps of the antrum can prolapse through the pylorus and present as solitary or multiple filling defects in the base of the duodenal bulb (Fig. 30-32*A*). These benign tumors are typically round or oval and have either a smooth or a slightly lobulated surface. Patients with prolapsed polyps are often anemic; abdominal pain is not infrequent. Most prolapsing antral polyps are adenomas. Ulceration within the lesion should suggest the diagnosis of leiomyoma. Like prolapsed antral mucosal folds, prolapsed antral tumors change location or completely reduce on serial films (Fig. 30-32*B*).

Any polypoid gastric tumor can pull a segment of stomach with it as it is pushed by peristalsis through the pylorus. In the resulting intussusception, the entire gastric wall is invaginated into the duodenum, not just the mucosa, as with prolapse of antral folds. Symptoms of gastric intussusception into the duodenum vary from acute obstruction and incarceration to more chronic gastrointestinal complaints. In addition to the radiographic appearance of an intraluminal duodenal mass, there can be shortening of the antrum, complete or incomplete gastric outlet obstruction, converging of distal gastric rugae, and compression of pyloric and duodenal folds.

BRUNNER'S GLAND ADENOMA

Brunner's gland adenomas can present as discrete filling defects in the bulb or second portion of the duodenum (Fig. 30-33). These "adenomas" probably represent localized areas of hypertrophy and hyperplasia rather than true neoplasms.

TUMORS OF VARIABLE MALIGNANT POTENTIAL

VILLOUS ADENOMA

Villous adenomas and carcinoid–islet cell tumors of the duodenum have a variable malignant potential; about half have histologic evidence of malignancy. Villous adenomas of the duodenum are unusual lesions that have a radiographic appearance similar to tumors of the same cell type in the colon (Fig. 30-34). Because the ampullary region is the most frequent location for duodenal villous adenomas, obstructive jaundice is the most common clinical presentation. Jaundice can be secondary to infiltrative growth into the ampulla or to exophytic growth physically blocking the common bile duct. Because the appearance of jaundice depends on the size of the villous adenoma and its relationship to the papilla, this physical finding can occur in benign lesions. The diffuse mucorrhea and potassium loss that is frequently associated with villous

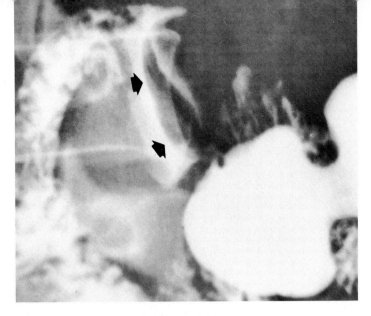

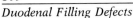

Fig. 30-29. Lipoma of the duodenal bulb. The soft consistency of the tumor allows it to conform its shape to the lumen of the bulb **(arrows).**

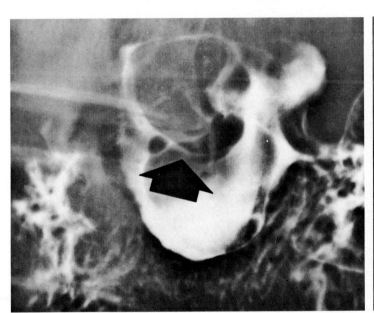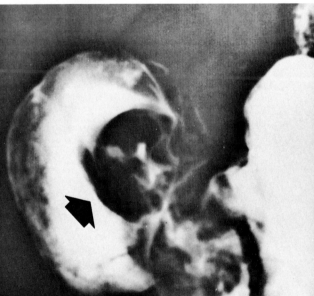

A B

Fig. 30-30. Lipoma of the duodenal bulb **(arrows).** Note the difference in the contour of the tumor between the two films.

adenoma of the colon and rectum is not seen with these duodenal lesions.

Villous adenomas of the duodenum appear radiographically as lobulated filling defects covered by fine networks of barium coating the interstices between the fine, frondlike projections of the tumor. Because of their soft consistency, villous adenomas can change contour on serial films. As with tumors of this cell type in the colon, there are no definite radiographic criteria with which to differentiate benign villous adenomas of the duodenum from lesions with early carcinomatous transformation.

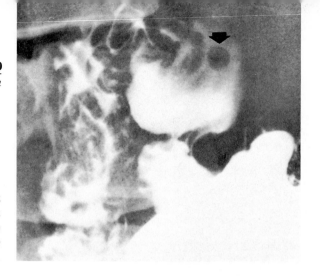

Fig. 30-31. Peutz–Jeghers syndrome. A hamartomatous polyp (**arrow**) mimics a smooth gas bubble in the duodenal bulb.

Fig. 30-32. Prolapsing antral polyp. (**A**) Prolapsed polyp presenting as a solitary filling defect (**arrows**) in the base of the duodenal bulb. (**B**) With reduction of the prolapse, the true origin of the polyp within the antrum becomes evident (**arrows**).

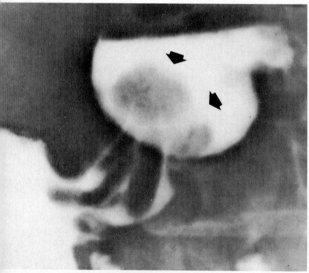

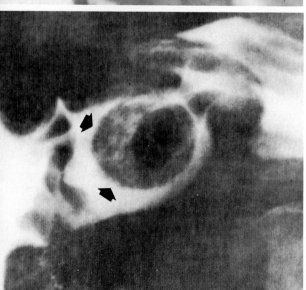

A
B

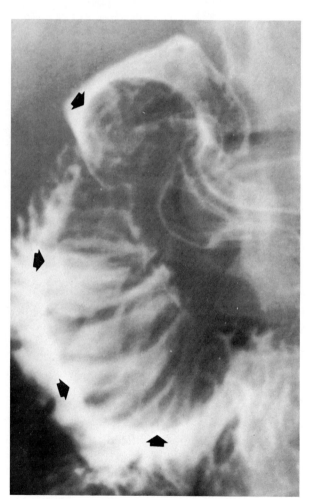

Fig. 30-33. Brunner's gland adenoma. A large filling defect (**arrows**) involves the duodenal bulb and sweep.

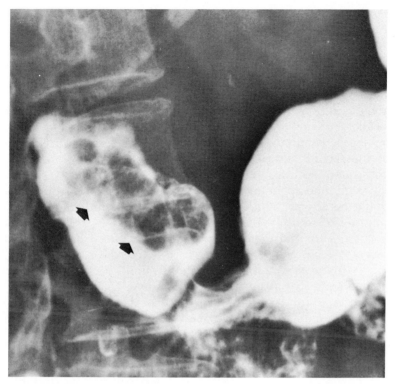

Fig. 30-34. Villous adenoma of the duodenal bulb. A bulky mass with irregular margins and barium may be seen entering the interstices in the tumor **(arrows).** Note the radiolucent defect in the antrum, which represents a benign gastric polyp.

Fig. 30-35. Carcinoid–islet cell tumor in the duodenal bulb **(arrow).**

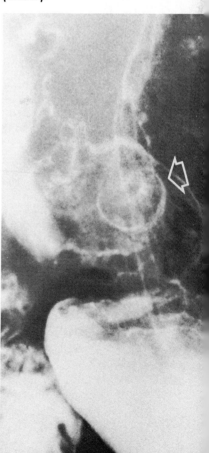

CARCINOID–ISLET CELL TUMOR

Carcinoid–islet cell tumors of the duodenum have morphologic and functional features of both carcinoid and islet cell tumors of the pancreas (Fig. 30-35). Both carcinoid and islet cell tumors appear to arise from a common neuroectodermal precursor that is related to the argentaffin cell. Clinically, progressive and intractable peptic ulceration or severe diarrhea is present in most patients. The patient frequently has a history of one or more operative procedures for ulcer disease. Carcinoid–islet cell tumors have remarkable endocrine activity; serotonin, insulin, and gastrinlike substances have been extracted from tumor tissue. Patients with these tumors may have multiple endocrine adenomatosis (parathyroid, pancreatic, and duodenal tumors) or evidence of neural ectodermal dysplasia.

Carcinoid–islet cell tumors are most commonly found in a submucosal location on the anterior or medial wall of the first or second portion of the duodenum proximal to the papilla. Although they are usually solitary, multiple tumors are occasionally present. Malignant tumors of this cell type often produce lymph node metastases in the region of the head of the pancreas.

MALIGNANT TUMORS

Primary duodenal malignancies are rare. Of all duodenal cancers, 80% to 90% are adenocarcinomas; most occur at or distal to the papilla. In addition to polypoid intraluminal masses (Fig. 30-36), adenocarcinomas can appear as annular constricting lesions with mucosal destruction and ulceration. Clinical symptoms vary according to the location of the lesion; they include obstructive jaundice, bowel obstruction, and hemorrhage. Carcinomas of the ampulla of Vater occur on the medial aspect of the second portion of the duodenum; they will be discussed in subsequent sections.

Sarcomas, primarily leiomyosarcomas, are rare duodenal lesions that generally present as lobulated intramural filling defects, often with central ulceration. Sinus tracts often extend into the necrotic central portion of the mass, which may be large, bulky, and primarily extramural in location.

Primary lymphoma of the duodenum is rare. It can present as a polypoid mass or as multiple small nodules that produce a cobblestone appearance simulating thickened mucosal folds.

Metastases can involve the duodenum by direct invasion from adjacent structures or by hematogenous spread. Gastric carcinoma or lymphoma can extend across the pylorus and produce contour deformities and filling defects in the duodenal bulb (Fig. 30-37). Carcinoma of the pancreas can cause ulcerating and constricting lesions that are indistinguishable from primary duodenal carcinoma (Fig. 30-38). Direct extension of primary malignancies of the gallbladder, colon, or kidney can produce a similar radiographic appearance. Rarely, retroperitoneal node involvement from distal tumors distorts or invades the duodenum. Duodenal filling defects with central necrosis and ulceration (bull's-eye lesions) suggest hematogenous metastases, most of which are due to melanoma (Fig. 30-39). Occasionally, metastases present as multiple filling defects simulating thickened mucosal folds (Fig. 30-40).

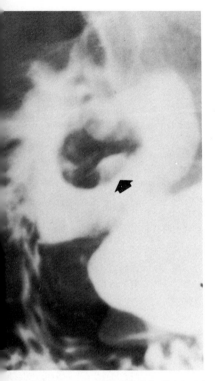

Fig. 30-36. Polypoid carcinoma of the duodenal bulb **(arrow).**

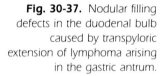

Fig. 30-37. Nodular filling defects in the duodenal bulb caused by transpyloric extension of lymphoma arising in the gastric antrum.

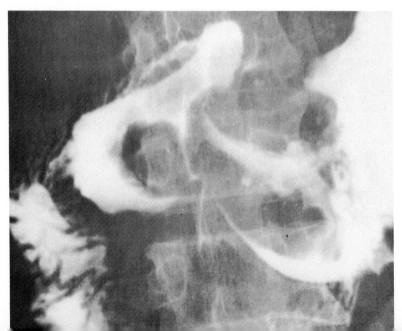

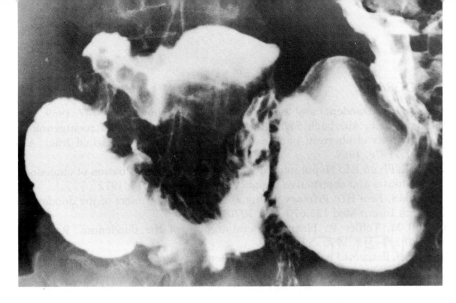

Fig. 30-38. Pancreatic carcinoma. There is an annular constriction of the proximal second portion of the duodenum. A large mass effect with spiculations involves most of the duodenal sweep.

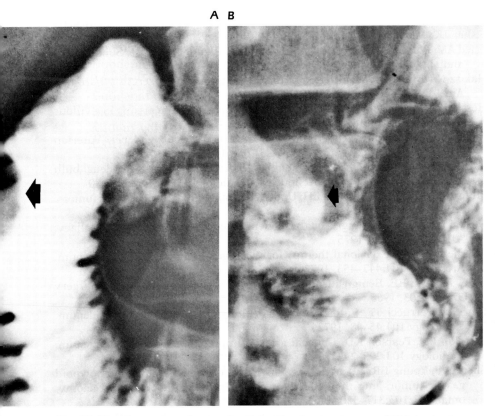

A B

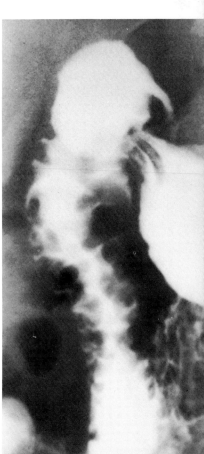

Fig. 30-39. Metastatic melanoma involving the duodenal sweep. **(A)** Intramural mass **(arrow)** on the lateral border of the descending duodenum. **(B)** Central ulceration **(arrow)** in the intramural mass suggests a hematogenous metastasis.

Fig. 30-40. Carcinoma of the lung metastatic to the duodenal sweep. Multiple filling defects simulate diffuse thickening of mucosal folds.

instances, the physical characteristics of the anomaly are such that the first symptoms do not occur until adulthood.

CONGENITAL OBSTRUCTION

DUODENAL ATRESIA

Duodenal atresia is *complete* obliteration of the intestinal lumen at the level of the duodenum (Fig. 31-1). The obstruction usually occurs distal to the ampulla of Vater, though the proximal duodenum is affected in 20% of cases. Duodenal atresia results from failure of the duodenum to recanalize between the 6th and 11th weeks of fetal life. The duodenum proximal to the atretic segment thus has a long time during which it can become dilated before birth. This is in contrast to other types of congenital obstruction that develop at a later stage in intrauterine life or are incomplete and therefore result in a lesser degree of proximal duodenal dilatation.

Duodenal atresia is the most common cause of congenital obstruction of the duodenum. In this condition, vomiting (usually containing bile) begins within a few hours of birth or following the first feeding. Because the obstruction is so high in the gastrointestinal tract, the frequent vomiting and consequent loss of fluids and electrolytes can cause rapid clinical deterioration unless a surgical diverting procedure is promptly performed. There is a higher than normal incidence of duodenal atresia in infants with Down's syndrome. Vertebral and rib

Fig. 31-1. Duodenal atresia. There is complete obstruction of the intestinal lumen at the level of the duodenum.

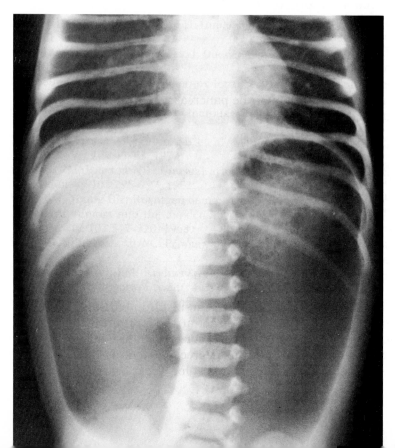

anomalies, intestinal malrotation, imperforate anus, and various urinary tract anomalies can be associated with duodenal atresia. However, since such anomalies can also occur in patients with annular pancreas, the presence of one or more of them in conjunction with congenital duodenal obstruction is of little help in differentiating between these two conditions.

The classic radiographic appearance of duodenal atresia is the "double bubble" sign (Fig. 31-2). Large amounts of gas are present in both a markedly dilated stomach (left bubble) and that portion of the duodenum that is proximal to the obstruction (right bubble). In duodenal atresia, there is a total absence of gas in the small and large bowel distal to the level of the complete obstruction. In high-grade but incomplete congenital stenosis of the duodenum, there is some gas in the bowel distal to the obstruction (Fig. 31-3).

ANNULAR PANCREAS

Annular pancreas is an anomalous ring of pancreatic tissue encircling the duodenal lumen usually at or above the level of the ampulla of Vater. The pancreas develops from two entirely distinct entodermal outgrowths (dorsal and ventral pancreas) that fuse to form a single organ. The ventral pancreatic bud is bilobed. The left bud usually degenerates, though it can persist and develop its own pancreatic lobe, which then grows around the left side of the duodenum to join the other two parts of the pancreas in the dorsal mesentery. Severe

Fig. 31-2. Duodenal atresia with double bubble sign. The left bubble **(open arrow)** represents air in the stomach; the right bubble **(solid arrow)** reflects duodenal gas. There is no gas in the small or large bowel distal to the level of the complete obstruction.

Fig. 31-3. Congenital duodenal stenosis. The presence of small amounts of gas distal to the obstruction indicates that the stenosis is incomplete.

Fig. 31-2   **Fig. 31-3**

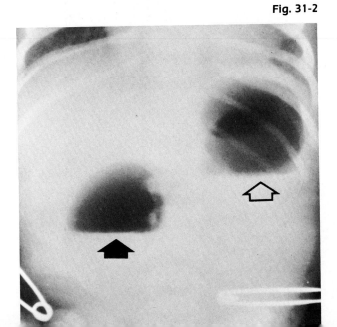
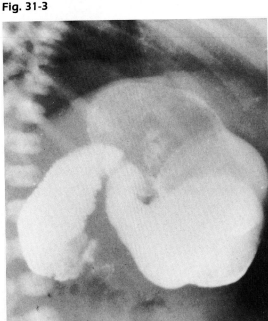

congenital anomalies of the gastrointestinal tract (*e.g.,* duodenal atresia, malrotation with bands, duodenal diaphragm) frequently coexist with annular pancreas; Down's syndrome is seen in about 30% of patients. Annular pancreas may be asymptomatic or produce symptoms consistent with varying degrees of duodenal obstruction.

Infants with symptomatic annular pancreas have the radiographic appearance of a double bubble sign (Fig. 31-4). Unlike duodenal atresia, annular pancreas almost always results in an *incomplete* obstruction. A small but recognizable amount of gas can be demonstrated within the bowel distal to the level of the high-grade duodenal stenosis. These tiny collections of gas distal to a partially obstructing annular pancreas can be easily missed. However, they must be carefully sought, since their presence excludes the possibility of duodenal atresia.

When symptoms arising from an annular pancreas are delayed until adulthood, some complicating condition must be suspected. Inflammatory edema of an annular pancreas can result in sufficient luminal narrowing to cause duodenal obstruction. Duodenal ulceration often accompanies symptomatic annular pancreas in adults, though it is unclear whether the ulcer precedes the duodenal obstruction or is a consequence of it.

The radiographic appearance of annular pancreas in adults is a notchlike defect on the lateral duodenal wall causing an eccentric narrowing of the lumen (Fig. 31-5). This appearance must be differentiated from a postbulbar ulcer (with deep incisura) or a malignant tumor, both of which can produce a similar deformity. Unlike the pattern seen with postbulbar disease, the duodenal mucosal folds in annular pancreas are intact, and no discrete ulcer crater can be identified. With malignant disease, the constriction is usually more irregular and involves a longer segment of the duodenum, and the mucosal pattern is destroyed through the area of constriction. Very rarely, pancreatic cancer develops in an annular pancreas and is indistinguishable from an intrinsic duodenal malignancy.

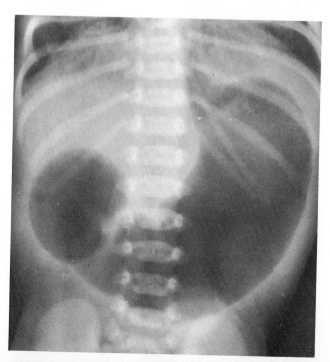

Fig. 31-4. Annular pancreas (infant). In this patient, there was complete duodenal obstruction and no evidence of distal gas.

DUODENAL DIAPHRAGM

Congenital duodenal diaphragms are weblike projections of the mucous membrane that occlude the lumen of the duodenum to varying degrees (Fig. 31-6). The majority of reported cases have occurred in the second part of the duodenum near the ampulla of Vater. Radiographically, the congenital duodenal diaphragm presents as a thin, radiolucent line extending across the lumen, often with proximal duodenal dilatation. Because the duodenal obstruction is incomplete, small amounts of gas are scattered through the more distal portions of the bowel. On rare occasions, the thin diaphragm balloons out distally, producing a rounded barium-filled, comma-shaped sac (intraluminal diverticulum).

MIDGUT VOLVULUS

Midgut volulus is an infrequent complication that occurs in patients with incomplete rotation of the bowel (Fig. 31-7). Normal rotation of the gut results in a broad mesenteric attachment of the small bowel that effectively precludes the development of a midgut volvulus. Incomplete rotation, however, leads to a narrow mesenteric attachment of the small bowel that can permit rotation around the axis of the superior mesenteric artery and result in a midgut volvulus. Although often an isolated finding, incomplete rotation coexists in about 20% of patients with congenital duodenal obstruction from duodenal atresia, annular pancreas, or duodenal diaphragm. Therefore, it is probably prudent to perform a barium enema in any newborn infant with congenital obstruction of the duodenum so as to demonstrate the position of the cecum and exclude the possibility of incomplete rotation of the gut

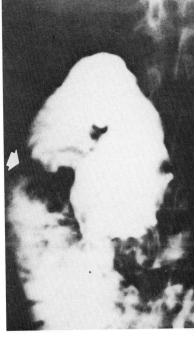

Fig. 31-5. Annular pancreas (adult). Extrinsic narrowing of the second portion of the duodenum **(arrow)** causes partial obstruction (large duodenal bulb). (Glazer GM, Margulis AR: Annular pancreas: Etiology and diagnosis using endoscopic retrograde cholangiopancreatography. Radiology 133:303–306, 1979)

Fig. 31-6. Duodenal diaphragm. There is high-grade stenosis of the second portion of the duodenum. The presence of gas in the bowel distal to the diaphragm indicates that the obstruction is not complete.

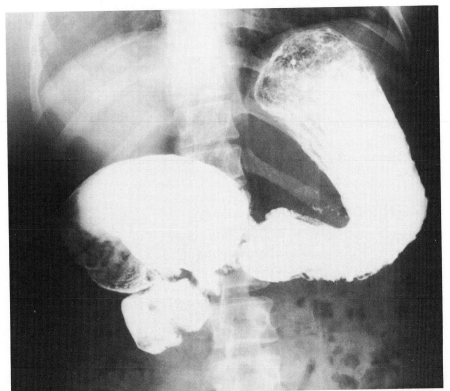

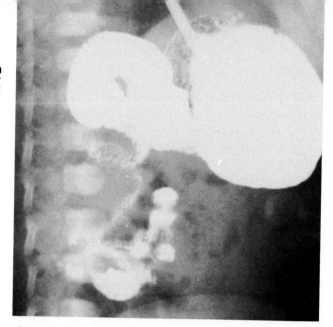

Fig. 31-7. *Midgut volvulus. There is duodenal obstruction and spiraling of the small bowel. (Swischuk LE: Emergency Radiology of the Acutely Ill or Injured Child. Baltimore, Williams & Wilkins, 1979)*

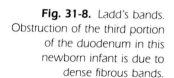

Fig. 31-8. *Ladd's bands. Obstruction of the third portion of the duodenum in this newborn infant is due to dense fibrous bands.*

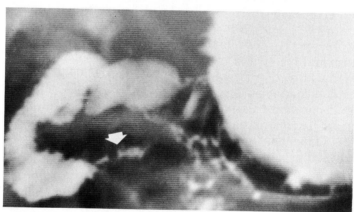

being a potential complicating factor. If the cecum is shown to be in an abnormal position in the midabdomen or on the left side, an upper gastrointestinal series is indicated to determine whether a midgut volvulus is the cause of the partial duodenal obstruction. The combination of a duodenojejunal junction (ligament of Treitz) located inferiorly and to the right of its expected position and a spiral course of bowel loops on the right side of the abdomen is diagnostic of midgut volvulus.

CONGENITAL PERITONEAL BANDS

Congenital peritoneal bands (Ladd's bands) can produce extrinsic duodenal obstruction in newborn infants (Fig. 31-8). These dense, fibrous bands extend from an abnormally placed, malrotated cecum or hepatic flexure over the anterior surface of the second or third portion of the duodenum to the right gutter and inferior surface of the liver. Obstruct-

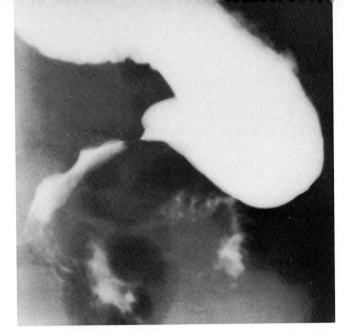

Fig. 31-9. Duodenal duplication cyst. An intramural mass causes high-grade stenosis of the duodenal sweep.

ing Ladd's bands can be an isolated process or be found in conjunction with malrotation, annular pancreas, preduodenal portal vein, or duplication of the duodenum. They cause episodes of acute obstruction or, more commonly, intermittent partial obstruction, which can be aggravated by food intake or change in position. Standing can result in tightening of the bands and increased symptoms; lying down often relaxes them.

DUPLICATION CYST

A duodenal duplication cyst is an uncommon spherical or tubular structure filled with serous fluid, mucus, or even bile (if the bile duct empties into the cyst). A duplication cyst is usually situated within the muscular layer of the duodenum but occasionally lies in a submucosal, subserosal, or even intramesenteric location. The cyst can encroach on the lumen of the duodenum and present as an intramural or extrinsic mass. Most duodenal duplications are asymptomatic and are found only incidentally at laparotomy during surgery for an unrelated problem. Extremely rarely, a duplication cyst causes high-grade stenosis or complete obstruction of the duodenum (Fig. 31-9).

INFLAMMATORY DISORDERS

POSTBULBAR ULCER

Postbulbar ulcers account for only a small percentage of all duodenal ulcers. Although they can be difficult to diagnose clinically or radiographically, it is important that they be recognized, because they may be the source of obstruction, pancreatitis, gastrointestinal hemorrhage, and atypical pain. The classic appearance of a postbulbar ulcer crater is a shallow, flat niche on the medial aspect of the second portion of the duodenum. The ulcer is usually accompanied by an incisura, an indrawing of the lateral wall of the duodenum caused by muscular spasm. In chronic ulceration or after healing of a postbulbar ulcer, the incisura may become a fixed and permanent stricture, producing a ringlike narrowing of the duodenum (Fig. 31-10). Although this pattern closely resembles the appearance in annular pancreas, the effaced, granular-appearing mucosa in the narrowed segment suggests healed ulceration.

CROHN'S DISEASE

Crohn's disease can cause narrowing and partial obstruction of the duodenum (Fig. 31-11). Although isolated duodenal involvement by this granulomatous process can occur, the disease is usually present elsewhere in the small bowel. The radiographic spectrum of Crohn's disease in the duodenum is similar to that in the ileum. In some patients, there are spiculated ulcers, linear ulcers, and a cobblestone appearance, usually associated with some narrowing. In others, there are long stenotic areas with effacement of the normal mucosal pattern (Fig. 31-12). These areas of narrowing tend to be fusiform and concentric (Fig. 31-13), unlike the puckering or "clover-leaf" type of deformity that is associated with duodenal ulcer disease (Fig. 31-14). In most cases of Crohn's disease of the duodenum, the stomach is also involved, resulting in a characteristic tubular or funnel-shaped narrowing of the antrum, pylorus, and proximal duodenum.

TUBERCULOSIS

Tuberculosis of the duodenum is extremely rare, even in patients with pulmonary or gastrointestinal disease. Isolated duodenal involvement has been reported, though tuberculosis of the duodenum is almost always associated with antral and pyloric disease. The radiographic pattern of nodular hyperplastic thickening of folds, diffuse ulceration, and luminal narrowing caused by a constricting inflammatory mass may be indistinguishable from Crohn's disease (Fig. 31-15). Caseation with abscess formation can lead to fistulas and the development of sinus tracts.

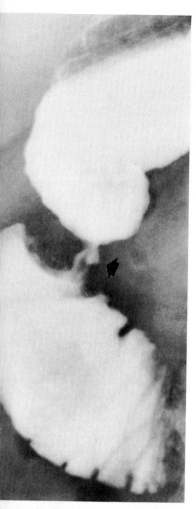

Fig. 31-10. Deep incisura, associated with a medial-wall postbulbar ulcer **(arrow)**, causing severe narrowing of the second portion of the duodenum.

Fig. 31-11. Crohn's disease. There is a tight stricture of the midportion of the descending duodenum **(arrow)**. ▶

Fig. 31-12. Crohn's disease. A long stenosis **(arrows)** involves the first and second portions of the duodenum with effacement of the normal mucosal pattern. ▶

Fig. 31-13. Crohn's disease. There is fusiform, concentric narrowing of the apical and postbulbar areas **(arrow)**. ▶

Fig. 31-14. Duodenal ulcer disease. A typical "clover-leaf" deformity is visible **(arrows)**. ▶

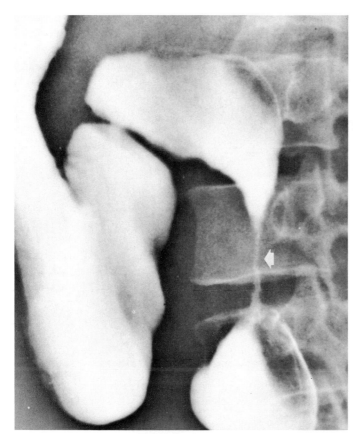

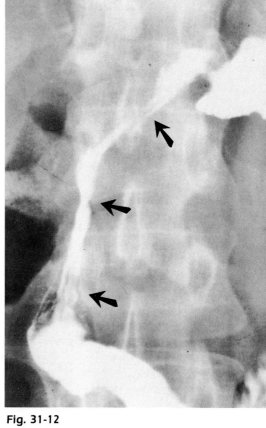

Fig. 31-11 **Fig. 31-12**

Fig. 31-13 **Fig. 31-14**

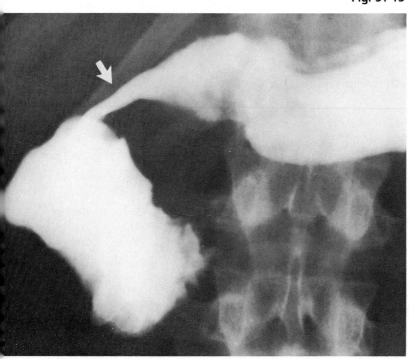

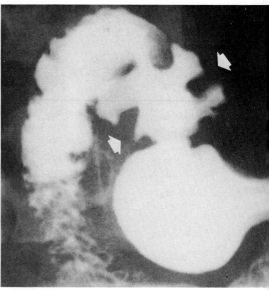

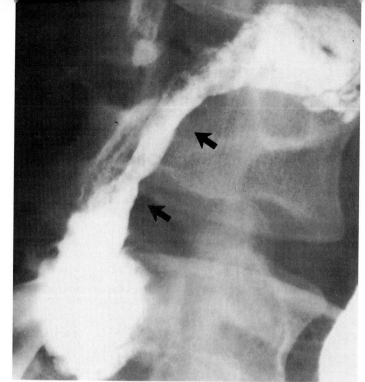

Fig. 31-15. Tuberculosis. There is narrowing of the second portion of the duodenum **(arrows)** with ulceration and diffuse mucosal irregularity.

Fig. 31-16. Strongyloidiasis. There is diffuse mucosal inflammation and ulceration with luminal narrowing.

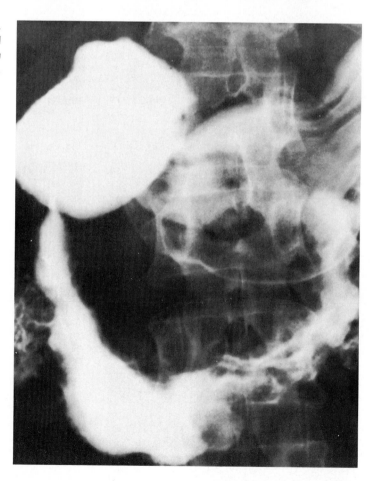

STRONGYLOIDIASIS / SPRUE

Strongyloidiasis involving the duodenum can also simulate Crohn's disease. Diffuse ulceration, mucosal inflammation, and abnormal peristalsis result in severe atony and duodenal dilatation. Fibrotic healing can lead to stenotic narrowing of the lumen (Fig. 31-16). Duodenal or jejunal ulceration in long-standing cases of nontropical sprue can cause multiple areas of stenosis and postobstructive dilatation of the duodenum.

PANCREATITIS / CHOLECYSTITIS

Severe acute inflammation of the pancreas can result in sufficient irritability and spasm to cause narrowing of the duodenal lumen. In addition, retroperitoneal inflammation due to acute pancreatitis can thicken the bowel wall and root of the mesentery in the space between the aorta and the superior mesenteric artery (aorticomesenteric angle), producing high-grade obstruction of the third portion of the duodenum. The postinflammatory fibrosis of chronic pancreatitis can cause narrowing and deformity of the second portion of the duodenum, with tapering stenosis, mucosal thickening, and spiculation (Fig. 31-17). A similar appearance involving the postbulbar area can be due to acute cholecystitis (Fig. 31-18).

Fig. 31-17. Chronic pancreatitis with acute exacerbation. The inflammatory mass narrows the second portion of the duodenum and causes marked mucosal edema and spiculation **(arrow).**

Fig. 31-18. Acute cholecystitis causing intense inflammation and narrowing of the adjacent portion of the duodenal sweep **(arrow).** The appearance simulates a malignant process.

Fig. 31-17   **Fig. 31-18**

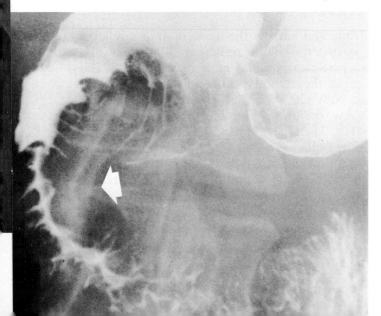

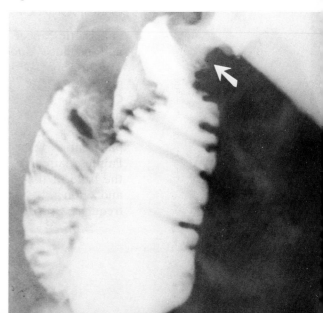

An enlarging pancreatic cancer can exert extrinsic pressure at any point along the duodenal sweep, resulting in a mass impression and "double-contour" effect. As the disease progresses, ulceration, stricture formation, and obstruction can occur. Pancreatic cancers can also involve the stomach, producing a typical indentation defect on the greater curvature of the gastric antrum (antral pad sign).

Differentiation of pancreatic cancer from pancreatitis can be difficult on barium examination. The presence of duodenal mucosal destruction suggests malignancy. However, pancreatic tumors can infiltrate the submucosa and produce stenosis without mucosal destruction (especially in the third portion of the duodenum). In patients with cancer of the head of the pancreas, a combination of tumor infiltration and neuromuscular irritation (wrap-around effect) can produce a fixed, partially obstructing lateral defect in the second portion of the duodenum.

OTHER MALIGNANCIES

Primary neoplasms of the duodenum, as well as metastases, can cause obstructive lesions of the duodenum and proximal duodenal dilatation. Adenocarcinomas, which constitute 80% to 90% of all duodenal malignancies, most commonly arise at or distal to the ampulla of Vater. Tumors in a periampullary location produce extrahepatic jaundice; those arising proximally or distally tend to cause bleeding, ulceration, or obstruction. The radiographic appearance of adenocarcinomas of the duodenum is similar to that associated with tumors of the same cell type arising at any level in the gastrointestinal tract. They most commonly present as annular constricting lesions with overhanging edges, nodular mucosal destruction, and frank ulceration (Fig. 31-22). Primary duodenal sarcomas, often with ulceration, also occur (Fig. 31-23). It is frequently impossible to differentiate primary duodenal malignancy from secondary neoplastic invasion of the duodenum by the extension of tumors arising in the pancreas, gallbladder, or colon.

Much of the duodenum is surrounded by groups of lymph nodes. The descending duodenum is encircled by peripancreatic lymph nodes; celiac and para-aortic nodes lie along the third portion of the duodenum. Metastatic enlargement of these nodes can produce a mass effect on the duodenal lumen with ulceration or obstructive narrowing. In the patient with a stenotic lesion of the third portion of the duodenum and a history of previous abdominal malignancy, the possibility of metastases to lymph nodes must be considered.

INTRAMURAL HEMATOMA

Because the duodenum is the most fixed portion of the small bowel, external blunt trauma predominantly affects this segment. Hemorrhage into the duodenal wall produces a tumorlike intramural mass that can become so large that it obstructs the lumen and results in proximal duodenal dilatation (Fig. 31-24). Intramural duodenal hematomas can also be, secondary to anticoagulant therapy or an abnormal bleeding diathesis.

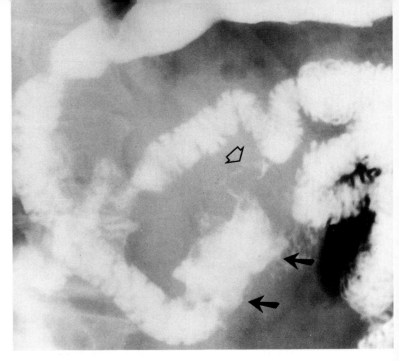

Fig. 31-23. Ulcerated fibrosarcoma of the third portion of the duodenum **(solid arrows)** causing luminal narrowing **(open arrow).**

Fig. 31-24. Intramural duodenal hematoma. This high-grade stenotic lesion **(arrow)** was seen in a young child who had been kicked in the abdomen by his father.

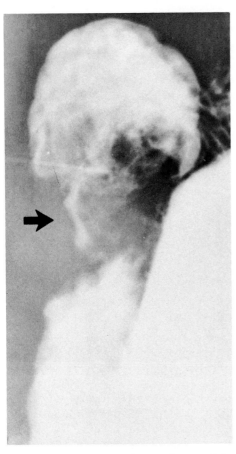

Fig. 31-22. Primary adenocarcinoma of the duodenum. Note the "apple-core" lesion **(arrow),** which is similar to primary carcinoma at other levels of the gastrointestinal tract.

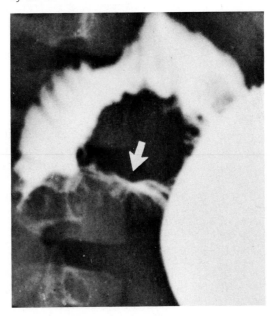

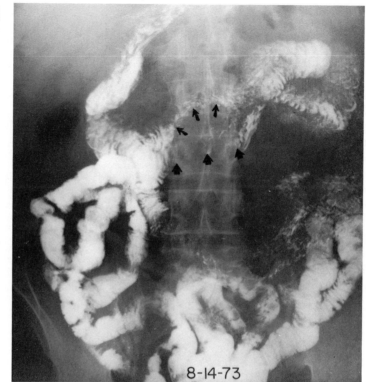

Fig. 31-25. Aorticoduodenal fistula causing extrinsic pressure on the third portion of the duodenum **(large arrows).** A jejunal loop is also slightly displaced **(small arrows).** (Wyatt GM, Rauchway MI, Spitz HB: Roentgen findings in aorto-enteric fistulae. AJR 126:714–722, 1976. Copyright 1976. Reproduced by permission)

Fig. 31-26. Radiation injury. This postbulbar duodenal stricture with irregular mucosa appeared 13 months after irradiation for an angiosarcoma of the right kidney. (Rogers LF, Goldstein HM: Roentgen manifestations of radiation injury to the gastrointestinal tract. Gastrointest Radiol 2:281–291, 1977).

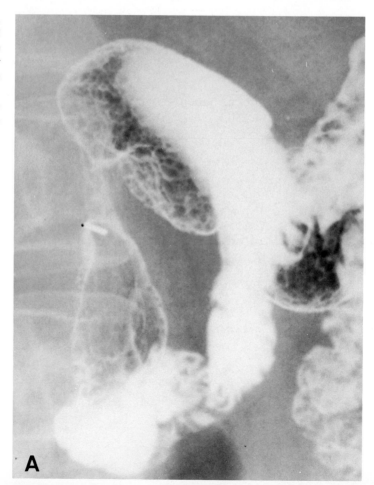

A

AORTICODUODENAL FISTULA

Aorticoduodenal fistula can occur primarily as a complication of abdominal aortic aneurysm or be secondary to placement of a prosthetic Dacron graft. Pressure necrosis of the third portion of the duodenum, which is fixed and apposed to the anterior wall of an aortic aneurysm, can lead to digestion of that wall by enteric secretions and a primary aorticoduodenal fistula. Secondary fistulas result from pseudoaneurysm formation with erosion into the adherent duodenum or dehiscence of the suture line due to infection caused by the leak of intestinal contents through the duodenum, the blood supply of which has been compromised at surgery. Aorticoduodenal fistula is an often fatal condition that presents clinically with abdominal pain, gastrointestinal bleeding, and a palpable, pulsatile mass.

Aorticoduodenal fistulas cause compression or displacement of the third portion of the duodenum by an extrinsic mass (Fig. 31-25). Central ulceration can also occur. On rare occasions, extraluminal contrast tracking along the graft into the paraprosthetic space outlines the wall of the abdominal aorta.

RADIATION INJURY

Duodenal changes can develop following radiation therapy to the upper abdomen. These primarily involve the second portion and vary from ulcerations to smooth strictures (Fig. 31-26).

SUPERIOR MESENTERIC ARTERY SYNDROME

The broad spectrum of conditions producing the superior mesenteric artery syndrome, which is characterized by obstruction of the third portion of the duodenum and proximal dilatation, is discussed in the next section.

BIBLIOGRAPHY

Bayless TM, Kapelowitz RF, Shelley WM et al: Intestinal ulceration: A complication of celiac disease. N Engl J Med 276:996–1002, 1967

Beranbaum SL: Carcinoma of the pancreas: A bidirectional roentgen approach. AJR 96:447–467, 1966

Berdon WE, Baker DH, Bull S et al: Midgut malrotation and volvulus: Which films are most helpful? Radiology 96:375–383, 1970

Eaton SB, Ferrucci JT: Radiology of the Pancreas and Duodenum. Philadelphia, WB Saunders, 1973

Faegenburg D, Bosniak M: Duodenal anomalies in the adult. AJR 88:642–657, 1962

Fonkalsrud EW, DeLorimier AA, Hays DM: Congenital atresia and stenosis of the duodenum: A review compiled from the members of the surgical section of the American Academy of Pediatrics. Pediatrics 43:79–83, 1969

Free EA, Gerald B: Duodenal obstruction in the newborn due to annular pancreas. AJR 103:321–329, 1968

Glazer GM, Margulis AR: Annular pancreas: Etiology and diagnosis using endoscopic retrograde cholangiopancreatography. Radiology 133:303–306, 1979

Hope JW, Gibbons JF: Duodenal obstruction due to annular pancreas with a differential diagnosis of other congenital lesions producing duodenal obstruction. Radiology 63:473–490, 1954

Ladd WE: Congenital obstruction of the duodenum. N Engl J Med 206:277–283, 1932

Lautin EM, Friedman AC: A complicated case of aortoduodenal fistula. Gastrointest Radiol 4:401–404, 1979

Louisy CL, Barton CJ: The radiological diagnosis of *Strongyloides stercoralis* enteritis. Radiology 98:535–541, 1971

McCort JJ: Roentgenographic appearance of metastases to the central lymph nodes of the superior mesenteric artery in carcinoma of the right colon. Radiology 60:641–646, 1953

Nelson SW: Some interesting and unusual manifestations of Crohn's disease ("regional enteritis") of the stomach, duodenum, and small intestine. AJR 107:86–101, 1969

Pratt AD: Current concepts of the obstructing duodenal diaphragm. Radiology 100:637–643, 1971

Simon M, Lerner MA: Duodenal compression by the mesenteric root in acute pancreatitis and inflammatory conditions of the bowel. Radiology 79:75–81, 1962

Thompson WM, Cockrill H, Rice RP: Regional enteritis of the duodenum. AJR 123:252–261, 1975

Wyatt GM, Rauchway MI, Spitz HB: Roentgen findings in aorto-enteric fistulae. AJR 126:714–722, 1976

32

DUODENAL DILATATION (SUPERIOR MESENTERIC ARTERY SYNDROME)

Disease Entities

Normal variant
Congenital small vascular angle or childhood growth spurt
Prolonged bed rest in supine position
  Body cast syndrome
  Whole-body burns
  Surgery
Loss of retroperitoneal fat
Multiple pregnancies with loss of muscle tone
Decreased duodenal peristalsis
  Smooth muscle or neuromuscular junction dysfunction
    Scleroderma
    Dermatomyositis/systemic lupus erythematosus
    Aganglionosis
    Chagas' disease
  Vagus or splanchnic nerve dysfunction
    Surgical or chemical vagotomy
    Neuropathy (diabetes, porphyria, thiamine deficiency)
  Inflammatory disorders
    Pancreatitis
    Cholecystitis
    Peptic ulcer disease
  Trauma
  Altered emotional states
Thickening of the bowel wall or root of the mesentery
  Crohn's disease
  Tuberculous enteritis
  Pancreatitis
  Peptic ulcer disease
  Strongyloidiasis
Metastatic lesions
Exaggerated lumbar lordosis
Abdominal aortic aneurysm
Aorticoduodenal fistula
Chronic idiopathic intestinal pseudo-obstruction

403

The transverse portion of the duodenum lies in a fixed position in a retroperitoneal location. It is situated in a closed compartment bounded anteriorly by the root of the mesentery, which carries the superior mesenteric vessel sheath (artery, vein, nerve), and posteriorly by the aorta and lumbar spine (at the L2-L3 level, where lumbar lordosis is most pronounced). Any factor that compresses or fills this compartment can favor the development of narrowing of the transverse duodenum with proximal duodenal dilatation and stasis (superior mesenteric artery syndrome). Regardless of the underlying cause, the radiographic pattern is similar.

Even in normal persons, there is often a transient delay of barium at the point at which the transverse duodenum crosses the spine (Fig. 32-1). This can be associated with mild, inconstant proximal duodenal dilatation (Fig. 32-2). Casts of the duodenum from cadavers with normal gastrointestinal tracts sometimes demonstrate grooves on the anterior and posterior duodenal walls, most likely secondary to impression by the superior mesenteric artery and aorta, respectively.

NARROWING OF AORTICOMESENTERIC ANGLE

Any process that tends to close the nutcrackerlike jaws of the aortico-mesenteric angle results in some degree of compression of the transverse portion of the duodenum. It is most common in asthenic persons, especially those who have lost substantial weight. This condition can be detected in children who have a congenitally small vascular angle or in children who are growing rapidly without a corresponding gain in weight. Prolonged bed rest or immobilization in the supine position (patients with body casts or whole-body burns or patients who are fixed in a position of hyperextension after spinal injury or surgery) causes

Fig. 32-1. Normal patient. There is a transient delay of barium at the point at which the transverse duodenum crosses the spine **(arrow).**

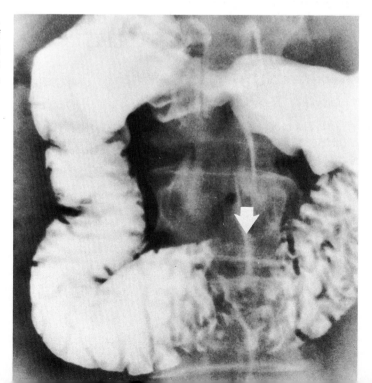

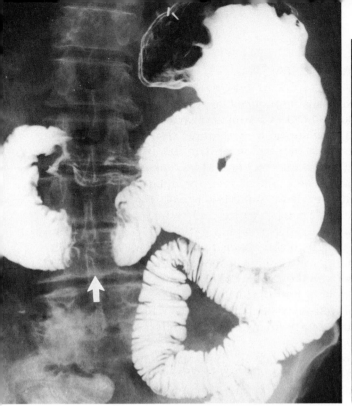

A B

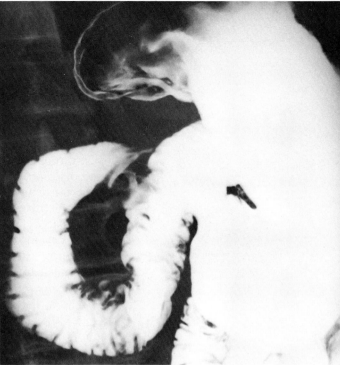

the superior mesenteric artery to fall back and anteriorly compress the transverse duodenum, resulting in relative duodenal obstruction (Fig. 32-3). In patients who lose weight and retroperitoneal fat because of a debilitating illness, the increased dragging effect of the mesenteric root narrows the aorticomesenteric compartment. Similary, conditions leading to relaxation of abdominal wall musculature (*e.g.,* multiple pregnancies) can obstruct the transverse duodenum.

Fig. 32-2. Normal patient. **(A)** A frontal projection shows apparent obstruction of the third portion of the duodenum **(arrow),** suggesting the superior mesenteric artery syndrome. **(B)** A right anterior oblique view obtained slightly later shows the duodenal sweep to be entirely normal, without any evidence of organic obstruction.

Fig. 32-3. Relative duodenal obstruction **(arrow)** in a bed-ridden patient who sustained a severe burn several weeks earlier.

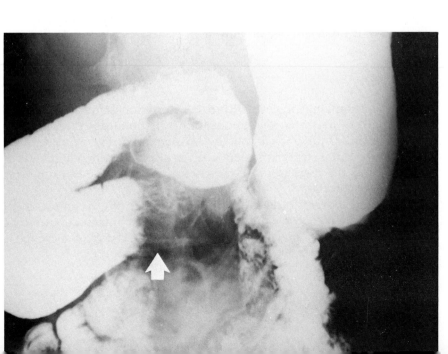

In patients with diseases causing reduced duodenal peristaltic activity, especially when they are placed in a supine position, the combination of lumbar spine, aorta, and superior mesenteric artery can constitute enough of a barrier to cause significant obstruction of the transverse duodenum. Muscular atrophy and intramural fibrosis in patients with scleroderma produce atony and dilatation of the duodenum as part of a diffuse process involving all of the small bowel (Fig. 32-4). Other collagen diseases, such as dermatomyositis and systemic lupus erythematosus, can cause the same radiographic pattern (Fig. 32-5). Aganglionosis, the absence of cells in Auerbach's plexus, is associated with a similar histologic finding in the distal esophagus and rectum and can result in pronounced proximal duodenal dilatation. In Chagas' disease, inflammatory destruction of intramural autonomic plexuses due to trypanosomes can lead to generalized gastrointestinal aperistalsis and dilatation. This most frequently involves the esophagus and colon but can also affect the duodenum.

As in other portions of the bowel, dysfunction of the vagus or splanchnic nerves can result in dilatation of the duodenum and the radiographic appearance of the superior mesenteric artery syndrome. This can occur after surgical vagotomy for peptic disease or following chemical vagotomy due to ingestion of such drugs as atropine, morphine, or Lomotil (diphenoxylate). Disordered duodenal motility with dilatation can also be seen in patients with neuropathies secondary to diabetes, porphyria, and thiamine deficiency.

Adynamic ileus caused by any acute upper abdominal inflammatory process can affect the duodenum and cause pronounced dilatation proximal to the midline barrier of normal structures (spine, aorta, superior mesenteric artery). This duodenal atony is seen in patients with acute pancreatitis, cholecystitis, and peptic ulcer disease. Adynamic ileus of the duodenum (as well as of the stomach) can occur in patients who have sustained severe trauma or acute burns. A controversial concept is the possible relationship of duodenal ileus to hysterical syndromes or other abnormal emotional states.

OTHER CAUSES

Any space-occupying process within the aorticomesenteric angle can also compress the transverse duodenum. Inflammatory thickening of the bowel wall or mesenteric root (*e.g.*, pancreatitis [Fig. 32-6], Crohn's disease, tuberculous enteritis, peptic ulcer disease, strongyloidiasis) or metastases to the mesentery or mesenteric nodes can lead to relative duodenal obstruction.

Increased lumbar lordosis diminishes the size of the compartment occupied by the transverse duodenum. This forces the duodenum to lie on a slightly convex surface, leading to a greater risk of mesenteric

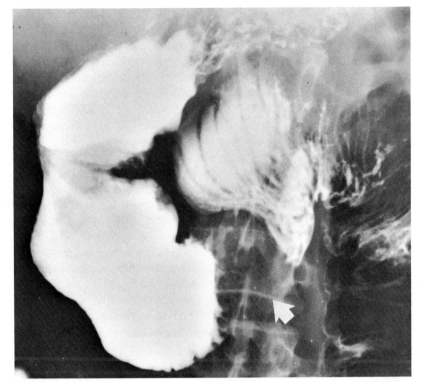

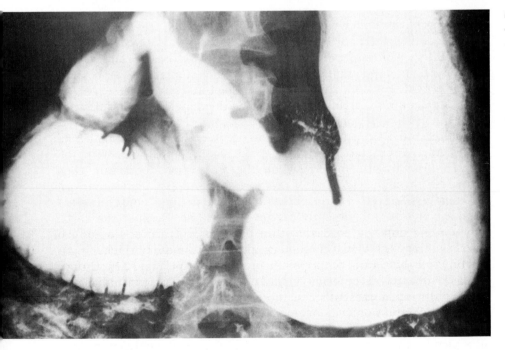

Fig. 32-4. Scleroderma. There is severe atony and dilatation of the duodenum proximal to the aorticomesenteric angle **(arrow)**.

Fig. 32-5. Systemic lupus erythematosus. Atony and dilatation of the proximal duodenum are indistinguishable from the pattern in scleroderma.

compression. A similar mechanism can occur when the transverse duodenum lies in a low position over the 4th lumbar vertebra.

A rare cause of relative obstruction of the transverse duodenum is an abdominal aortic aneurysm (Fig. 32-7). This etiology should be suspected whenever duodenal stasis first occurs in an elderly patient with arteriosclerosis, especially if plain radiographs demonstrate calcification of a dilated aorta in this region. After reconstructive arterial surgery, aorticoduodenal fistulas can cause partial obstruction of the third portion of the duodenum.

Severe dilatation of the duodenum mimicking the superior mesenteric artery syndrome has been described as the first manifestation of chronic idiopathic intestinal pseudo-obstruction (Fig. 32-8). As this disease of unknown etiology progresses, more segments of the small bowel become dilated; dilatation can eventually involve the colon and stomach.

Symptoms attributed to the superior mesenteric artery syndrome include epigastric or periumbilical pain, which typically occurs several hours after eating and is relieved by a prone or knee–chest position. Bilious vomiting is also a common complaint. High-grade obstruction of the transverse duodenum can lead to emaciation and nutritional deficiency, with such striking loss of weight that a provisional diagnosis of malignancy is made.

RADIOGRAPHIC FINDINGS

Regardless of the underlying pathologic mechanism, the radiographic appearance is almost identical in all patients with the superior mesenteric artery syndrome. Pronounced dilatation of the first and second portions of the duodenum (and frequently the stomach) is associated with a vertical, linear extrinsic pressure defect in the transverse portion of the duodenum overlying the spine. The duodenal mucosal folds are intact but compressed. For the superior mesenteric artery syndrome to be differentiated from an organic obstruction, the patient should be turned to a prone, left decubitus, or knee–chest position. With the traction drag by the mesentery on the transverse duodenum thus decreased (through widening of the aorticomesenteric angle), barium can usually be seen to promptly pass the "obstruction," confirming the diagnosis of superior mesenteric artery syndrome. Because the aorticomesenteric angle is not reduced in patients with thickening of the bowel wall or root of the mesentery, postural change provides much less relief of duodenal compression. In these conditions, relative duodenal obstruction is primarily related to the clinical activity of the inflammatory process. If there is no emptying of the duodenum with change in position or evidence of intra-abdominal inflammation, the possibility of an organic duodenal obstruction (*e.g.*, metastases to the mesentery, direct spread of carcinoma of the body of the pancreas) must be excluded.

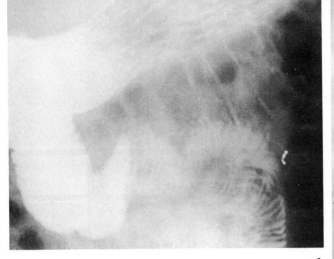

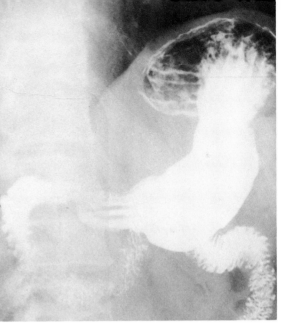

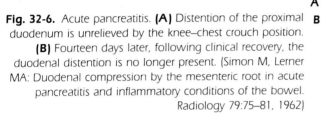

A

B

Fig. 32-6. Acute pancreatitis. **(A)** Distention of the proximal duodenum is unrelieved by the knee–chest crouch position. **(B)** Fourteen days later, following clinical recovery, the duodenal distention is no longer present. (Simon M, Lerner MA: Duodenal compression by the mesenteric root in acute pancreatitis and inflammatory conditions of the bowel. Radiology 79:75–81, 1962)

Fig. 32-7. Abdominal aortic aneurysm. **(A)** Relative obstruction of the third portion of the duodenum **(arrow)** with proximal dilatation. **(B)** A plain radiograph demonstrates calcification of the abdominal aortic aneurysm **(arrows),** which is causing the extrinsic impression and partial obstruction.

A B

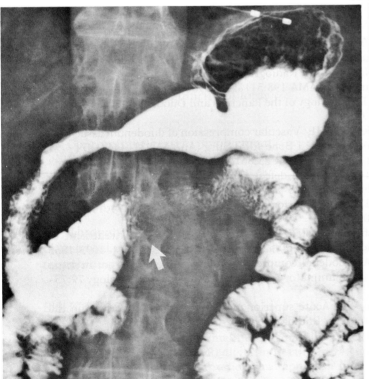

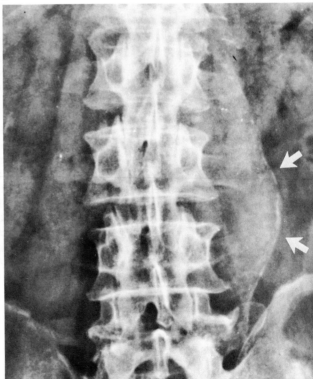

33

SMALL BOWEL OBSTRUCTION

Mechanical small bowel obstruction occurs whenever there is an intrinsic or extrinsic blockage of the normal flow of bowel contents. Without medical therapy, complete small bowel obstruction has about a 60% mortality rate. Prompt diagnosis and institution of optimal treatment, as well as recognition of the importance of replacing fluid and electrolytes and maintaining an adequate circulating blood volume, can reduce the mortality rate to less than 5%. The classic symptoms of small bowel obstruction include crampy abdominal pain, bloating, nausea, vomiting, and decreased stool output. Diffuse abdominal tenderness and peritoneal signs are common. An abdominal examination usually reveals distention and increased, high-pitched bowel sounds with rushes and tinkles. However, it is extremely important to remember that the typical clinical signs and symptoms can be absent, even in a high-grade small bowel obstruction. In patients with fluid-filled loops containing little or no gas, there can be little abdominal distention; bowel sounds can be normal or diminished because there are no gas bubbles to gurgle. Absence of bowel sounds late in the course of obstruction can be due to the inability of the fatigued bowel to contract effectively or to associated peritonitis.

RADIOGRAPHIC FINDINGS

Distended loops of small bowel containing gas and fluid can usually be recognized within 3 hr to 5 hr of the onset of complete obstruction. Almost all gas proximal to a small bowel obstruction represents swallowed air. In the upright or lateral decubitus view, the interface between gas and fluid forms a straight horizontal margin (Fig. 33-1). Gas–fluid levels are occasionally present normally. However, more than two gas–fluid levels in the small bowel is generally considered to be   **413**

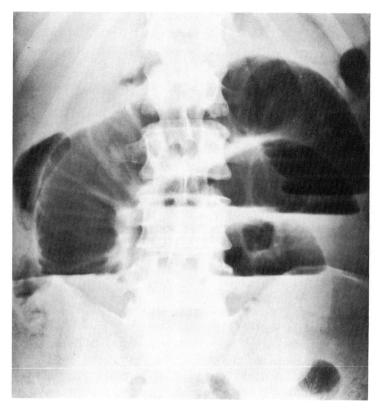

Fig. 33-1. Small bowel obstruction. The interfaces between gas and fluid form straight horizontal margins within small bowel loops proximal to the obstruction.

Fig. 33-2. Small bowel obstruction. Gas–fluid levels are at different heights within the same loop **(arrows).**

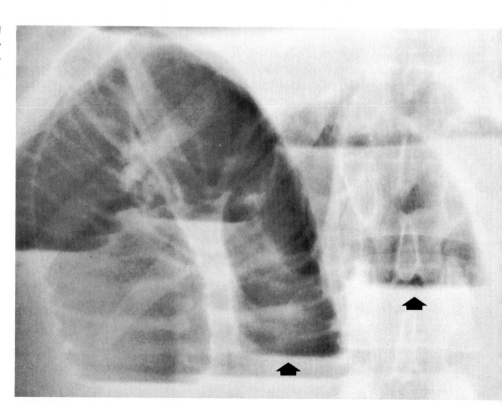

abnormal. The presence of gas–fluid levels at different heights in the same loop has traditionally been considered excellent evidence for mechanical obstruction (Fig. 33-2). Unfortunately, this pattern can also be demonstrated in some patients with adynamic ileus rather than mechanical obstruction (Fig. 33-3).

Abdominal radiographs in patients with mechanical obstruction usually demonstrate large quantities of gas within distended loops of bowel (Fig. 33-4). The small bowel is capable of huge distention and can become so enlarged as to be almost indistinguishable from colon. To make the critical differentiation between small and large bowel obstruction, it is essential to determine which loops of bowel contain abnormally large amounts of gas. Small bowel loops generally occupy the more central portion of the abdomen, whereas colonic loops are positioned laterally around the periphery of the abdomen or inferiorly in the pelvis (Fig. 33-5). Gas within the lumen of the small bowel outlines the valvulae conniventes, which completely encircle the bowel (Fig. 33-6). In contrast, colonic haustral markings occupy only a portion of the transverse diameter of the bowel. Valvulae conniventes are finer and closer together than colonic haustra. In the jejunum, simple distention, no matter how severe, will not completely efface these mucosal folds.

Fig. 33-3. Adynamic ileus in a patient with acute appendicitis. Although mechanical obstruction was suggested by gas–fluid levels at different heights in the same loop, no evidence of obstruction was found at surgery.

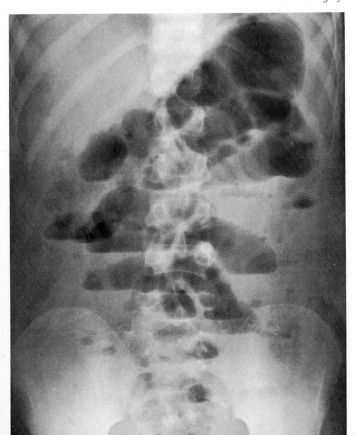

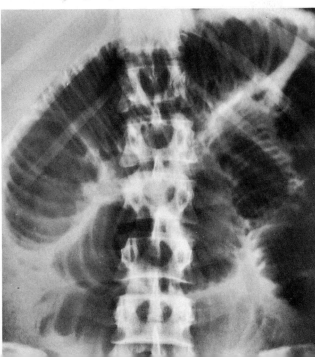

Fig. 33-4. Small bowel obstruction. Gas-filled loops of small bowel are greatly distended.

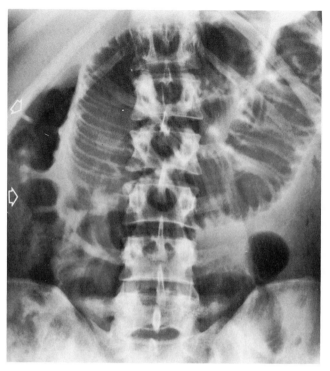

Fig. 33-5. Small bowel obstruction. The dilated loops of small bowel occupy the central portion of the abdomen, with the nondilated cecum and ascending colon positioned laterally around the periphery of the abdomen **(arrows).**

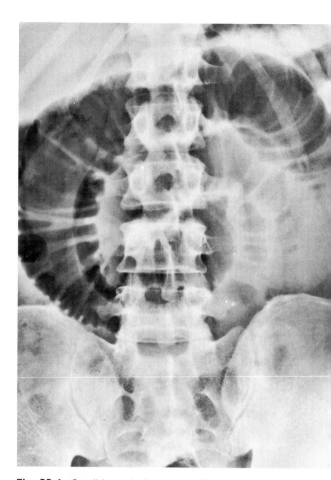

Fig. 33-6. Small bowel obstruction. Gas within the lumen of the bowel outlines the valvulae conniventes, which completely encircle the bowel.

Fig. 33-7. Jejunal obstruction. The few dilated loops of small bowel are located in the left upper abdomen.

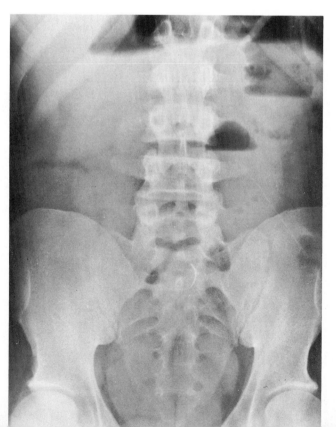

The site of obstruction can usually be predicted with considerable accuracy if the number and position of dilated bowel loops are analyzed. The presence of a few dilated loops of small bowel located high in the abdomen (in the center or slightly to the left) indicates an obstruction in the distal duodenum or jejunum (Fig. 33-7). Involvement of more small bowel loops suggests a lower obstruction (Fig. 33-8). As additional loops are affected, they appear to be placed one above the other, upward and to the left, producing a characteristic "stepladder" appearance (Fig. 33-9). This inclined direction is due to fixation of the mesentery, which extends from the right iliac fossa to the upper pole of the left kidney. The point of obstruction is always distal to the lowest loop of dilated bowel.

In patients with complete mechanical small bowel obstruction, little or no gas is found in the colon (Fig. 33-10). This is a valuable differential point between mechanical obstruction and adynamic ileus, in which gas is seen within distended loops throughout the bowel. Small amounts of gas or fecal accumulations may be present in the colon if an examination is performed within the first few hours of the onset of symptoms. The presence of gas in the colon in the late stages of a complete small bowel obstruction can be the result of putrefaction or represent air introduced during administration of an enema. In patients with an incomplete small bowel obstruction, some gas can pass into the colon, though the caliber of the distended small bowel will be far larger than the normal or decreased width of the colon. The presence of large amounts of gas in the colon effectively eliminates the diagnosis of small bowel obstruction.

Fig. 33-8. Low small bowel obstruction. The involvement of multiple small bowel loops extends to the right lower quadrant. **(A)** Supine and **(B)** upright views.

A B

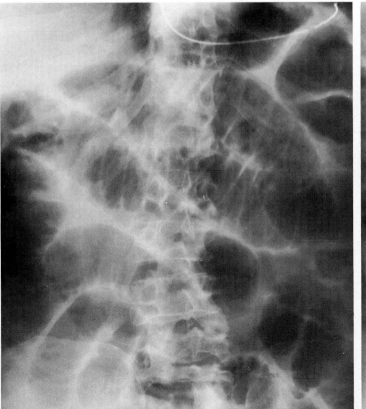
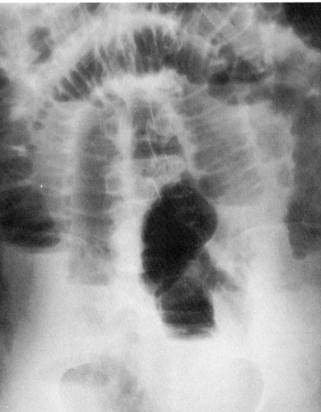

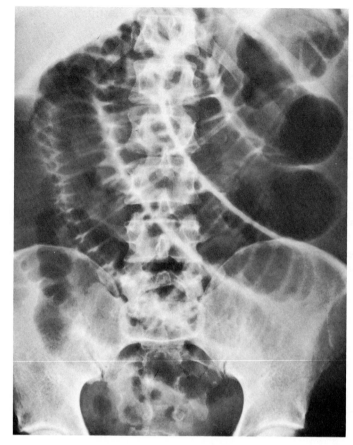

Fig. 33-9. Low small bowel obstruction. The dilated loops of gas-filled bowel appear to be placed one above the other, upward and to the left, producing a characteristic stepladder appearance.

Fig. 33-10. Small bowel obstruction. **(A)** Supine and **(B)** upright views demonstrate large amounts of gas in dilated loops of small bowel but only a single, small collection of gas **(arrow)** in the colon.

A B

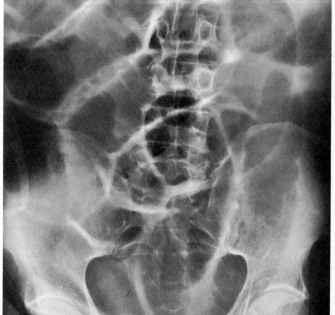

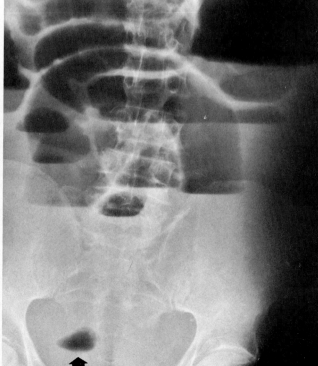

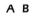

An analysis of the position and amount of abdominal gas can be difficult to make on a single examination; serial observations are often extremely valuable. If gas-filled loops are the result of obstruction, the amount of intraluminal gas and the degree of bowel distention will increase rapidly over several hours.

Small amounts of gas in obstructed loops of bowel can produce the characteristic "string-of-beads" appearance of small gas bubbles in an oblique line (Fig. 33-11). This sign apparently depends on a combination of fluid-filled bowel and peristaltic hyperactivity. Although often considered diagnostic of mechanical obstruction, the string-of-beads sign occasionally appears in adynamic ileus secondary to inflammatory disease.

The bowel proximal to an obstruction can contain no gas but be completely filled with fluid (Fig. 33-12). This pattern is seen in patients who swallow little air or have it removed by effective gastric suction. Large quantities of fluid produce sausage-shaped water-density shadows that can be difficult to diagnose. This pseudotumor, consisting of a large soft-tissue density combined with gaseous distention of the intestine proximal to it, is very likely to represent a strangulation obstruction.

CONTRAST EXAMINATION

Plain abdominal radiographs are occasionally not sufficient for a distinction to be made between small and large bowel obstruction. In these instances, a contrast examination is required. A carefully performed barium enema will document or eliminate the possibility of large bowel obstruction. If it is necessary to determine the precise site of small bowel obstruction, barium can be administered in either a

Fig. 33-11. Small bowel obstruction. Two examples of the string-of-beads appearance (arrows).

A B

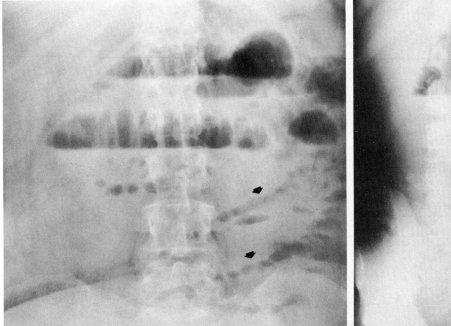
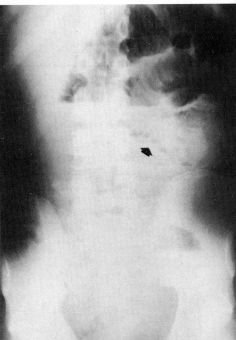

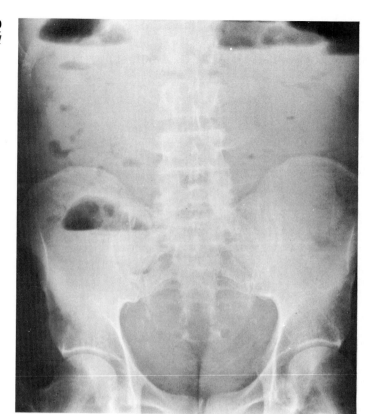

Fig. 33-12. Distal small bowel obstruction. Most of the loops of small bowel proximal to the point of obstruction are filled with fluid and contain only a very small amount of gas.

Fig. 33-13. Antegrade administration of barium demonstrating the precise site of a small bowel obstruction. A radiolucent gallstone **(arrow)** is causing the distal ileal obstruction.

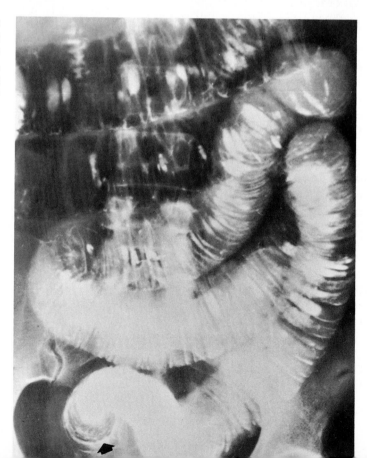

retrograde or an antegrade manner. A retrograde examination of the small bowel can be successfully performed in about 90% of patients. Radiographs of the small bowel can be obtained once the colon is emptied. Oral barium, *not* water-soluble agents, is the most effective contrast for demonstrating the site of small bowel obstruction. The large amount of fluid proximal to a small bowel obstruction keeps the mixture fluid, so that the trapped barium does not harden or increase the degree of obstruction. Barium is far superior to water-soluble agents in evaluating a small bowel obstruction. The density of barium permits visualization far into the intestine (Fig. 33-13), unlike aqueous agents, which are lost to sight because of dilution and absorption. In addition, the problem of electrolyte imbalance due to the hyperosmolality of water-soluble contrast agents may be significant. However, it is important to remember that oral barium should not be used unless the colon has been excluded as the site of mechanical obstruction; the piling up of hardened barium proximal to a distal colonic obstruction entails some risk. Obviously, if plain radiographs clearly demonstrate a mechanical small bowel obstruction, any contrast examination is superfluous.

STRANGULATED OBSTRUCTION

Strangulation of bowel refers to interference with the blood supply associated with an obstruction that is not necessarily complete. In a closed-loop obstruction, both the afferent and the efferent limbs of a loop of bowel become obstructed. Examples of this type of obstruction include volvulus, incarcerated hernia, and loops of small bowel trapped by an adhesive band or passing through an abnormal loop in the mesentery. This is a clinically dangerous form of obstruction, since the continuous outpouring of fluid into the enclosed space can raise the intraluminal pressure and rapidly lead to occlusion of the blood supply to that segment of bowel. Because venous pressure is normally lower than arterial pressure, blockage of venous outflow from the strangulated segment occurs before obstruction of the mesenteric arterial supply. Ischemia can rapidly cause necrosis of the bowel with sepsis, peritonitis, and a potentially fatal outcome.

Strangulation of the bowel can lead to other serious complications. High-grade small bowel obstruction results in an enormous increase in the bacterial population in the stagnant, obstructed segment. Because there is no absorption from this distended bowel, the bacteria-laden fluid within the obstructed segment is of little danger to the patient. If strangulation leads to frank hemorrhagic infarction and gangrenous bowel, intestinal contents can pass into the peritoneal cavity even if no gross perforation is evident. Bacteria can then become absorbed into the systemic circulation and cause severe toxicity and a fatal outcome. Severe hemorrhage into the lumen of the bowel, bowel wall, and peritoneal cavity can be fatal depending on the length of the strangulated segment.

Strangulation of an obstructed loop of small bowel is often difficult to diagnose radiographically. Several signs, though not pathognomonic of strangulated obstruction, are found often enough with strangulation to be an indication for immediate therapy.

An obstructed closed loop bent on itself assumes the shape of a coffee bean, the doubled width of the apposed bowel walls resembling the cleft of the bean. The points of fixation and the length of the involved segment determine whether the loop will bend on itself. Additional evidence of strangulation is a bowel wall that is smooth and featureless because of flattening of the valvulae by edema or hemorrhage. A similar appearance can be seen in the twisted portion of the colon in sigmoid volvulus.

The involved segment of bowel in a closed-loop obstruction is usually filled with fluid and presents radiographically as a tumorlike mass of water density (Fig. 33-14). The outline of this pseudotumor is easier to detect if there is gas distention of bowel above the obstruction than if there are no gas-distended loops. The pseudotumor sign must be differentiated from the fluid-filled loops that are seen in simple mechanical obstruction. In closed-loop obstruction, the pseudotumor sign reflects a loop that is fixed and remains in the same position on multiple projections. This is probably due to the combination of fixation of the bowel loop at both ends and vascular compromise, which prevents the normal tendency of bowel to change configuration and position. When an abdominal mass is apparent radiographically but cannot be palpated, the radiologist must be alerted to the possibility of a strangulated loop of bowel.

The absence of gas proximal to a strangulating obstruction sometimes results in a normal-appearing abdomen on plain radiographs. In

Fig. 33-14. Pseudotumor. **(A)** Supine film showing fluid-filled loops as a tumorlike density in the midabdomen with a polycyclic outline indenting adjacent gas-containing loops **(arrows)**. **(B)** Upright film showing fluid levels in the pseudotumor **(arrows)**. (Bryk D: Strangulating obstruction of the bowel: A reevaluation of radiographic criteria. AJR 130:835–843, 1978. Copyright 1978. Reproduced by permission)

A B

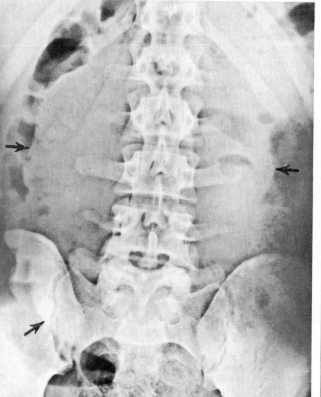 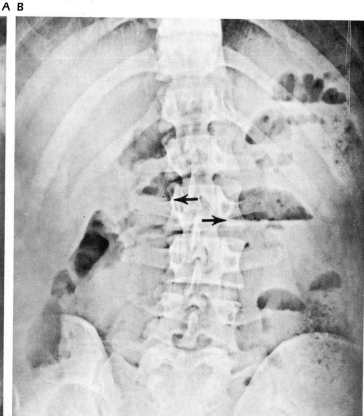

the patient with clinical signs of obstruction, a film of the abdomen showing no abnormality should alert the radiologist to search very closely for subtle signs of strangulation.

Complications of strangulation obstruction can be detected radiographically. Exudate and free fluid in the peritoneal cavity can cause separation of adjacent loops of bowel and shifting fluid density in the abdomen and pelvis. Frank perforation produces free gas, which can be demonstrated on upright or lateral decubitus views. If necrosis develops, gas can be found in the wall of the involved loop of bowel or in the portal venous system.

CAUSES OF SMALL BOWEL OBSTRUCTION

Extrinsic bowel lesions
  Adhesions
    Previous surgery
    Previous peritonitis
  Hernias
    External
    Internal
  Extrinsic masses
    Neoplasm
    Abscess
  Volvulus
  Congenital bands
Luminal occlusion
  Tumor
  Gallstone
  Foreign body
Bezoar
Intussusception
Meconium ileus
Intrinsic lesions of the bowel wall
  Strictures
    Neoplastic
    Inflammatory
    Chemical
    Anastomotic
    Radiation-induced
    Amyloid
  Vascular insufficiency
    Arterial occlusion
    Venous occlusion
  Congenital atresia or stenosis

EXTRINSIC BOWEL LESIONS

Fibrous adhesions caused by previous surgery or peritonitis account for almost 75% of all small bowel obstructions (Fig. 33-15). Because the right lower quadrant and pelvis are the site of most abdominal inflammatory processes and a majority of operative procedures, small bowel obstructions due to adhesions most frequently occur in the ileum. In patients with mechanical obstruction, the abdomen should be examined for evidence of surgical scars. Adhesions can produce obstruction by kinking or angulating bowel loops or by forming bands of tissue that compress the bowel.

External hernias (inguinal, femoral, umbilical, incisional) are the second most frequent cause of mechanical small bowel obstruction (Fig. 33-16). Indeed, the risk of intestinal obstruction is a major reason for the decision to electively repair external hernias. The inguinal and obturator foramen areas should always be closely evaluated on abdominal radiographs of patients with mechanical small bowel obstruction. Greater soft-tissue density on one side than the other or tapering of a bowel loop toward the groin should suggest an inguinal or femoral hernia as the underlying cause.

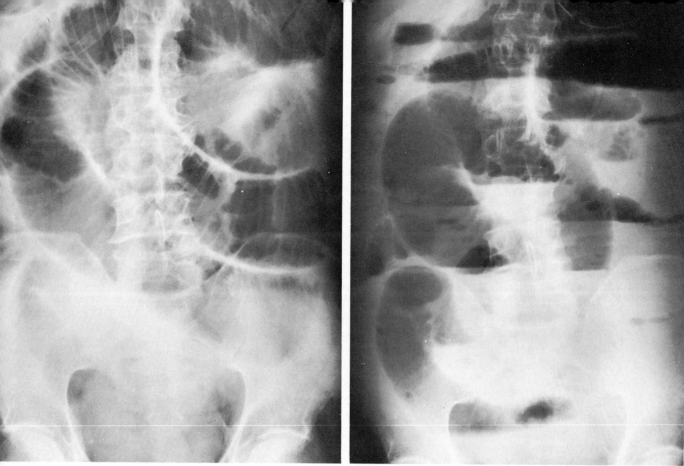

Fig. 33-15. Small bowel obstruction due to adhesions from previous surgery. **(A)** Supine and **(B)** upright views.

A B

Fig. 33-16. Small bowel obstruction caused by an inguinal hernia in a child.

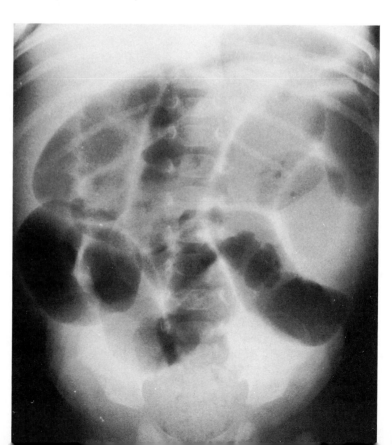

Internal hernias result from congenital abnormalities or surgical defects within the mesentery. If a loop of small bowel is trapped within the mesenteric defect, obstruction can result. More than half of all internal abdominal hernias are paraduodenal, mostly on the left. In this condition, small bowel loops are packed together and displaced under the transverse colon to the left of the midline. In the much less common herniation of small bowel through the foramen of Winslow, abnormal loops are seen along the lesser curvature medial and posterior to the stomach.

Neoplasms (Fig. 33-17) or inflammatory disease (Fig. 33-18) involving the bowel wall or mesentery can cause extrinsic compression and small bowel obstruction. In small intestinal volvulus, anomalies of the mesentery with defective fixation of bowel permit abnormal rotation. Twisting of the bowel about itself results in kinking and mechanical obstruction, frequently with occlusion of the blood supply to that intestinal segment. Another type of volvulus occurs when a segment of the intestine is fixed by adhesions and thus acts as a pivot for other portions of the small bowel to rotate about. In children, congenital fibrous bands are a not uncommon cause of extrinsic mechanical small bowel obstruction.

LUMINAL OCCLUSION

Large polypoid tumors, either benign or malignant, can occlude the bowel lumen and produce small bowel obstruction. Gallstones, foreign bodies, and bezoars can obstruct the small bowel if they are sufficiently large to be trapped and block the lumen. The combination of small bowel obstruction and gas in the biliary tree from a cholecystoenteric

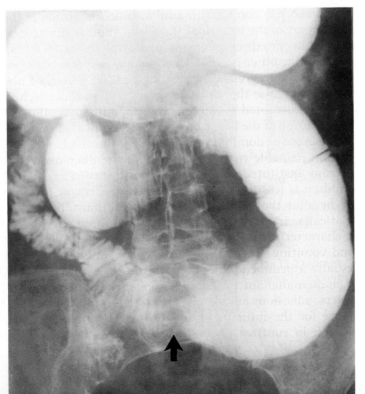

Fig. 33-17. Small bowel obstruction due to carcinoma of the jejunum. Antegrade administration of barium shows pronounced dilatation of the duodenum and proximal jejunum to the level of the annular constricting tumor **(arrow).**

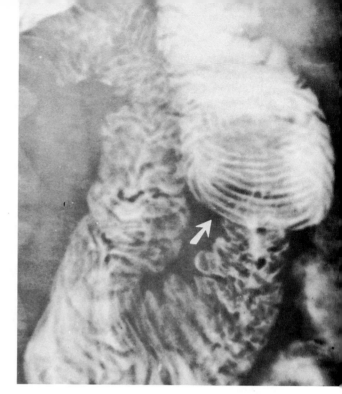

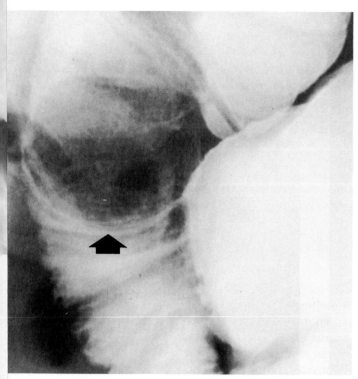

Fig. 33-22. Intermittent small bowel obstruction caused by an inverting Meckel's diverticulum. The Meckel's diverticulum presents as a large filling defect in the distal ileum **(arrow)**.

Fig. 33-23. Small bowel obstruction caused by a jujunojejunal intussusception. Note the characteristic coiled-spring appearance **(arrow)**.

Fig. 33-24. Meconium ileus causing small bowel obstruction.

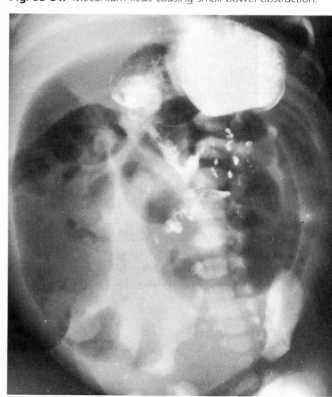

always occur without any apparent anatomic etiology. Radiographically, an intussusception produces the classic coiled-spring appearance of barium trapped between the intussusceptum and surrounding portions of bowel (Fig. 33-23).

Meconium Ileus

Meconium ileus is a cause of distal small bowel obstruction in infants, in whom the thick and sticky meconium cannot be readily propelled through the bowel (Fig. 33-24). The excessive viscidity of the meconium is due to the absence of normal pancreatic and intestinal gland secretions during fetal life. Meconium ileus is frequently associated with fibrocystic disease of the pancreas (mucoviscidosis). The unusually viscid intestinal contents in infants with meconium ileus present radiographically as a bubbly or frothy pattern superimposed on numerous dilated loops of small bowel. On barium enema examination, the colon is seen to have a very small caliber (microcolon), since it has not been used during fetal life.

INTRINSIC LESIONS OF THE BOWEL WALL

Strictures due to intrinsic abnormalities of the bowel wall can produce small bowel obstruction. Such strictures can be caused by constricting primary or metastatic neoplasms, or by inflammatory processes, such as Crohn's disease, tuberculous enteritis, and parasitic infections. Unusual causes include chemical irritation, such as from enteric-coated potassium chloride tablets, which produce ulceration and subsequent fibrosis; postoperative strictures at the level of previous small bowel anastomosis; complications of radiation therapy; and massive deposition of amyloid.

Intestinal ischemia, whether arterial or venous, can heal with intense fibrosis, which may lead to stenosis and small bowel obstruction. Intramural hematomas, due to either abdominal trauma or complications of anticoagulant therapy, can be large enough to occlude the intestinal lumen.

Congenital Atresia or Stenosis

Congenital jejunal (Fig. 33-25) or ileal (Fig. 33-26) atresia or stenosis is a major cause of mechanical small bowel obstruction in infants and young children. In children with obstruction of the jejunum or proximal ileum, distention of the proximal small bowel makes the diagnosis readily apparent on plain radiographs. In jejunal atresia, the characteristic "triple bubble" sign (stomach, duodenum, proximal jejunum) can often be demonstrated (Fig. 33-27). With lower ileal obstruction, on the other hand, it may be difficult to determine whether the dilated intestinal loops seen on plain radiographs represent large or small bowel. A barium enema may be necessary for this differentiation to be made.

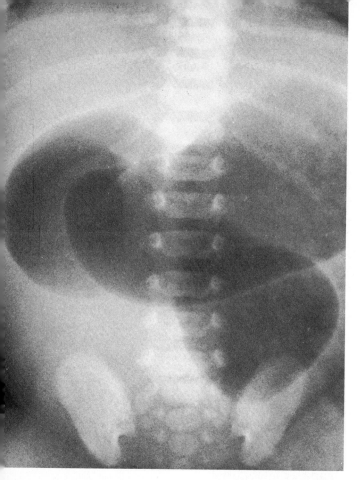

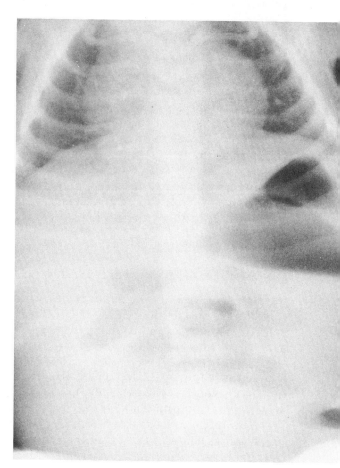

Fig. 33-25. Jejunal atresia. Dilatation of only proximal small bowel loops indicates a jejunal lesion.

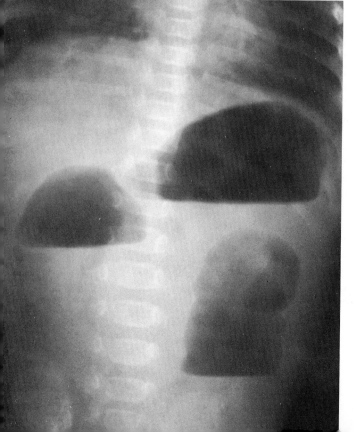

Fig. 33-26. Ileal atresia. Dilated loops of gas- and fluid-filled small bowel extend to the left lower quadrant.

Fig. 33-27. Jejunal atresia. Note the characteristic triple bubble sign (stomach, duodenum, proximal jejunum).

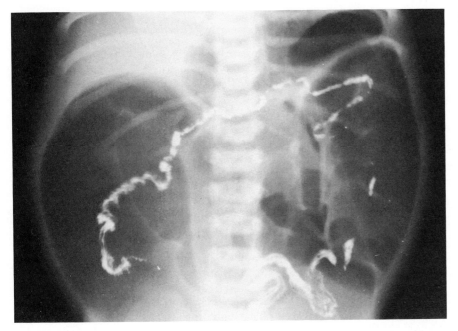

Fig. 33-28. Ileal atresia with microcolon. Barium enema examination shows the colon to be thin and ribbonlike. Note the markedly distended loops of small bowel extending to the point of obstruction in the lower ileum.

In ileal atresia, little or no small bowel contents reach the colon during fetal life, and the colon therefore remains thin and ribbonlike (Fig. 33-28). This microcolon appearance is most pronounced in infants with complete low small bowel obstructions. It is progressively less marked in babies with higher obstructions, in whom some intestinal secretions have reached the colon. Infants with duodenal atresia often have colons of normal caliber.

Meconium peritonitis is a complication of small bowel atresia. This condition develops *in utero* and is presumed to be the result of a proximal perforation that permits meconium to pass into the peritoneal cavity and incite an inflammatory reaction. Meconium peritonitis frequently causes calcifications, which are usually evident at birth. These calcifications can appear as small flecks scattered throughout the abdomen, curvilinear densities on the serosa of the bowel wall, or larger conglomerates of calcium along the inferior surface of the liver or concentrated in the flanks.

Small Bowel

Berdon WE, Baker DH, Santulli TV et al: Microcolon in newborn infants with intestinal obstruction. Radiology 90:878–885, 1968

Bryk D: Functional evaluation of small bowel obstruction by successive abdominal roentgenograms. AJR 116:262–275, 1972

Bryk D: Strangulating obstruction of the bowel. A re-evaluation of radiographic criteria. AJR 130:835–843, 1978

Levin B: Mechanical small bowel obstruction. Semin Roengenol 8:281–297, 1973

Leonidas J, Berdon WE, Baker DH et al: Meconium ileus and its complications. AJR 108:598–609, 1970

Louw JH: Jejunoileal atresia and stenosis. J Pediatr Surg 1:8–23, 1966

Margulis AR, Burhenne HJ: Alimentary Tract Roentgenology. St. Louis, C.V. Mosby, 1973

Miller RE: The technical approach to the acute abdomen. Semin Roentgenol 13:267–275, 1973

Miller RE, Brahme F: Large amounts of orally administered barium for obstruction of the small intestine. Surg Gynecol Obstet 129:1185–1188, 1969

Nelson SW, Christoforidis AJ: The use of barium sulfate suspension in the diagnosis of acute diseases of the small intestine. AJR 104:505–521, 1968

Rigler LG, Pogue WL: Roentgen signs of intestinal necrosis. AJR 94:402–409, 1965

Schwartz SS: The differential diagnosis of intestinal obstruction. Semin Roentgenol 8:323–338, 1973

Shauffer IA, Ferris EJ: The mass sign in primary volvulus of the small intestine in adults. Radiology 84:374–378, 1965

Strauss S, Rubinstein ZJ, Shapira Z et al: Food as a cause of small intestinal obstruction: A report of five cases without previous gastric surgery. Gastrointest Radiol 2:17–20, 1977

Tomchik FS, Wittenberg J, Ottinger LW: The roentgenographic spectrum of bowel infarction. Radiology 96:249–260, 1970

Williams JL: Fluid-filled loops in intestinal obstruction. AJR 88:677–686, 1962

Williams JL: Obstruction of the small intestine. Radiol Clin North Am 2:21–31, 1964

ADYNAMIC ILEUS

34

Adynamic ileus is a common disorder of intestinal motor activity in which fluid and gas do not progress normally through a nonobstructed small and large bowel. A variety of neural, humoral, and metabolic factors can precipitate reflexes that inhibit intestinal motility. The clinical appearance of patients with adynamic ileus varies from minimal symptoms to generalized abdominal distention with a marked decrease in the frequency and intensity of bowel sounds. The radiographic hallmark of adynamic ileus is retention of large amounts of gas and fluid in a dilated small and large bowel (Fig. 34-1). Unlike the appearance in mechanical small bowel obstruction (Fig. 34-2), the entire small and large bowel in adynamic ileus appear almost uniformly dilated with no demonstrable point of obstruction. Concomitant distention of the gas-filled stomach, an infrequent occurrence with mechanical small bowel obstruction, is often seen in patients with adynamic ileus (especially if it is secondary to peritonitis).

CAUSES

Surgical procedure
Peritonitis
Medication
Electrolyte imbalance
Metabolic disorder
Abdominal trauma
Retroperitoneal hemorrhage
Gram-negative sepsis; shock
Renal or ureteral calculus
Acute chest disease (pneumonia, myocardial infarction, congestive heart failure)
Mesenteric vascular occlusion

Fig. 34-1. Adynamic ileus. Large amounts of gas and fluid are retained in loops of dilated small and large bowel. The entire small and large bowel appear almost uniformly dilated with no demonstrable point of obstruction.

Fig. 34-2. Mechanical small bowel obstruction. **(A)** Supine and **(B)** upright views demonstrate only a few dilated, gas-filled loops of small bowel proximal to the point of obstruction. This is unlike the general dilatation of the entire small and large bowel seen in adynamic ileus.

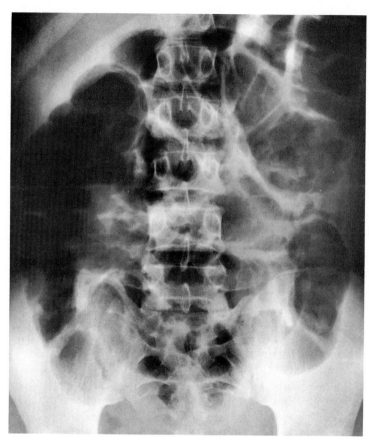

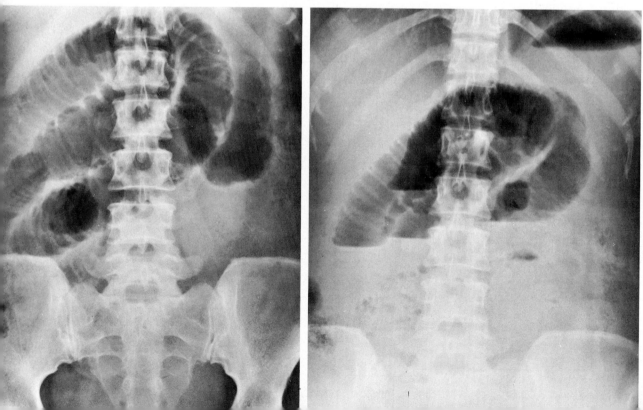

A B

SURGICAL PROCEDURE

Adynamic ileus occurs to some extent in almost every patient who undergoes abdominal surgery (Fig. 34-3). Although the precise etiology is unclear, postoperative ileus may be related to drying of the bowel while it is outside the peritoneal cavity, excessive traction on the bowel or its mesentery, or even mere handling of the bowel during operation. Gas–fluid levels may not be seen in postoperative ileus, even though the bowel loops are markedly dilated. Postoperative adynamic ileus usually resolves spontaneously or clears with the aid of intubation and suction. However, if the ileus progresses and bowel loops become greatly distended, intestinal rupture and pneumoperitoneum can result.

PERITONITIS

Dilated loops of large and small bowel with multiple gas–fluid levels is a common appearance in patients with peritonitis (Fig. 34-4). As the motor activity of the intestine decreases, the gas–fluid levels in each loop tend to stand at the same height, in contrast to mechanical obstruction, in which the gas–fluid levels in the same loop are often seen at different heights. Peritonitis is a likely cause of adynamic ileus whenever there is associated blurring of the mucosal pattern and intestinal edema, evidence of free peritoneal fluid, restricted diaphragmatic movement, or pleural effusion. Even without peritonitis, gastroenteritis or enterocolitis can present as generalized adynamic ileus (Fig. 34-5).

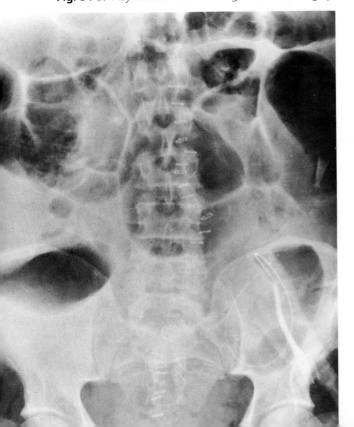

Fig. 34-3. Adynamic ileus following abdominal surgery.

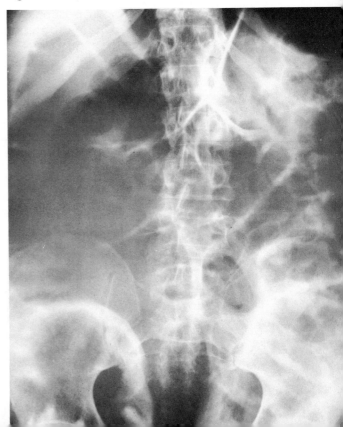

Fig. 34-4. Adynamic ileus in a patient with peritonitis.

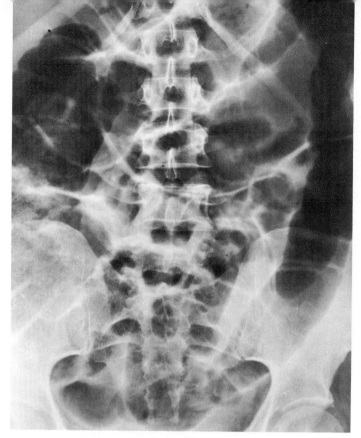

Fig. 34-5. Adynamic ileus in a patient with severe gastroenteritis but without peritonitis.

Some intra-abdominal inflammatory processes can cause both a mechanical block and adynamic ileus. Both conditions may be present at the same time and produce a confusing appearance. For example, an acute periappendiceal abscess can cause true mechanical obstruction in addition to the characteristic adynamic ileus seen in patients with appendicitis. Clinical correlation, serial radiographs, and even a barium enema examination may be necessary to establish the diagnosis.

MEDICATION

Many drugs with muscarinic (atropine-like) effects can produce a radiographic pattern of adynamic ileus (Fig. 34-6). In addition to atropine, this appearance can be caused by morphine, Lomotil (diphenoxylate), L-dopa, barbiturates, and other sympathomimetic agents.

ELECTROLYTE IMBALANCE

Electrolyte imbalances can lead to adynamic ileus by interfering with normal ionic movements during contractions of the smooth muscle of the large and small bowel. Hypokalemia (Fig. 34-7) is the most common electrolyte imbalance to cause this pattern, but adynamic ileus can also be seen in patients with hypochloremia and in persons with calcium or magnesium abnormalities. Hormonal deficits, such as hypothyroid-

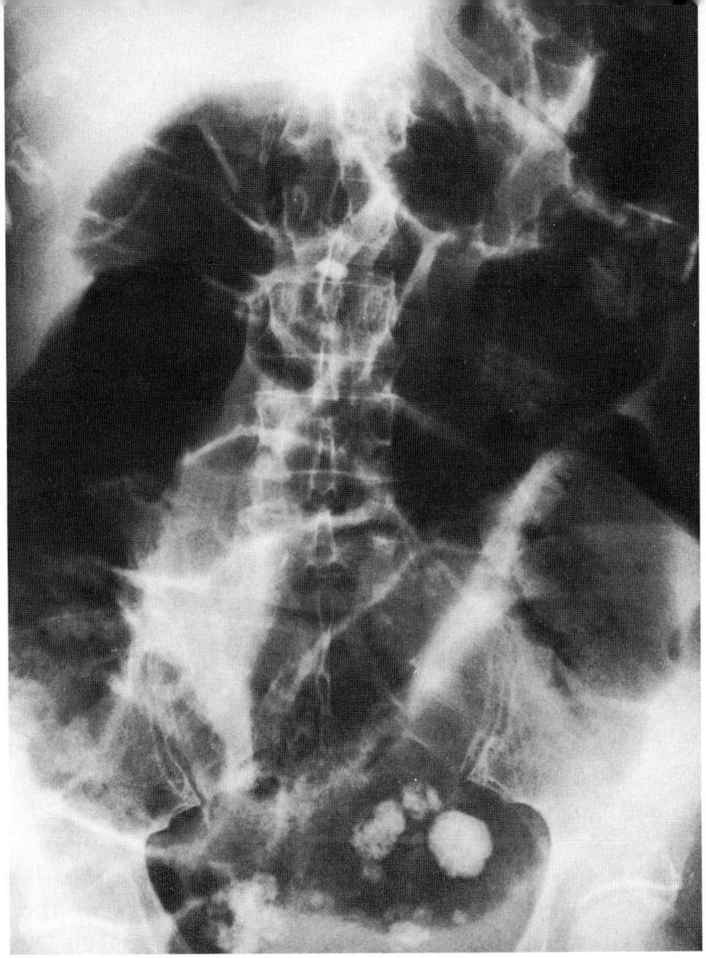

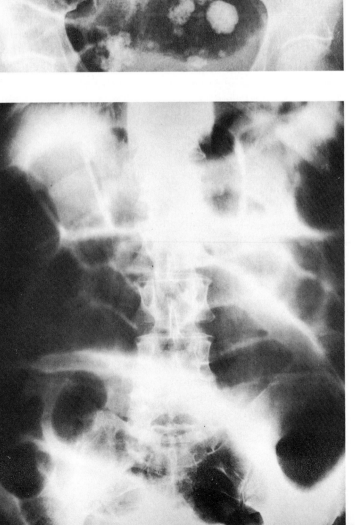

Fig. 34-6. Adynamic ileus in a patient on L-dopa therapy (atropine-like effect).

Fig. 34-7. Adynamic ileus in a patient with severe hypokalemia.

ism and hypoparathyroidism, can present a similar radiographic appearance.

OTHER CAUSES

Abdominal trauma, retroperitoneal hemorrhage, and spinal or pelvic fractures can also result in adynamic ileus. Generalized gram-negative sepsis, shock, and hypoxia are often associated with decreased intestinal motility, as is the colicky pain due to the passage of renal or ureteral stones. Generalized dilatation of the small and large bowel can be seen in patients with acute chest diseases such as pneumonia, myocardial infarction, and congestive heart failure. Vascular occlusion resulting in mesenteric ischemia and infarction often causes segmental or generalized adynamic ileus.

VARIANTS

LOCALIZED ILEUS

An isolated distended loop of small or large bowel reflecting a localized adynamic ileus (sentinel loop) is often associated with an adjacent acute inflammatory process. The portion of the bowel involved can offer a clue to the underlying disease. Localized segments of the jejunum or transverse colon are frequently dilated in patients with acute pancreatitis (Fig. 34-8). Similarly, the hepatic flexure of the colon can be distended in acute cholecystitis (Fig. 34-9), the terminal ileum can be dilated in acute appendicitis, the descending colon can be distended in acute diverticulitis, and dilated loops can be seen along the course of the ureter in acute ureteral colic (Fig. 34-10).

COLONIC ILEUS

Some patients demonstrate selective or disproportionate gaseous distention of the large bowel without an organic obstruction (colonic ileus) (Fig. 34-11). Massive distention of the cecum, which is often horizontally oriented, characteristically dominates the radiographic appearance. There is often much more gas in the right and transverse colon than in the rectum, sigmoid, and descending colon.

Although the pathogenesis of colonic ileus is not known, it is probably related to an imbalance between sympathetic and parasympathetic innervation to the large bowel. Colonic ileus usually accompanies or follows an acute abdominal inflammatory process or abdominal surgery, but it can also occur with any of the etiologic factors associated with adynamic ileus (Figs. 34-12, 34-13).

The clinical presentation of colonic ileus simulates that of mechanical obstruction of the colon. Because colonic ileus usually represents acute dilatation of a previously normal colon, it tends to appear radiographically as pronounced dilatation of part or all of the large

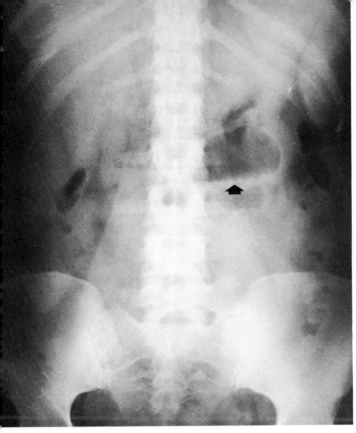

Fig. 34-8. Localized ileus **(arrow)** in a patient with acute pancreatitis.

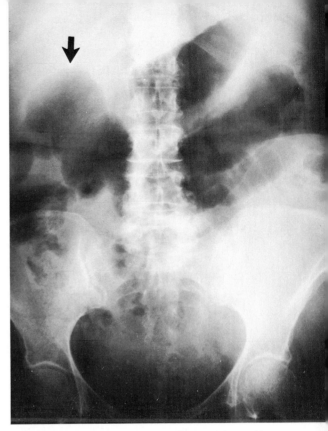

Fig. 34-9. Localized ileus **(arrow)** in a patient with acute cholecystitis.

Fig. 34-10. Localized ileus in a patient with acute ureteral colic. The **arrow** points to the impacted ureteral stone.

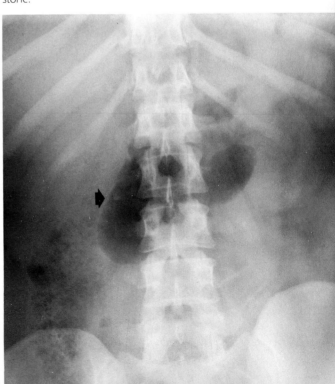

bowel with preserved haustrations, thin, well-defined septae, and smooth inner colonic contours. In colonic obstruction, in contrast, mucosal edema, adherent fecal matter, and secretions result in an accentuation of haustrations with numerous, closely packed septations; loss or shallowness of haustrations; large amounts of fecal retention; thickened, ill-defined, irregular septae; and a ragged inner colonic contour. Nevertheless, it can often be difficult to distinguish between colonic ileus and obstruction on plain abdominal radiographs. A barium enema examination is usually necessary to exclude the possibility of an obstructing lesion.

ADYNAMIC ILEUS SIMULATING MECHANICAL OBSTRUCTION

Disease Entities

Chronic idiopathic intestinal pseudo-obstruction
Pelvic surgery
Urinary retention
Pancreatitis
Acute intermittent porphyria
Ceroidosis
Neonatal adynamic ileus
   Systemic
   Chemical/hormonal
   Abdominal

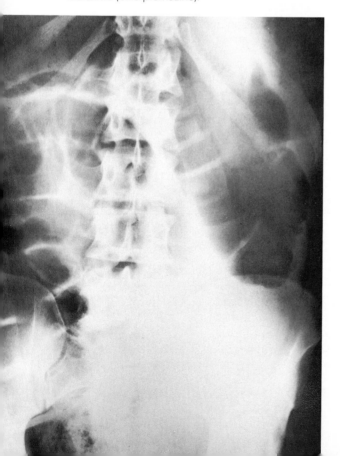

Fig. 34-11. Colonic ileus related to an overdose of Thorazine (chlorpromazine).

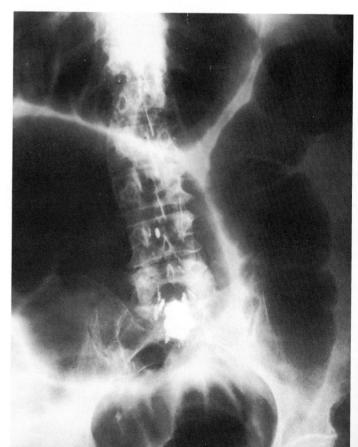

Fig. 34-12. Colonic ileus in a patient with severe diabetes and hypokalemia.

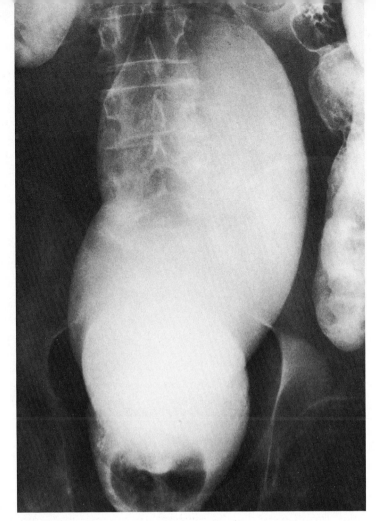

Fig. 34-13. Colonic ileus in a patient on Cogentin (benztropine) therapy. Barium enema examination reveals a massively dilated colon without any point of obstruction.

CHRONIC IDIOPATHIC INTESTINAL PSEUDO-OBSTRUCTION

Chronic idiopathic intestinal pseudo-obstruction is a rare condition in which there is pronounced distention of the bowel (especially the small intestine) mimicking intestinal obstruction without a demonstrable obstructive lesion (Fig. 34-14). A disease of unknown etiology, chronic idiopathic intestinal pseudo-obstruction may be related to an intrinsic smooth muscle lesion or an abnormality of the intramural nerve plexuses. Recognition of the true nature of this nonobstructive condition is essential if the patient is to be prevented from undergoing an unnecessary laparotomy.

PELVIC SURGERY

An unusual type of adynamic ileus simulating reversible small bowel obstruction can develop after transabdominal hysterectomy or other pelvic surgery, especially when the procedure involves manipulation of the small bowel. Typically, the patient becomes distended and begins

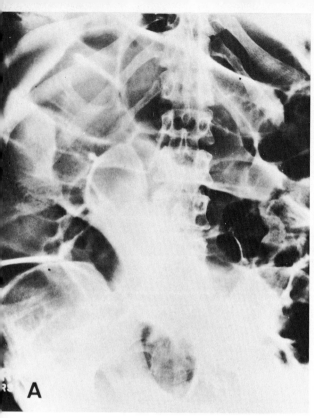 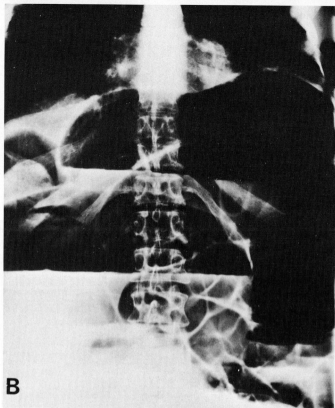

Fig. 34-14. *Idiopathic intestinal pseudo-obstruction.* **(A)** *Supine and* **(B)** *upright views show a massively dilated stomach and small and large bowel with nondifferential gas–fluid levels in all three portions of the gastrointestinal tract. (Teixidor HS, Heneghan MA: Idiopathic intestinal pseudo-obstruction in a family. Gastrointest Radiol 3:91–95, 1978)*

vomiting between the second and fifth postoperative days. Bowel sounds are hyperactive, and plain abdominal radiographs demonstrate the classic appearance of small bowel obstruction. This phenomenon is probably related to impeded peristalsis due to local paralysis of the small bowel secondary to inflammation or manipulation. Although the radiographic picture is typical of high-grade mechanical small bowel obstruction, surgery is seldom required. If the patient can be kept comfortable by intestinal intubation for a few days, the signs and symptoms of obstruction invariably disappear.

URINARY RETENTION AND PANCREATITIS

Adynamic ileus simulating bowel obstruction can be secondary to urinary retention. Emptying of the distended bladder can result in complete disappearance of symptoms. Adynamic ileus mimicking bowel obstruction can also be seen in patients with acute pancreatitis (Fig. 34-15).

ACUTE INTERMITTENT PORPHYRIA

Acute intermittent porphyria is a familial metabolic disease characterized by attacks of severe, colicky, abdominal pain in association with obstipation. Clinical and radiographic symptoms and signs often lead to the erroneous diagnosis of bowel obstruction (Fig. 34-16). Although many patients are operated upon for this reason, no organic obstruction

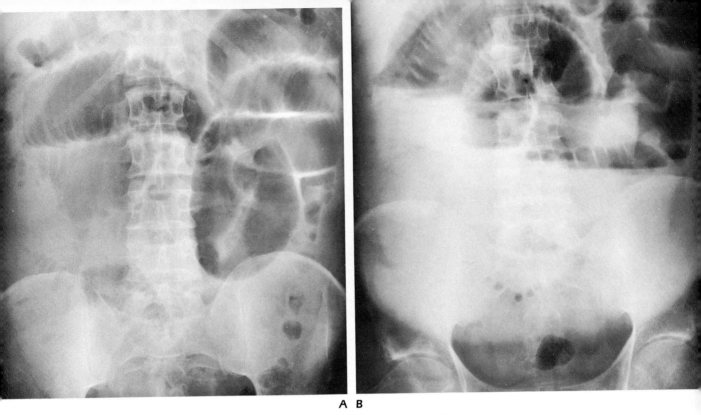

A B

Fig. 34-15. Adynamic ileus mimicking mechanical obstruction in a patient with pancreatitis. **(A)** Supine and **(B)** upright views.

Fig. 34-16. Adynamic ileus simulating mechanical obstruction in a patient with acute intermittent porphyria. **(A)** Supine and **(B)** upright views.

A B

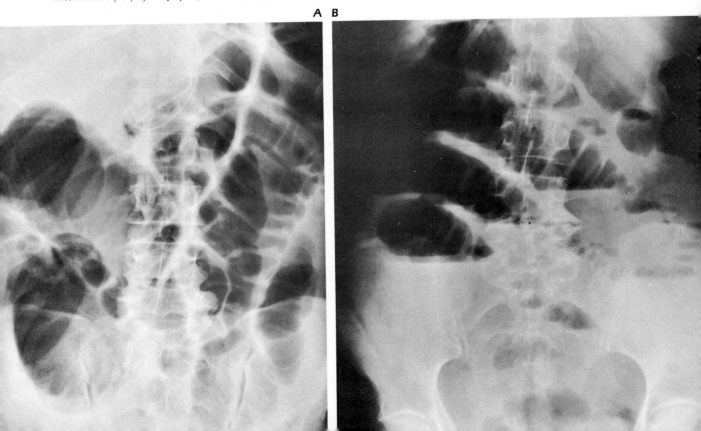

is found. The diagnosis is usually made from the chance observation that the urine becomes dark on exposure to light or on the basis of the development of characteristic neurologic symptoms, which lead to a search for the presence of abnormal porphyrins in the urine and feces.

CEROIDOSIS

Ceroidosis is the diffuse accumulation of a brown lipofuscin pigment in the muscularis propria of the gastrointestinal tract (brown bowel syndrome). It is not a primary disease but rather an irreversible consequence of long-standing malabsorption and prolonged depletion of vitamin E. The progressive dilatation and hypomotility of the entire gastrointestinal tract demonstrated by radiographic studies (Fig. 34-17) is probably related to infiltration of ceroid pigment in the smooth muscle cells with resulting functional impairment. As with chronic idiopathic pseudo-obstruction, the correct diagnosis of ceroidosis is essential to prevent unnecessary bowel resection for a nonexistent obstruction.

NEONATAL ADYNAMIC ILEUS

In neonates and young children, adynamic ileus can predominantly affect the small bowel, producing a radiographic appearance resembling mechanical intestinal obstruction (Fig. 34-18). In most cases, adynamic ileus results from nongastrointestinal ailments such as septicemia, hormonal or chemical deficits, hypoxia-induced vasculitis, or the respiratory distress syndrome. Intestinal infection, peritonitis, mesenteric thrombosis, and infusion of fluid into an umbilical venous line can produce a similar radiographic appearance.

Fig. 34-17. Ceroidosis. **(A)** Barium study showing dilatation of the stomach, duodenum, and proximal jejunum with thickening of valvulae conniventes. **(B)** Follow-up 8½ hr later showing barium still in the diffusely dilated jejunum and proximal ileum. Thickening of valvulae conniventes is again apparent. (Boller M, Fiocchi C, Brown CH: Pseudo-obstruction in ceroidosis. AJR 127:277–279, 1976. Copyright 1976. Reproduced by permission)

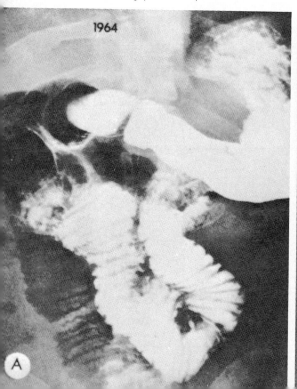

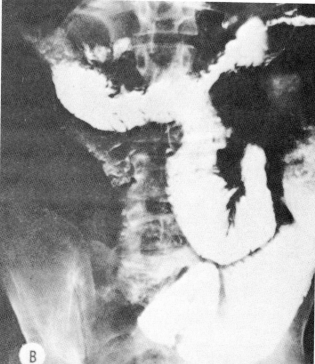

BIBLIOGRAPHY

Boller M, Fiocchi C, Brown CH: Pseudo-obstruction in ceroidosis. AJR 127:277–279, 1976

Bryk D, Soong KY: Colonic ileus and its differential roentgen diagnosis. AJR 101:329–337, 1967

Franken EA, Smith WL, Smith JA: Paralysis of the small bowel resembling mechanical intestinal obstruction. Gastrointest Radiol 5:161–167, 1980

Hohl RD, Nixon RK: Myxedema ileus. Arch Intern Med 115:145–150, 1965

Legge DA, Wollaeger EE, Carlson HC: Intestinal pseudo-obstruction in systemic amyloidosis. Gut 11:764–767, 1970

Meyers MA: Colonic ileus. Gastrointest Radiol 2:37–40, 1977

Moss AA, Goldberg HI, Brotman M: Idiopathic intestinal pseudo-obstruction. AJR 115:312–317, 1972

Schuffler MD, Rohrmann CA, Templeton FE: The radiographic manifestations of idiopathic intestinal pseudo-obstruction. AJR 127:729–736, 1976

Seaman WB: Motor dysfunction of the gastrointestinal tract. AJR 116:235–244, 1972

Treacy WL, Bunting WL, Gambill EE et al: Scleroderma presenting an obstruction of the small bowel. Mayo Clin Proc 37:607–616, 1962

Fig. 34-18. Adynamic ileus resembling mechanical intestinal obstruction in a child. Vasculitis with localized paralysis of the jejunum is seen in a 3-year-old girl with mucocutaneous lymph node syndrome. **(A)** The plain film shows that the proximal jejunum is dilated disproportionately with respect to the remainder of the bowel. **(B)** An antegrade barium study confirmed the jejunal dilatation, but contrast passed slowly into a normal-caliber bowel without an abrupt transition of caliber. (Franken EA, Smith WL, Smith JA: Paralysis of the small bowel resembling mechanical intestinal obstruction. Gastrointest Radiol 5:161–167, 1980)

A **B**

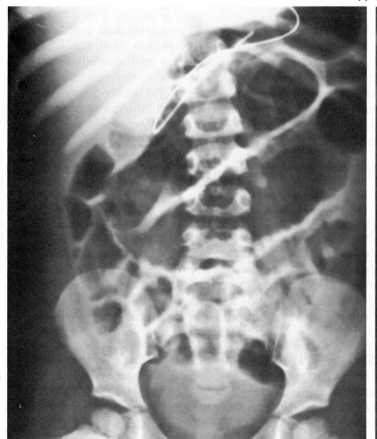 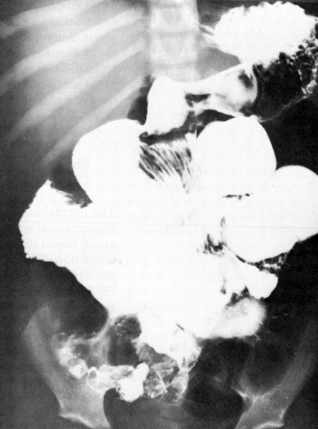

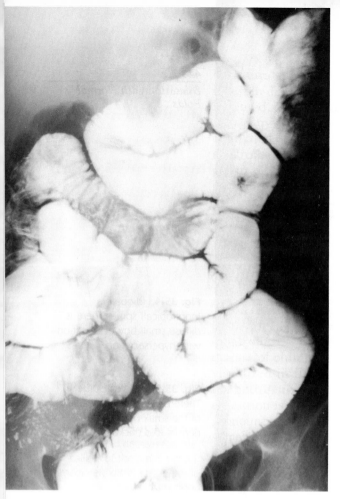

Fig. 35-6. Idiopathic (nontropical) sprue. There is diffuse dilatation of the entire small bowel with pronounced hypersecretion.

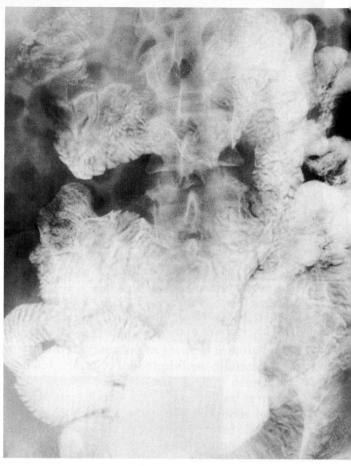

Fig. 35-7. Idiopathic (nontropical) sprue. The barium in the dilated loops of small bowel has a coarse, granular appearance due to hypersecretion.

indicative of sprue or other malabsorption disorders. In recent years, however, the use of nondispersible barium with suspending agents has all but eliminated these radiographic signs.

An excessive amount of fluid in the bowel lumen (hypersecretion) is a constant phenomenon in patients with sprue. This fluid may represent either excessive movement of water into the lumen or deficient absorption of water by the deranged mucosa. As a result of hypersecretion, gas–fluid levels are occasionally seen on upright films. The barium in the small bowel has a coarse, granular appearance (Fig. 35-7), unlike barium in the normal intestine, which has a homogeneous quality.

The *"moulage"* sign describes a radiographic appearance of the jejunum in sprue. The French term means "moulding" or "casting" and refers to the smooth contour and unindented margins of barium-filled small bowel loops. This tubular appearance in sprue is probably due to atrophy and effacement of the jejunal mucosal folds.

Intussusception is a not uncommon finding in patients with sprue (Fig. 35-8). The diagnosis is based on the typical findings of a localized filling defect with stretched and thin valvulae conniventes overlying it (coiled-spring appearance). Because the intussusceptions in sprue are

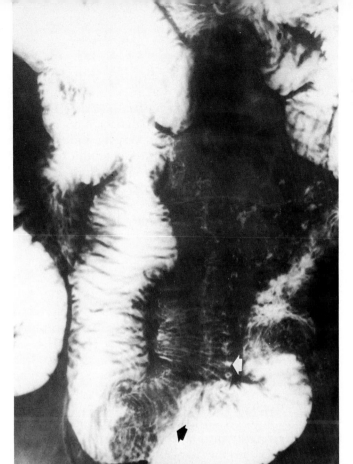

Fig. 35-8. Intussusception **(arrows)** in idiopathic (nontropical) sprue. Note the characteristic coiled-spring appearance.

transient and nonobstructing, they are often missed on a single examination.

The diagnosis of sprue is made by jejunal biopsy, which demonstrates flattening, broadening, coalescence, and sometimes complete atrophy of intestinal villi. A characteristic finding of idiopathic sprue and celiac disease of children is dramatic clinical and histologic improvement after the patient has been placed on a diet free from gluten (the water-insoluble protein fraction of cereal grains). The radiographic and jejunal biopsy findings in tropical sprue are identical to those seen in idiopathic sprue. However, clinical improvement in tropical sprue follows folic acid or antibiotic therapy rather than gluten withdrawal.

LYMPHOMA

Diffuse intestinal lymphoma may complicate long-standing sprue, and this complication should be considered whenever a patient with sprue shows a sudden refractoriness to treatment or develops fever, bowel perforation, or hemorrhage. Primary diffuse intestinal lymphoma is rare in the Western world but relatively frequent in adolescents and young adults in populations native to Middle Eastern countries. Symptoms and signs of intestinal malabsorption are a prominent feature, and the radiographic findings may be indistinguishable from sprue. More commonly, lymphoma produces thickening of the bowel wall, displacement of intestinal loops, and extraluminal masses, any of which can be superimposed on the classic sprue pattern. There is also a significantly increased incidence of small bowel and esophageal carcinoma in those patients (especially males) with long-established sprue who have not adhered strictly to a gluten-free diet.

CONNECTIVE TISSUE DISEASE

The connective tissue diseases, particularly scleroderma, can also cause the malabsorption syndrome and the radiographic pattern of dilated small bowel with normal folds (Fig. 35-9). The small bowel can be affected at any time during the course of scleroderma; however, skin changes, joint symptoms, or the appearance of Raynaud's phenomenon usually precede changes in the small bowel. In scleroderma, smooth muscle atrophy and deposition of connective tissue in the submucosal, muscular, and serosal layers result in hypomotility of the small bowel and an extremely prolonged transit time. Although dilatation is often most marked in the duodenum proximal to the site at which the transverse portion passes between the aorta and superior mesenteric artery, the entire small bowel can be diffusely involved (Fig. 35-10). In scleroderma, there is frequently a relative decrease in the distance between the valvulae conniventes for any given degree of small bowel dilatation. This "hide-bound" sign of folds that are abnormally packed together despite bowel dilatation (Fig. 35-11) is in sharp contrast to the

Fig. 35-9. Scleroderma causing the malabsorption syndrome and the radiographic pattern of dilated small bowel with normal folds.

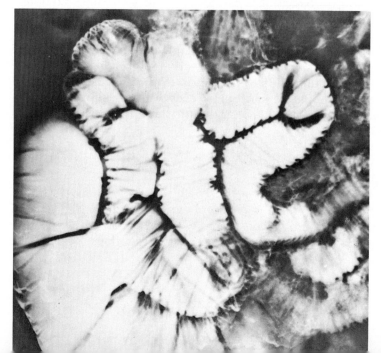

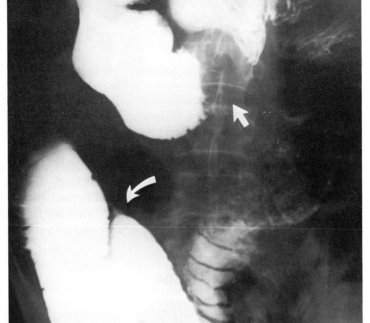

Fig. 35-10. Scleroderma. There is diffuse dilatation of distal small bowel loops **(curved arrow)** in addition to severe dilatation of the duodenum proximal to the site at which the transverse portion passes between the aorta and superior mesenteric artery **(straight arrow).**

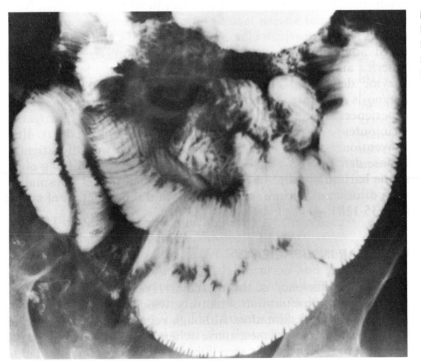

Fig. 35-11. Scleroderma. For the degree of dilatation, the small bowel folds are packed strikingly close together ("hidebound" pattern).

infarction will not occur. In these cases, the relative degrees of damage and healing give rise to a variety of radiographic findings (Fig. 37-4).

Bleeding into the bowel wall secondary to ischemic mesenteric vascular disease classically produces the radiographic pattern of regular thickening of small bowel folds. Other manifestations of bowel ischemia include ulceration, thumbprinting, sacculation, and stricture formation.

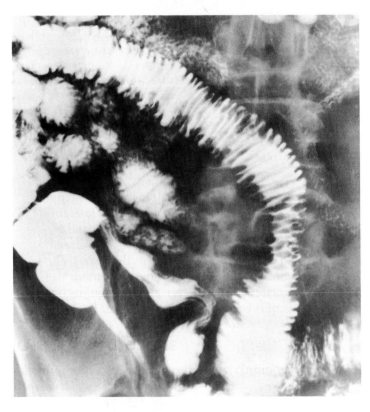

Fig. 37-3. Bleeding into the bowel wall and mesentery due to an overdose of Coumadin (warfarin). In addition to regular thickening of folds, note the separation and uncoiling of bowel loops.

Fig. 37-4. Small bowel ischemia. **(A)** Segmental ischemia in a picket-fence pattern of regular thickening of small bowel folds **(arrows)**. **(B)** Complete resolution of the ischemic process following conservative therapy.

A B

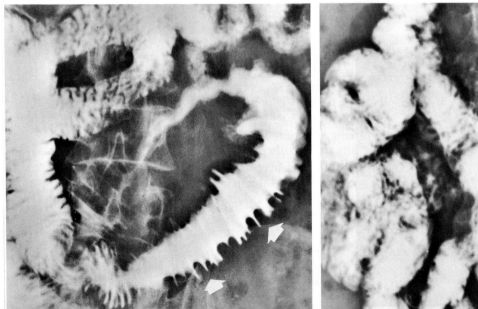
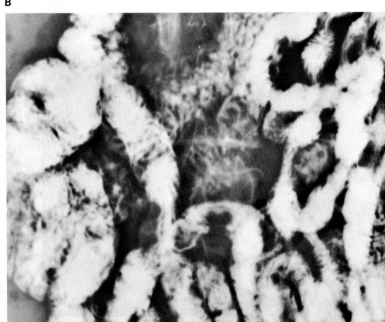

VASCULITIS

Vasculitis can compromise the blood supply to a segment of the small bowel and cause ischemic or hemorrhagic changes in the bowel wall. In systemic connective tissue diseases (rheumatoid arthritis, polyarteritis nodosa, systemic lupus erythematosus, dermatomyositis), a necrotizing vasculitis can involve small arteries, arterioles, and veins in the bowel wall (Fig. 37-5). In severe cases, massive bleeding, multiple infarctions, and perforation may also occur.

Thromboangiitis obliterans, which is usually found in relatively young men who are heavy smokers, is generally considered to be a peripheral vascular disease. However, this condition can also affect the gastrointestinal tract and produce inflammation of the mesenteric vessels, resulting in ischemic changes in the bowel wall and regular thickening of small bowel folds.

The Henoch–Schönlein syndrome is an acute arteritis characterized by purpura, nephritis, abdominal pain, and joint pain. The disease tends to be self-limited and frequently develops several weeks after a streptococcal infection. Like other causes of vasculitis, Henoch–Schönlein purpura causes a radiographic pattern of regular thickening of small bowel folds (Fig. 37-6). Large amounts of edema and hemorrhage can lead to scalloping, thumbprinting, and dilution of contrast. Henoch–Schönlein purpura can also affect the colon, causing circumferential submucosal lesions with marked luminal narrowing simulating carcinoma.

HEMOPHILIA

Hemophilia is an inherited (sex-linked recessive) anomaly of blood coagulation that appears clinically only in males. Patients with this disease have a decreased or absent serum concentration of antihemophilic globulin and suffer a life-long tendency for spontaneous hemorrhage. Bleeding into the intestinal wall is more frequently found in the small bowel than in the colon. The extent of bleeding is variable, and either a short or a long segment of small bowel can display the radiographic appearance of regular thickening of folds.

IDIOPATHIC THROMBOCYTOPENIC PURPURA

Acute idiopathic thrombocytopenic purpura typically presents with the sudden onset of severe purpura 1 to 2 weeks after a sore throat or upper respiratory infection in an otherwise healthy child. The manifestations of acute idiopathic thrombocytopenic purpura include extensive petechial hemorrhages and gingival, gastrointestinal, and genitourinary bleeding. In more than 80% of patients, this disorder is self-limited and clears spontaneously within 2 weeks.

Unlike the acute form, chronic idiopathic thrombocytopenic purpura occurs primarily in young female adults. The disease usually has

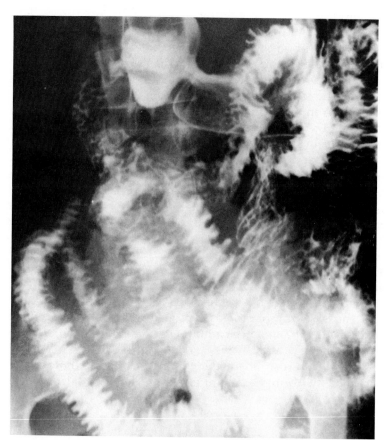

Fig. 37-5. Systemic lupus erythematosus causing ischemic and hemorrhagic changes in the bowel wall and the radiographic pattern of regular thickening of small bowel folds.

Fig. 37-6. Henoch–Schönlein purpura causing regular thickening of small bowel folds.

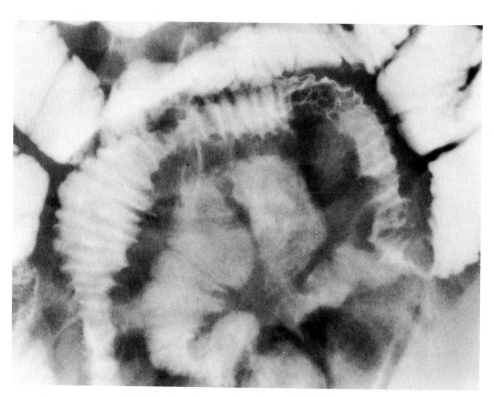

an insidious onset, with a relatively long history of easy bruising and menorrhagia. Because most patients with this condition have a circulating platelet autoantibody that develops without underlying disease or significant exposure to drugs, chronic idiopathic thrombocytopenic purpura is generally considered to be an autoimmune disorder. Although steroid therapy leads to complete recovery in some patients, splenectomy is required in most cases. This can result in long-term and even permanent remission, presumably due to removal of a major site of platelet destruction as well as elimination of a major source of synthesis of platelet antibodies.

Hemorrhage into the small bowel caused by either acute or chronic idiopathic thrombocytopenic purpura produces characteristic uniform, regular thickening of mucosal folds in the affected intestinal segment (Fig. 37-7).

TRAUMA

Intramural hemorrhage secondary to trauma can present as localized, regular thickening of small bowel folds. In children, intramural hemorrhage is most commonly seen in boys who suffer abdominal injuries in athletics. In adults, small bowel contusion may occur after automobile accidents, especially in persons wearing seat belts. In addition to regular thickening of folds, traumatic small bowel hemorrhage can result in the formation of an intramural hematoma, a mass lesion that can narrow and even obstruct the lumen.

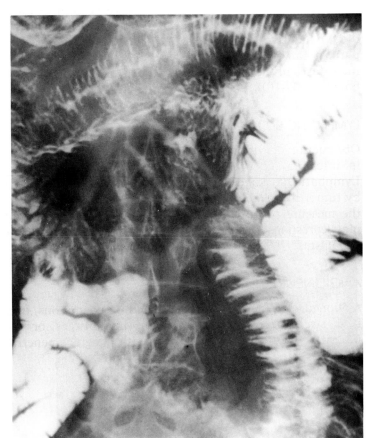

Fig. 37-7. Chronic idiopathic thrombocytopenic purpura. Hemorrhage into the wall of the small bowel causes regular thickening of mucosal folds.

tract. Diffuse intestinal edema in a patient (especially a child or young adult) with no evidence of liver, kidney, or heart disease should suggest the diagnosis of intestinal lymphangiectasia.

ABETALIPOPROTEINEMIA

Abetalipoproteinemia is a rare, recessively inherited disease manifested clinically by malabsorption of fat, progressive neurologic deterioration, and retinitis pigmentosa. An inability to produce the apoprotein moiety of the beta-lipoprotein leads to failure to transport lipid material out of the intestinal epithelial cell. This results in fat malabsorption, with no plasma beta-lipoproteins and markedly reduced serum levels of cholesterol, phospholipids, carotenoids, and vitamin A. Acanthocytosis, a thorny appearance of the red blood cells, is a characteristic finding. Jejunal biopsy reveals accumulation of foamy lipid material in the cytoplasm of intestinal epithelial cells, a pathognomonic lesion.

Abetalipoproteinemia presents radiographically as small bowel dilatation with mild to moderate thickening of mucosal folds (Fig. 37-13). Although most marked in the duodenum and jejunum, fold thickening is present throughout the small bowel. The folds may be uniformly thickened, demonstrate an irregular, more disorganized appearance, or even have a nodular pattern.

OTHER CAUSES

Regular thickening of small bowel mucosal folds can occur in the early phase of eosinophilic enteritis, when the considerable edema that

Fig. 37-13. Abetalipoproteinemia. There is regular thickening of folds in the jejunum with less marked changes in the ileum. Dilution and mild dilatation are also present. (Weinstein MA, Pearson KD, Agus SG: Abetalipoproteinemia. Radiology 108:269–273, 1973)

Fig. 37-14. Amyloidosis. There is relatively regular thickening of small bowel folds in this patient with clinical malabsorption. (Legge DA, Carlson HC, Wallaeger EE: Roentgenologic appearance of systemic amyloidosis involving gastrointestinal tract. AJR 110:406–412, 1970. Copyright 1970. Reproduced by permission)

Fig. 37-14

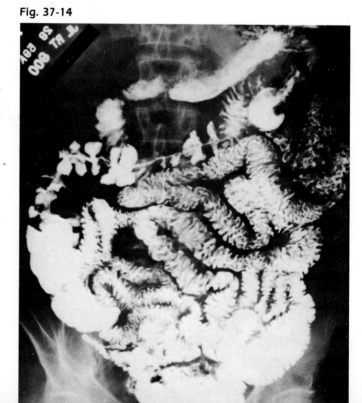

Fig. 37-13

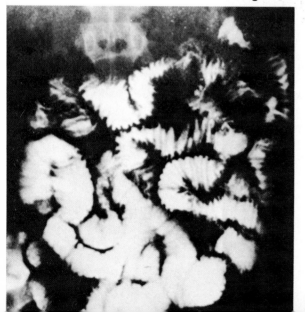

accompanies the eosinophilic infiltrate has not yet extended through the bowel wall. As the disease progresses and infiltration becomes more extensive, the more characteristic distorted, irregular thickening of small bowel folds is seen. Amyloid involvement of the small bowel can cause symmetric thickening of folds due to vasculitis, infiltration, and edema (Fig. 37-14). In patients with pneumatosis intestinalis involving the small bowel, the technical impossibility of demonstrating the outer walls of the radiolucent gas cysts can produce an appearance simulating regular thickening of small bowel folds.

BIBLIOGRAPHY

Dodds WJ, Spitzer RM, Friedland GW: Gastrointestinal roentgenographic manifestations of hemophilia. AJR 110:413–416, 1970

Ellis K, McConnell DJ: Hereditary angioneurotic edema involving the small intestine. Radiology 92:518–519, 1969

Ghahremani GG, Meyers MA, Farman J et al: Ischemic disease of the small bowel and colon associated with oral contraceptives. Gastrointest Radiol 2:221–228, 1977

Handel J, Schwartz S: Gastrointestinal manifestations of the Schönlein–Henoch syndrome. AJR 78:643–652, 1957

Khilnani MT, Marshak RH, Eliasoph J et al: Intramural intestinal hemorrhage. AJR 92:1061–1071, 1964

Kumpe DA, Jaffe RB, Waldman TA et al: Constrictive pericarditis and protein-losing enteropathy: An imitator of intestinal lymphangiectasia. AJR 124:365–373, 1975

MacPherson RI: The radiologic manifestations of Henoch–Schoenlein purpura. J Can Assoc Radiol 25:275–281, 1974

Marshak RH, Khilnani MT, Eliasoph J et al: Intestinal edema. AJR 101:379–387, 1967

Marshak RH, Lindner AE, Maklansky D: Ischemia of the small intestine. Am J Gastroenterol 66:309–400, 1976

Marshak RH, Wolf BS, Cohen N et al: Protein-losing disorders of the gastrointestinal tract: Roentgen features. Radiology 77:893–906, 1961

Mueller CF, Morehead R, Alter AJ et al: Pneumatosis intestinalis in collagen disorders. AJR 115:300–305, 1972

Olmsted WW, Madewell JE: Lymphangiectasia of the small intestine: Description and pathophysiology of the roentgenographic signs. Gastrointest Radiol 1:241–243, 1976

Pearson KD, Buchignani JS, Shimkin PM et al: Hereditary angioneurotic edema of the gastrointestinal tract. AJR 116:256–261, 1972

Schwartz S, Boley S, Schultz L et al: A survey of vascular diseases of the small intestine. Semin Roentgenol 1:178–218, 1966

Shimkin PM, Waldmann TA, Krugman RL: Intestinal lymphangiectasia. AJR 110:827–841, 1970

Weinstein MA, Pearson KD, Agus SG: Abetalipoproteinemia. Radiology 108:269–273, 1973

Wiot JF: Intramural small intestinal hemorrhage—A differential diagnosis. Semin Roentgenol 1:219–233, 1966

Giardia lamblia is a protozoan parasite harbored by millions of asymptomatic individuals throughout the world. Clinically significant infestations occur predominantly in children, postgastrectomy patients, and travelers to endemic areas (*e.g.*, Leningrad, India, and the Rocky Mountains of Colorado). The infection is apparently acquired through drinking water. Clinical symptoms range from a mild gastroenteritis to a severe, protracted illness with profuse diarrhea, cramping, malabsorption, and weight loss. In children, the disease can cause a chronic malabsorption syndrome that appears identical to celiac sprue. A striking association has been noted between giardiasis and the gastrointestinal immunodeficiency syndromes.

The irregular, distorted, thickened small bowel mucosal folds in giardiasis are most apparent in the duodenum and jejunum (Fig. 38-2). Diffuse mucosal inflammation, along with proliferative changes in the mucosal glands, edema of the lamina propria, and widespread infiltration by inflammatory cells, results in irregularly tortuous folds that present a distinctly nodular appearance when seen on end. Hypersecretion and hypermotility (rapid transit time) are also frequently noted. The lumen of the bowel is often narrowed because of spasm. When giardiasis complicates an immunodeficiency state, the irregularly thickened folds can be superimposed on a pattern of multiple tiny filling defects characteristic of nodular lymphoid hyperplasia.

An unequivocal diagnosis of *Giardia lamblia* infestation can be made through identification of the characteristic cysts in the stool. However, these cysts may be absent from the stool even in patients with severe disease. In such patients, the organism may be found only in smears of the jejunal mucus or by careful examination of the intervillous spaces on stained sections of a small bowel biopsy. Irradication of the parasite after treatment with Atabrine (quinacrine) or Flagyl (metronidazole) results in a return of the small bowel pattern to normal.

LYMPHOMA

Intestinal lymphoma can either originate in the small bowel (primary) or be a manifestation of a disseminated lymphomatous process that affects many organs (secondary). In either case, the disease can be localized to a single intestinal segment, be multifocal, or diffusely involve most of the small bowel (Fig. 38-3). In primary lymphoma, the neoplasm arises in the lamina propria or lymph follicles and is localized to one segment in about 75% of patients. The disease is most frequent in the ileum, where the greatest amount of lymphoid tissue is present. Tumor destruction of the overlying epithelium causes ulceration. Isolated or multifocal polypoid tumor masses can develop and, if large enough or acting as the leading edge of an intussusception, can even

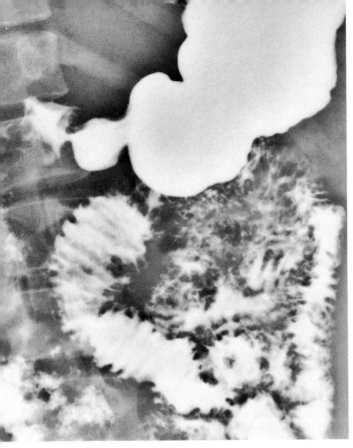

Fig. 38-2. Giardiasis. Irregular fold thickening is most prominent in the proximal small bowel.

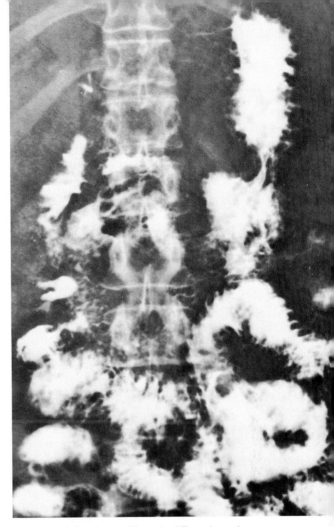

Fig. 38-3. Lymphoma. There is diffuse, irregular thickening of small bowel folds with mesenteric involvement and separation of bowel loops.

Fig. 38-4. Lymphoma. In addition to the generalized, irregular thickening of small bowel folds, there is segmental circumferential infiltration by tumor causing a constricting napkin-ring lesion **(arrow).**

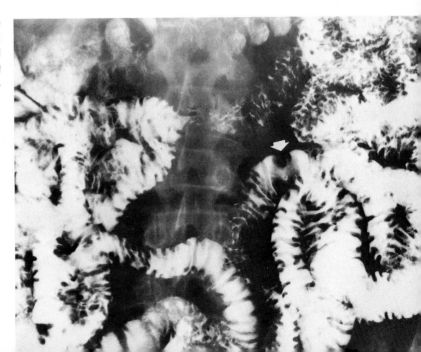

obstruct the intestinal lumen. At times, the bowel wall becomes circumferentially infiltrated, resulting in a constricting napkin-ring lesion (Fig. 38-4). Neoplastic involvement of the adjacent mesentery and lymph nodes is common.

Approximately 25% of patients with disseminated lymphoma are found at autopsy to have small bowel involvement. A majority have multifocal intestinal lesions. Unlike the situation in primary intestinal lymphoma, the small bowel involvement in most patients with disseminated lymphoma is merely incidental; specific gastrointestinal symptoms are frequently absent.

A classic radiographic appearance of primary intestinal lymphoma is infiltration of the bowel wall with thickening or obliteration of mucosal folds (Fig. 38-5). Segmental constriction of the bowel is less commonly noted. If lymphoma produces large masses in the bowel that necrose and cavitate, the central core may slough into the bowel lumen and produce aneurysmal dilatation of the bowel (Fig. 38-6).

AMYLOIDOSIS

Small intestinal involvement occurs in at least 70% of cases of generalized amyloidosis. Amorphous, eosinophilic amyloid is deposited in and around the walls of small blood vessels and between muscle fibers of the muscularis mucosa and major muscular layers. As deposition of amyloid increases, the entire bowel wall can become involved and appear as a rigid tube. Occlusion of small blood vessels can cause ischemic enteritis with ulceration, intestinal infarction, and hemorrhage. The deposition of amyloid in the muscular layers produces impairment of peristaltic activity. Symptoms include dysphagia, gastric retention, constipation or diarrhea, and intestinal obstruction. Muscular deposition combined with ischemia can cause mucosal atrophy leading to erosion and ulceration. As the bowel wall thickens, the lumen becomes increasingly narrow; even complete obstruction can occur. Generalized deposition of amyloid can also result in a protein-losing enteropathy and malabsorption.

Amyloidosis can be primary and occur without any antecedent disease. More commonly, amyloidosis is secondary to some chronic inflammatory or necrotizing process (*e.g.*, tuberculosis, osteomyelitis, ulcerative colitis, rheumatoid arthritis, malignant neoplasm), multiple myeloma, or hereditary diseases such as familial Mediterranean fever.

The diagnosis of amyloidosis requires demonstration of the characteristic eosinophilic material in affected intestinal tissues. Rectal biopsy has long been considered the most convenient diagnostic procedure in patients with generalized amyloidosis. More recently, peroral jejunal biopsy has proved to be a safe procedure with an equivalently high accuracy rate. Radiographically, amyloidosis is characterized by sharply demarcated thickening of folds throughout the small bowel

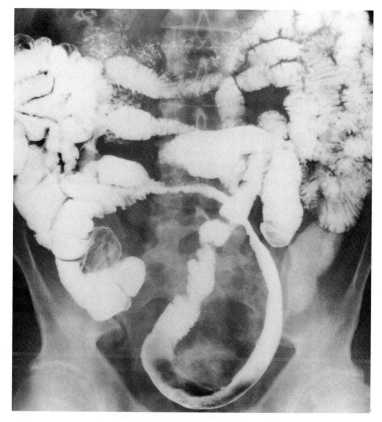

Fig. 38-5. Primary intestinal lymphoma. There is smooth narrowing of a segment of ileum with obliteration of mucosal folds. The elongated bowel loop is displaced around a large suprapubic mass.

Fig. 38-6. Aneurysmal lymphoma. Localized dilatation of a segment of small bowel **(arrows)** on two separate examinations is due to sloughing of the necrotic central core of the neoplastic mass.

A B

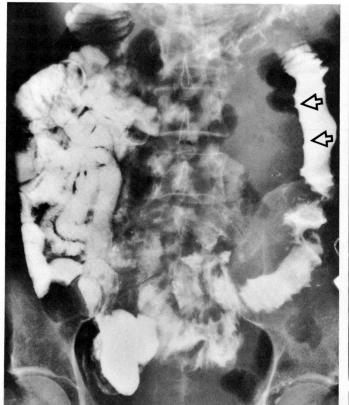
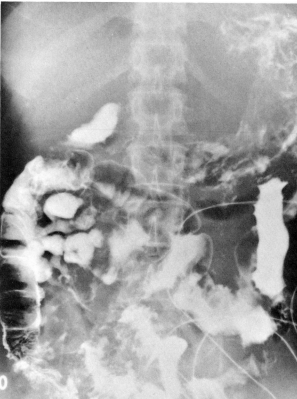

(Fig. 38-7). The folds can be symmetric and present a uniform appearance or be irregular, with nodularity and tumorlike defects. The appearance of prominent ileal folds resembling valvulae conniventes of the jejunum (jejunization) should suggest amyloidosis as the underlying disorder.

EOSINOPHILIC ENTERITIS

Diffuse infiltration of the small bowel by eosinophilic leukocytes produces the thickened folds seen in eosinophilic enteritis (Fig. 38-8). The jejunum is most prominently involved, though the entire small bowel is sometimes affected. Concomitant eosinophilic infiltration of the stomach is common. Involvement of the mucosa and lamina propria initially results in regular thickening of small bowel folds. More extensive, transmural involvement causes irregular fold thickening, angulation, and a saw-toothed contour of the small bowel. This can be associated with rigidity of the bowel and hyperplastic mesenteric nodes that simulate Crohn's disease. However, peripheral eosinophilia and the typical history of gastrointestinal symptoms related to the ingestion of specific foods usually permit differentiation between these two entities.

Fig. 38-7. Amyloidosis. There is irregular thickening of small bowel folds.

Fig. 38-8. Eosinophilic enteritis. Irregular thickening of folds primarily involves the jejunum. No concomitant involvement of the stomach is identified.

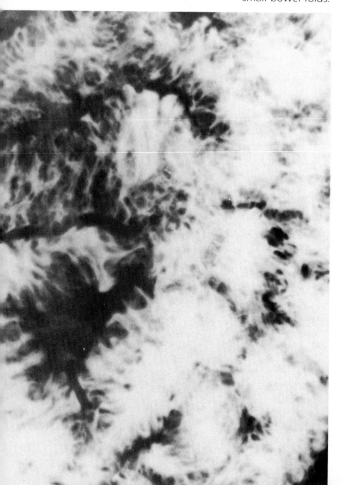

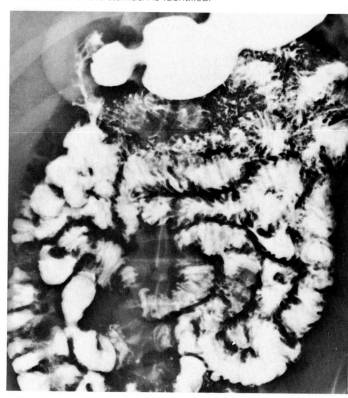

CROHN'S DISEASE

Although Crohn's disease most often involves the terminal ileum, it can affect any part of the alimentary canal. The process is frequently discontinuous, with diseased segments of bowel separated by apparently healthy portions. In Crohn's disease, there is diffuse transmural inflammation with edema and infiltration of lymphocytes and plasma cells in all layers of the gut wall. Ulceration is common, and intramural tracking within the submucosal and muscular layers is not infrequent. Fistulas are created when deep ulcerations burrow through the serosa into adjacent loops of bowel. They can extend to the colon, bladder, and even the skin or can end blindly in intraperitoneal or retroperitoneal abscess cavities or in the mesentery.

The clinical spectrum of Crohn's disease is broad, ranging from an indolent course with unpredictable exacerbations and remissions to severe diarrhea and an acute abdomen. Extraintestinal complications (large joint migratory polyarthritis, ankylosing spondylitis, sclerosing cholangitis) occur with a higher frequency than normal in patients with Crohn's disease. In the genitourinary system, infections can result from enterovesical fistulas, hydronephrosis can develop from ureteral obstruction due to involvement of the ureter in the granulomatous inflammatory process, and renal oxalate stones can be caused by increased absorption of dietary oxalate and consequent hyperoxaluria. Almost one-third of all patients hospitalized for Crohn's disease eventually develop a small bowel obstruction. Fistula formation is seen in at least half of patients with chronic Crohn's disease, and chronic indurated rectal fissures and fistulas with associated perirectal abscesses occur in about one-third. After surgical resection of an involved segment of small bowel, there is a high incidence of Crohn's disease recurring adjacent to the anastamosis.

RADIOGRAPHIC FINDINGS

The earliest small bowel changes in Crohn's disease include irregular thickening and distortion of the valvulae conniventes due to submucosal inflammation and edema (Fig. 38-9). Transverse and longitudinal ulcerations can separate islands of thickened mucosa and submucosa, leading to a characteristic rough cobblestone appearance. Rigid thickening of the entire bowel wall produces pipelike narrowing (Fig. 38-10). Continued inflammation and fibrosis can result in a severely narrowed, rigid segment of small bowel in which the mucosal pattern is lost ("string" sign) (Fig. 38-11). When several areas of small bowel are diseased, involved segments of varying length are often sharply separated from radiographically normal segments ("skip" lesions) (Fig. 38-12).

Loops of small bowel involved with Crohn's disease often appear to be separated from one another due to thickening of the bowel wall (Fig. 38-13). Mass effects on involved loops can be produced by adjacent

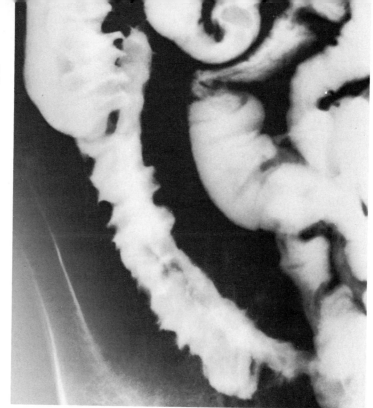

Fig. 38-9. Crohn's disease. There is irregular thickening of the valvulae conniventes in the terminal ileum.

Fig. 38-10. Crohn's disease. There is severe segmental narrowing in the jejunum **(arrows).** The jejunum shows pronounced involvement, although there is no clear evidence of terminal ileal disease.

Fig. 38-11. String sign in Crohn's disease. The mucosal pattern is lost in a severely narrowed, rigid segment of the terminal ileum **(arrows).**

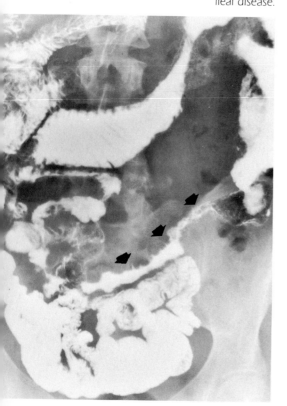

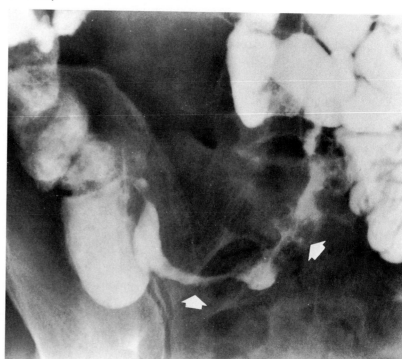

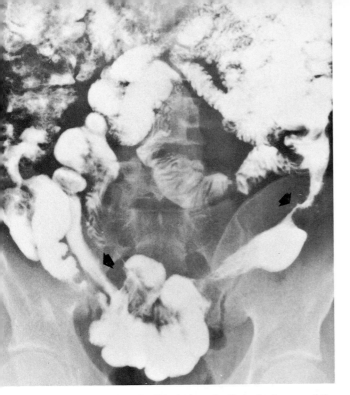 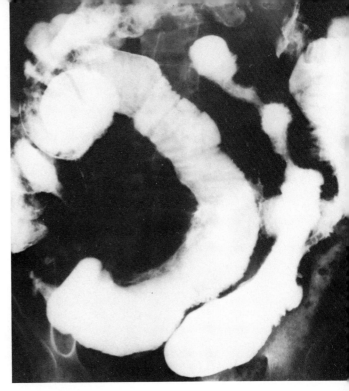

Fig. 38-12. Skip lesions in Crohn's disease of the small bowel. The **arrows** point to widely separated areas of disease.

Fig. 38-13. Crohn's disease. Marked separation of bowel loops is due to thickening of the bowel wall and mesenteric involvement.

abscesses, thickened indurated mesentery, or enlarged and matted lymph nodes. Irregular strictures are not uncommon (Fig. 38-14). Localized perforations and fistulas from the small bowel to other visceral organs can sometimes be demonstrated.

TUBERCULOSIS

Tuberculous involvement of the small bowel can produce a radiographic pattern indistinguishable from Crohn's disease (Fig. 38-15). Tuberculosis tends to be more localized than Crohn's disease and predominantly affects the ileocecal region.

HISTOPLASMOSIS

Although histoplasmosis is primarily a benign, self-limited pulmonary disease caused by the fungus *Histoplasma capsulatum*, it can rarely cause a systemic or disseminated disease that affects the gastrointestinal tract. Symptoms include nausea, vomiting, diarrhea, abdominal colic, anorexia, and weight loss. A protein-losing enteropathy has been described with this disease; generalized lymphadenopathy may mimic malignancy. Infiltration of enormous numbers of *Histoplasma*-laden macrophages into the lamina propria, accompanied by intense villous edema, produces irregularly thickened and distorted small bowel folds (Fig. 38-16). When seen on end, the folds appear as innumerable filling defects varying in size from sandlike pinpoints to nodules >2 mm in diameter. Focal stenotic lesions may closely resemble neoplastic disease.

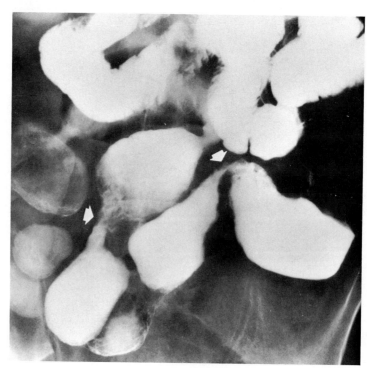

Fig. 38-14. Crohn's disease. Irregular strictures **(arrows)** alternate with areas of dilated small bowel.

Fig. 38-15. Tuberculosis. Irregular thickening of folds, segmental narrowing, and separation of bowel loops produce a pattern indistinguishable from Crohn's disease.

Fig. 38-16. Histoplasmosis. There is irregular thickening and distortion of folds throughout the small bowel.

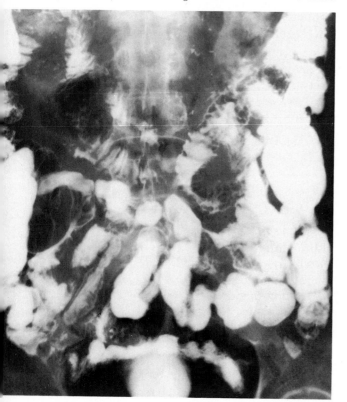

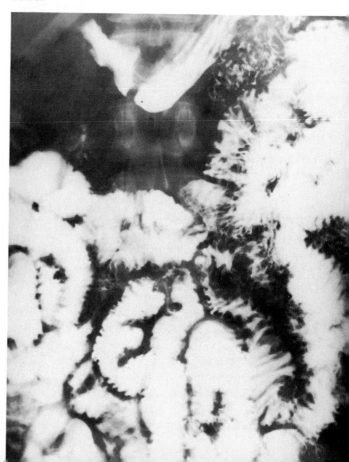

MASTOCYTOSIS

Systemic mastocytosis is characterized by mast cell proliferation in the reticuloendothelial system and skin (urticaria pigmentosa). Because the lamina propria of the intestinal mucosa is an important component of the reticuloendothelial system, involvement of the small bowel by mastocytosis is not uncommon. Infiltration of lymph nodes and hepatosplenomegaly are frequent; sclerotic bone lesions can also occur. The episodic release of histamine from mast cells causes such symptoms as pruritus, flushing, tachycardia, asthma, and headaches. Nausea, vomiting, abdominal pain, and diarrhea are common gastrointestinal complaints. The incidence of peptic ulcers is high (presumably because of histamine-mediated acid secretion), and malabsorption occurs not infrequently.

Mast cell infiltration into the lamina propria produces the radiographic appearance of generalized irregular, distorted, thickened folds (Fig. 38-17). At times, a diffuse pattern of sandlike nodules is seen. Urticaria-like lesions of the gastric and intestinal mucosa have also been described.

STRONGYLOIDIASIS

Strongyloides stercoralis is a round worm that exists in warm, moist climates in areas in which there is frequent fecal contamination of the soil. When parasitic females of the species are swallowed, they invade the mucosa and produce an infection that predominantly involves the proximal small bowel but can affect any part of the gastrointestinal tract from the stomach to the anus. Mild intestinal disease is often asymptomatic, but severe symptoms of abdominal pain, nausea, vomiting, weight loss, and fever can occur. Severe diarrhea and steatorrhea can mimic acute tropical sprue.

Radiographically, strongyloidiasis produces irritability and irregular thickening of the mucosal folds of the duodenum and proximal

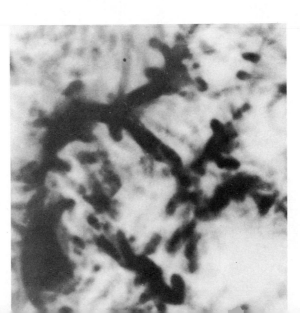

Fig. 38-17. Mastocytosis. Irregular, distorted, thickened folds are visible.

jejunum. Severe infestation can involve the entire small and large bowel. A definitive diagnosis requires detection of the worms or larvae in duodenal secretions.

YERSINIA ENTEROCOLITICA

Yersinia enterocolitica is a gram-negative rod resembling *Escherichia coli*. In children, *Yersinia* infections most frequently cause acute enteritis with fever and diarrhea; in adolescents and adults, acute terminal ileitis or mesenteric adenitis simulating appendicitis more commonly occurs. *Yersinia* usually causes a focal disease involving short segments of the terminal ileum, though it can also affect the colon and rectum.

Coarse, irregular thickening of small bowel mucosal folds is the most common radiographic pattern with *Yersinia* infection (Fig. 38-18*A*). Nodular filling defects and ulceration are also seen (Fig. 38-18*B*). Densely packed nodules surrounded by deep ulcerations can produce a pattern resembling the cobblestone appearance of Crohn's disease. Pathologically, acute and chronic nonspecific inflammatory changes are seen in the mucosa. During the healing phases of the disease, the mucosal thickening decreases and tiny filling defects appear (follicular ileitis). These can persist for months following an acute *Yersinia* infection.

Fig. 38-18. Yersinia enterocolitis. **(A)** Numerous small nodules, marked edema, and moderate narrowing of the lumen combine to give the terminal ileum an appearance of irregularly thickened folds. **(B)** Nodular pattern. (Ekberg O, Sjostrom B, Brahme F: Radiological findings in Yersinia ileitis. Radiology 123:15–19, 1977)

A B

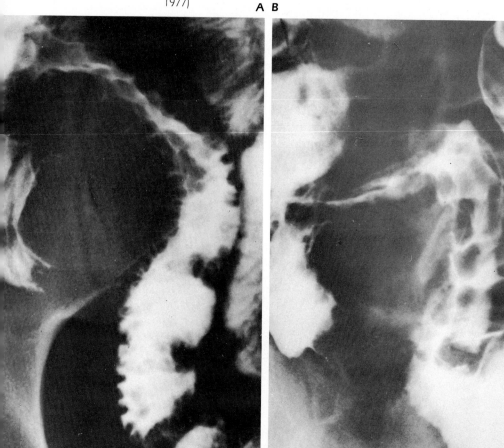

TYPHOID FEVER

Irregular thickening and nodularity of the mucosal folds is effectively limited to the terminal ileum in patients with typhoid fever (Fig. 38-19A). This acute, often severe illness, caused by *Salmonella typhosa*, is transmitted by bacterial contamination of food and water by human feces. Once in the gastrointestinal tract, the organisms are phagocytized by lymphoid tissue, particularly in the Peyer's patches of the terminal ileum. The organisms multiply there and produce raised plaques, which appear as thickened mucosal folds. Necrosis of the overlying mucosa causes ulceration. After treatment, the small bowel usually returns to normal (Fig. 38-19B), though healing with fibrosis and stricture can occur.

Typhoid fever must be distinguished radiographically from Crohn's disease of the terminal ileum. Ileal involvement in typhoid fever is symmetric; skip areas and fistulas do not occur. In addition, most patients with typhoid fever have clinical and radiographic evidence of splenomegaly.

ALPHA CHAIN DISEASE

Alpha chain disease is a disorder of immunoglobulin peptide synthesis and assembly of IgA. Major gastrointestinal symptoms, which include diarrhea and malabsorption, are possibly related to the inability of a defective secretory IgA system to prevent bacteria from penetrating the intestinal epithelial cells. The lamina propria is infiltrated by mono-nuclear cells (predominantly plasma cells), causing distorted villous

Fig. 38-19. Typhoid fever. **(A)** Thickened, coarse mucosal folds and marginal irregularity of the terminal ileum. **(B)** After therapy, the ileum returns to normal. (Francis RS, Berk RN: Typhoid fever. Radiology 112:583–585, 1974)

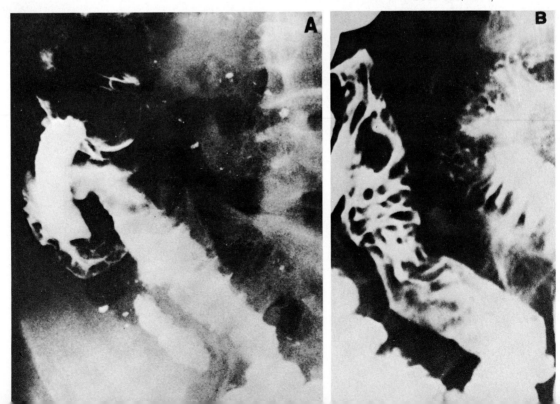

architecture and a radiographic pattern of coarsely thickened, irregular mucosal folds. A diffuse pattern of small nodules is occasionally seen.

ABETALIPOPROTEINEMIA

Abetalipoproteinemia is a rare, recessively inherited disease characterized by malabsorption of fat, progressive neurologic deterioration, and retinitis pigmentosa. In addition to producing regular thickening of small bowel folds, abetalipoproteinemia can also cause moderate disorganization of the mucosal fold pattern (Fig. 38-20A) or a nodular or cobblestone pattern of folds (Fig. 38-20B).

A B

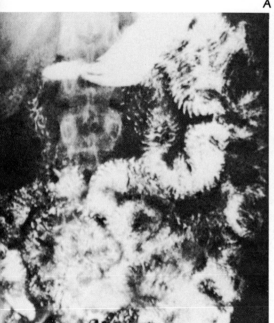 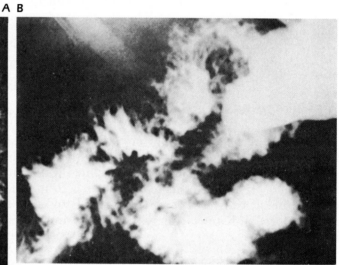

Fig. 38-20. Abetalipoproteinemia. **(A)** Moderately disorganized fold pattern. **(B)** Nodular or cobblestone pattern of folds in the duodenum and jejunum. (Weinstein MA, Pearson KD, Agus SG: Abetalipoproteinemia. Radiology 108:269–273, 1973)

Balikian JP, Nassar NT, Shamma'A NH et al: Primary lymphomas of the small intestine including the duodenum: A roentgen analysis of 29 cases. AJR 107:131–141, 1969

Bank S, Trey C, Gans I et al: Histoplasmosis of the small bowel with "giant" intestinal villi and secondary protein-losing enteropathy. Am J Med 39:492–501, 1965

Clemett AR, Fishbone G, Levine RJ et al: Gastrointestinal lesions in mastocytosis. AJR 103:405–412, 1968

Clemett AR, Marshak RH: Whipple's disease: Roentgen features and differential diagnosis. Radiol Clin North Am 7:105–111, 1969

Fisher CH, Oh KS, Bayless TM et al: Current perspectives on giardiasis. AJR 125:207–217, 1975

Francis RS, Berk RN: Typhoid fever. Radiology 112:583–585, 1974

Goldberg HI, O'Kieffe D, Jenis EH et al: Diffuse eosinophilic enteritis. AJR 119:342–351, 1973

Legge DA, Carlson HC, Wollaeger EE: Roentgenologic appearance of systemic amyloidosis involving the gastrointestinal tract. AJR 110:406–412, 1970

Margulis AR, Burhenne HJ: Alimentary Tract Roentgenology. St. Louis, C.V. Mosby, 1973

Marshak RH, Lindner AE: Radiology of the Small Intestine. Philadelphia, WB Saunders, 1976

Marshak RH, Ruoff M, Lindner AE: Roentgen manifestations of giardiasis. AJR 104:557–560, 1968

Olmsted WW, Reagin DE: Pathophysiology of enlargement of the small bowel fold. AJR 127:423–428, 1976

Philips RL, Carlson HC: The roentgenographic and clinical findings in Whipple's disease. AJR 123:268–273, 1975

Reeder MM, Hamilton LC: Radiologic diagnosis of tropical diseases of the gastrointestinal tract. Radiol Clin North Am 7:57–81, 1969

Rice RP, Roufail W, Reeves RJ: The roentgen diagnosis of Whipple's disease (intestinal lipodystrophy) with emphasis on improvement following antibiotic therapy. Radiology 88:295–301, 1967

Robbins AH, Schimmel EM, Rao KC: Gastrointestinal mastocytosis: Radiologic alterations after ethanol ingestion. AJR 115:297–299, 1972

Shimkin PM, Waldmann TA, Krugman RL: Intestinal lymphangiectasia. AJR 110:827–841, 1970

Vantrappen G, Agg HO, Ponette E et al: *Yersinia* enteritis and enterocolitis: Gastroenterological aspects. Gastroenterology 72:220–227, 1977

Vessal K, Dutz W, Kohout E et al: Immunoproliferative small intestinal disease with duodenojejunal lymphoma: Radiologic changes. AJR 135:491–497, 1980

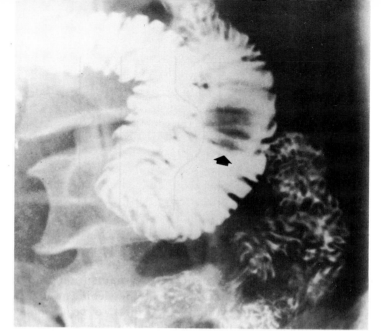

Fig. 39-2. Small intramural leiomyoma of the jejunum. An intramural filling defect **(arrow)** is visible on the <u>en face</u> view. (Good CA: Tumors of the small intestine. AJR 89:685–705, 1963. Copyright 1963. Reproduced by permission)

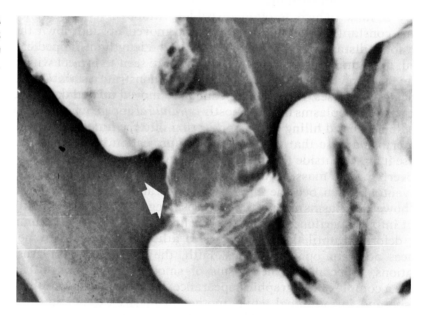

Fig. 39-3. Adenoma. A smooth polypoid mass **(arrow)** fills most of the lumen of the terminal ileum.

the jejunum. Leiomyomas arise as subserosal or submucosal lesions but can extend intraluminally and become pedunculated. Although the surface of a leiomyoma exhibits a rich blood supply, the central portion of the tumor is often virtually avascular and tends to undergo central necrosis and ulceration causing gastrointestinal hemorrhage. A leiomyoma with a large intraluminal component can be the leading point of an intussusception.

Many leiomyomas project from the serosal surface and are detectable radiographically only when they are large enough to displace adjacent barium-filled loops of small bowel. An intramural leiomyoma is seen in profile as a characteristic broad filling defect, its base wider than its projection into the lumen. Intraluminal tumors often lead to intussusception if they are located in the jejunum or ileum but almost never do so when they are situated in the duodenum. Retention of barium in a superficial mucosal ulceration that communicates with a relatively deep pit in the tumor is a finding that is characteristic of leiomyoma.

ADENOMA

Adenomas are the second most common benign small bowel neoplasms (Fig. 39-3). They can be found throughout the small bowel but are most frequent in the ileum. Most adenomas are single, well-circumscribed polyps, though multiple lesions do occur. These polyps are usually intraluminal and pedunculated and are therefore prone to act as the leading point of an intussusception.

LIPOMA

Lipomas are the third most frequent benign tumors of the small bowel (Fig. 39-4). Although most are found in the distal ileum and ileocecal valve area, they can occur anywhere in the small bowel. Lipomas arise in the submucosa but tend to protrude into the lumen. On barium studies, lipomas characteristically appear as intraluminal filling defects with a smooth surface and a broad base of attachment indicating their intramural origin. The fatty consistency of these tumors permits them to be easily deformed by palpation. Pedunculated lipomas can be associated with intussusception.

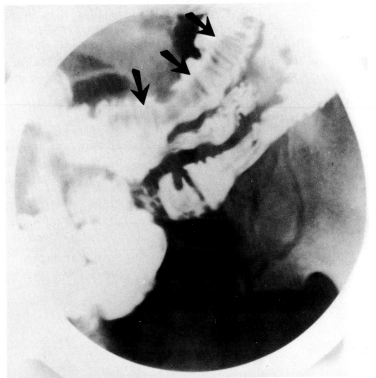

Fig. 39-4. Lipoma. A long pedunculated tumor produces an intraluminal filling defect. (Good CA: Tumors of the small intestine. AJR 89:685–705, 1963. Copyright 1963. Reproduced by permission)

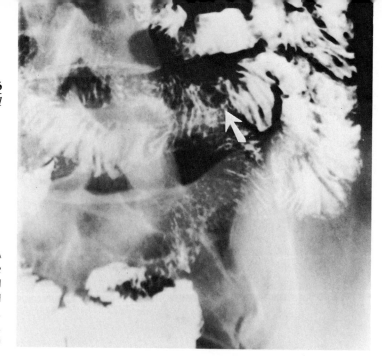

Fig. 39-5. Hemangioma. A filling defect **(arrows)** may be seen in the jejunum. (Good CA: Tumors of the small intestine. AJR 89:685–705, 1963. Copyright 1963. Reproduced by permission)

HEMANGIOMA

Hemangiomas are tumors composed of endothelium-lined, blood-containing spaces (Fig. 39-5). Though far less common than other benign small bowel tumors, hemangiomas are clinically important because of their propensity for bleeding. Less than 25% of hemangiomas are solitary tumors. Most are relatively sessile lesions that are frequently missed on barium studies because of their small size and easy compressibility. The uncommon demonstration of phleboliths in the wall of an involved segment is a pathognomonic sign of hemangioma. Some authors do not distinguish between hemangiomas (true tumors) and telangiectasias (dilatation of existing vascular structures). Telangiectasias can be associated with several abnormalities, the best known of which is the Osler–Weber–Rendu syndrome, in which there is a familial history of repeated hemorrhage from the nasopharynx and gastrointestinal tract and multiple telangiectatic lesions involving the nasopharyngeal, buccal, and gastrointestinal mucosa.

NEUROFIBROMA

Neurofibromas are unusual tumors of the small bowel that most frequently occur in the ileum. Most arise in the subserosal layer (presumably from Auerbach's plexus) and present as pedunculated masses growing in an extraluminal direction along the antimesenteric border. Neurofibromas originating in the muscularis or submucosa tend to grow toward the lumen and cause well-demarcated polypoid filling defects. Neurofibromas can ulcerate, and, if the crater is large or irregular, malignancy is likely.

MALIGNANT NEOPLASMS

Primary small bowel malignancies can present as solitary filling defects. Although a given type of primary tumor can be found anywhere in the small bowel, carcinomas tend to cluster around the ligament of Treitz, whereas sarcomas occur more frequently in the ileum. Like benign tumors, a malignant lesion with a large intraluminal component can be the leading point of an intussusception.

CARCINOMA

Adenocarcinomas are the most common malignant tumors of the small bowel. They tend to be aggressively invasive and extend rapidly around the circumference of the bowel, inciting a fibrotic reaction and luminal narrowing that soon cause obstruction (Fig. 39-6). Occasionally, adenocarcinomas of the small bowel appear as broad-based intraluminal masses; extremely rarely, they present as pedunculated polyps.

LYMPHOMA

One of the many appearances of small bowel lymphoma is a discrete polypoid mass that is often large and bulky and has irregular ulcerations (Fig. 39-7). If there is no substantial intramural extension, the intraluminal mass can be drawn forward by peristalsis to form a pseudopedicle and even become the lead point of an intussusception. Displacement of adjacent loops of bowel is common, as are mesenteric impressions and a diffuse desmoplastic response.

SARCOMA

Leiomyosarcomas are most often large, bulky, irregular lesions usually more than 5 cm in diameter (Fig. 39-8). Like benign leiomyomas, leiomyosarcomas have a tendency for central necrosis and ulceration

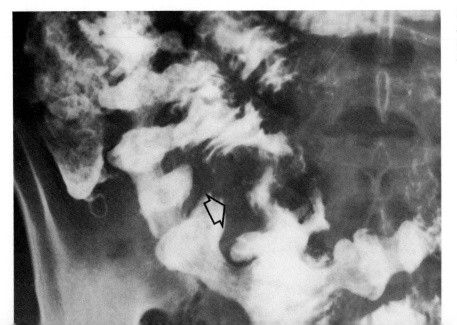

Fig. 39-6. Primary adenocarcinoma of the ileum **(arrow)** appearing as an annular constricting lesion.

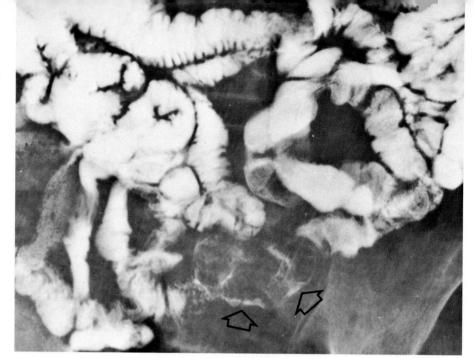

Fig. 39-7. Lymphoma. Note the large, bulky, irregular lesion **(arrows)**.

Fig. 39-8. Leiomyosarcoma. Note the large, bulky, irregular lesion **(arrow)**.

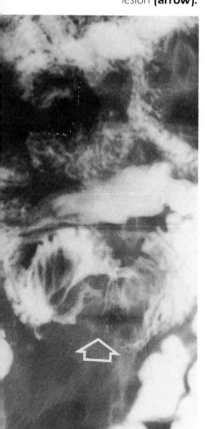

leading to massive gastrointestinal hemorrhage and the radiographic appearance of an umbilicated lesion. Because more than two-thirds of leiomyosarcomas primarily project into the peritoneal cavity, the major manifestation of this type of tumor is displacement of adjacent, uninvolved, barium-filled loops of small bowel.

METASTASES

Metastases to the small intestine (especially from such primaries as melanoma, lung, kidney, and breast) can appear as single intraluminal or intramural small bowel masses (Figs. 39-9, 39-10). However, most metastases to the small bowel are multiple. Single metastatic lesions that present as huge cavitary lesions with irregular, amorphous ulcerations can simulate leiomyosarcoma or lymphoma. Metastases are often masked by the spread of tumor to the adjoining mesentery or by a reactive desmoplastic response.

CARCINOID TUMOR

Carcinoid tumors are the most common primary neoplasms of the small bowel (Fig. 39-11). The "rule of one-third" has been applied to small bowel carcinoids: they account for one-third of gastrointestinal carcinoid tumors, one-third of them show metastases, one-third present with a second malignancy, and about one-third are multiple. Although carcinoids of the small bowel can occur at any site, they are most frequently seen in the ileum.

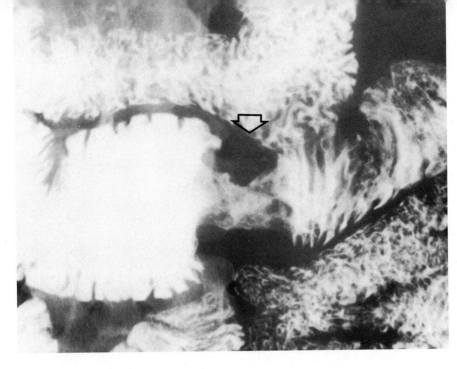

Fig. 39-9. Adenocarcinoma of the lung metastatic to the jejunum **(arrow)**.

The characteristic carcinoid syndrome consists of skin flushing and diarrhea as well as cyanosis, asthmatic attacks, and lesions of the tricuspid and pulmonic valves. The clinical symptoms are due to circulating serotonin produced by the carcinoid tumor. Because serotonin released into the portal venous system is inactivated in the liver, the carcinoid syndrome is seen almost exclusively in patients with liver metastases (Fig. 39-12), in whom serotonin is released directly into the systemic circulation without being inactivated. The primary tumor site in almost all patients with carcinoid syndrome is the small intestine; however, only a minority of small bowel lesions present with this endocrine syndrome.

Small carcinoids present as sharply defined, small submucosal lesions. At this stage of development, they are usually asymptomatic

Fig. 39-10. Hypernephroma metastatic to the jejunum. **(A)** Full and **(B)** coned views show the multilobulated nodular mass **(arrow)** in the proximal jejunum.

A B

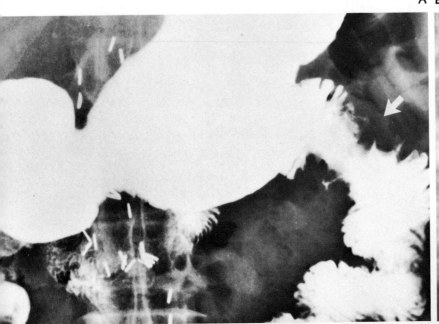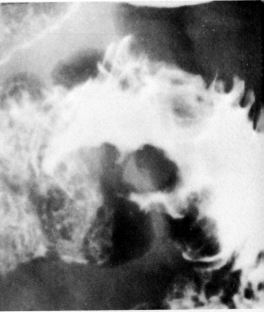

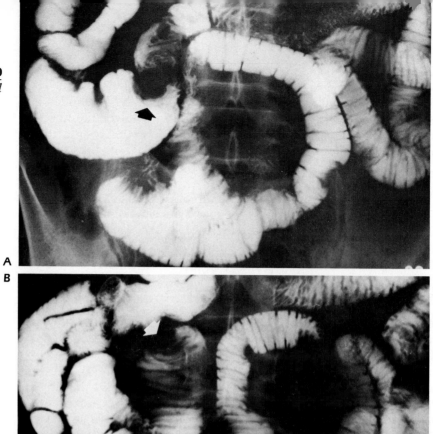

A

B

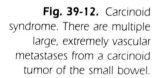

Fig. 39-11. Carcinoid tumor. Two views show the polypoid filling defect **(arrows).**

Fig. 39-12. Carcinoid syndrome. There are multiple large, extremely vascular metastases from a carcinoid tumor of the small bowel.

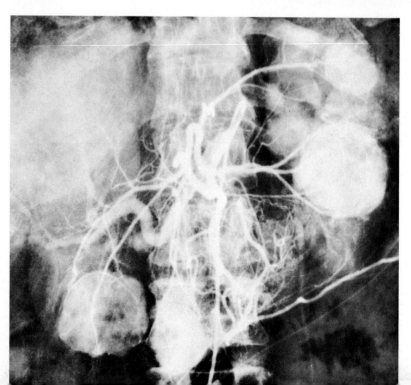

and are rarely detected on routine small bowel examination. Most carcinoids tend to grow extraluminally, infiltrating the bowel wall, lymphatic channels, and eventually the regional lymph nodes and mesentery. Local release of serotonin leads to hypertrophic muscular thickening and intense desmoplastic response, which results in the characteristic radiographic appearance of separation, fixation, and angulation of intestinal loops and diffuse luminal narrowing (Fig. 39-13).

The presence of metastases from carcinoid tumors is directly related to the size of the primary lesion. Metastases are rare in primary tumors of under 1 cm; they are seen in half of tumors between 1 cm and 2 cm in size and in about 90% of primary lesions larger than 2 cm.

GALLSTONE ILEUS

The combination of a filling defect in the ileum or jejunum, mechanical small bowel obstruction, and gas or barium in the biliary tree is virtually pathognomonic of gallstone ileus (Fig. 39-14). In this condition, which primarily occurs in elderly women, a large gallstone enters the small bowel by way of a fistula from the gallbladder or common bile duct to the duodenum. As the stone temporarily lodges at various levels in the small bowel, intermittent symptoms of abdominal cramps, nausea, and vomiting can simulate a recurrent partial obstruction. Complete obstruction develops when the gallstone finally reaches a portion of bowel too narrow to allow further progression. This usually occurs in the ileum, which is the narrowest segment of the small bowel. Far less commonly, a gallstone enters the colon (either by traversing the entire small bowel or by passing directly through a cholecystocolonic fistula). However, gallstone obstruction of the colon is unusual because of the

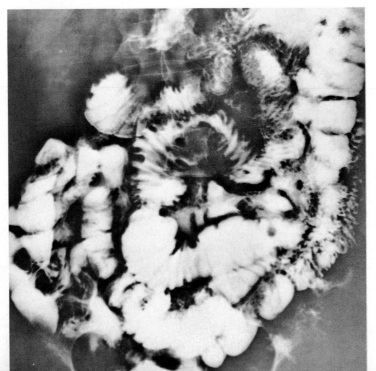

Fig. 39-13. Carcinoid tumor. Separation, fixation, and angulation of intestinal loops and diffuse luminal narrowing are caused by the intense desmoplastic response incited by the tumor.

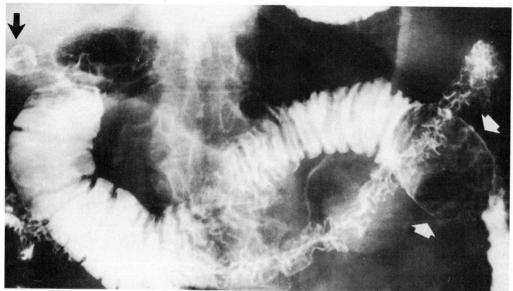

A

Fig. 39-14. Two patients with gallstone ileus. Obstructing stones **(white arrows)** are present, and there is evidence of barium in the biliary tree **(black arrows).**

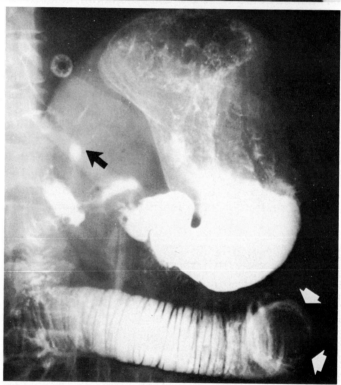

B

large size of the lumen. When it does occur, the obstructing stone usually lodges in a segment that has been narrowed by another disease process (*e.g.*, chronic sigmoid diverticulitis).

On plain abdominal radiographs, the demonstration of an opaque gallstone in the small bowel associated with typical findings of small bowel obstruction and gas in the biliary tree is sufficient for the diagnosis of gallstone ileus to be made. If a barium examination is performed, the obstructing gallstone may appear as a lucent filling defect, and contrast is often seen in the biliary ductal system.

OTHER CAUSES

Several unusual conditions can produce solitary filling defects in the small bowel that are indistinguishable from primary neoplasms. In premenopausal women with pelvic endometriosis, a polypoid lesion in the small bowel can represent an endometrioma. In patients from endemic areas or nonnatives who have spent time in the tropics, a filling defect in the region of the ileocecal valve can represent a pseudotumor caused by invasion of the gut wall by roundworms (*Ascaris* or *Strongyloides*) or a bolus of ascaris worms in the intestinal lumen. An inflammatory pseudotumor, similar to the far more common eosinophilic granuloma in the stomach, can present as a localized, predominantly submucosal mass in the small bowel. Large inflammatory pseudotumors produce polypoid masses, which can lead to intussusception. A duplication cyst can appear radiographically as a solitary intramural filling defect. Duplication cysts tend to change in contour with external pressure and can be associated with vertebral abnormalities. They occasionally communicate with the small bowel lumen and fill with contrast. Rarely, an inverted Meckel's diverticulum appears as a characteristic oblong filling defect in the distal ileum (Fig. 39-15).

Fig. 39-15. Inverted Meckel's diverticulum and intussuscepted jejunal polyp. **(A)** Initial examination of the small bowel demonstrates an intussuscepted polypoid mass in the distal jejunum **(arrows).** **(B)** An inverted Meckel's diverticulum was identified in the terminal ileum. (Freeny PC, Walker JH: Inverted diverticula of the gastrointestinal tract. Gastrointest Radiol 4:57–59, 1979)

A B

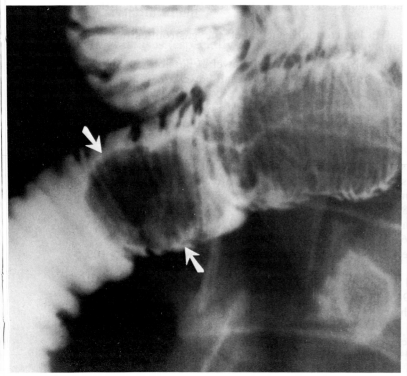

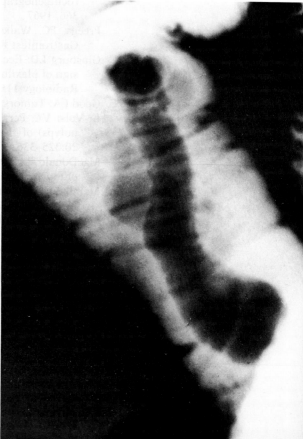

43

SEPARATION OF SMALL BOWEL LOOPS

Disease Entities

Processes that thicken or infiltrate the bowel wall or mesentery
  Crohn's disease
  Tuberculosis
  Intestinal hemorrhage or mesenteric vascular occlusion
  Whipple's disease
  Amyloidosis
  Lymphoma
  Primary carcinoma of the small bowel
  Radiation-induced enteritis
  Carcinoid tumor
  Neurofibromatosis of the small bowel
Ascites
  Hepatic cirrhosis
  Peritonitis
  Congestive failure/constrictive pericarditis
  Peritoneal carcinomatosis
  Primary or metastatic disease of the lymphatic system
Neoplasms
  Primary tumors of the peritoneum
  Primary tumors of the mesentery
  Metastases (peritoneal carcinomatosis)
Intraperitoneal abscess
Retractile mesenteritis
Retroperitoneal hernia

THICKENING OR INFILTRATION OF THE BOWEL WALL OR MESENTERY

Any process that infiltrates or thickens the bowel wall or mesentery can produce the radiographic appearance of separation of small bowel loops. A classic example of this mechanism is Crohn's disease of the small bowel (Fig. 43-1). In this condition, transmural inflammation results in thickening of all layers of the small bowel wall. The mesentery is markedly thickened, fatty, and edematous; mesenteric nodes are enlarged, firm, and often matted together to form an irregular mass (Fig. 43-2). Narrowing of the bowel lumen further enhances the radiographic appearance of separation of small bowel loops (Fig. 43-3). A similar appearance of irregular narrowing and separation of loops can be due to tuberculosis involving the small bowel (Fig. 43-4).

In patients with intestinal hemorrhage or mesenteric vascular occlusion, bleeding into the bowel wall or mesentery causes separation of bowel loops (Fig. 43-5). Thickening of the mesentery, infiltration of the bowel wall, and enlargement of mesenteric lymph nodes cause separation of small bowel loops in patients with Whipple's disease (Fig. 43-6) and amyloidosis. In primary lymphoma of the small bowel, diffuse submucosal infiltration combined with mesenteric involvement produce the appearance of separated bowel loops (Fig. 43-7). Primary carcinoma of the small bowel (Fig. 43-8) infrequently presents a similar pattern.

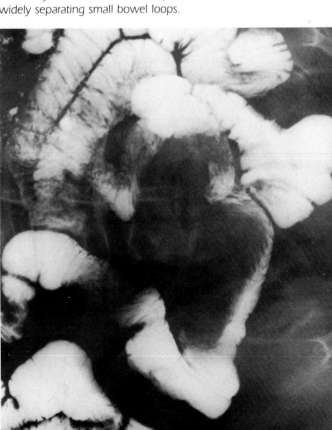

Fig. 43-2. Crohn's disease. Marked thickening of the mesentery and mesenteric nodes produces a lobulated mass widely separating small bowel loops.

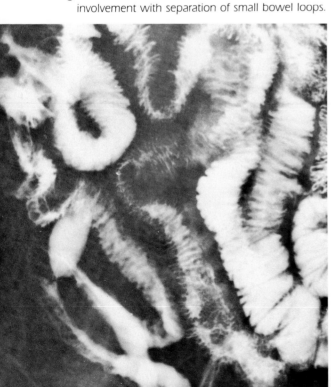
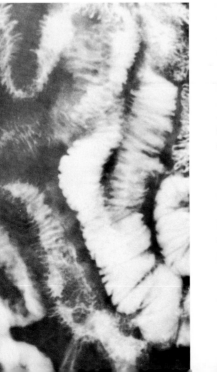

Fig. 43-1. Crohn's disease. There is diffuse mesenteric involvement with separation of small bowel loops.

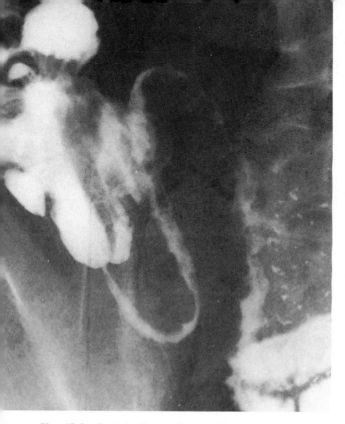

Fig. 43-3. Crohn's disease. Severe narrowing of the lumen enhances the radiographic appearance of separation of bowel loops.

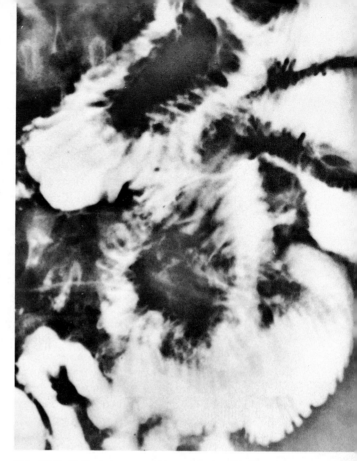

Fig. 43-4. Tuberculous enteritis and peritonitis. There is separation of bowel loops, irregular narrowing, fold thickening, and angulation.

Fig. 43-5. Intestinal hemorrhage. This patient, who was on Coumadin (warfarin) therapy, shows radiographic evidence of bleeding into the bowel wall and mesentery.

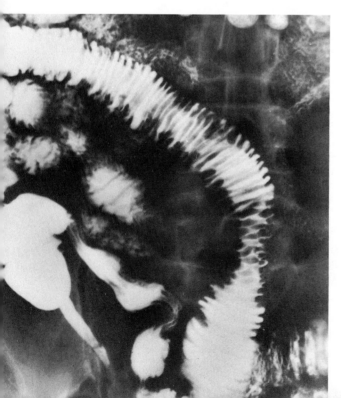

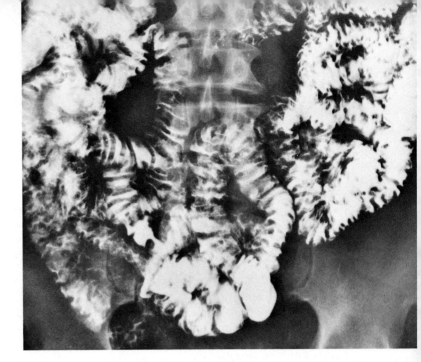

Fig. 43-7. Lymphoma. Submucosal infiltration and mesenteric involvement produce a pattern of generalized irregular fold thickening and separation of bowel loops.

Fig. 43-8. Primary adenocarcinoma of the jejunum. Separation of bowel loops is visible in the region of the tumor mass.

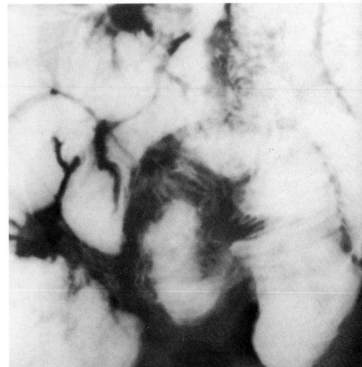

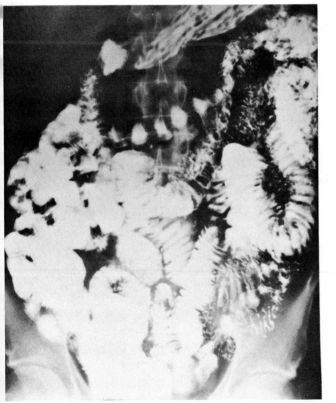

Fig. 43-6. Whipple's disease. Separation of bowel loops containing grossly distorted, irregular folds. (Phillips RL, Carlson HC: The roentgenographic and clinical findings in Whipple's disease. AJR 123:268–273, 1975. Copyright 1975. Reproduced by permission)

RADIATION INJURY

Clinically significant radiation damage to the gastrointestinal tract can occur following radiotherapy to the abdomen (Fig. 43-9). This radiation injury is thought to be secondary to an endarteritis with vascular occlusion and bowel ischemia. Radiographic manifestations include shallow ulceration of the mucosa, submucosal thickening with straightening of folds, and nodular filling defects. Thickening of the bowel wall due to submucosal edema and fibrosis is an almost universal finding in radiation enteritis and leads to separation of adjacent small bowel loops.

CARCINOID TUMOR

Carcinoid tumors initially appear as sharply defined, small submucosal lesions. As they develop, most carcinoids tend to grow extraluminally, infiltrating the bowel wall, lymphatic channels, and eventually regional lymph nodes and the mesentery. Local release of serotonin causes hypertrophic muscular thickening and severe fibroblastic proliferation, which lead to diffuse luminal narrowing and separation of intestinal loops with external compression and localized abrupt angulation (Fig. 43-10). The presence of one or several intramural nodules coexisting with severe intestinal kinking and a bizarre pattern of small bowel loops is characteristic of carcinoid tumors (Fig. 43-11).

Fig. 43-9. Radiation enteritis and mesenteritis. Thickening of the bowel wall and multiple nodular masses cause separation of small bowel loops. The patient had received 7000 rad for treatment of metastatic carcinoma of the cervix.

Fig. 43-10. Carcinoid tumor. Separation of bowel loops, luminal narrowing, and fibrotic tethering of mucosal folds are evident.

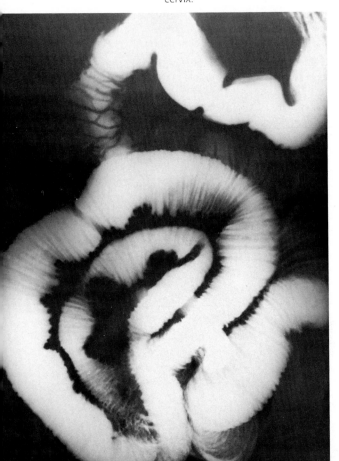

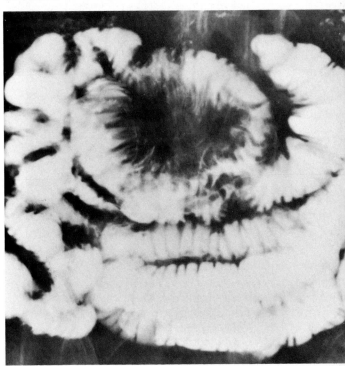

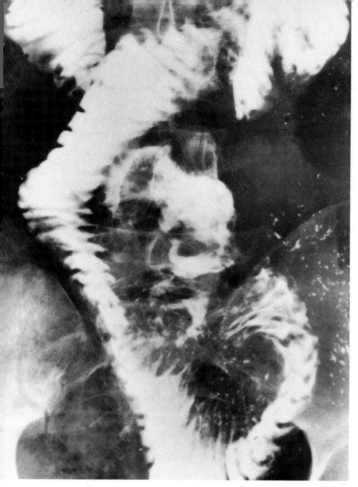

Fig. 43-11. Carcinoid tumor. An intense desmoplastic reaction incited by the tumor causes kinking and angulation of the bowel and separation of small bowel loops in the midabdomen.

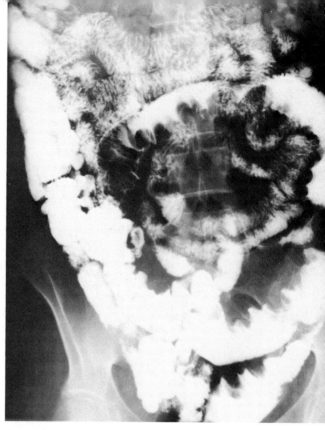

Fig. 43-12. Neurofibromatosis (von Recklinghausen's disease). The mesentery is thickened, and there is separation of small bowel loops. Multiple polypoid filling defects are present along the mesenteric side of the small bowel. (Ginsburg LD: Eccentric polyposis of the small bowel. Radiology 116:561–562, 1975)

NEUROFIBROMATOSIS

Plexiform neurofibromatosis, a manifestation of von Recklinghausen's disease, consists of the enlargement of many nerve trunks in a given area. When the disease involves the small bowel, multiple polypoid filling defects and thickening of the mesentery cause separation of loops. A characteristic finding in this disorder is eccentric polyposis of the small bowel, the defects being seen entirely on the mesenteric side (Fig. 43-12).

ASCITES

The accumulation of ascitic fluid in the peritoneal cavity can be caused by abnormalities in venous pressure, plasma colloid osmotic pressure, hepatic lymph formation, splanchnic lymphatic drainage, renal sodium and water excretion, or subperitoneal capillary permeability. In almost 75% of patients with ascites, the underlying disease is hepatic cirrhosis, in which there is elevated portal venous pressure and a decreased serum albumin level. Extrahepatic portal venous obstruction can also produce ascites, though it rarely does so in the absence of liver disease or hypoalbuminemia. The permeability of subperitoneal capillaries is increased in a broad spectrum of inflammatory and neoplastic diseases. Large amounts of intraperitoneal fluid are seen in patients with peritonitis secondary to infectious processes such as bacterial infection, tuberculosis, typhoid fever, and various fungal and parasitic infestations. Altered capillary permeability is most likely responsible for the development of ascites in patients with peritoneal carcinomatosis, as well as in patients with myxedema, ovarian disease, and allergic vasculitis. Primary or metastatic diseases of the lymphatic system can obstruct lymphatic vessels or the thoracic duct and produce ascites by blocking the normal splanchnic lymphatic drainage.

Large amounts of ascitic fluid are easily detectable on plain abdominal radiographs as a general abdominal haziness ("ground-glass" appearance) and increased density that shifts to the pelvis on upright films (Fig. 43-13). Smaller amounts of fluid (800–1000 ml) may widen the flank stripe and obliterate the right lateral inferior margin of the liver (hepatic angle). On barium examination, the presence of ascitic fluid is seen to cause separation of small bowel loops.

NEOPLASMS

PERITONEAL TUMORS

Primary neoplasms of the peritoneum (mesotheliomas) are extremely rare. They are usually seen in middle-aged to elderly persons, predominantly men. Like tumors of the same cell type involving the pleura, peritoneal mesotheliomas appear to be closely related to exposure to asbestos. In addition to having a large bulk, peritoneal mesotheliomas are associated with severe ascites, which contributes to the separation of small bowel loops. Metastatic mesothelioma from a lung primary can produce a similar radiographic appearance (Fig. 43-14).

MESENTERIC TUMORS

Primary tumors of the mesentery are also rare. Almost two-thirds of mesenteric tumors are benign, primarily fibromas or lipomas. Many are discovered incidentally during operations for other diseases. Most primary malignant tumors of the mesentery are fibrosarcomas or leiomyosarcomas arising from the smooth muscle of mesenteric blood vessels. They can grow to an extremely large size before producing symptoms or metastasizing. Malignant lymphoid tumors of the mesentery are rare lesions that can be locally infiltrative and cause separation of bowel loops (Fig. 43-15). Mesenteric lymphoid tumors can also be benign and present with systemic manifestations such as fever, leukocytosis, hyperglobulinemia, and anemia. Rather than true lymphoid neoplasms, these benign lesions probably represent giant lymph node hyperplasia secondary to an inflammatory or infectious process.

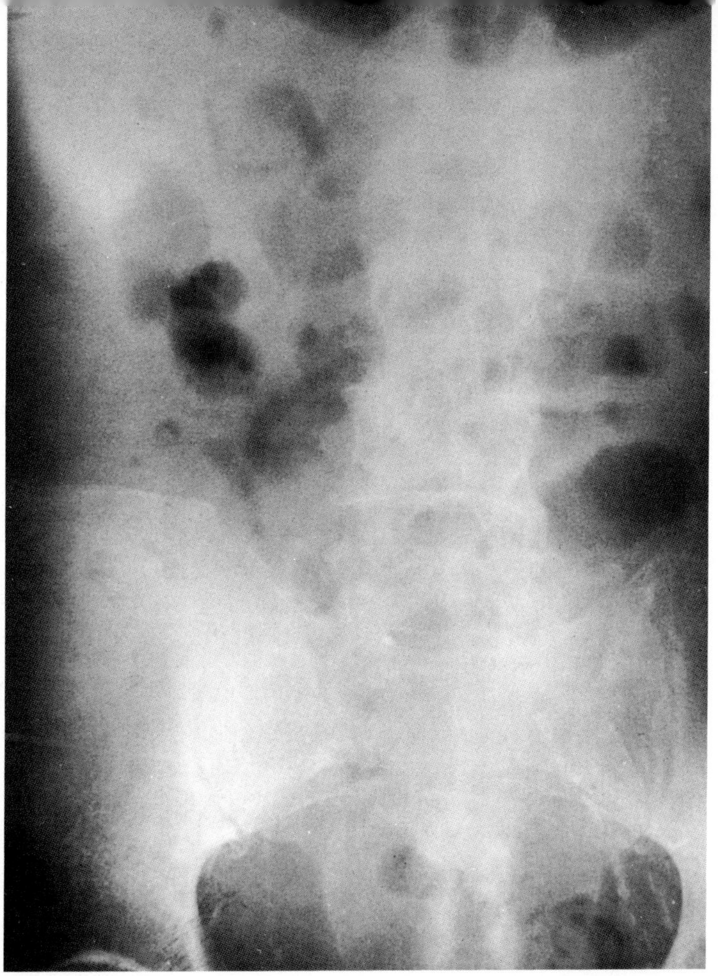

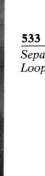

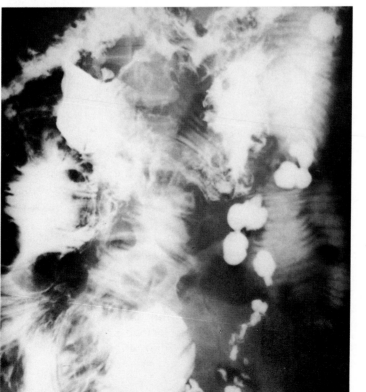

Fig. 43-13. Ascites. Note the general abdominal haziness ("ground-glass" appearance).

Fig. 43-14. Metastatic mesothelioma to the small bowel from a lung primary. Separation of bowel loops is evident, with multiple intrinsic and extrinsic nodular masses and areas of annular constriction and ulceration.

Intraperitoneal seeding occurs as a result of tumor cells floating freely in ascitic fluid and implanting themselves on peritoneal surfaces. Metastatic tumors to the peritoneum commonly occur in the terminal stages of cancer of the intraperitoneal organs (Fig. 43-16), most being due to adenocarcinoma (Fig. 43-17). Neoplasms of the ovary and stomach are especially prone to widespread seeding of the peritoneal surfaces. However, a variety of mesenchymal tumors (Fig. 43-18), lymphoma, and leukemia can also infiltrate the peritoneum. Major areas of intraperitoneal seeding include the pouch of Douglas at the rectosigmoid junction; the right lower quadrant at the lower end of the small bowel mesentery; the left lower quadrant along the superior border of the sigmoid mesocolon and colon; and the right pericolic gutter lateral to the cecum and ascending colon. Metastases to the peritoneum usually produce large volumes of ascites, and the diagnosis of intraperitoneal carcinomatosis can often be made by cytologic examination of aspirated ascitic fluid. In addition to separation of intestinal loops by ascites, peritoneal carcinomatosis can cause mesenteric masses, nodular impressions, or angulated segments of small bowel. Stretching and fixation of mucosal folds transverse to the longitudinal axis of the bowel lumen (transverse stretch) is reported to be highly indicative of secondary neoplastic involvement of the small bowel.

Fig. 43-15. Primary lymphangioma of the small bowel and mesentery. Diffuse mesenteric infiltration causes prominent nodularity and separation of bowel loops.

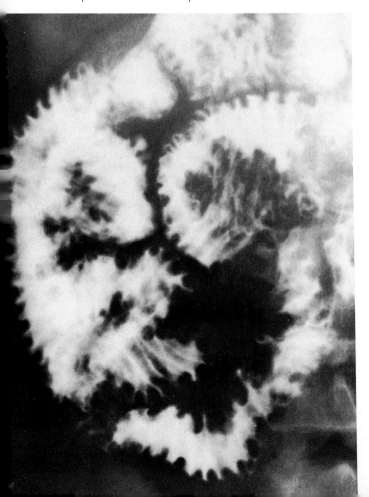

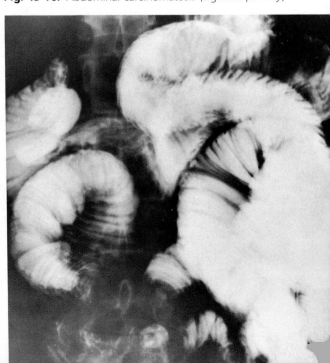

Fig. 43-16. Abdominal carcinomatosis (sigmoid primary).

INTRAPERITONEAL ABSCESS

Intraperitoneal abscesses are localized collections of pus that can follow either generalized peritonitis or a more localized intra-abdominal disease process or injury. The location of intraperitoneal abscesses depends on the site of the primary underlying disease. For example, appendicitis leads to abscesses in the right pericolic gutter and pelvis, and sigmoid diverticulitis produces abscesses in the left pericolic gutter and pelvis. Pancreatitis and perforated gastric or duodenal ulcers lead to abscesses in the lesser sac, whereas Crohn's disease generally results in abscesses in the center of the peritoneal cavity. Radiographically, intraperitoneal abscesses appear as soft-tissue masses displacing and separating small bowel loops. A critical radiographic sign of an intraperitoneal abscess is the presence of extraluminal bowel gas, which can appear as discrete, round lucencies, multiple small lucencies ("soap bubbles"), or linear radiolucent shadows that follow fascial planes. Localized ileus (sentinel loop) is often seen adjacent to an intraperitoneal abscess, though this is a nonspecific finding.

RETRACTILE MESENTERITIS

Retractile mesenteritis is a disease characterized by fibro-fatty thickening and sclerosis of the mesentery. A poorly understood condition, it

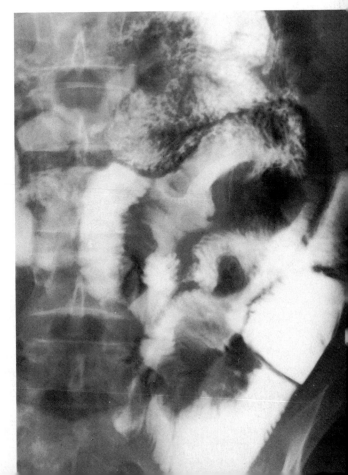

Fig. 43-18. Leiomyosarcoma of the ileum metastatic to the small bowel and mesentery. Multiple nodular masses cause separation of small bowel loops.

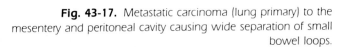

Fig. 43-17. Metastatic carcinoma (lung primary) to the mesentery and peritoneal cavity causing wide separation of small bowel loops.

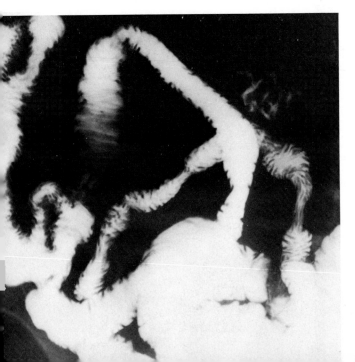

probably represents a slowly progressive mesenteric inflammatory process. Three major pathologic features are usually present to some extent: fibrosis, inflammation, and fatty infiltration. When fibrosis is the dominant feature, the disease is known as retractile mesenteritis. When fatty infiltration is the most prominent feature, the condition is called lipomatosis or isolated lipodystrophy of the mesentery. Mesenteric panniculitis is the term used whenever chronic inflammation is the major pathologic feature. For all practical purposes, these three different terms describe the same process, or perhaps different stages of a single disease.

The small bowel mesentery is the usual site of origin of retractile mesenteritis, though the sigmoid mesentery can also be affected. The radiographic appearance is that of a diffuse mesenteric mass that separates and displaces small bowel loops (Fig. 43-19). When prominent fibrosis causes adhesions and retractions, the bowel tends to be drawn into a central mass with kinking, angulation, and conglomeration of adherent loops (Fig. 43-20).

RETROPERITONEAL HERNIA

Retroperitoneal hernias occur in fossae formed by peritoneal folds and are generally found in paraduodenal, paracecal, or intersigmoidal locations. The herniated portion of intestine is almost always a part of the small bowel. Although the loops of bowel within the hernia sac

Fig. 43-19. Retractile mesenteritis. Separation of small bowel folds remained constant on successive studies. (Clemett AR, Tracht DG: The roentgen diagnosis of retractile mesenteritis. AJR 107:787, 1969. Copyright 1969. Reproduced by permission)

Fig. 43-20. Marked separation of bowel loops with segmental dilatation and abrupt angulation of the mid-small bowel associated with indentations on the concave border. The more severely involved bowel was arranged distally in a spiral pattern of continuous curves smoothly narrowed on the inside of the loop. (Aach RD, Kahn LJ, Frech RS: Obstruction of the small intestine due to retractile mesenteritis. Gastroenterology 54:594–598, 1968)

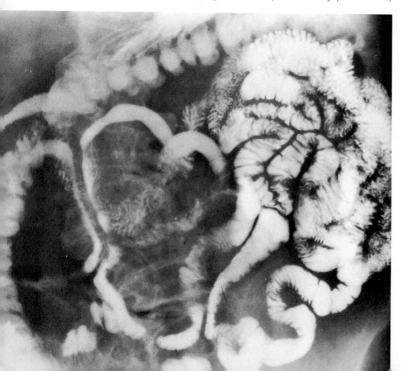

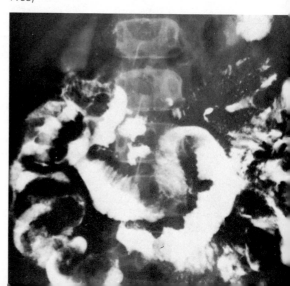

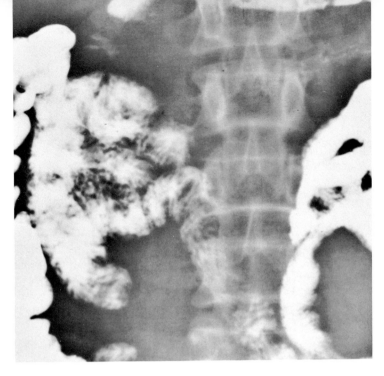

Fig. 43-21. Right
paraduodenal hernia. The
loops of bowel crowded
together in the hernia sac are
widely separated from other
segments of small bowel that
remain free in the peritoneal
cavity.

appear to be crowded closely together in a small, confined space, they
are widely separated from those segments of small bowel that remain
free in the peritoneal cavity (Fig. 43-21).

BIBLIOGRAPHY

Aach RD, Kahn LI, Frech RS: Obstruction of the small intestine due to retractile
    mesenteritis. Gastroenterology 54:594–598, 1968

Balikian JP, Nassar NT, Shamma'A NH et al: Primary lymphomas of the small
    intestine including the duodenum: A roentgen analysis of 29 cases. AJR
    107:131–141, 1969

Balthazar EJ: Carcinoid tumors of the alimentary tract: Radiographic diagnosis.
    Gastrointest Radiol 3:47–56, 1978

Banner MP, Gohel VK: Peritoneal mesothelioma. Radiology 129:637–640, 1978

Clemett AR, Marshak RH: Whipple's disease: Roentgen features and differential
    diagnosis. Radiol Clin North Am 7:105–111, 1969

Clemett AR, Tracht DG: The roentgen diagnosis of retractile mesenteritis. AJR
    107:787, 1969

Khilnani MT, Marshak RH, Eliasoph J et al: Intramural intestinal hemorrhage.
    AJR 92:1061–1071, 1964

Legge DA, Carlson HC, Wollaeger EE: Roentgenologic appearance of systemic
    amyloidosis involving the gastrointestinal tract. AJR 110:406–412, 1970

Marshak RH, Lindner AE: Radiology of the Small Intestine. Philadelphia, WB
    Saunders, 1976

Marshak RH, Lindner AE, Maklansky DM: Lymphoreticular disorders of the
    gastrointestinal tract: Roentgenographic features. Gastrointest Radiol 4:103–
    120, 1979

Rogers LF, Goldstein HM: Roentgen manifestations of radiation injury to the
    gastrointestinal tract. Gastrointest Radiol 2:281–291, 1977

Smith SJ, Carlson HC, Gisvold JJ: Secondary neoplasms of the small bowel.
    Radiology 125:29–33, 1977

Tedeschi CG, Botta GC: Retractile mesenteritis. N Engl J Med 266:1035–1040,
    1962

44

SMALL BOWEL DIVERTICULA AND PSEUDODIVERTICULA

Disease Entities

True diverticula
  Duodenal
  Jejunal
  Meckel's
  Ileal
Pseudodiverticula
  Giant duodenal ulcer
  Peptic disease
  Intraluminal diverticula
  Scleroderma
  Crohn's disease
  Lymphoma
  Communicating ileal duplication

DUODENAL DIVERTICULA

Diverticula of the duodenum are incidental findings in 1% to 5% of barium examinations of the upper gastrointestinal tract. They are acquired lesions consisting of a sac of mucosal and submucosal layers herniated through a muscular defect, and they fill and empty by gravity as a result of pressures generated by duodenal peristalsis. Although most commonly found along the medial border of the descending duodenum in the periampullary region (Fig. 44-1), diverticula frequently arise in the third (Fig. 44-2) and fourth portions of the duodenum (30%–40%) and can even occur on the lateral border of the descending duodenum (Fig. 44-3).

538

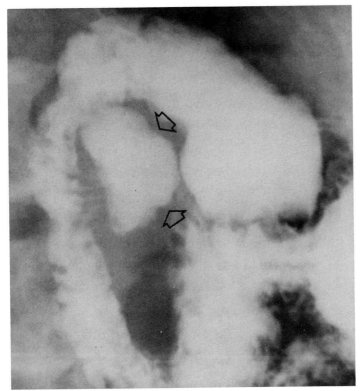

Fig. 44-1. Diverticulum **(arrows)** arising from the second portion of the duodenum.

Fig. 44-2. Diverticulum arising from the third portion of the duodenum **(solid arrow).** Of incidental note is an adenomatous polyp **(open arrow)** in the second portion of the duodenum.

Fig. 44-3. Diverticulum arising on the lateral aspect of the duodenum at the junction of the second and third portions **(arrow).**

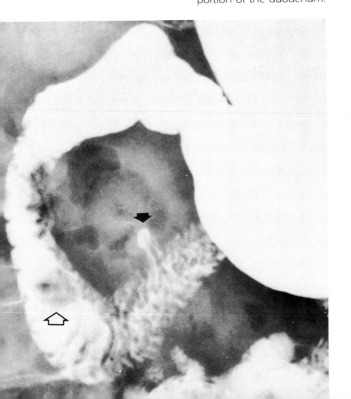

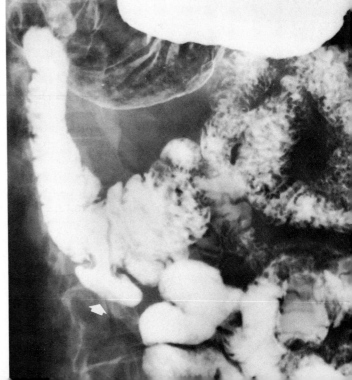

On barium examinations, duodenal diverticula typically have a smooth rounded shape, are often multiple, and generally change configuration during the course of the study. The lack of inflammatory reaction (spasm, distortion of mucosal folds) permits a duodenal diverticulum to be differentiated from a postbulbar ulcer. Bizarre multilobulated diverticula (racemose) occasionally occur (Fig. 44-4). Filling defects representing inspissated food particles, blood clots, or gas can be identified in a duodenal diverticulum (Fig. 44-5); these are inconstant and may change in appearance or disappear during observation.

Although the overwhelming majority of duodenal diverticula are asymptomatic, serious complications can develop. Duodenal diverticulitis mimics numerous abdominal diseases (cholecystitis, peptic ulcer disease, pancreatitis) and is a diagnosis of exclusion. Complications of inflammation of duodenal diverticula include hemorrhage, perforation, abscesses, and fistulas. Because duodenal diverticula are retroperitoneal structures, perforation occurs without signs of peritonitis and with no free intraperitoneal gas. The most common radiographic finding of a perforated duodenal diverticulum is retroperitoneal gas localized to the area surrounding the duodenum and the upper pole of the right kidney. A very large diverticulum occasionally causes symptoms of partial upper gastrointestinal obstruction.

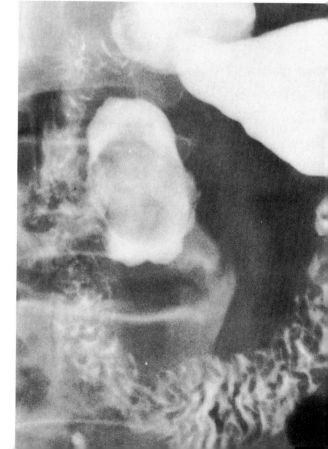

Fig. 44-5. Irregular filling defect representing a blood clot within a duodenal diverticulum in a patient with severe upper gastrointestinal bleeding.

Fig. 44-4. Bizarre multilobulated diverticulum (racemose).

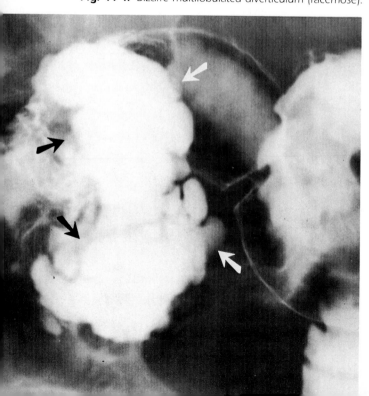

Anomalous insertion of the common bile duct and pancreatic duct into a duodenal diverticulum can be demonstrated in about 3% of carefully performed T-tube cholangiograms (Fig. 44-6). This anatomic arrangement appears to interfere with the normal emptying mechanism of the ductal systems and predisposes to obstructive biliary and pancreatic disease. The absence of an ampullary sphincter mechanism permits spontaneous reflux of barium from the diverticulum into the common bile duct, and this can be a cause of ascending infection.

Duodenal diverticula occasionally become very large and present on plain abdominal radiographs as confusing collections of gas. Because diverticula on the medial wall are usually limited in size by surrounding pancreatic tissue, these "giant" diverticula tend to arise laterally (Fig. 44-7). A gas-filled giant duodenal diverticulum may be incorrectly interpreted as an abscess, dilated cecum, colonic diverticulum, or pseudocyst of the pancreas.

GIANT DUODENAL ULCER

Giant duodenal ulcers occasionally mimic diverticula arising from the first portion of the duodenum. In contrast to the vast majority of ulcers, which are small and involve only a small portion of the duodenal bulb,

Fig. 44-6. (A) Operative cholangiogram and **(B)** corresponding line drawing. These illustrations clearly demonstrate the insertion of the common bile duct and pancreatic duct into the dome of a small duodenal diverticulum. (Nelson JA, Burhenne HJ: Anomalous biliary and pancreatic duct insertion into duodenal diverticula. Radiology 120:49–52, 1976)

A B

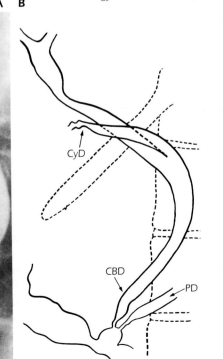

Fig. 44-7. Giant diverticulum **(arrows)** arising laterally from the junction of the first and second portions of the duodenum.

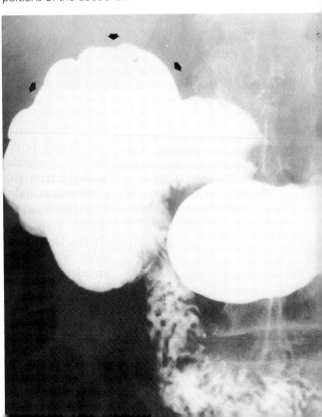

spasm of the circular muscles opposite the ulcer, a mechanism similar to that of an incisura opposite a gastric or postbulbar ulcer. The degree of deformity is not directly related to ulcer size; small ulcers may produce large deformities, and huge ulcers may produce little alteration in bulb contour.

INTRALUMINAL DIVERTICULA

An intraluminal duodenal diverticulum is a sac of duodenal mucosa originating in the second portion of the duodenum near the papilla of Vater (Fig. 44-13). Formation of the diverticulum in adults from a congenital duodenal web or diaphragm appears to be due to purely mechanical factors, such as forward pressure by food and strong peristaltic activity. When filled with barium, the intraluminal duodenal diverticulum appears as a fingerlike sac separated from contrast in the duodenal lumen by a radiolucent band representing the wall of the diverticulum ("halo sign"). When empty of barium, it can simulate a pedunculated polyp. Complications of intraluminal duodenal diverticula include retention of food and foreign bodies and partial duodenal obstruction. Increased intraluminal pressure can cause reflux of duodenal contents into the pancreatic duct and an acute attack of pancreatitis.

JEJUNAL DIVERTICULA

Jejunal diverticula are herniations of mucosa and submocosa through muscular defects at points of entrance of blood vessels on the mesenteric side of the small bowel (Fig. 44-14). These thin-walled outpouchings lack muscular components and are atonic; they are filled and emptied by the activity of adjacent bowel. The most common complication of jejunal diverticulosis is the blind loop syndrome, in which the population of bacteria within the stagnant diverticula becomes so large as to cause steatorrhea with increased numbers of bowel movements, malabsorption, anemia, and weight loss. Most symptomatic patients have multiple diverticula; however, the development of complications of bacterial overgrowth has been reported in a few patients with a single large jejunal diverticulum.

Jejunal diverticulitis is a rare complication. The larger size and wider necks of jejunal as opposed to colonic diverticula may mitigate against the inspissation of bowel contents and obstruction of the diverticular opening, thereby decreasing the incidence of inflammatory disease. Radiographically, jejunal diverticulitis can present as incomplete jejunal obstruction, an omental mass displacing jejunal loops, leakage of barium into an adjacent mesenteric abscess, or extrinsic serosal changes involving the transverse colon.

Jejunal diverticulosis is one of the leading gastrointestinal causes of pneumoperitoneum without peritonitis or surgery. It is postulated that gas passes through small perforations in the wall of the diverticula

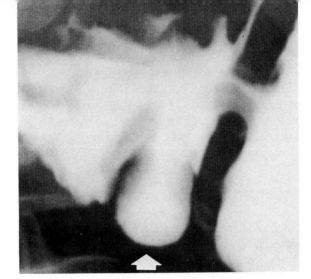

Fig. 44-12. Pseudodiverticulum of the duodenal bulb. Exaggerated outpouching **(arrow)** of the inferior recess, which is located at the base of the bulb and is related to duodenal ulcer disease.

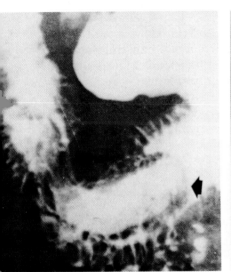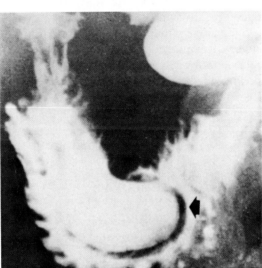

A B

Fig. 44-13. Intraluminal duodenal diverticulum. "Halo" sign **(arrow)** seen with the diverticulum **(A)** partially and **(B)** completely filled. (Laudan JCH, Norton GI: Intraluminal duodenal diverticulum. AJR 90:756–760, 1963. Copyright 1963. Reproduced by permission)

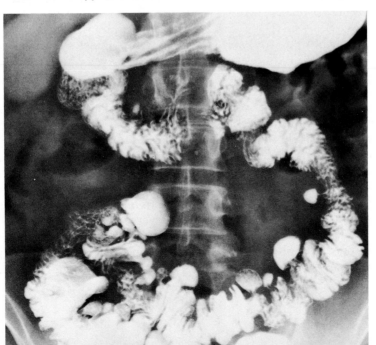

Fig. 44-14. Jejunal diverticulosis.

during periods of hyperperistalsis. Although the perforations are so small that gas can pass through them, the intestinal contents are filtered free of fecal matter, so peritonitis does not develop. Other rare complications of jejunal diverticulosis include bleeding (usually chronic), enterolith formation, and impaction of a foreign body, which can ultimately result in perforation with peritonitis.

PSEUDODIVERTICULA OF THE JEJUNUM OR ILEUM

Sacculation of the small bowel in scleroderma can simulate jejunal diverticulosis (Fig. 44-15). These pseudodiverticula are the result of smooth muscle atrophy and fibrosis accompanied by vascular occlusion. They involve only one wall of the bowel and have an appearance similar to the characteristic sacculation in the colon in patients with scleroderma.

Radiographically, pseudodiverticula due to scleroderma are large sacs with squared, broad bases that resemble colonic haustra. Sacculations are readily differentiated from true diverticula of the small bowel, which have narrow necks and are usually smaller.

Pseudodiverticula can also be demonstrated in Crohn's disease (Fig. 44-16) and lymphoma. In the former, the pseudodiverticula are associated with strictures and characteristic mucosal changes; in the latter, the aneurysmal dilatation is fusiform and not restricted to one wall.

MECKEL'S DIVERTICULA

Meckel's diverticulum is the most frequent congenital anomaly of the intestinal tract, having an incidence of 1% to 4% in autopsy reports (Fig. 44-17). The diverticula are blind outpouchings representing the rudimentary omphalomesenteric duct (embryonic communication between the gut and yolk sac), which is normally obliterated between the

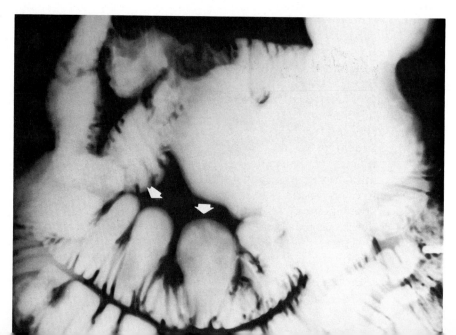

Fig. 44-15. Sacculations of the small bowel **(arrows)** in scleroderma simulating jejunal diverticulosis (pseudodiverticula).

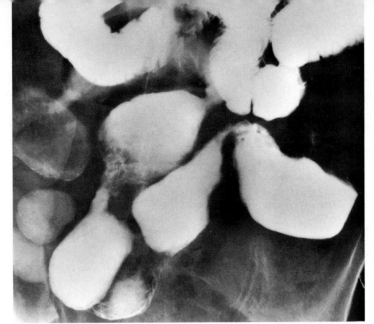

Fig. 44-16. Sacculations of the small bowel in Crohn's disease simulating intestinal diverticulosis.

fifth and seventh weeks of gestation. Meckel's diverticulum usually arises within 100 cm of the ileocecal valve (average, 80–85 cm). It opens into the antimesenteric side of the ileum, unlike other diverticula, which arise on the mesenteric side of the small bowel.

In most patients, Meckel's diverticulum remains asymptomatic throughout life. Of persons presenting with complications, a majority are under 2 years of age, and more than one-third are less than 1 year. In children, the most common symptom of Meckel's diverticulum is bleeding. Usually copious and painless, the bleeding is almost invariably the result of ulceration of ileal mucosa adjacent to heterotopic gastric mucosa in the diverticulum. Because this ectopic gastric mucosa has an affinity for pertechnetate, radionuclide imaging can be helpful in demonstrating the lesion. In adults, the most common symptom is intestinal obstruction, which can be due to invagination and intussusception of the diverticulum (Fig. 44-18), volvulus, inflammation, or adhesions.

Inflammation in a Meckel's diverticulum can produce a clinical picture indistinguishable from acute appendicitis. Resultant stenosis of the neck of the diverticulum or a valvelike flap of mucosa arising from the margin can prevent adequate drainage from the diverticulum. Stasis can precipitate changes in the acid–base balance, causing the development of faceted calculi. Neoplasms in Meckel's diverticula have been reported; free perforation with peritonitis is rare.

Despite the relative frequency of Meckel's diverticula, preoperative radiographic demonstration is unusual. If a diverticulum is not large, it can be difficult to distinguish from normal loops of small bowel unless careful compression films are obtained. Failure to demonstrate a diverticulum on routine small bowel examination can be due to stenosis of the opening, filling of the diverticulum with intestinal contents or feces, muscular contractions, or rapid emptying and small size of the diverticulum. The use of enteroclysis (antegrade small bowel enema) has been reported to greatly improve the detection rate.

Fig. 44-17. Meckel's diverticulum **(arrows)** arising from the distal ileum.

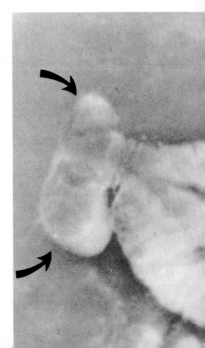

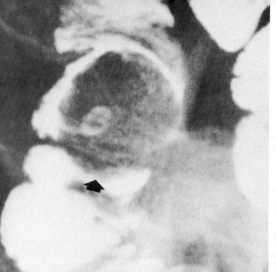

A B

Fig. 44-18. (A) <u>En face</u> and
(B) profile views of an
ulcerated lipoma arising from a
Meckel's diverticulum and
causing an intussusception
(arrows).

A Meckel's diverticulum appears radiographically as an outpouching arising from the antimesenteric side of the distal ileum. The mouth of the sac is wide, often equal to the width of the intestinal lumen itself (Fig. 44-19). Demonstration of a mucosal triangular plateau or triradiate fold pattern indicating the site of exit of the omphalomesenteric duct should lead to the correct diagnosis. Filling defects in the diverticulum, irregularity, or distortion of a segment strongly suggests the presence of ectopic gastric mucosa in the diverticulum (Fig. 44-20).

ILEAL DIVERTICULA

Diverticula are less common in the ileum than in the proximal segments of the small bowel. They are generally small and can be multiple. Most ileal diverticula lie in the terminal portion near the ileocecal valve (Fig. 44-21), unlike Meckel's diverticula, which are more proximally situated and generally much larger.

Although diverticula in the terminal ileum resemble those in the sigmoid colon, complications of these distal small bowel diverticula

Fig. 44-19. Meckel's
diverticulum **(arrow)** with a
small diverticulum (area of
increased density) arising from
it. Note the mouth of the
diverticular sac, the width of
which is approximately equal
to the width of the intestinal
lumen.

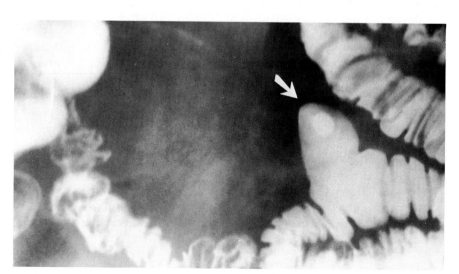

are rare. Acute ileal diverticulitis probably results from irritation or occlusion of the diverticulum by food particles or a foreign body. The clinical symptoms are usually indistinguishable from those of acute appendicitis. Localized abscess formation or generalized peritonitis can result, and postinflammatory fibrosis can cause partial small bowel obstruction.

COMMUNICATING ILEAL DUPLICATION

A communicating ileal duplication can be confused with a Meckel's diverticulum. This rare tubular lesion has an axis parallel to that of the bowel loop. Like ileal diverticula, communicating duplications are differentiated from Meckel's diverticula in that they lie on the mesenteric border and do not demonstrate a junctional fold pattern.

BIBLIOGRAPHY

Bothen NF, Ekloff O: Diverticula and duplications (enterogenous cysts) of stomach and duodenum. AJR 96:375–381, 1966

Dalinka MK, Wunder JF: Meckel's diverticulum and its complications with emphasis on roentgenologic demonstration. Radiology 106:295–298, 1973

Dunn V, Nelson JA: Jejunal diverticulosis and chronic pneumoperitoneum. Gastrointest Radiol 4:165–168, 1979

Eaton SB, Berke RA, White AF: Preoperative diagnosis of common bile duct entering a duodenal diverticulum. AJR 107:43–46, 1969

Eisenberg RL, Margulis AR, Moss AA: Giant duodenal ulcers. Gastrointest Radiol 2:347–353, 1978

Faulkner JW, Dockerty MB: Lymphosarcoma of the small intestine. Surg Gynecol Obstet 95:76–84, 1952

Fisher JK, Fortin D: Partial small bowel obstruction secondary to ileal diverticulitis. Radiology 122:321–322, 1977

Giustra PE, Killoran PJ, Root JA et al: Jejunal diverticulitis. Radiology 125:609–611, 1977

Loudan JCH, Norton GI: Intraluminal duodenal diverticulum. AJR 90:756–760, 1963

Maglinte DDT, Elmore MF, Isenberg M et al: Meckel diverticulum: Radiologic demonstration by enteroclysis. AJR 134:925–932, 1980

Millard JR, Ziter FMH, Slover WP: Giant duodenal diverticula. AJR 121:334–337, 1974

Nelson JA, Burhenne HJ: Anomalous biliary and pancreatic duct insertion into duodenal diverticula. Radiology 120:49–52, 1976

Nosher JL, Seaman WB: Association of intraluminal duodenal diverticulum with acute pancreatitis. Radiology 115:21–22, 1975

Ohba S, Fakuda A, Kohno S et al: Ileal duplication and multiple intraluminal diverticula: Scintigraphy and barium meal. AJR 136:992–994, 1981

Queloz JM, Woloshin HJ: Sacculation of the small intestine in scleroderma. Radiology 105:513–515, 1972

White AF, Oh KS, Weber AL et al: Radiologic manifestations of Meckel's diverticulum. AJR 118:86–94, 1973

Wolfe RD, Pearl MJ: Acute perforation of duodenal diverticulum with roentgenographic demonstration of localized retroperitoneal emphysema. Radiology 104:301–302, 1972

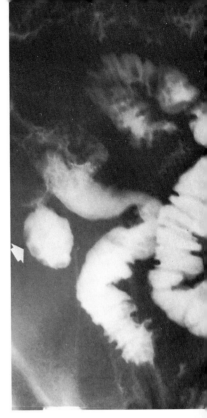

Fig. 44-20. Ectopic gastric mucosa appearing as multiple filling defects **(arrow)** in a Meckel's diverticulum.

Fig. 44-21. Ileal diverticula. Note that these diverticula are near the ileocecal valve, unlike Meckel's diverticula, which are situated more proximally.

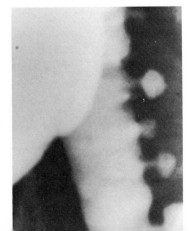

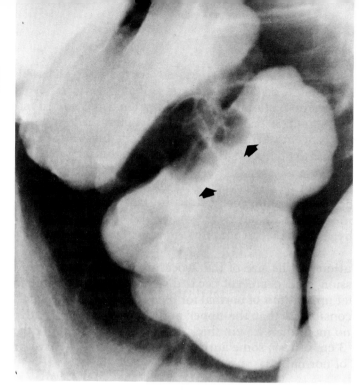

Fig. 45-6. Lipomatosis of the ileocecal valve. Although the valve is lobulated, the surface remains completely smooth (arrows).

may be due to the enlarged valve causing intermittent episodes of chronic intussusception and bowel obstruction.

Lipomatosis of the ileocecal valve appears radiographically as a smooth, masslike enlargement that is sharply demarcated from the surrounding bowel mucosa (Fig. 45-5). The valve can be lobulated and slightly irregular due to contraction of the muscularis, but the surface remains smooth (Fig. 45-6), and the valve is changeable in size and shape. If barium can be refluxed back into the terminal ileum, demonstration of the characteristic stellate appearance of the ileal mucosa on the *en face* view reveals that the process is benign. The stellate pattern indicates that the muscularis is intact and not infiltrated with tumor, since it is contraction of this tissue that presumably causes the wrinkling of the overlying mucosa.

BENIGN TUMORS

LIPOMA

The most common benign neoplasm of the ileocecal valve is a lipoma, which presents as a sharply circumscribed, smooth, rounded mass arising from either lip of the valve (Fig. 45-7). In contrast to lipomatous infiltration, lipomas of the ileocecal valve have a true capsule and are confined to only one portion of the valve. Their appearance, like that of tumors of this cell type elsewhere in the bowel, may change on serial films, reflecting their soft consistency (Fig. 45-8). Lipomas of the ileocecal valve are rarely of clinical significance unless they become so large as to cause substantial bleeding or episodes of intussusception.

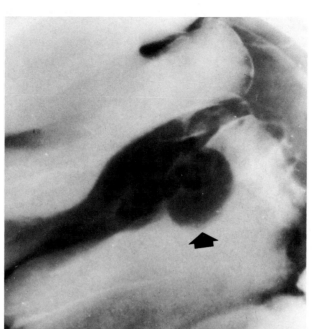

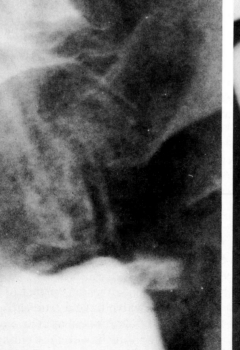

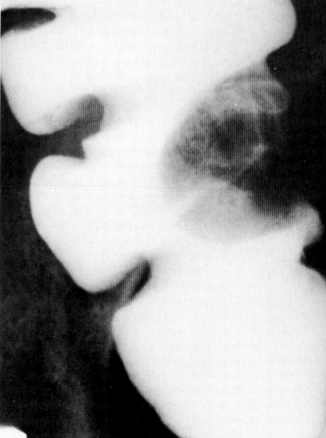

A B

Fig. 45-7. Lipoma of the ileocecal valve. A sharply circumscribed, smooth, rounded mass arises from the lower lip of the valve **(arrow)**.

Fig. 45-8. Lipoma of the ileocecal valve. Note the change in appearance on serial views.

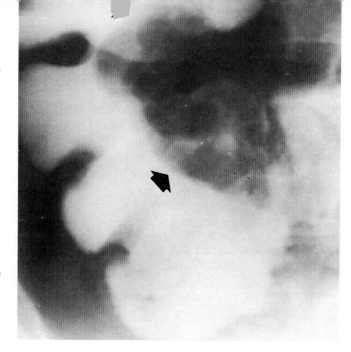

Fig. 45-9. Villous adenoma of the ileocecal valve. This large benign tumor has a moderately irregular surface **(arrows).**

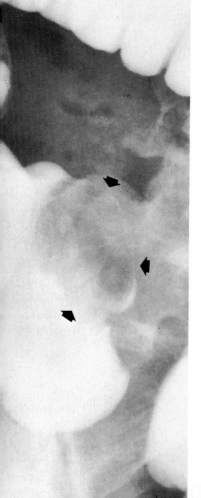

ADENOMA / VILLOUS ADENOMA

Adenomatous polyps and villous adenomas (Fig. 45-9) are rare benign tumors arising from the ileocecal valve. The surface of these tumors is usually shaggy and irregular, in contrast to the invariably smooth, though often lobulated, contours of lipomas and fatty infiltration of the ileocecal valve.

CARCINOID TUMOR

Carcinoid tumors of the ileocecal valve often arise centrally within the lumen of the valve (*i.e.*, within the terminal ileum itself) rather than from either the upper or the lower lip (Fig. 45-10). One characteristic feature of these tumors is the corrugated appearance of the adjacent cecal wall, which most likely reflects edema and spasm of the wall due to plugging of lymphatics by the tumor cells. However, this feature is not specific for carcinoid tumors; it can also be produced by inflammatory lesions in the cecum.

Fig. 45-10. Carcinoid tumor of the ileocecal valve **(arrows).** The tumor, which measured 5 cm in diameter, is contained within the lumen of the valve. A few small nodules on the colonic surface of the valve are not visible in this radiograph. Because a carcinoid tumor may cause smooth, symmetric enlargement of the valve, it is important that the terminal ileum be visualized whenever a prominent, nonpliable valve is encountered. (Short WF, Smith BD, Hoy RJ: Roentgenologic evaluation of the prominent or the unusual ileocecal valve. Med Radiogr Photogr 52:2–26, 1976)

MALIGNANT TUMORS

ADENOCARCINOMA

About 2% of adenocarcinomas of the colon arise from the ileocecal valve (Fig. 45-11). Pronounced lobulation, asymmetry, rigidity, or eccentricity of the ileocecal valve is highly indicative of a malignant tumor (Fig. 45-12). Although they are usually broad-based, irregular polypoid masses, carcinomas of the ileocecal valve can be surprisingly smooth and well-demarcated and indistinguishable from benign lesions. Villous adenocarcinomas frequently present as large, irregular masses with the typical frondlike shaggy surface that is characteristic of these tumors elsewhere in the bowel (Fig. 45-13). Because of the fluid consistency of the ileal contents, obstruction caused by carcinoma of the ileocecal valve usually appears late. Nevertheless, obstruction is a frequent complication that can be the result of occlusion of the intestinal lumen either by growth of the tumor or by intussusception of the malignant mass.

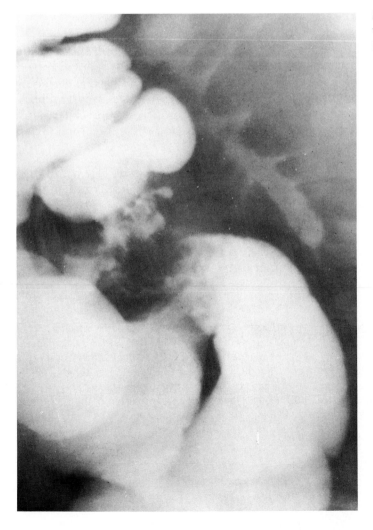

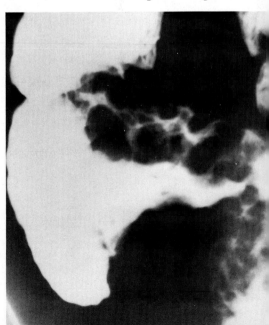

Fig. 45-11. Adenocarcinoma of the ileocecal valve. Note the prominent dilatation of the small bowel proximal to this partially obstructing lesion.

Fig. 45-12. Adenocarcinoma of the ileocecal valve. Note that the mass is rigid and irregular.

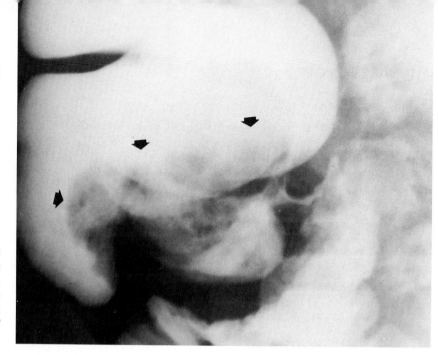

Fig. 45-13. Villous adenocarcinoma of the ileocecal valve. This large, irregular mass **(arrows)** with a typical frondlike shaggy surface is characteristic of this type of tumor elsewhere in the bowel.

LYMPHOMA

Lymphoma can present as a polypoid mass arising from the region of the ileocecal valve (Fig. 45-14). It can have a diffusely nodular appearance or be seen as a bulky, ulcerating lesion. Unlike carcinoma, lymphoma often involves the terminal ileum. Because lymphoma typically causes little desmoplastic reaction, the tumor can reach a large size before causing obstructive narrowing of the intestinal lumen.

Fig. 45-14. Lymphoma involving the ileocecal valve, ascending colon, cecum, and terminal ileum. The irregular nodularity and diffuse involvement seen in this radiograph are common features of lymphoma. (Short WF, Smith BD, Hoy, RJ: Roentgenologic evaluation of the prominent or the unusual ileocecal valve. Med Radiogr Photogr 52:2–26, 1976)

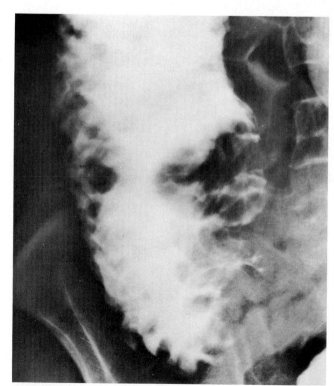

INFLAMMATORY DISORDERS

Inflammatory diseases involving the terminal ileum and cecum, especially Crohn's disease and ulcerative colitis, can affect the ileocecal valve. In Crohn's disease, extensive panenteric lymphedema frequently produces valvular enlargement, which can be in the form of direct inflammatory enlargement, lipomatous infiltration, or solitary or multiple well-encapsulated lipomas (Fig. 45-15). Small sinus tracts traversing the valve strongly suggest Crohn's disease. In ulcerative colitis (backwash ileitis), the ileocecal valve is often rigid and irregular but usually not enlarged. Indeed, it tends to be thin, patulous, and fixed in an open position (Fig. 45-16). A similar wide-open appearance of the ileocecal valve can be seen in patients with prolonged cathartic abuse.

Thickening of the ileocecal valve is not uncommon in patients with tuberculosis and amebiasis. In tuberculosis, concomitant ileal changes (mucosal ulceration and nodularity, mural rigidity, luminal narrowing, fistulas) are often seen (Fig. 45-17). In amebiasis, in contrast, the terminal ileum is not involved (Fig. 45-18). Typhoid fever, anisakiasis (Fig. 45-19), schistosomiasis, and actinomycosis can also alter the appearance of the ileocecal valve. These inflammatory processes sometimes produce radiographic patterns that are difficult to distinguish from more common conditions, such as Crohn's disease or ulcerative colitis.

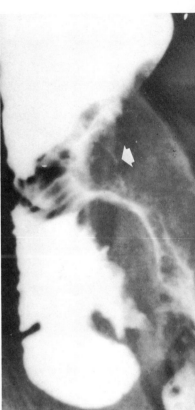

Fig. 45-15. Crohn's disease involving the ileocecal valve. Note the fistula **(arrow)** traversing the thickened upper lip of the ileocecal valve. (Short, WF, Smith BD, Hoy, RJ: Roentgenologic evaluation of the prominent or the unusual ileocecal valve. Med Radiogr Photogr 52:2–26, 1976)

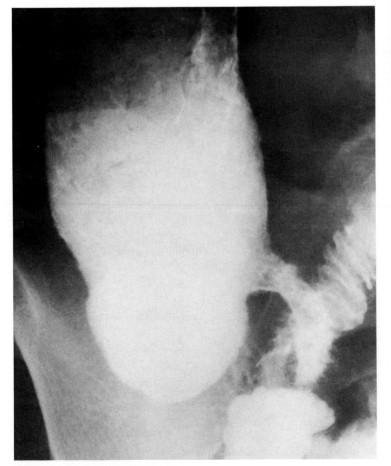

Fig. 45-16. Ulcerative colitis. The ileocecal valve is gaping, and there are inflammatory changes in the terminal ileum (backwash ileitis).

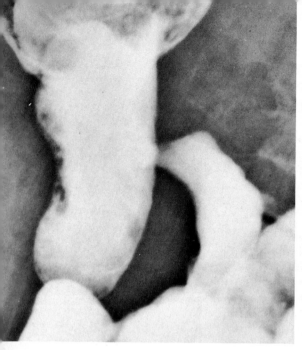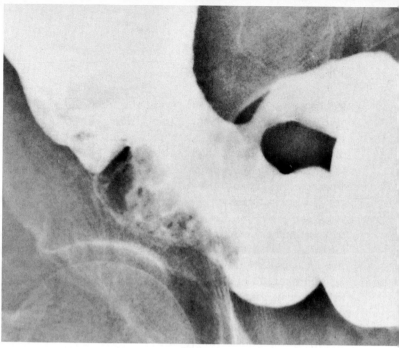

A B

Fig. 45-17. Tuberculosis of the terminal ileum and ileocecal valve. Two views demonstrate a coned cecum, thickening of the ileocecal valve, and mucosal irregularity of the terminal ileum.

Fig. 45-19. Anisakiasis of the ileocecal region. There is irregular thickening of the ileocecal valve with mucosal edema and luminal narrowing in the cecum.

Fig. 45-18. Amebiasis of the ileocecal valve and cecum. Note that the terminal ileum is not involved.

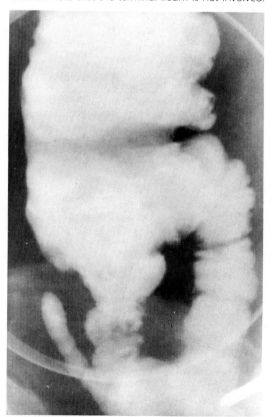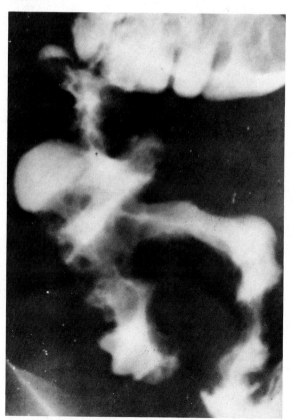

PROLAPSE

Prolapse of ileal mucosa through the lips of the ileocecal valve is an unusual cause of apparent valve enlargement and an intracecal mass (Fig. 45-20A). This phenomenon, which is similar to the extension of gastric mucosa across the pylorus into the base of the duodenal bulb, is an asymptomatic condition probably related to lipomatous infiltration of the valve. The prolapsed tissue produces smooth enlargement of the ileocecal valve, causing an appearance that is indistinguishable from lipomatosis. Extensive prolapse can simulate a benign or malignant tumor arising from the valve. The correct diagnosis of ileal prolapse can be made if it is shown by appropriate compression that the mass arises between the lips of the ileocecal valve and that there is barium in the center of the mass representing the ileal lumen. If there is substantial change in the volume of a valve on serial films and if this change is clearly not attributable to differences in compression or distention of the cecum, ileal prolapse is probably the cause of the apparent enlargement of the ileocecal valve (Fig. 45-20B).

Prolapsing neoplasms of the terminal ileum are rare causes of prominence of the ileocecal valve. Like prolapsing normal ileal mucosa, a prolapsing ileal neoplasm presents in the region of the ileocecal valve as a mass that changes size and shape during barium enema examination. The pressure of the barium column may force the tumor back across the valve, demonstrating the true origin of the lesion to be in the terminal ileum.

Retrograde prolapse of the ileocecal valve results when redundant mucosa produces prominence of the lips of the valve, which is seen as a filling defect within the cecum (Fig. 45-21A). With manual palpation or the hydrostatic pressure of the barium column, this prominent ileocecal valve prolapses in a retrograde fashion to produce a tapered defect of the terminal ileum (Fig. 45-21B,C). The pliability and changeability of the defect indicates that it represents a benign condition.

Fig. 45-20. Prolapse of the ileocecal valve. **(A)** Spot films showing a large papillary-shaped valve. Note the smooth, polypoid lobulation of the upper lip **(arrows)**. **(B)** Radiograph made a few minutes later. The valve is much smaller and has a classic spindle shape. Marked change in the volume of a valve that is not attributable to differences in compression or distention of the large intestine is probably the best evidence of prolapse. Note that the smooth, polypoid lobulation of the upper lip **(bottom arrow)** is localized but changeable. An appearance such as this should suggest the possibility of a tumor, particularly a lipoma. Note also the small polyp **(top arrow)** of the ascending colon. Follow-up studies over the next 2 years showed no change in the ileocecal valve. (Short WF, Smith BD, Hoy RJ: Roentgenologic evaluation of the prominent or the unusual ileocecal valve. Med Radiogr Photogr 52:2–26, 1976)

A B

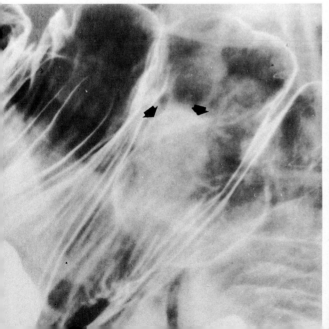
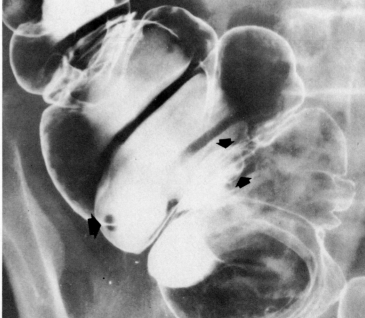

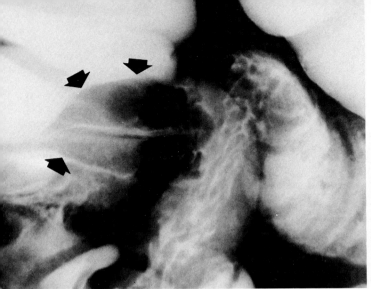

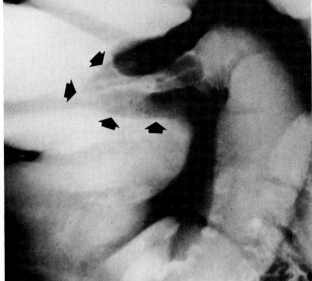

A B
C

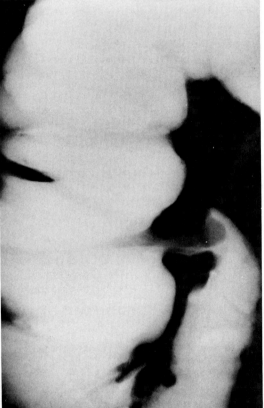

Fig. 45-21. Retrograde prolapse of the ileocecal valve on serial films from a barium enema examination. **(A)** Nondistended colon. Note the filling defect within the cecum **(arrows)**. **(B)** and **(C)** Distention of the cecum by the barium column. **(B)** The ileocecal valve **(arrows)** prolapses in a retrograde manner and **(C)** finally produces an entirely extracecal defect of the terminal ileum. (Hatten HP, Mostowycz L, Higihara PF: Retrograde prolapse of the ileocecal valve. AJR 128:755–757, 1977. Copyright 1977. Reproduced by permission)

Fig. 45-22. Massive enlargement of the ileocecal valve due to lymphoid hyperplasia. Barium enema reveals a persistent smooth mass (4 cm) in the area of the ileocecal valve. (Selke AC, Jona JZ, Belin RP: Massive enlargement of the ileocecal valve due to lymphoid hyperplasia. AJR 127:518–520, 1976. Copyright 1976. Reproduced by permission)

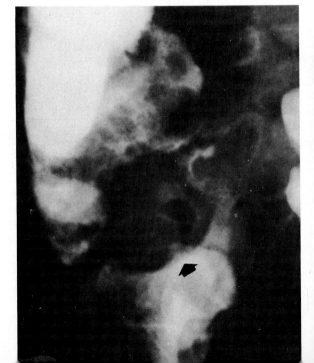

INTUSSUSCEPTION

Intussusception of the distal ileum into the cecum can present as a discrete mass arising from the region of the ileocecal valve. The distensibility of the colon can permit intussusception of numerous ileal loops, producing the characteristic "coiled-spring" appearance on barium enema examination. With relatively fixed intussusceptions, orally administered barium may only demonstrate the long, very narrow central channel of the intussuscepted small bowel. This appearance suggests some degree of vascular insufficiency and a possible surgical emergency. After reduction of an ileocolic intussusception, there may be temporary generalized thickening of the ileocecal valve due to edema from mechanical trauma sustained during the intussusception.

LYMPHOID HYPERPLASIA

Although most cases of benign lymphoid hyperplasia of the small bowel and colon present as multiple small papillary lesions, massive enlargement of the ileocecal valve has also been reported in this condition (Fig. 45-22). Lymphoid hyperplasia occurs primarily in children and is presumed to be a response to nonspecific inflammation.

BIBLIOGRAPHY

Berk RN, Davis GB, Cholhaffy EB: Lipomatosis of the ileocecal valve. AJR 119:323–328, 1973

Boquist L, Bergdahl L, Andersson A: Lipomatosis of the ileocecal valve. Cancer 29:136–140, 1972

Calenoff L: Rare ileocecal lesions. AJR 110:343–351, 1970

Carlson HC: Small intestinal intussusception. An easily misunderstood sign. AJR 110:338–339, 1970

Fleischner FG, Bernstein C: Roentgen—anatomical studies of the normal ileocecal valve. Radiology 54:43–58, 1950

Hatten HP, Mostowycz L, Hagihara PF: Retrograde prolapse of the ileocecal valve. AJR 128:755–757, 1977

Hinkel CL: Roentgenological examination and evaluation of the ileocecal valve. AJR 68:171–182, 1952

Kabakian HA, Nassar NT, Nasrallah SM: Roentgenographic findings in typhoid fever. AJR 125:198–206, 1975

Lasser EC, Rigler LG: Observations on the structure and function of the ileocecal valve. Radiology 63:176–183, 1954

Lasser EC, Rigler LG: Ileocecal valve syndrome. Gastroenterology 28:1–16, 1955

Richman RH, Lewicki AM: Right ileocolitis secondary to anisakiasis. AJR 119:329–331, 1973

Rubin S, Dann DS, Ezekial C et al: Retrograde prolapse of the ileocecal valve. AJR 87:706–708, 1962

Schnur MJ, Seaman WB: Prolapsing neoplasms of the terminal ileum simulating enlarged ileocecal valves. AJR 134:1133–1136, 1980

Selke AC, Jona JZ, Belin RP: Massive enlargement of the ileocecal valve due to lymphoid hyperplasia. AJR 127:518–520, 1976

Short WF, Smith BD, Hoy RJ: Roentgenologic evaluation of the prominent or unusual ileocecal valve. Med Radiogr Photogr 52:2–26, 1976

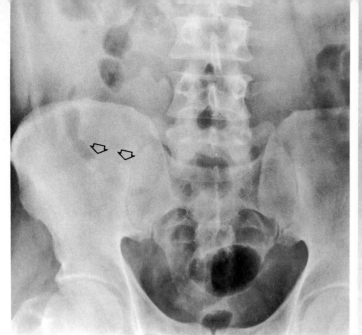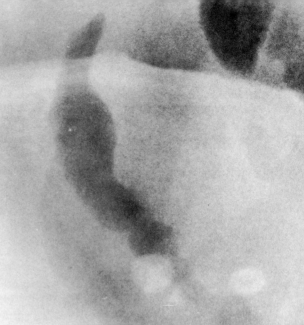

A B

Fig. 46-6. Appendicoliths in a patient with acute appendicitis and a periappendiceal abscess. **(A)** Full and **(B)** coned views show that the appendicoliths **(arrows)** lie in an abscess outside of the gas-filled appendix.

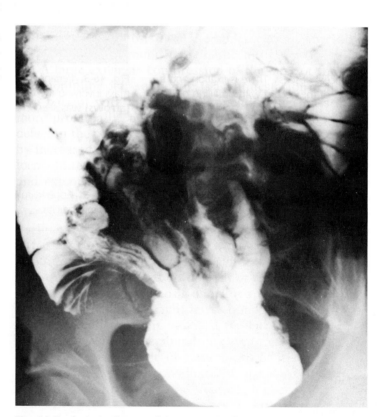

Fig. 46-7. Crohn's disease of the appendix. Pressure film from a barium enema examination reveals a large extrinsic mass impinging upon the cecal tip and medial cecal wall. Note the normal mucosa and the distensibility of the terminal ileum. (Threatt B, Appelman H: Crohn's disease of the appendix presenting as acute appendicitis. Radiology 110:313–317, 1974)

acute onset of abdominal pain and a palpable right lower quadrant mass simulating acute appendicitis. Barium enema examination generally demonstrates a large extrinsic mass impinging upon the cecal tip and medial cecal wall (Fig. 46-7). The terminal ileum is distensible and has a normal mucosal pattern.

INVERTED APPENDICEAL STUMP

An inverted appendiceal stump following appendectomy produces a filling defect in the tip of the cecum at the base of the appendix that may be seen on barium studies (Fig. 46-8). The mass is usually small and localized but can be very prominent for several weeks after surgery until postoperative edema and inflammation subside (Fig. 46-9). The surface of an inverted stump deformity is generally smooth but can be lobulated or irregular. Although an inverted appendiceal stump is essentially asymptomatic, recognition of the entity is essential, because the radiographic appearance can be indistinguishable from a neoplasm at the base of the cecum (Fig. 46-10). A smooth cecal defect in the expected site of the appendix in a patient with a history of previous appendectomy is presumptive evidence for the diagnosis of an inverted appendiceal stump. A negative history of appendectomy, however, does not exclude the diagnosis of appendiceal stump, since many patients have had appendectomies incidental to other surgery without being aware of it. If the cecal defect is large or irregular, colonoscopy or surgical intervention is necessary to exclude the possibility of a neoplastic process.

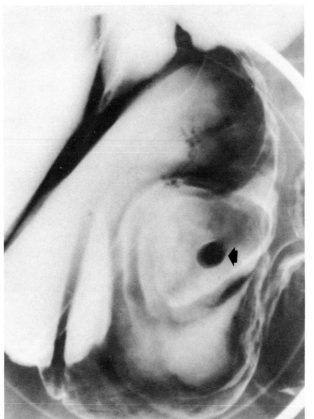

Fig. 46-8. Inverted appendiceal stump **(arrow)** following appendectomy.

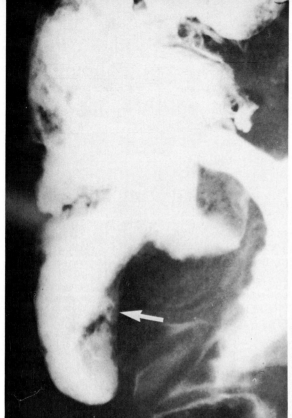
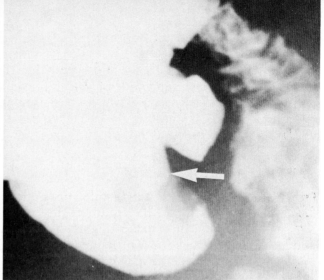
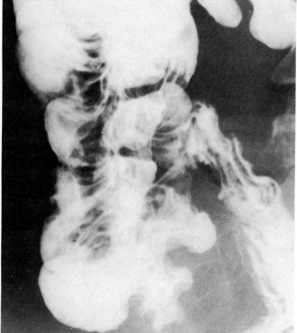

A B
C

Fig. 46-9. Development of an appendiceal stump. **(A)** Two days after appendectomy, there is a 3 × 5-cm deformation of the medial aspect of the cecum **(arrow)**. Note the typical, somewhat eccentrically located umbilication. **(B)** Five weeks after the operation, the defect has diminished, and the umbilicus is more prominent **(arrow)**. **(C)** After 9 months, there is only a slight deformation of the cecum. (Ekberg O: Cecal changes following appendectomy. Gastrointest Radiol 2:57–60, 1977)

Fig. 46-10. Inverted appendiceal stump. In this patient, the mass **(arrow)** is large and irregular, simulating a neoplasm at the base of the cecum.

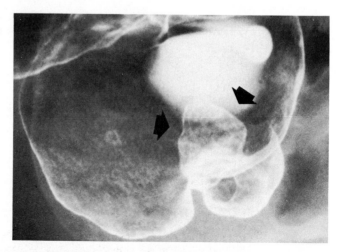

MUCOCELE

Mucocele of the appendix is an uncommon benign condition in which there is cystic dilatation of the appendix. Most mucoceles are believed to result from proximal luminal obstruction (caused by a fecalith, foreign body, tumor, adhesions, or volvulus), which leads to accumulation of mucus distally in the distended appendix. A few authors suggest that the lesion represents a mucinous cystadenoma arising within the appendix.

Most mucoceles of the appendix are found incidentally during abdominal radiography, at laparotomy, or on portmortem examination. Some patients with mucoceles complain of recurrent vague lower abdominal discomfort; physical examination may reveal a right lower quadrant mass. Significant symptoms are infrequent and reflect complications such as secondary infection or intussusception of the lesion.

Plain radiographs of the abdomen may demonstrate a mottled or rimlike calcification around the periphery of an appendiceal mucocele. This calcification occurs infrequently but is helpful in establishing the diagnosis. On barium enema examination, a mucocele presents as a sharply outlined smooth-walled, broad-based filling defect indenting the lower part of the cecum, usually on its medial side (Fig. 46-11). There is typically nonfilling of the appendix, though a few cases have been reported in which barium has entered the mucocele through what was probably a recanalized lumen.

Rupture of a mucocele of the appendix (or ovary) can lead to the development of pseudomyxoma peritonei, a condition characterized by epithelial implants on the peritoneal surface with massive accumulation of gelatinous ascites. Acute, sharp abdominal pain can occur at the time of rupture of the mucocele; this event is often associated with straining. Radiographic demonstration of a sudden decrease in the size of a mucocele may indicate that rupture has occurred. Rarely, a mucocele causes ureteral or ileal obstruction, becomes inflamed, twists on itself, or intussuscepts.

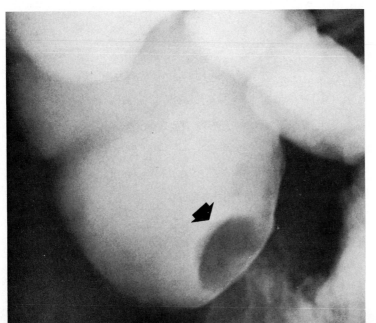

Fig. 46-11. Mucocele of the appendix. A smooth, broad-based filling defect **(arrow)** indents the lower part of the cecum. There is no filling of the appendix with barium.

MYXOGLOBULOSIS

Myxoglobulosis is a rare type of mucocele of the appendix that is composed of many round or oval translucent globules mixed with mucus. The globules vary from 0.1 cm to 1.0 cm in size and are said to resemble tapioca or fish eggs. Like simple mucoceles of the appendix, myxoglobulosis is usually asymptomatic. Radiographically, myxoglobulosis can present as a smooth extramucosal mass impressing on the cecum and associated with nonfilling of the appendix, a pattern indistinguishable from simple mucocele (Fig. 46-12A). The most characteristic features of myxoglobulosis are calcified rims about the periphery of the individual globules. Unlike appendiceal calculi, the calcified spherules in myxoglobulosis usually are annular and nonlaminated, shift within the mucocele, and can layer in the upright position. In contrast to simple mucoceles, in which calcification involves only the wall, the individual globules within the lumen in myxoglobulosis are calcified (Fig. 46-12B).

INTUSSUSCEPTION

Primary appendiceal intussusception is an infrequent occurrence in which the appendix invaginates into the cecum and simulates a cecal tumor (Fig. 46-13). It can present as an acute surgical emergency or as a subacute recurring condition. Intussusception of the appendix can also be asymptomatic and may be noted only during a barium enema examination (Fig. 46-14).

Fig. 46-12. Myxoglobulosis of the appendix. **(A)** A mass effect on the medial wall of the cecum with distortion but no destruction of cecal folds is seen on barium enema examination. **(B)** Typical calcifications of myxoglobulosis. (Felson B, Wiot JF: Some interesting right lower quadrant entities. Radiol Clin North Am 7:83–95, 1969)

A   B

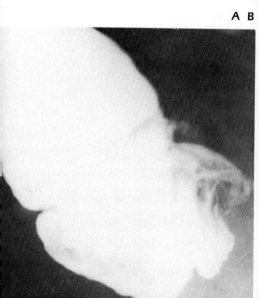
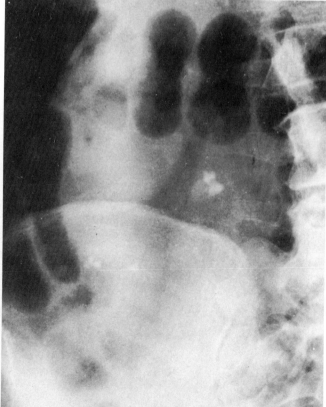

Intussusception is probably caused by increased and abnormal peristalsis of the appendix. This may be related either to an attempt of the organ to extrude an intraluminal abnormality (foreign body, fecalith, polyp, parasite) or to intramural disease (mucocele, tumor, endometriosis, lymphoid follicles).

On barium enema examination, intussusception of the appendix produces an oval, round, or fingerlike filling defect projecting from the medial wall of the cecum. The appendix is not visible.

An intussusception of the appendix demonstrated by barium enema can reduce itself completely during the course of a single examination or be reduced on a subsequent study. After reduction occurs, the cecum and appendix appear radiographically to be entirely normal. Patients with this condition are asymptomatic, and the cause of reducible partial intussusception of a normal appendix is unknown.

BENIGN NEOPLASMS

Although tumors of the appendix can be demonstrated in about 6% of surgical and autopsy specimens, these lesions are rarely diagnosed radiographically because of their small size or the frequent complication of appendicitis. The most common appendiceal neoplasm is the carcinoid tumor, which arises from the argentaffin cells of the crypts of Lieberkuhn. Of all carcinoids, 90% arise in the distal ileum or appendix; of all tumors of the appendix, 90% are carcinoids. These lesions are almost always benign and rarely metastasize or cause the carcinoid syndrome. Most carcinoids are discovered in appendices removed incidentally at surgery for another procedure or because of acute appendicitis. Appendiceal carcinoids tend to obstruct the lumen and cause acute appendicitis. This permits such a tumor to be diagnosed relatively early, thereby greatly decreasing the incidence of metastases.

Fig. 46-13. Primary appendiceal intussusception. Lobulated, fingerlike filling defect **(arrows)** projects into the cecum and simulates a cecal tumor.

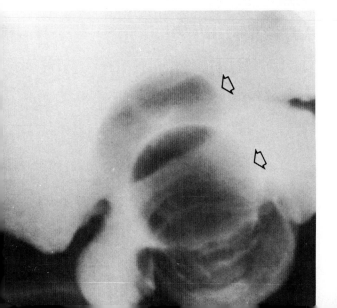

Fig. 46-14. Primary appendiceal intussusception **(arrow).** Following reduction, the cecum and appendix appeared normal on a subsequent barium enema examination.

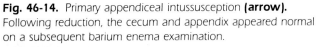
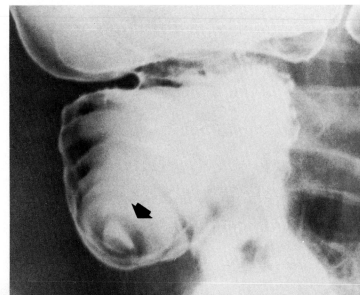

Other benign tumors of the appendix include leiomyomas, neuromas, and lipomas. Like carcinoids, these small tumors are generally incidental findings in surgical specimens and are rarely diagnosed by barium studies.

MALIGNANT NEOPLASMS

Adenocarcinoma of the appendix usually arises in the distal third of the appendix, where it frequently results in luminal obstruction and secondary acute appendicitis. The preoperative diagnosis of adenocarcinoma of the appendix is rarely made. In half of the reported cases, patients were initially thought to have acute appendicitis.

Radiographic demonstration of appendiceal carcinoma is unusual. When visualized, these tumors generally present as extrinsic masses deforming and displacing the cecum. If the tumor is extensive enough, the acute angle formed between the mass and the adjacent cecal wall can mimic an intramural (Fig. 46-15) or even an intraluminal (Fig. 46-16) cecal mass. Calcification is occasionally detected in the tumor on plain abdominal radiographs.

METASTASES

A localized defect on the medial aspect of the cecum below the ileocecal valve can represent a metastatic lesion (Fig. 46-17). Metastases in the right lower quadrant producing such defects are most commonly

Fig. 46-15. Adenocarcinoma arising from the base of the appendix and projecting into the cecal lumen **(arrow)**. Note the sharply defined lobulated contour and acute angle, characteristic of an intrinsic lesion, that are formed by the mass and the adjacent wall of the cecum. (Stiehm WD, Seaman WB: Radiographic aspects of primary carcinoma of the appendix. Radiology 108:275–278, 1973)

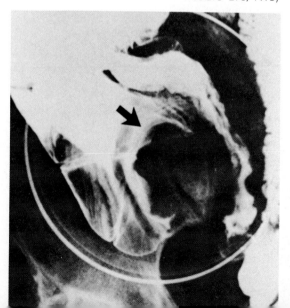

Fig. 47-16. Adenocarcinoma of the appendix. The extensive tumor produces a large mass **(arrows)** that mimics an intraluminal cecal neoplasm.

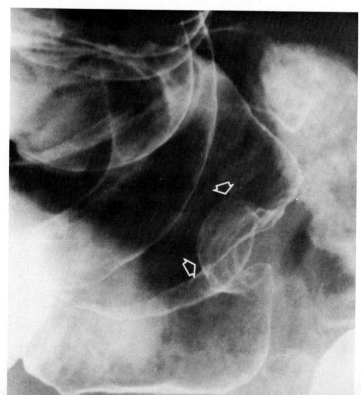

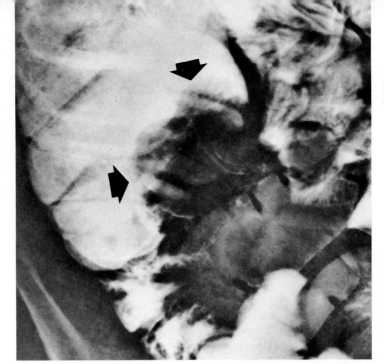

Fig. 46-17. Carcinoma of the pancreas metastatic to the cecum. There is a localized extrinsic pressure defect **(arrows)** on the medial and inferior aspects of the cecum and no filling of the appendix.

secondary to a primary neoplasm in the ovary, colon, stomach, or pancreas. The relatively common association of primary pancreatic carcinoma with a prominent right lower quadrant metastatic mass is due to the typical routes of spread of this malignancy. The origin of the mesentery near the inferior margin of the pancreas and its insertion in the region of the ileocecal valve provide a pathway for the spread of pancreatic carcinoma to the right lower quadrant of the abdomen. This is analogous to the pattern seen in acute pancreatitis, in which extravasated enzymes dissecting between the leaves of the mesentery cause abscess formation in the ileocecal area. These secondary abscesses can produce a medial cecal deformity identical to that seen in patients with metastatic pancreatic carcinoma. Metastatic spread by intraperitoneal seeding often demonstrates preferential flow along the root of the small bowel mesentery toward the right lower quadrant and then upward in the right pericolic gutter; this can cause extrinsic impressions in the region of the ileocecal junction or the lateral and posterior aspects of

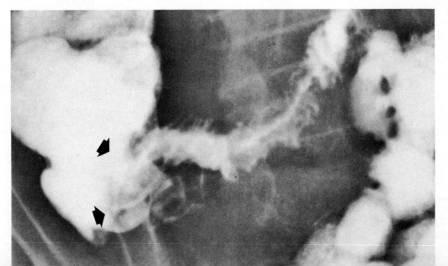

Fig. 46-18. Crohn's disease. This irregular mass on the medial aspect of the cecum **(arrows)** was seen in a patient with extensive disease of the terminal ileum.

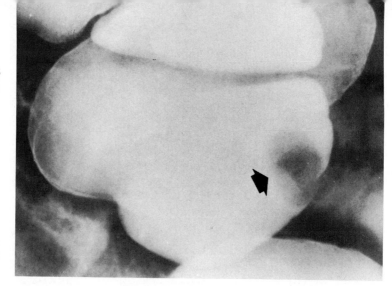

Fig. 46-19. Benign adenomatous polyp **(arrow)** in the cecum.

the cecum, respectively. In middle-aged or elderly patients with non-specific abdominal complaints and no clinical evidence of inflammatory disease in the right lower quadrant, the presence of a localized defect on the medial aspect of the cecum should raise the possibility of metastatic carcinoma.

GENERAL COLONIC LESIONS

Fig. 46-20. Development of a cecal carcinoma. **(A)** Small, smooth impression on the medial wall of the cecum **(arrow)** that was noted only in retrospect. **(B)** One year later, the malignant mass is irregular **(solid arrow),** and the tumor has spread to irregularly narrow the appendix **(open arrow).**

Numerous conditions described in detail in other sections can produce filling defects in the barium-filled cecum. These include inflammatory masses (Fig. 46-18), especially ameboma, benign (Fig. 46-19) and malignant (Fig. 46-20, 46-21) primary cecal neoplasms, and ileocolic intussusception (Fig. 46-22). Several unusual entities, however, can cause masses or contour deformities that either primarily involve the cecum or have a specific radiographic appearance when the cecum is affected.

A B

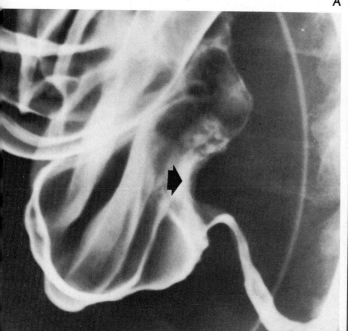
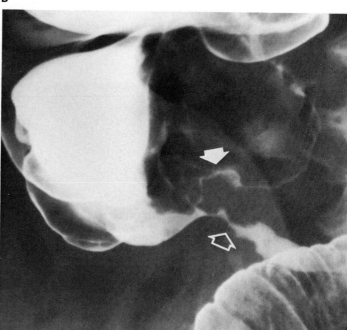

ILEOCECAL DIVERTICULITIS

Diverticulitis of the ileocecal area can result in a localized mural abscess in the wall of the colon that presents radiographically as a smooth, eccentric mass that is sharply demarcated from the adjacent colonic wall (Fig. 46-23). Extraluminal barium is occasionally seen as a small fleck in a fistula or in an abscess cavity. Both cecal and ileal diverticula are uncommon. Because the major symptom of acute diverticulitis in the ileocecal area is generalized abdominal pain that eventually localizes to the right lower quadrant, the preoperative diagnosis is almost always acute appendicitis. A major reason for these errors in diagnosis is that cecal diverticulitis often occurs in young patients (up to 50% of cases develop in persons under the age of 30) who are generally not considered to suffer from complications of diverticular disease. A barium enema in patients with diverticulitis of the ileocecal area sometimes demonstrates complete filling of the appendix, excluding the presence of acute appendicitis. A correct preoperative diagnosis of cecal diverticulitis is of great importance, since it may permit medical treatment rather than immediate surgical intervention.

SOLITARY BENIGN ULCER OF THE CECUM

A smooth mass in the base of the cecum can be due to granulation tissue caused by the healing of a solitary benign ulcer of the cecum. In

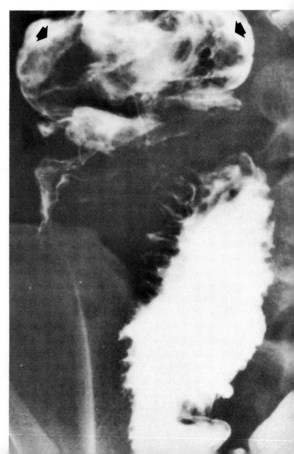

Fig. 46-22. Ileocolic intussusception due to pseudolymphoma of the distal ileum. A large mass **(arrows)** is visible at the base of the cecum. There are inflammatory (pseudoneoplastic) changes in the distal ileum.

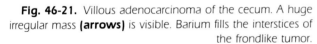

Fig. 46-21. Villous adenocarcinoma of the cecum. A huge irregular mass **(arrows)** is visible. Barium fills the interstices of the frondlike tumor.

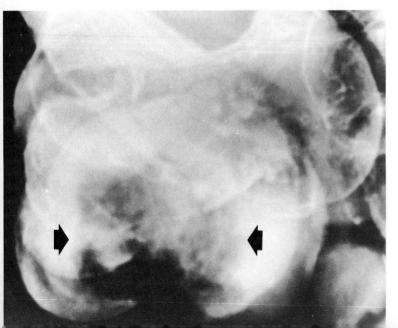

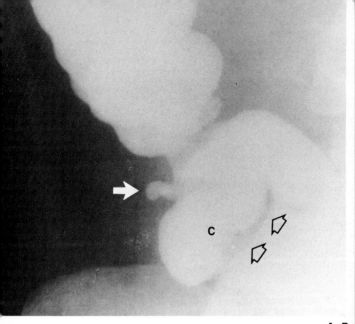

A B

Fig. 46-23. Cecal diverticulitis in a 24-year-old man. **(A)** Solitary cecal diverticulum **(white arrow)** surrounded by an intramural mass. The mucosa over the mass is intact and not ulcerated. The terminal ileum **(black arrows)** is not displaced from the cecum (C). **(B)** Postevacuation spot film demonstrates the cecal diverticulum **(white arrow)** and normal filling of the appendix **(black arrows).** (Norfray JF, Givens JD, Sparberg MS et al: Cecal diverticulitis in young patients. Gastrointest Radiol 5:379–382, 1980)

Fig. 46-24. Adherent fecalith. A tumorlike mass **(arrows)** is visible in the cecum of a patient with cystic fibrosis.

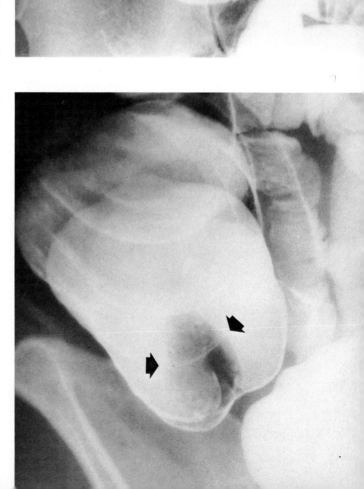

this rare disease, which is of uncertain etiology, the ulcer itself is infrequently visible on barium enema examination. The adjacent inflammatory reaction can be so intense that it simulates a discrete tumor mass. Localized irritability, hypermotility, spasm, and stricture can also be present. Because of the danger of perforation, surgical resection of the cecum is usually performed.

ADHERENT FECALITH

The sticky fecal material that is found in patients with cystic fibrosis can form a persistent tumorlike mass in the colon, particularly in the cecum (Fig. 46-24). This can produce a filling defect on barium enema examination that often persists on repeat studies over an interval of several weeks. Palpable adherent fecaliths in cystic fibrosis can simulate colonic neoplasms; associated tenderness can suggest acute appendicitis. Occasionally, an adherent fecalith can be the leading point of an intussusception.

ENDOMETRIOSIS

Endometriosis can present as an intramural, extramucosal lesion of the cecum with a smooth surface and sharp margins (Fig. 46-25). The mucosa overlying the lesion usually remains intact. Cecal endometriosis rarely causes the fibrotic compression and kinking of the colon that are characteristic of the disease in the sigmoid region.

Fig. 46-25. Endometriosis of the cecum. Note the intramural extramucosal lesion **(arrows).** The mucosa over the mass is stretched but preserved. (Felson B, Wiot JF: Some interesting right lower quadrant entities. Radiol Clin North Am 7:83–95, 1969)

A B

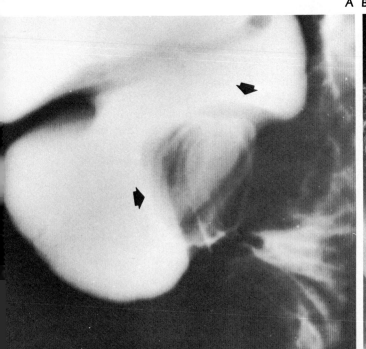
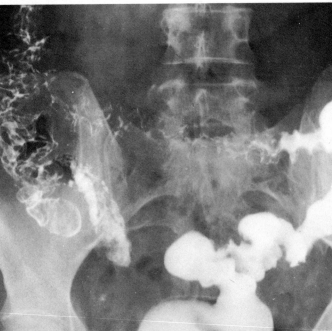

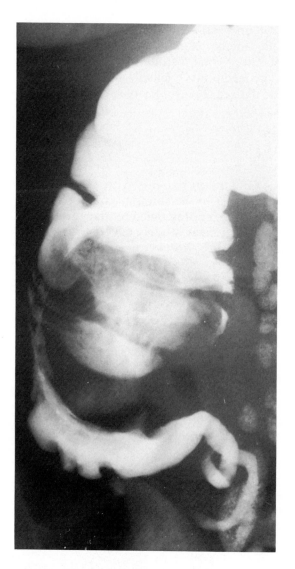

Fig. 46-26. Burkitt's lymphoma. A huge mass fills essentially the entire cecum.

BURKITT'S LYMPHOMA

Burkitt's lymphoma is a distinct childhood tumor of the reticuloendothelial system. The disease predominantly affects African children and is characterized by swelling and bony lesions of the mandible and maxilla. A tumor histologically indistinguishable from the African variety is being increasingly reported in North American children. Most of these children, unlike their African counterparts, have demonstrated some involvement of the gastrointestinal tract, predominantly masses in the ileocecal area (Fig. 46-26), which often cause intussusception or obstruction.

Alford BA, Coccia PF, L'Heureux PR: Roentgenographic features of American Burkitt's lymphoma. Radiology 124:763–770, 1977

Bachman AL, Clemett AR: Roentgen aspects of primary appendiceal intussusception. Radiology 101:531–538, 1971

Beneventano TC, Schein CJ, Jacobson HG: The roentgen aspects of some appendiceal abnormalities. AJR 96:344–360, 1966

Benninger GW, Honig LJ, Fein HD: Nonspecific ulceration of the cecum. Am J Gastroenterol 55:594–601, 1971

Berk RN, Lee FA: The late gastrointestinal manifestations of cystic fibrosis of the pancreas. Radiology 106:377–381, 1973

Collins DC: Seventy-one thousand human appendix specimens. A final report summarizing 40 years' study. Am J Proctol 14:365–381, 1963

Douglas NJ, Cameron SJ, Nixon MV et al: Intussusception of a mucocele of the appendix. Gastrointest Radiol 3:97–100, 1978

Felson B, Wiot JF: Some interesting right lower quadrant entities. Myxoglobulosis of the appendix, ileal prolapse, diverticulitis, lymphoma, endometriosis. Radiol Clin North Am 7:83–95, 1969

Figiel LS, Figiel SJ: Barium examination of cecum in appendicitis. Acta Radiol 57:469–480, 1962

Freedman E, Radwin MH, Linsman JF: Roentgen simulation of polypoid neoplasms by invaginated appendicele stumps. AJR 75:380–385, 1956

Ghosh BC, Huvos AG, Whiteley HW: Pseudomyxoma peritonei. Dis Colon Rectum 15:420–425, 1972

Gibbs NM: Mucinous cystadenocarcinoma of vermiform appendix with particular reference to mucocele and pseudomyxoma peritonei. J Clin Pathol 26:413–421, 1973

Gorske K: Intussusception of the proximal appendix into the colon. Radiology 91:791, 1968

Howard RJ, Ellis CM, Delaney JP: Intussusception of the appendix simulating carcinoma of the cecum. Arch Surg 101:520–522, 1970

Joffe N: Medial cecal defect associated with metastatic pancreatic carcinoma. Radiology 111:297–300, 1974

Marshak RH, Gerson A: Mucocele of the appendix. Am J Dig Dis 5:49–54, 1960

Norfray JF, Givens JD, Sparberg MS et al: Cecal diverticulitis in young patients. Gastrointest Radiol 5:379–382, 1980

Otto RE, Ghislandi EV, Lorenzo GA et al: Primary appendiceal adenocarcinoma. Am J Surg 120:704–707, 1970

Ponka JL: Carcinoid tumors of the appendix. Report of 35 cases. Am J Surg 126:77–83, 1973

Schey WL: Use of barium in the diagnosis of appendicitis in children. AJR 118:95–103, 1973

Soter CS: The contribution of the radiologist to the diagnosis of acute appendicitis. Semin Roentgenol 8:375–388, 1973

Stiehm WD, Seaman WB: Roentgenographic aspects of primary carcinoma of the appendix. Radiology 108:275–278, 1973

Threatt B, Appelman H: Crohn's disease of the appendix presenting as acute appendicitis. Radiology 110:313–317, 1974

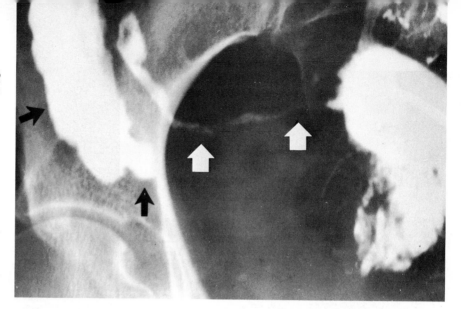

Fig. 47-4. Crohn's disease. There is incomplete filling of the terminal ileum ("string sign"; **right arrows**) in a patient with rigid narrowing of the cecum **(left arrows)**.

TUBERCULOSIS

The coned cecum is a characteristic finding of intestinal tuberculosis. Healing of acute tuberculous inflammation of the terminal ileum and cecum results in shortening and narrowing of the purse-shaped cecum. This is most marked opposite the ileocecal valve, where there can be a broad, deep indentation. Further progression of this process causes straightening and rigidity of the ileocecal valve. The terminal ileum can appear to empty directly into the stenotic ascending colon with nonopacification of the fibrotic, contracted cecum (Stierlin's sign, Fig. 47-5). In contrast to those in Crohn's disease, the lesions in tuberculosis tend to have more irregular contours and coarser mucosal markings, and involvement of the colon is usually more prominent than that of the terminal ileum (Fig. 47-6). The majority of patients in the western hemisphere who have gastrointestinal tuberculosis also have pulmonary tuberculous disease, with typical symptoms of cough, fever, night sweats, hemoptysis, anorexia, and weight loss. Without concomitant pulmonary involvement, however, differentiation between tuberculosis and Crohn's disease can be extremely difficult.

AMEBIASIS

The cecum is involved in about 90% of cases of chronic amebiasis. In the early stages of the disease, small, shallow ulcers produce an irregular bowel margin and finely granular mucosa (Fig. 47-7). With continued inflammation and fibrosis, the lumen of the cecum concentrically narrows until it has assumed a cone-shaped configuration (Fig. 47-8). The ileocecal valve often appears to move downward, sometimes lying close to the cecal tip. In contrast to Crohn's disease and tuberculosis, in which terminal ileum involvement is the rule, the terminal ileum in amebic colitis is usually normal. In amebiasis, the ileocecal valve is

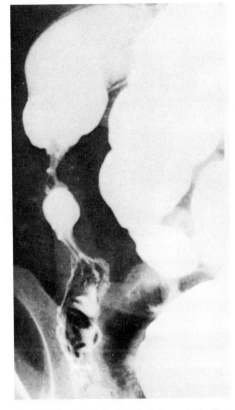

Fig. 47-5. Stierlin's sign in tuberculosis. The terminal ileum appears to empty directly into the stenotic ascending colon with nonopacification of the fibrotic, contracted cecum. (Carrera GF, Young S, Lewicki AM: Intestinal tuberculosis. Gastrointest Radiol 1:147–155, 1976)

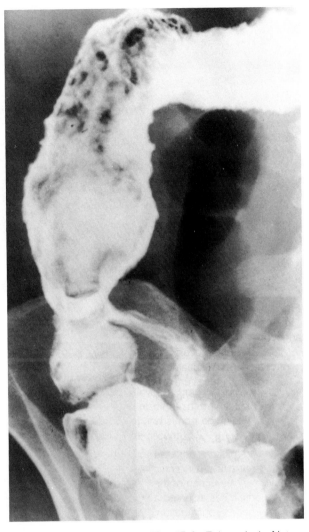

Fig. 47-6. Tuberculosis. Note that the ulcerative process primarily involves the ascending and transverse colon and essentially spares the terminal ileum, unlike the usual appearance in Crohn's disease.

almost invariably thickened, rigid, and fixed in an open position, permitting free reflux into the terminal ileum; this is in contrast to tuberculosis, in which reflux is infrequent because of intense ileocecal spasm. The combination of a coned cecum, an intact terminal ileum, and skip lesions in the colon is highly suggestive of amebic infection. The diagnosis is made by demonstration of *Entamoeba histolytica* in the stool or rectal biopsy. However, a negative stool examination or rectal biopsy does not rule out amebiasis; similarly, the presence of amebas in the stool does not exclude the possibility of other ulcerative diseases of the colon. Laparotomy as a means for diagnosis or for resection of the lesion is dangerous and is contraindicated in untreated patients. One differential point is the dramatic change in radiographic appearance seen within 2 weeks of the institution of antiamebic therapy (Fig. 47-7*B*).

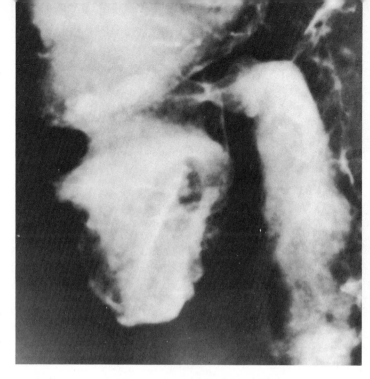

Fig. 47-17. <u>Yersinia enterocolitica.</u> Conical narrowing and irregular margins of the cecum are present with mild inflammatory changes in the terminal ileum.

Most cases appear to be related to infection secondary to potent antimetabolite therapy, with cecal predilection for progressive ulceration and invasion by enteric organisms. Hemorrhage or direct leukemic infiltration is a much less common cause of this radiographic pattern.

BIBLIOGRAPHY

Avritchir Y, Perroni AA: Radiological manifestations of small intestinal South American blastomycosis. Radiology 127:607–609, 1978

Balikian JR, Uthman SM, Khorui NF: Intestinal amebiasis. AJR 122:245–256, 1974

Berk RN, Lasser EC: Radiology of the Ileocecal Area. Philadelphia, WB Saunders, 1975

Carrera GF, Young S, Lewicki AM: Intestinal tuberculosis. Gastrointest Radiol 1:147–155, 1976

Del Fava RL, Cronin TG: Typhlitis complicating leukemia in an adult: Barium enema findings. AJR 129:347–348, 1977

Ekberg O: Cecal changes following appendectomy. Gastrointest Radiol 2:57–60, 1977

Kolawole PM, Lewis EA: Radiologic observations on intestinal amebiasis. AJR 122:257–265, 1974

Lockhart–Mummery HE, Morson BC: Crohn's disease of the large intestine. Gut 5:493–509, 1964

Moss JD, Knauer CM: Tuberculous enteritis. Gastroenterology 65:959–966, 1973

Werbeloff L, Novis BH, Bank S et al: The radiology of tuberculosis of the gastrointestinal tract. Br J Radiol 46:329–336, 1973

PART SEVEN

COLON

ULCERATIVE LESIONS OF THE COLON

48

Disease Entities

Ulcerative colitis
Crohn's colitis
Ischemic colitis
Specific infections
  Protozoan
    Amebiasis
    Schistosomiasis
  Bacterial
    Shigellosis
    Salmonellosis
    Tuberculous colitis
    Gonorrheal proctitis
    Staphylococcal colitis
    Yersinia colitis
    Campylobacter fetus colitis
  Fungal
    Histoplasmosis
    Mucormycosis
    Actinomycosis
    Candidiasis
  Viral
    Lymphogranuloma venereum
    Herpes zoster
    Cytomegalovirus
  Helminthic
    Strongyloidiasis
Pseudomembranous colitis
  Postantibiotic colitis
  Postoperative colitis
  Uremia
  Large bowel obstruction
  Hypoxia
Radiation injury
Caustic colitis
Pancreatitis
Malignancy
  Primary carcinoma
  Metastases
  Leukemic infiltration
Amyloidosis
Inorganic mercury poisoning
Behcet's syndrome
Diverticulosis/diverticulitis
Solitary rectal ulcer syndrome
Nonspecific benign ulceration of the colon

Ulcerative inflammation of the colon or rectum is a nonspecific response to a host of harmful agents and processes. In many cases, an ulcerating colitis can be attributed to a specific infectious disease, systemic disorder, or toxic agent. However, in a large group of patients, a precise cause cannot be determined. Most of these "nonspecific" inflammatory diseases of the colon are generally placed into one of two categories: ulcerative colitis or Crohn's disease. Although radiographic and pathologic criteria have been established for distinguishing between these two processes, there is a substantial overlap in practice. In at least 10% of colectomy specimens for ulcerating colitis, it is impossible to distinguish between ulcerative colitis and Crohn's disease even with careful gross inspection and multiple microscopic sections. Features of ulcerative colitis and Crohn's disease often coexist, making a precise histologic diagnosis difficult. Such cases can be termed "unclassified colitis" or "colitis, type unknown."

ULCERATIVE COLITIS

Ulcerative colitis is primarily a disease of young adults, the peak incidence being in persons between 20 and 40 years of age. The disease may be first diagnosed at an older age; a second peak incidence has been reported in persons in their sixth and seventh decades. These patients are reputed to have a higher mortality rate than younger persons and often require surgical therapy. It has been suggested, however, that many cases of "ulcerative" colitis in elderly patients actually represent an ischemic process secondary to occlusive vascular disease. This hypothesis is based on the clinical onset and post-treatment course of the disease, which often closely simulate ischemic colitis, and the difficulty in separating the various forms of ulcerating colitis on radiographic or pathologic grounds.

Although the etiology of ulcerative colitis is unknown, current theory points to a hypersensitivity and autoimmune mechanism as the most likely cause of the disease. Evidence for this theory includes the relatively frequent association of ulcerative colitis with connective tissue diseases (rheumatoid arthritis, rheumatic fever, systemic lupus erythematosus), increased serum gamma-globulin in some cases, the response of the disease to steroid and immunosuppressive drugs, and the demonstration of circulating antibodies to colon extract in some patients with ulcerative colitis. Other suggested causes of ulcerative colitis include infection, destructive enzymes and surface irritants, exogenous antigens (food allergies), and psychosomatic or emotional factors.

Ulcerative colitis is not a distinct histopathologic entity. Most of the features of the disease can be seen in other inflammations of the colon of known cause. Therefore, the diagnosis of ulcerative colitis requires a combination of clinical, radiographic, and pathologic criteria. These include the course of the disease, extent and distribution of the anatomic lesions, and exclusion of other forms of ulcerating colitis caused by specific infectious or toxic agents, or associated with systemic diseases.

Except in rare instances, ulcerative colitis is an inflammatory disease confined to the mucosa and, to a lesser extent, to the adjacent submucosa. The deeper muscular layers and serosa of the colon are usually not involved; the process does not extend to regional lymph nodes (except perhaps as a nonspecific reactive hyperplasia). A characteristic microscopic finding in ulcerative colitis is the crypt abscess, which reflects necrosis of the crypt epithelium with extension of polymorphonuclear infiltrate into the crypt. It is associated with a more chronic inflammatory infiltrate and vascular engorgement in the adjacent submucosa. Although often considered pathognomonic of ulcerative colitis, crypt abscess formation can be seen in any infectious colitis and in ischemic disease.

CLINICAL SYMPTOMS AND COURSE

Ulcerative colitis is highly variable in severity, clinical course, and ultimate prognosis. The onset of the disease, as well as subsequent exacerbations, can be insidious or abrupt. Symptoms range from small amounts of rectal bleeding (simulating hemorrhoids) to prominent diarrhea with colonic hemorrhage and prostration. A characteristic feature of ulcerative colitis is alternating periods of remission and exacerbation. Most patients (up to 75%) have intermittent episodes of symptoms with complete remission between attacks. Of the remainder, about half have one attack and no subsequent symptoms and the same number have continuous symptoms without any remission.

A majority of patients have mild ulcerative colitis that is often segmental in distribution and usually involves just the distal colon. In less than 10% of patients, ulcerative colitis presents as an acute fulminating process. Patients with this form of the disease have severe diarrhea, fever, systemic toxicity, and electrolyte depletion or hemorrhage. They also have a far higher incidence than usual of severe complications, such as toxic megacolon and free perforation into the peritoneal cavity.

EXTRACOLONIC MANIFESTATIONS

Extracolonic manifestations of ulcerative colitis are relatively common and include spondylitis, peripheral arthritis, iritis, skin disorders (erythema nodosum, pyoderma gangrenosum), and various liver abnormalities. It is unclear whether these concomitant conditions represent the host's systemic response to the agent causing the colonic disease, a complication of the colonic lesion, or a general abnormality of the autoimmune mechanism. The extracolonic manifestations of ulcerative colitis appear to have little relation to the severity, extent, or duration of bowel disease.

Up to 20% of patients with ulcerative colitis have some form of arthritis: spondylitis, peripheral arthritis, or coincidental rheumatoid arthritis. Spondylitis, which is seen as symmetric involvement of the sacroiliac joints (Fig. 48-1), is closely associated with the presence of

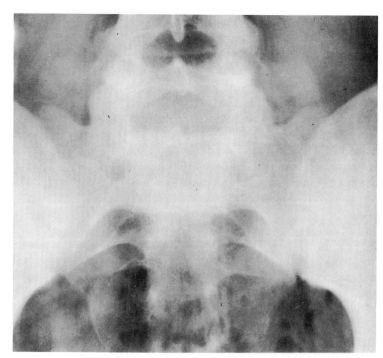

Fig. 48-1. Spondylitis in a patient with ulcerative colitis. Note the symmetric involvement of the sacroiliac joints.

Fig. 48-2. Plain abdominal radiographs in two patients with ulcerative colitis. **(A)** Nodular protrusions of hyperplastic mucosa and the loss of haustral markings involve essentially the entire sigmoid colon. **(B)** Featureless transverse colon with complete loss of normal haustration.

A   B

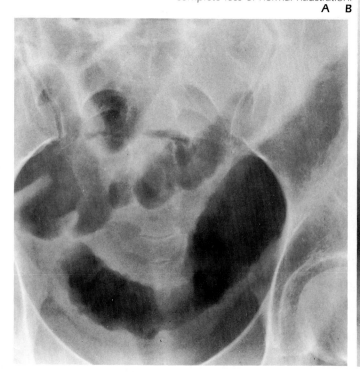 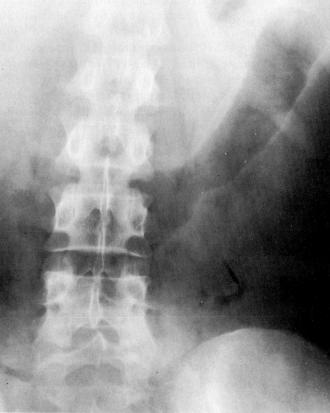

the tissue histocompatibility antigen HLA-B27. The peripheral arthritis almost always occurs at the same time or after the onset of the colitis. When the arthritis antedates the onset of colitis, it usually flares up again during subsequent exacerbations of colonic disease. The peripheral arthritis associated with ulcerative colitis tends to be migratory and to involve large joints. Because joint cartilage and bony apposition are generally unaffected, there often is no residual damage.

The most characteristic liver disorder associated with ulcerative colitis is pericholangitis. The term is used to describe inflammation not only about the bile ducts but also involving the connective tissue around the hepatic artery and portal vein (portal triad). Fatty infiltration of the liver, chronic active hepatitis, and primary sclerosing cholangitis are not infrequently seen.

Patients with ulcerative colitis also appear to have a relatively high incidence of thrombotic complications. Although this predisposition to thromboembolism may be due to venous stasis secondary to dehydration and immobilization, a tendency toward hypercoagulability has been demonstrated and suggested as a causative factor.

The major complication of ulcerative colitis is the high risk of carcinoma of the colon. This is an especially virulent malignancy that often appears as a filiform stricture and is difficult to detect radiographically at an early stage. Unlike Crohn's colitis, free perforation of the colon and toxic megacolon are relatively common in ulcerative colitis, whereas fistula formation is rare.

RADIOGRAPHIC FINDINGS

In the radiographic evaluation of a patient with known or suspected ulcerative colitis, plain abdominal radiographs are essential (Fig. 48-2). Large nodular protrusions of hyperplastic mucosa, deep ulcers outlined by intraluminal gas, or polypoid changes with a loss of haustral markings suggest the diagnosis. Plain abdominal radiographs can also demonstrate evidence of toxic megacolon or free intraperitoneal gas, contraindications to barium enema examination in patients with acute colitis.

Preparation of the colon prior to a barium enema in a patient with suspected or known ulcerative colitis is controversial. Although a clean colon is desirable, some authors report complications after the use of routine purgatives and sizable enemas. If time permits, the safest preparation is several days of a clear liquid diet with gentle, small-volume enemas the night before and the morning of the examination.

Ulcerative colitis has a strong tendency to begin in the rectosigmoid (Fig. 48-3). Although by radiographic criteria alone the rectum appears normal in about 20% of patients with ulcerative colitis (Fig. 48-4), proctosigmoidoscopy can detect rectosigmoid involvement in about 95% of patients with active disease, especially when minimal or equivocal endoscopic findings are corroborated by rectal biopsy. Therefore, true rectal sparing (no disease seen on barium enema, colonoscopy, or biopsy) should suggest the possibility of another etiology for an

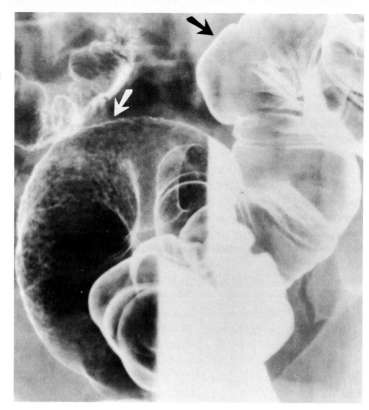

Fig. 48-3. Ulcerative colitis primarily involving the rectosigmoid. The distal rectosigmoid mucosa **(white arrow)** is finely granular, compared to the normal-appearing mucosa **(black arrow)** in the more proximal colon.

Fig. 48-4. Ulcerative colitis with true rectal sparing. In this unusual case, there was no evidence of rectal involvement on barium enema, colonoscopy, or biopsy.

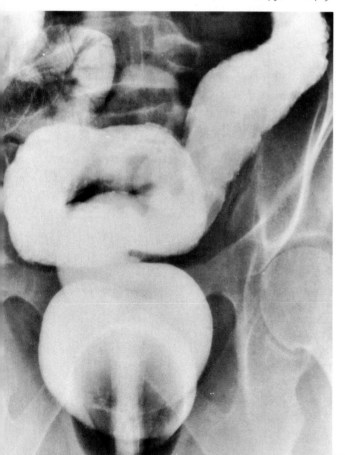

Fig. 48-5. Diffuse ulcerative colitis involving the entire colon. Note the gaping ileocecal valve.

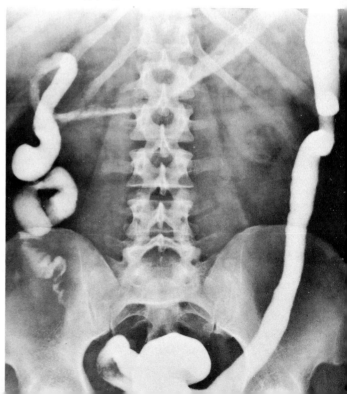

ulcerating colitis. Although ulcerative colitis not infrequently spreads to involve the entire colon (Fig. 48-5), isolated right colon disease with a normal left colon does not occur.

Terminal ileum involvement can be demonstrated in about 10% to 25% of patients with ulcerative colitis. In this backwash ileitis, minimal inflammatory changes involve a short segment of terminal ileum (Fig. 48-6). In backwash ileitis, unlike Crohn's disease, narrowing and rigidity are almost invariably absent, and sinus tracts or fistulas are very infrequent.

On double-contrast studies, the earliest detectable radiographic abnormality in ulcerative colitis is fine granularity of the mucosa corresponding to the hyperemia and edema seen endoscopically (Figs. 48-7, 48-8). Once superficial ulcers develop, small flecks of adherent barium produce a stippled mucosal pattern (Fig. 48-9).

On full-column examination, an early finding in ulcerative colitis is a hazy or fuzzy quality of the bowel contour that is related to edema, excessive mucus, and tiny ulcerations (Fig. 48-10). Ulcerations can cause the margin of the barium-filled colon to be serrated, or they can appear as small spicules extending from the mucosa on postevacuation films. It is essential that these hazy, asymmetric, nonuniform ulcerations be distinguished from innominate lines, tiny spicules that mimic ulcerations but are symmetric and sharply defined (Fig. 48-11). These pseudoulcers are a transient finding representing barium penetration into normal grooves that are present on the surface of the colonic mucosa.

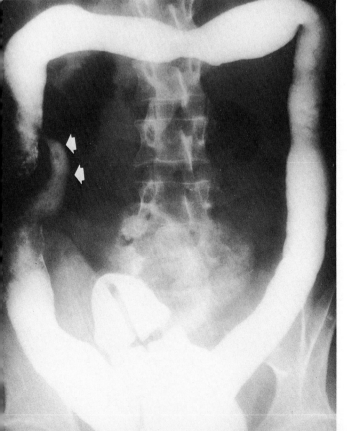

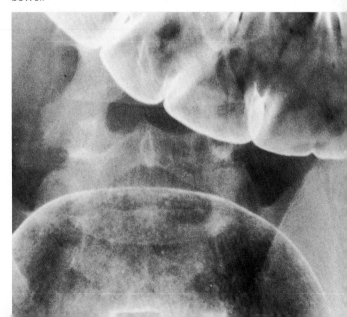

Fig. 48-6. Backwash ileitis **(arrows)** in ulcerative colitis. Note the shortening and rigidity of the colon and the gaping ileocecal valve.

Fig. 48-7. Early ulcerative colitis. Note the fine granularity of the mucosa in the sigmoid (lower loop of bowel) compared to the normal pattern in the upper loop of bowel.

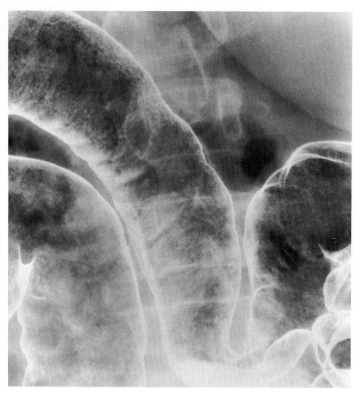

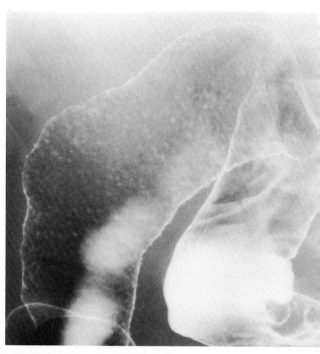

Fig. 48-8. Early ulcerative colitis. Fine granularity of the mucosa reflects the hyperemia and edema that are seen endoscopically.

Fig. 48-9. Early ulcerative colitis. Note the stippled mucosal pattern.

Fig. 48-10. Early ulcerative colitis. The hazy quality of the bowel contour is due to edema, excessive mucus, and tiny ulcerations.

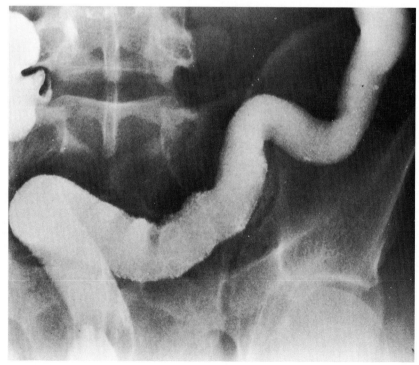

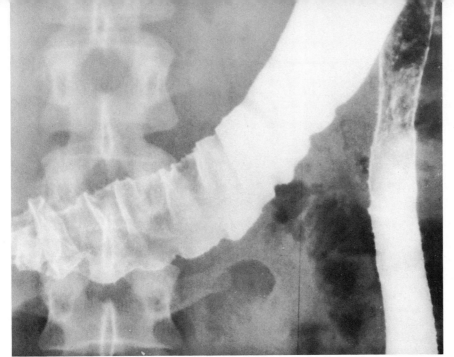

Fig. 48-11. Innominate lines. A transient finding, these tiny spicules mimicking ulcerations are symmetric and sharply defined.

Mucosal edema results in thickening of colonic folds and a coarsely granular appearance. There may be flattening and squaring of the normally smoothly rounded haustral markings. Although loss of haustral markings, particularly in the left colon, is often considered a sign of ulcerative colitis, it is a nonspecific appearance that is commonly seen in normal persons.

The postevacuation film is frequently of great value in the detection of early changes of ulcerative colitis. Unlike the fine crinkled pattern of criss-crossing thin mucosal folds seen in the normal colon, the folds in ulcerative colitis become thickened, indistinct, and coarsely nodular and tend to course in a longitudinal direction (Fig. 48-12). The thin coating of barium on the surface appears finely stippled because of countless tiny ulcers, which cause numerous spikelike projections when seen in profile (Fig. 48-13).

As the disease progresses, marginal ulcerations become deeper, reflecting penetration into the mucosal layer (Fig. 48-14). Although the ulcers can assume a wide variety of sizes and shapes and be discrete and widely separated, they are usually somewhat monotonous in appearance and symmetrically distributed around the circumference of the bowel wall. The ulcerative process extends into the relatively vulnerable submucosa but is limited by the resistant, more deeply lying muscle. This leads to lateral undermining beneath the relatively resistant mucous membrane and the characteristic radiographic appearance of "collar-button" ulcers, a nonspecific pattern that can be seen in numerous forms of ulcerating colitis. Areas of undermining ulceration eventually join together in an interlacing network. Further extension produces large areas that are essentially denuded of mucosa and submucosa. The remaining scattered islands of edematous mucosa and

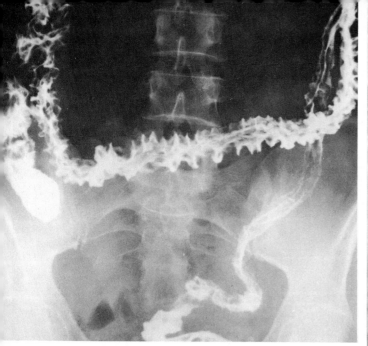
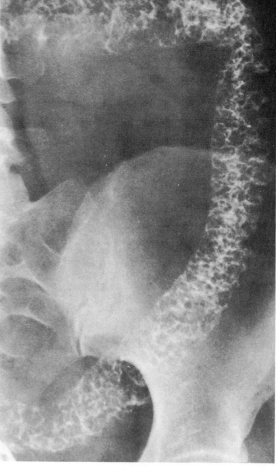

A B

Fig. 48-12. Postevacuation films in two patients with ulcerative colitis. **(A)** The mucosal folds, predominantly in the descending colon, are thickened and indistinct and course in a longitudinal direction. **(B)** Coarse nodular folds.

Fig. 48-13. Ulcerative colitis. This postevacuation film shows coarse mucosal folds with numerous spikelike projections causing a finely stippled pattern.

Fig. 48-14

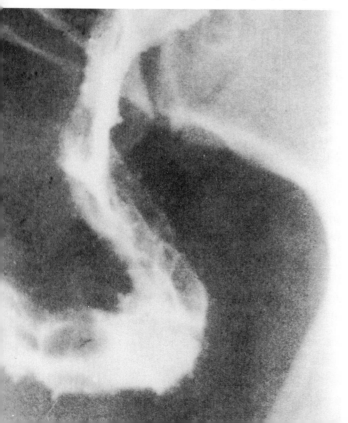

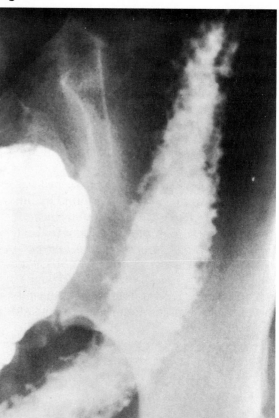

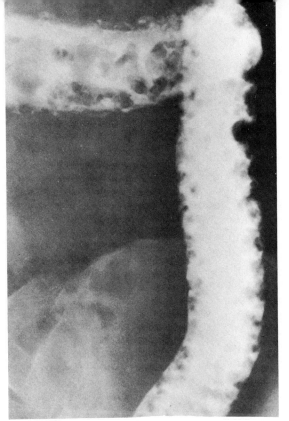

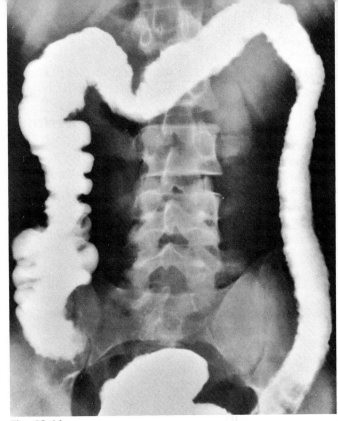

Fig. 48-15

Fig. 48-16

Fig. 48-15. Ulcerative colitis. Multiple filling defects (pseudopolyps) represent islands of edematous mucosa and re-epithelialized granulation tissue in a sea of ulcerations.

Fig. 48-16. Chronic ulcerative colitis. Fibrosis and muscular spasm cause shortening and rigidity of the colon with a loss of haustral markings.

re-epithelialized granulation tissue cause a pattern of multiple discrete filling defects (pseudopolyps) (Fig. 48-15). As the inflammatory process enters a chronic stage, fibrosis and muscular spasm cause progressive shortening and rigidity of the colon (Fig. 48-16; see also Fig. 48-6). This tubular appearance, combined with atrophy of the colonic mucosa, leads to the characteristic "lead-pipe" configuration of chronic ulcerative colitis.

In patients with mild ulcerative colitis, there is good correlation between the extent of disease on barium enema and clinical severity. In persons with moderate or severe disease, however, the tendency is for fewer radiographic changes to be demonstrated than would be anticipated clinically. With colonoscopy used as a reference standard,

◀ **Fig. 48-14.** Ulcerative colitis. Progression of the disease results in deep ulceration ("collar-button" ulcers) into the mucosal layer.

the routine barium enema examination clearly underestimates the activity of the inflammatory process.

CROHN'S COLITIS

Crohn's disease of the colon is identical to the same pathologic process involving the small bowel. Therefore, Crohn's colitis is a far better term for the disease than "granulomatous" colitis. In addition, the term granulomatous is imprecise, since about half of patients with Crohn's disease of the colon do not demonstrate granuloma formation.

Crohn's colitis is a chronic inflammatory disease of the colon that occurs primarily in adolescents and young adults. Although the etiology of the disease is unknown, genetic factors, transmissible infectious agents, and autoimmune phenomena have been suggested as causative factors. The proximal portion of the colon is most frequently involved; concomitant disease of the terminal ileum is seen in up to 80% of patients (Fig. 48-17). Involvement of multiple, noncontiguous segments of colon (skip lesions) not infrequently occurs (Fig. 48-18). Although Crohn's disease is generally considered a disease of the right side of the colon, rectal involvement is not uncommon and can be seen in 30% to 50% of cases. Nevertheless, demonstration of a normal rectal mucosa on sigmoidoscopy in a patient with nonspecific chronic inflammatory bowel disease should suggest Crohn's colitis as a likely diagnosis.

The major pathologic abnormalities in Crohn's disease of the colon include penetrating ulcers or fissures, confluent linear ulcers, a discontinuous segmental pattern, and a thickened bowel wall. Microscopically, there is transmural inflammation, in contrast to the inflammation limited to the mucosa and submucosa that is seen in patients with ulcerative colitis. Although granulomas can be demonstrated in only about half of patients with Crohn's disease of the colon, they are virtually a specific histopathologic feature in that they are not seen in patients with ulcerative colitis.

CLINICAL SYMPTOMS

The clinical hallmark of Crohn's disease of the colon is diarrhea, a symptom that is more distressing, more intense, and an earlier complaint in this condition than in ulcerative colitis. Gross bleeding is rare in Crohn's disease of the colon, in contrast to ulcerative colitis. Abdominal pain is a common manifestation of Crohn's colitis; it is generally crampy and colicky and is usually confined to the lower quadrants, particularly on the right side. Insidious weight loss is frequent, presumably due to contiguous ileal disease preventing normal absorption of bile acids. Perianal or perirectal abnormalities (fissures, hemorrhoids, abscesses, fistulas) occur at some point during the course of disease in half of all patients with Crohn's colitis. Indeed, about 10% of patients first present with one or more of these clinical problems. Enterocutaneous or intestinal fistulas can develop, usually arising from matted or adherent loops of diseased small bowel.

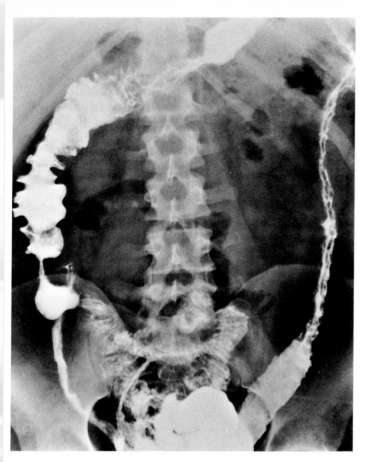

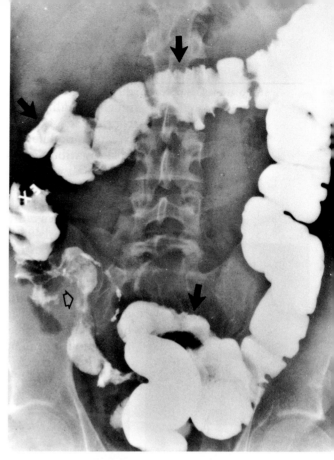

Fig. 48-17. Crohn's colitis. In addition to the diffuse colonic disease, there is severe involvement of much of the distal ileum.

Fig. 48-18. Crohn's colitis. Areas of involved colon in the ascending, transverse, and sigmoid regions **(solid arrows)** are separated by normal-appearing segments. Note the inflammatory changes affecting the distal ileum **(open arrow)**.

The extraintestinal complications of Crohn's disease of the colon are similar to those of ulcerative colitis but occur much less frequently. Concomitant disease of the terminal ileum results in an increased incidence of biliary and renal stones. Deficient absorption of bile salts distorts the ratio of bile salts to cholesterol and predisposes to the development of cholesterol stones in the gallbladder. Excessive oxalate absorption in patients with Crohn's disease leads to hyperoxaluria and a tendency to form oxalate stones in the kidney.

Segmental resection of Crohn's disease of the colon, like that of disease involving the ileum, is associated with a high rate of recurrence (50% or more) at the anastomotic site. Therefore, surgery is usually deferred as long as possible in favor of medical treatment.

RADIOGRAPHIC FINDINGS

The earliest radiographic findings of Crohn's disease of the colon are seen on double-contrast examinations. Isolated, tiny, discrete erosions (aphthoid ulcers) appear as punctate collections of barium with a thin

age of 50 and many have a history of prior cardiovascular disease. Ischemic colitis occasionally occurs in persons younger than 50, especially women taking birth control pills. Colonic ischemia is reported to be a complication in about 2% of aortoiliac reconstructions, and it probably affects many more patients who demonstrate only mild or transient symptoms.

The extent and severity of ischemic colitis vary widely. Mesenteric occlusive disease can lead to extensive infarction of the colon with gangrene or perforation. More frequently, there is localized or segmental ischemia with no evidence of large vessel obstruction; in these cases, the pathophysiologic event is presumed to be regional alterations in the vasa recta of the colonic wall. Particularly vulnerable areas of the colon are the "watershed" regions between two adjacent major arterial supplies: the splenic flexure (superior and inferior mesenteric arteries) and the rectosigmoid area (inferior mesenteric and internal iliac arteries) (Fig. 48-23). Because rectal collaterals tend to be extensive, ischemia generally spares the rectum, and proctoscopy is usually negative.

Unlike ulcerative colitis or Crohn's disease of the colon, ischemic colitis (except for the infrequent fulminant variety) tends to follow a short, generally mild clinical course. The radiographic abnormalities often resolve within a few weeks of the acute onset of abdominal pain, and they rarely recur. Post-ischemic strictures, which are uncommon, tend to develop within a month of the acute event.

RADIOGRAPHIC FINDINGS

The radiographic (and pathologic) appearance of ischemic colitis depends on the phase of the process during which the patient is examined. Because the mucosa is the layer most dependent on intact vascularity, fine superficial ulceration associated with inflammatory edema is the earliest radiographic sign of ischemic colitis. This causes the outer margin of the barium-filled colon to appear serrated, simulating ulcerative colitis (Fig. 48-24). As the disease progresses, deep penetrating ulcers, pseudopolyposis, and "thumbprinting" can be demonstrated. In most cases, the radiographic appearance of the colon returns to normal (Fig. 48-25), though stricturing with proximal dilatation does occur.

In patients with suspected ischemic colitis, mechanical factors such as volvulus and carcinoma must be sought as possible precipitating factors. An extensive ischemic lesion can distract the radiologist, preventing detection of a coexisting malignancy. Bleeding disorders, arteritis, and intravascular occlusion in patients with sickle cell disease can also result in an ischemic colitis pattern.

The differentiation of ischemic colitis from ulcerative colitis and Crohn's disease of the colon can be extremely difficult on radiographic or pathologic examination alone. In such cases, the clinical presentation and subsequent course can be the only basis for making a diagnosis. The characteristic acute episode of abdominal pain and bleeding, the rapid progression of radiographic findings, and the low rate of recurrence usually permit ischemic colitis to be readily distinguished from such conditions as ulcerative colitis and Crohn's disease of the colon, which are typically more indolent, chronic, and recurring.

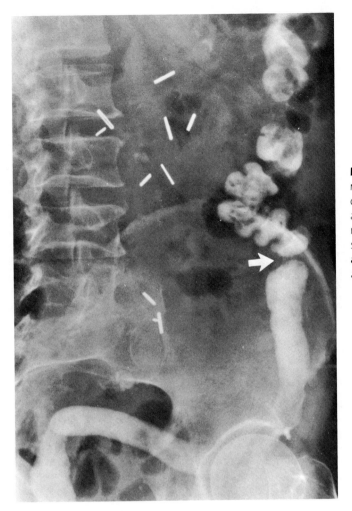

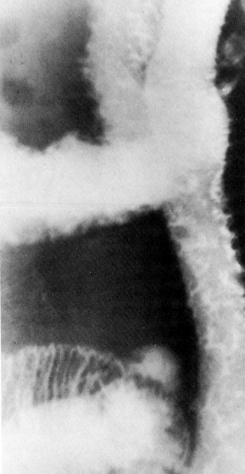

Fig. 48-23. Chronic ischemic colitis of the rectosigmoid and lower descending colon. The condition developed following abdominal aneurysm repair with sacrifice of the inferior mesenteric artery. The pattern is featureless, similar to that in chronic ulcerative colitis. The **arrow** points to the site of abrupt change in the appearance of the colon.

Fig. 48-24. Ischemic colitis. Superficial ulcers and inflammatory edema produce a serrated outer margin of the barium-filled colon simulating ulcerative colitis.

A B

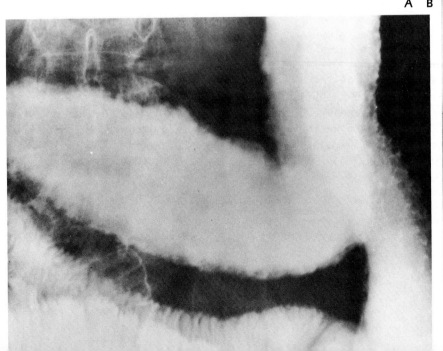

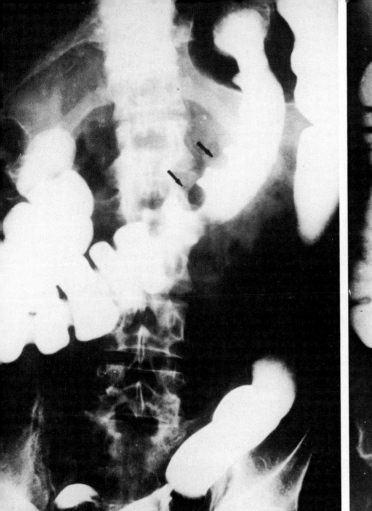 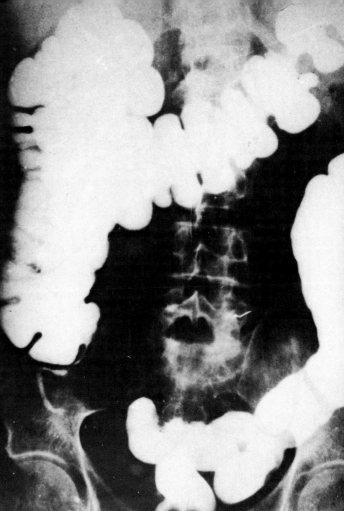

A B

Fig. 48-25. Reversibility of ischemic colitis in an elderly male admitted with abdominal cramps of 3 days' duration and rectal bleeding. **(A)** "Thumbprinting" **(arrows)** along the superior aspect of the transverse colon. **(B)** Repeat study 2 days later. The colon now appears normal. (Schwartz S, Boley S, Lash J et al: Roentgenologic aspects of reversible vascular occlusion of the colon and its relationship to ulcerative colitis. Radiology 90:625–635, 1963)

AMEBIASIS

Infectious diseases involving the colon can present the radiographic pattern of an ulcerating colitis. The most prevalent of these diseases is amebiasis, which is caused by a protozoan that lives and develops in the colon of humans. Amebiasis can present as a segmental process, with skip lesions simulating Crohn's disease, or as a diffuse colitis mimicking ulcerative colitis (Fig. 48-26). It is estimated that 20% of the world's population harbor amebae, though only about 5% of these individuals demonstrate clinical disease. Although the protozoan is most common in tropical countries, it is frequently found in nontropical areas. Indeed, about 5% of the population of the United States is probably infested with the parasite.

Amebiasis begins as a primary infection of the colon that is acquired by the ingestion of food or water contaminated by amebic cysts. The amebae tend to settle in areas of stasis and thus primarily affect the cecum and, to a lesser extent, the rectosigmoid and the hepatic and splenic flexures. The patient is asymptomatic (in a carrier state) until the protozoan actually invades the wall of the colon. Penetration of the bowel wall by the organism incites an inflammatory reaction that leads to a broad clinical spectrum. Some patients, however, remain symptom-free for months or years. Many patients with amebic colitis are acutely ill, complaining of frequent diarrhea, blood and mucus in the stools, and cramping abdominal pain that tends to be located in the right lower quadrant. Others have only mild abdominal discomfort and intermittent diarrhea. The most common extracolonic complication of amebiasis is hepatic abscess, which is seen in about one-third of patients with amebic dysentery. Hepatic abscesses are also frequently found without clinical colonic disease. In about 90% of patients, properly obtained stool specimens are adequate for the diagnosis of amebic colitis. A hemagglutination or ameba precipitin test is positive in a high percentage of patients with the disease.

RADIOGRAPHIC FINDINGS

In the early stages of amebic colitis, superficial ulcerations are super-imposed on a pattern of mucosal edema or nodularity, spasm, and loss of the normal haustral pattern (Fig. 48-27). The cecum is the primary

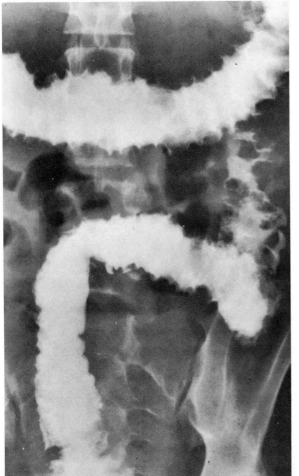

Fig. 48-26. Amebic colitis. Diffuse ulceration and mucosal edema mimic ulcerative colitis.

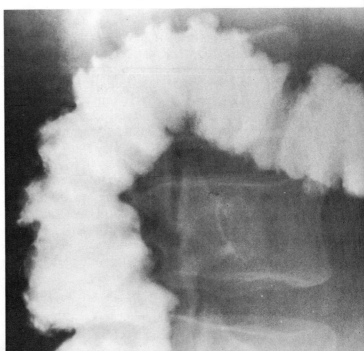

Fig. 48-27. Amebic colitis. There is ulceration, mucosal edema, and loss of the normal haustral pattern.

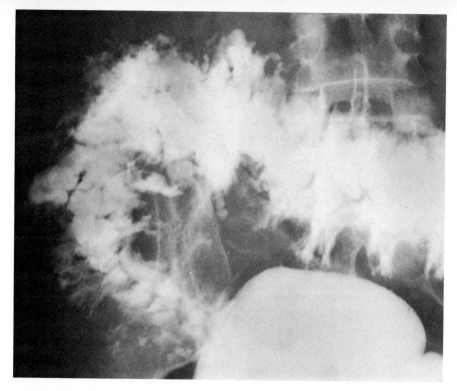

Fig. 48-28. Amebic colitis. Deep, penetrating ulcers produce a bizarre appearance.

site of involvement in up to 90% of patients with clinical disease. Fibrosis due to secondary infection and long-sustained spasm often produces a characteristic cecal deformity (cone-shaped cecum). Scattered areas of segmental involvement can occur, especially in the rectosigmoid, and generalized severe colitis sometimes develops. Deep penetrating ulcers (Fig. 48-28), pseudopolyps, cobblestoning, and thumbprinting can also be demonstrated; multiple skip lesions are frequent. Complications of amebic colitis include perforation, sinuses, fistulas, and pericolic abscesses.

Because amebiasis rarely affects the ileum, the presence of concomitant ileal disease (especially if it is extensive) favors Crohn's disease as the underlying etiology. If disease is limited to the colon, the demonstration of transverse and longitudinal ulcers, eccentric involvement of the colonic wall, or extensive fistula formation should suggest Crohn's disease rather than amebiasis. When colon inflammation is diffuse and simulates ulcerative colitis, the presence of multiple skip areas makes amebic colitis the more likely diagnosis.

SCHISTOSOMIASIS

In schistosomiasis, the sharp terminal or lateral spines of the eggs of the blood flukes, together with the muscular action of the colon wall, permit the parasite to penetrate the colonic mucosa and stimulate an inflammatory response. Because of the predilection of the adult worms to enter the inferior mesenteric vein and discharge their eggs there, the descending and sigmoid colon are most frequently affected. However, any portion of the colon can be involved. The mucosa is edematous and demonstrates tiny ulcerations or mural spiculations that simulate the appearance of ulcerative colitis. On double-contrast studies, a diffuse granular pattern can be seen. Spasm, disturbed motility, and a loss of haustral pattern are common. During this acute stage of the disease, the diagnosis of schistosomiasis is readily made by detection of ova in freshly passed stools. As the disease progresses, formation of discrete granulomas produces the more characteristic radiographic pattern of multiple small filling defects in the barium column.

BACTERIAL INFECTIONS

SHIGELLOSIS / SALMONELLOSIS

Shigellosis (bacillary dysentery) and salmonellosis (food poisoning, typhoid fever) are acute or chronic inflammatory bowel diseases caused by gram-negative, non-spore-forming bacilli of the *Enterobacteriaceae* family. *Shigella* organisms predominantly involve the colon; salmonellosis mainly affects the terminal ileum, though colon changes are also seen. Although they are generally considered to be tropical diseases, the distribution of *Shigella* and *Salmonella* is worldwide; they not infrequently occur in low socioeconomic groups in the United States (especially in California and Texas). Overcrowding and poor sanitary conditions, particularly in warm, humid climates, predispose to the spread of infection. In well-developed countries with good sanitation, outbreaks of small epidemics of dysentery tend to occur in schools, military barracks, prisons, and mental asylums. Debility, exhaustion, weakness, and malnutrition predispose to development of the disease.

Shigellae and salmonellae enter the bowel in food and drink that have been contaminated by infected fecal material. Acute and chronic carriers serving as cooks or processors of food and milk are important sources of contamination. In tropical countries in which human excrement is used as fertilizer, uncooked vegetables and salads can cause infection. Another major source of infection is flies that have eaten or walked in stools contaminated with the organisms. In addition, many household pets are known to harbor and excrete salmonellae.

Shigella organisms penetrate the colonic mucosa and grow rapidly, liberating exo- and endotoxins that cause inflammation of the colon and rectum. Mucosal edema and submucosal infiltration are associated with an outpouring of mucoid and blood-streaked exudate, which fills the lumen of the gut. As necrotic tissue sloughs, shallow, ragged ulcers remain, partially or completely encircling the bowel. In salmonellosis, the organisms also penetrate the wall of the small bowel, invading the lymphoid tissues of Peyer's patches and the solitary lymph follicles and thereby gaining access to the blood stream by way of the thoracic duct. The characteristic pathologic lesions of typhoid fever are found primarily in lymphatic tissue of the distal small bowel. Deep ulcerations can cause perforation and peritonitis. The systemic infection in salmonellosis can lead to focal liver necrosis, cholecystitis, and involvement of the lungs and kidney.

Bacillary dysentery has a short incubation period, usually 2 to 3 days but occasionally as long as 1 week. Diarrhea is the most characteristic sign. In acute, fulminating infection, abdominal pain is severe, and profuse diarrhea can result in life-threatening fluid loss and electrolyte imbalance.

The symptoms and signs of salmonellosis vary from acute gastroenteritis to severe septicemia. In typical "food poisoning," there is sudden onset of fever, nausea, vomiting, and diarrhea that occurs after a very short incubation period, often as little as 12 hr. In most cases, the disease is self-limited, and there is complete recovery in 4 to 5 days. In the classic form of typhoid fever, there is the insidious onset of malaise, frontal headache, muscular aches, and joint pain. After a week, the fever becomes high and continuous; apathy, toxemia, and delirium may become prominent. Complications such as massive intestinal bleeding, perforation, and circulatory failure can be fatal.

Radiographic Findings

Patients with suspected salmonellosis seldom undergo a barium enema examination, since the symptoms are acute and suggest the underlying self-limited condition. However, when performed, the barium enema

Fig. 48-29. Salmonellosis. Diffuse, fine ulcerations simulate ulcerative colitis.

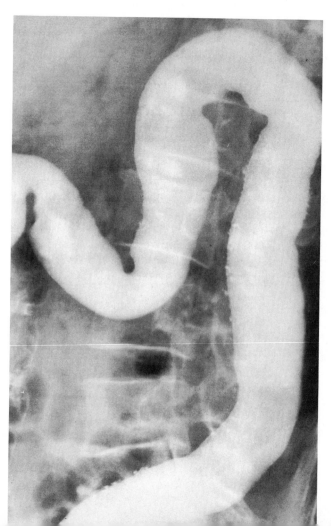

may demonstrate diffuse, fine ulcerations (Fig. 48-29) and irregular thickening of folds on postevacuation views (Fig. 48-30). In acute bacillary dysentery due to shigellosis, a barium enema examination generally cannot be tolerated. If an examination is performed, severe spasm of the colon may prevent complete filling. When a barium enema examination is successful, the radiographic appearance is related to the severity and stage of colon involvement. The acute, severe form is a pancolitis characterized by deep "collar-button" ulcers, intense spasm, and mucosal edema. In less severe disease, superficial ulcerations with coarse, nodular, edematous folds can involve the entire colon or be segmental in distribution, primarily affecting the rectum and sigmoid and, less commonly, the descending portion (Fig. 48-31). Nonspecific findings, such as spasm, haustral distortion, and excess fluid, usually accompany the mucosal changes.

Radiographic differentiation between salmonellosis and shigellosis is frequently impossible in the colon. Involvement of the terminal ileum, however, strongly suggests salmonellosis as the correct diagnosis. Because it can be impossible to distinguish between these diseases and other forms of ulcerating colitis, bacteriologic investigation is often required for a specific diagnosis. It is critical that the precise causative agent be identified, since steroid therapy, often used to treat noninfectious forms of colitis, is obviously contraindicated in these infectious processes.

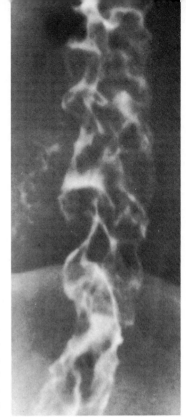

Fig. 48-30. Salmonellosis. A postevacuation film demonstrates ulceration and irregular thickening of mucosal folds.

Fig. 48-31. Shigellosis. Mucosal edema and ulceration primarily involve the rectosigmoid. Note the fistulous tract **(arrow).**

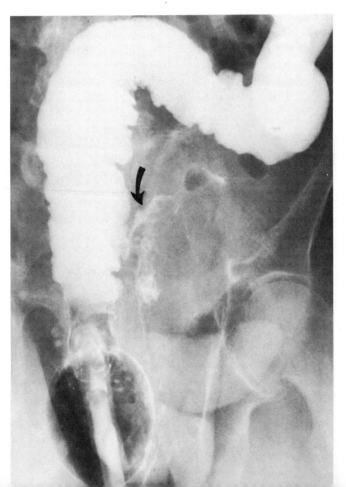

Colonic tuberculosis predominantly affects the cecum, and concomitant disease in the distal ileum is usually seen. The ascending and transverse colon can also be involved (Fig. 48-32), though almost invariably in continuity with the cecum. Occasionally, tuberculosis is segmental and occurs elsewhere in the colon, primarily in the sigmoid.

Radiographically, gastrointestinal tuberculosis closely simulates Crohn's disease. The correct diagnosis is often not made before surgery, especially since recognizable pulmonary tuberculosis is frequently not present. In addition, because acutely ill patients can be anergic to skin test antigens, a negative tuberculin skin test is often seen in patients with active gastrointestinal disease.

The majority of cases of tuberculosis of the colon in the United States are caused by *Mycobacterium tuberculosis;* coexistent pulmonary disease can often be demonstrated radiographically. In areas in which cattle are diseased and milk is not pasteurized, *Mycobacterium bovis* can be the etiologic agent. In patients with this form of tuberculosis, intestinal disease is usually associated with a normal chest radiograph.

Tuberculosis of the colon can be asymptomatic or produce a spectrum of nonspecific complaints such as weight loss, fever, anorexia, right lower quadrant pain, and diarrhea. The primary tuberculous lesion of the gastrointestinal tract originates within the lymphatic structures of the submucosa and is covered by a normal overlying mucosa. A combination of caseous necrosis and ischemia leads to sloughing of the mucosa and development of an ulcer. In early stages of the disease, superficial or deep mucosal ulcerations can sometimes be identified radiographically, though intense spasm and irritability often make adequate filling of the involved portion of the colon impossible. Progressive inflammatory changes, fibrosis, and lymphatic obstruction cause the colon wall to become thickened and rigid.

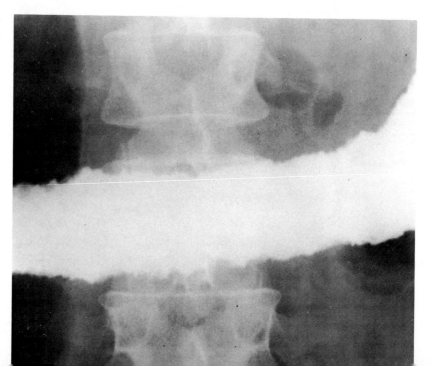

Fig. 48-32. Tuberculosis. Fine ulcerations diffusely involve the transverse colon.

GONORRHEAL PROCTITIS

Gonorrheal proctitis in men is almost always the result of anal intercourse; in women, most cases are believed to be secondary to genitoanal spread. Most patients with rectal gonorrhea have no symptoms and are discovered only by the meticulous tracing of sexual contacts and a high index of suspicion. To differentiate gonorrheal proctitis from other ulcerative diseases, Gram staining and selective culturing of the purulent exudate must be performed. The symptoms associated with gonorrheal proctitis are similar to those of other forms of ulcerative proctitis and include rectal burning, itching, purulent anal discharge, and blood and mucus in the stools. Barium enema examination is normal in most patients with gonorrheal proctitis. Infrequently, mucosal edema and ulceration confined to the rectum can be demonstrated. Gonorrheal proctitis responds promptly to specific antibiotic therapy.

STAPHYLOCOCCAL COLITIS

Postantibiotic staphylococcal diarrhea occurs after a course of orally administered broad-spectrum antibiotics, usually tetracycline. The disease is most common among hospitalized patients and is caused by antibiotic-resistant strains that enter the gastrointestinal tract by way of the nasopharyngeal route and grow profusely in the intestine once the population of normal intestinal flora has been significantly reduced by oral antibiotics. Staphylococcal enteritis can produce only mild, self-limited diarrhea. In severe disease, nausea, vomiting, and profuse diarrhea can occur. Mild staphylococcal enteritis subsides rapidly once the antibiotic to which the organism is resistant is discontinued and the normal intestinal flora is allowed to return. In severe enteritis, it may be necessary to administer an antibiotic to which the *Staphylococcus* is sensitive. Although barium enema examinations are rarely performed in patients with staphyloccoccal enterocolitis, they can demonstrate the characteristic features of a generalized ulcerating colitis (Fig. 48-33).

YERSINIA COLITIS

Yersinia enterocolitica is a gram-negative bacillus that has been increasingly implicated as a cause of ileitis and colitis in children. Fever, diarrhea, and sometimes blood in the stools are the predominant presentations in infants; a pattern simulating appendicitis can be seen in older children. Barium enema examination can demonstrate multiple small colonic ulcerations similar to those seen in Crohn's colitis (Fig. 48-34).

CAMPYLOBACTER FETUS COLITIS

Campylobacter fetus, subspecies jejuni, has recently been recognized as a common human enteric pathogen (Fig. 48-35). Indeed, in a recent

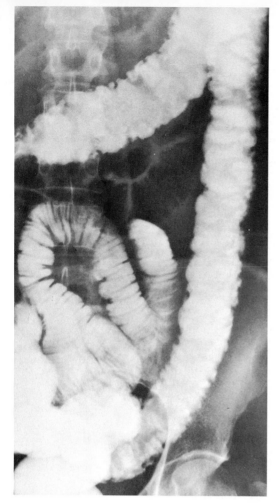

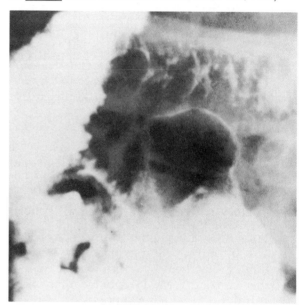

Fig. 48-33. Postantibiotic staphylococcal infection. The features are typical of a severe ulcerating colitis.

Fig. 48-34. Yersinia colitis. A coned view of the right colon shows marked irregularity of the mucosa and transmural thickening. (Lackman R, Soong J, Wishon G et al: Yersinia colitis. Gastrointest Radiol 2:133–135, 1977)

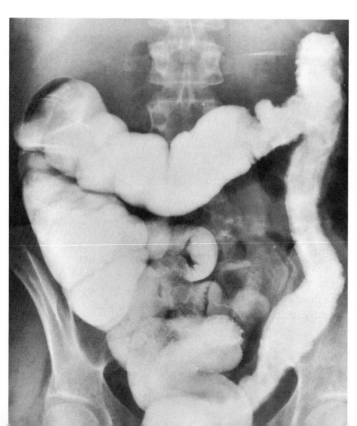

Fig. 48-35. Colitis caused by Campylobacter fetus. The radiographic pattern is indistinguishable from ulcerative colitis. Cultures and immunologic studies were necessary for proper diagnosis.

series, this organism was the most common cause of specific infectious colitis. Patients with this disease typically present with the acute onset of diarrhea, abdominal pain, fever, and constitutional symptoms. Proctoscopy demonstrates an inflamed mucosa with bloody exudate and numerous polymorphonuclear leukocytes on fecal smear. *Campylobacter* colitis is usually self-limited; in protracted or severe cases, antibiotic therapy (erythromycin) may be required.

It has been postulated that single episodes of acute colitis formerly attributed to ulcerative colitis may have been caused by *Campylobacter fetus*. Therefore, in patients presenting with acute colitis, *Campylobacter* infection should be ruled out with appropriate cultures and immunologic studies before the diagnosis of ulcerative colitis is made.

FUNGAL INFECTIONS

Histoplasmosis, mucormycosis, actinomycosis, and candidiasis are among the fungal diseses that infrequently involve the colon. They usually occur in chronically ill, debilitated patients and can either arise in the bowel or spread from another site in the body. Fungal invasion of the walls of the bowel and blood vessels produces an intense localized inflammatory reaction. The bowel wall appears irritable and spastic, and the mucosal folds are thickened and irregular. Mucosal ulcerations can occasionally be identified. The correct diagnosis of fungal disease involving the colon is rarely made before operation or postmortem examination.

VIRAL INFECTIONS

LYMPHOGRANULOMA VENEREUM

Lymphogranuloma venereum is a venereal disease that is especially common in the tropics. It is caused by a large virus closely related to the organisms that produce psittacosis and trachoma. The disease is transmitted almost exclusively through sexual contact. The rectal form of the disease is most prevalent in women, though it is being found with increasing frequency in homosexual men. Lymphogranuloma venereum in men usually appears as a primary genital sore followed by purulent inflammation of inguinal lymph nodes (bubo formation). In women, the primary lesion occurs in the vagina or cervix, where it often goes undetected. In up to 25% of patients, however, the rectum is the predominant site of disease.

The major symptom of lymphogranuloma venereum involving the colon is bleeding. Mucopurulent rectal discharge, diarrhea, low-grade fever, perianal fistulas, and recurrent abscesses can also be present. As rectal stricturing increases, constipation and crampy lower abdominal pain can develop. The diagnosis of lymphogranuloma venereum can be confirmed by the Frei intradermal skin test or the complement fixation test, or by recovery of the virus from the blood, feces, or bubos.

The rectum is the first and usually the only portion of the colon involved in lymphogranuloma venereum (Fig. 48-36). The pathologic changes result from viral invasion and blockage of the rectal lymphatics which, together with secondary infection, lead to rectal edema and cellular infiltrate in the submucosa and muscularis. In the early stages of lymphogranuloma venereum, as in all forms of ulcerating colitis, the bowel is spastic and irritable with boggy and edematous mucosa and multiple shaggy ulcers. Fistulas and sinus tracts of varying length are frequently present. As the disease progresses, the classic pattern of rectal stricture develops.

HERPES ZOSTER

Rarely, herpes zoster causes small ulcerations in a narrowed portion of colon, a radiographic pattern similar to that of a segmental ulcerating colitis. This corresponds to the ulcerative cutaneous changes that sometimes follow the more characteristic vesicular skin lesions. The short length of the colonic lesion and the typical clinical history and skin lesions should suggest the correct diagnosis.

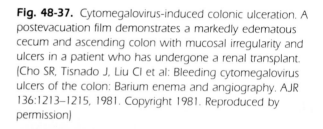

Fig. 48-37. Cytomegalovirus-induced colonic ulceration. A postevacuation film demonstrates a markedly edematous cecum and ascending colon with mucosal irregularity and ulcers in a patient who has undergone a renal transplant. (Cho SR, Tisnado J, Liu CI et al: Bleeding cytomegalovirus ulcers of the colon: Barium enema and angiography. AJR 136:1213–1215, 1981. Copyright 1981. Reproduced by permission)

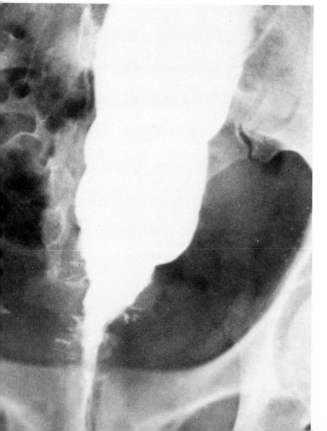

Fig. 48-36. Lymphogranuloma venereum. There is a long rectal stricture with multiple deep ulcers. (Dreyfuss JR, Janower ML: Radiology of the Colon. Baltimore, Williams & Wilkins, 1980)

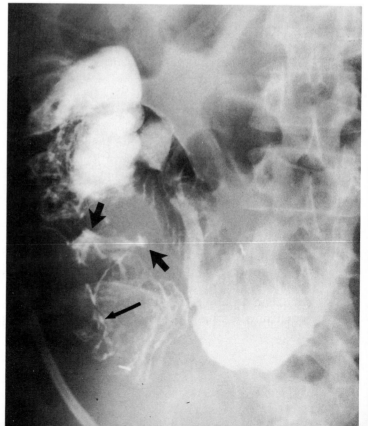

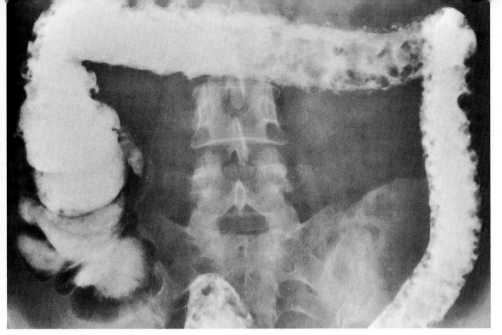

Fig. 48-38. Strongyloidiasis. Diffuse ulcerating colitis is present with deep and shallow ulcers and pronounced mucosal edema.

CYTOMEGALOVIRUS

Cytomegalovirus-induced colonic ulcers are the most important cause of severe lower gastrointestinal bleeding in renal transplant recipients in whom immunosuppressive therapy has been initiated (Fig. 48-37). Early diagnosis and prompt surgical intervention are essential in the management of this often fatal complication. Cytomegalovirus usually involves the cecum, causing mucosal ulceration with severe local inflammation. Besides the inflammatory change caused by the cytomegalovirus infection itself, an associated vasculitis contributes to prominent local edema, which can appear radiographically as luminal narrowing, thumbprinting, or even tumorlike defects.

STRONGYLOIDIASIS

Severe colitis is an extremely unusual manifestation of infestation by *Strongyloides stercoralis*. Invasion of the bowel wall by larvae of this nematode results in a diffuse ulcerating colitis characterized by both small and large ulcers, mucosal edema, and the loss of haustral markings (Fig. 48-38). Colonic infection is often associated with overwhelming sepsis, hemorrhage, and death, though healing with stricture formation can occur.

PSEUDOMEMBRANOUS COLITIS

Pseudomembranous colitis is a spectrum of entities that are potentially serious complications of antibiotic therapy, surgery, uremia, and large bowel obstruction. It most often occurs following the administration of well-established drugs such as tetracycline, penicillin, and ampicillin, or after treatment with newer wide-spectrum antibiotics, such as clindamycin and lincomycin. Pseudomembranous colitis most commonly arises after oral antibiotic therapy, though it can also develop following intravenous administration. Whether the antibiotic-associated pseudomembranous colitis is related to a change in the normal bacterial flora of the colon or to a direct toxic action of the drug itself has been a controversial question. The theory that a resistant strain of a specific organism causes pseudomembranous colitis is supported by recent studies demonstrating the presence of *Clostridium difficile* in the the stools of a high percentage of patients with this condition. This bacterium elaborates a cytotoxic substance that destroys human cells in culture and produces a severe enterocolitis when injected into the cecum of animals. Clinical symptoms can be identified within 1 day to 1 month (average, 2 weeks) after the initiation of antibiotic therapy. Most patients recover uneventfully after withdrawal of the offending antibiotic and the institution of adequate fluid and electrolyte replacement. However, there is an overall mortality rate in this condition of about 15%.

The clinical hallmark of pseudomembranous colitis is debilitating, severe diarrhea with or without blood. Indeed, this complication should be suspected in any patient receiving antibiotics who suddenly experiences copious diarrhea and signs of abdominal cramps, tenderness, or peritonitis. At proctosigmoidoscopy, there is the characteristic appearance of a friable, edematous mucosa with yellow–green exudate and white, patchy, raised 1-mm to 6-mm plaquelike lesions scattered over the mucosal surface. A confluent, purulent pseudomembrane, histologically composed of mucus, fibrin, leukocytes, and bacteria, can often be observed enveloping the entire mucosal surface.

RADIOGRAPHIC FINDINGS

Plain abdominal radiographs in severe cases of pseudomembranous colitis can demonstrate moderate, diffuse gaseous distention of the

Fig. 48-39. Pseudomembranous colitis. A plain abdominal radiograph demonstrates wide transverse bands of thickened colonic wall **(arrows)**. (Stanley RJ, Melson GL, Tedesco FJ et al: Plain film findings in severe pseudomembranous colitis. Radiology 118:7–11, 1976)

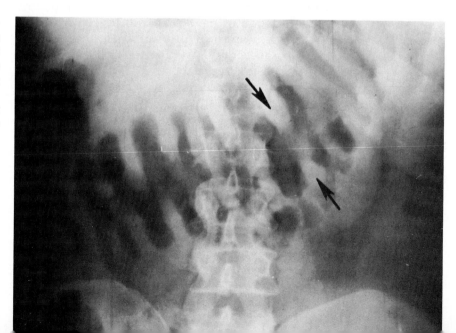

colon. The haustral markings are edematous and distorted, with wide transverse bands of thickened colonic wall (Fig. 48-39). Barium enema examination is contraindicated in patients with severe pseudomembranous colitis. In mild cases, or as the condition subsides, a low-pressure barium enema study can be performed with caution. The barium column appears shaggy and irregular because of the pseudomembrane and superficial necrosis (Fig. 48-40). Multiple flat, raised lesions may be distributed circumferentially about the margin of the colon (Fig. 48-41). Mucosal ulcerations simulating other forms of ulcerating colitis are frequently seen. In many cases, however, this serrated outline actually represents barium interposed between the plaquelike membranes rather than true ulceration with surrounding edema.

A fulminant and often fatal type of pseudomembranous colitis characterized by profuse, occasionally bloody diarrhea, dehydration, shock, and toxemia, occasionally occurs in the absence of antibiotic therapy. This nonspecific disorder has multiple etiologies, the most common being postoperative states, uremia (uremic colitis) (Fig. 48-42), colitis proximal to a large bowel obstruction, and any cause of severe hypoxia.

Fig. 48-41. Pseudomembranous colitis. The pseudomembranes appear as multiple flat, raised lesions distributed circumferentially about the margin of the colon.

Fig. 48-40. Pseudomembranous colitis. The barium column has a shaggy and irregular appearance because of the pseudomembrane and superficial necrosis with mucosal ulceration.

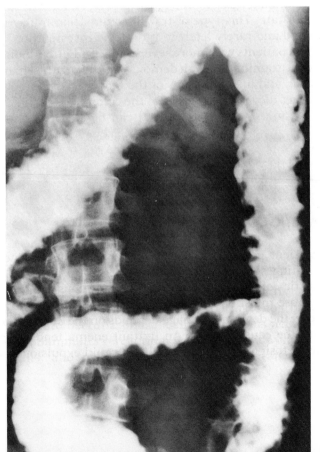

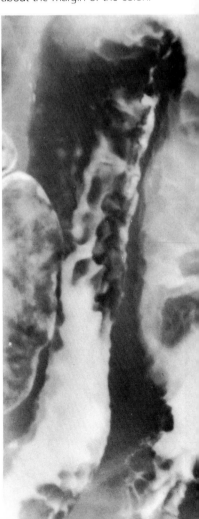

INORGANIC MERCURY POISONING

Poisoning with inorganic mercury can cause intestinal hemorrhage and ulceration of the colon. The clinical history and concomitant renal involvement should permit differentiation of this condition from other forms of ulcerating colitis.

BEHCET'S SYNDROME

Behcet's syndrome is an uncommon multiple-system disease characterized by ulcerations of the buccal and genital mucosa, occular inflammation, and a variety of skin lesions. Colonic involvement associated with diarrhea, abdominal pain, and bleeding occasionally occurs. In several reported cases, multiple discrete ulcers grossly simulating peptic ulcers of the stomach and duodenum were seen in an otherwise normal-appearing colon. In other patients, diffuse mucosal thickening and ulceration have involved large segments of the colon and terminal ileum but spared the rectum (Fig. 48-53). The ulcers in Behcet's syndrome tend to be larger than those in Crohn's colitis. Patients with colitis due to Behcet's disease have a high incidence of perforation and hemorrhage, both of which are life-threatening complications.

DIVERTICULOSIS / DIVERTICULITIS

Rarely, small diverticula projecting from the colon are confused with the serrated colonic margin in a patient with ulcerative colitis. In almost every instance, however, the appearance of diverticula as sac-like outpouchings with short necks, often associated with deep criss-crossing ridges of thickened circular muscle (sawtooth pattern), is easy to distinguish from true ulceration (Fig. 48-54). In diverticulitis, extrav-

Fig. 48-53. Colitis in Behcet's syndrome. **(A)** Barium enema examination demonstrates extensive involvement of all of the large bowel except for the rectosigmoid and hepatic flexure regions. The affected mucosa is nodular, ulcerated, and thickened secondary to granulomatous disease. **(B)** Enlarged view of the splenic flexure shows deep, circular ulcerations of uniform size and multiple nodular mucosal lesions. (Goldstein SJ, Crooks DJM: Colitis in Behcet's syndrome. Radiology 128:321–323, 1978)

A B

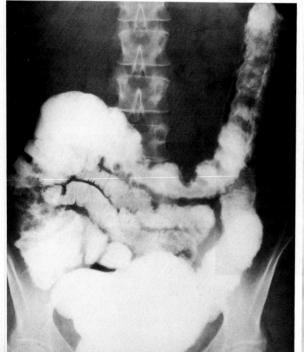
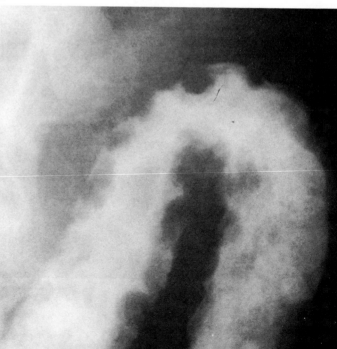

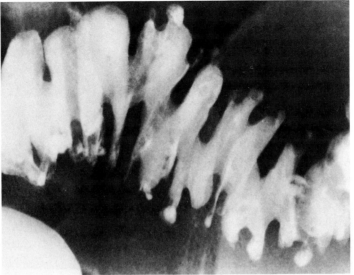

Fig. 48-54. Diverticulosis. The small diverticula clearly represent saclike outpouchings with short necks rather than diffuse ulcerations.

asated contrast material arising as a tiny projection from the top of a perforated diverticulum can simulate an acute ulceration. Ulcerative or Crohn's colitis and diverticular disease of the colon can coexist. In these cases, fine ulcerations within and about the diverticula are often demonstrated.

SOLITARY RECTAL ULCER SYNDROME

The solitary rectal ulcer syndrome is a distinct clinical entity occurring mainly in young patients complaining of rectal bleeding. Constipation or diarrhea can occur; pain is an inconstant feature. Solitary and occasionally multiple ulcers occur predominantly on the anterior or anterolateral aspects of the rectum. Although the precise etiology is unclear, the ulcers may be secondary to partial rectal mucosal prolapse and traumatic ulceration related to pelvic muscle discoordination during defecation.

The earliest radiographic and pathologic change in this condition is nodularity of the rectal mucosa (preulcerative phase) (Fig. 48-55). This is followed by the development of ulcerations that are usually single but may be of various sizes and shapes and occur within 15 cm of the anal verge and near a valve of Houston. Long-standing ulceration produces progressive fibrosis leading to rectal stricture. When either ulceration or stricturing is present, differentiation of the solitary rectal ulcer syndrome from inflammatory bowel disease or malignancy can be difficult.

NONSPECIFIC BENIGN ULCERATION OF THE COLON

Nonspecific ulceration of the colon is a diagnosis of exclusion that is rarely made preoperatively. Although several etiologies have been

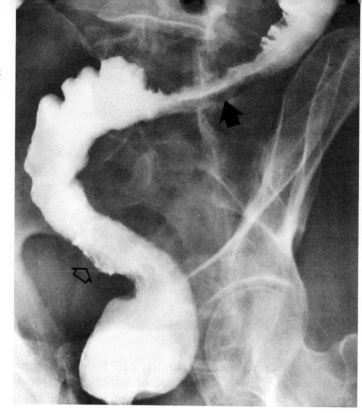

Fig. 49-2. Chronic ulcerative colitis. A benign stricture is visible in the sigmoid colon **(solid arrow).** Note the ulcerative changes in the upper rectum and proximal sigmoid colon **(open arrow).**

Radiographically, a stricture due to ulcerative colitis has a typically benign appearance with a concentric lumen, smooth contours, and fusiform, pliable, tapering margins (Fig. 49-3). Occasionally, the stricture is somewhat eccentric and has irregular contours, simulating a malignancy. Although the bowel proximal to a benign stricture can be slightly dilated, obstruction is rare, and the colon usually empties well on evacuation. Because carcinoma in patients with ulcerative colitis can have a radiographic appearance indistinguishable from a benign stricture, colonoscopy or surgery is frequently required to make this differentiation.

CROHN'S COLITIS

In Crohn's disease of the colon, deep ulceration and transmural inflammation with thickening of the bowel wall produce multiple irregular stenotic segments and strictures. Narrowing and stricture formation occur frequently and early in the course of Crohn's colitis, in contrast to ulcerative colitis. Patients with chronic disease may develop a "lead-

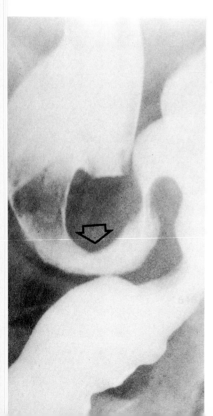

Fig. 49-3. Chronic ulcerative colitis. A benign rectosigmoid stricture with a smooth contour and tapering margins **(arrow)** is evident.

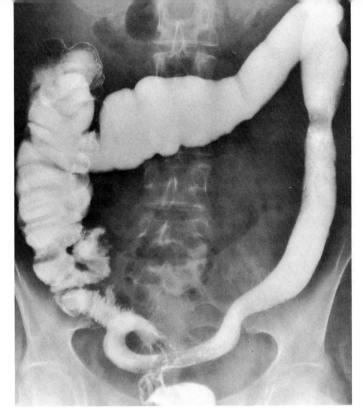 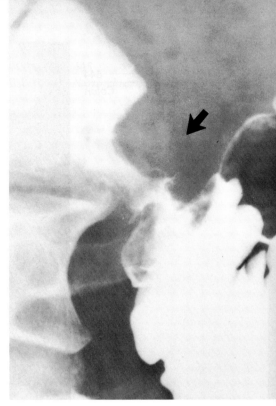

Fig. 49-4. Chronic Crohn's colitis. Foreshortening and loss of haustrations involving the colon distal to the hepatic flexure simulate the appearance of chronic ulcerative colitis.

Fig. 49-5. Chronic Crohn's colitis. A benign stricture with overhanging edges in the transverse colon simulates carcinoma **(arrow)**.

pipe" colon identical to that seen in ulcerative colitis (Fig. 49-4). Occasionally, an eccentric stricture with a suggestion of overhanging edges can make it difficult to exclude the possibility of carcinoma (Fig. 49-5). In most instances, however, characteristic features of Crohn's disease elsewhere in the colon (deep ulcerations, pseudopolyposis, skip lesions, sinus tracts, fistulas) clearly indicate the correct diagnosis.

ISCHEMIC COLITIS

During the healing phase of ischemic colitis, marked fibrosis of the submucosal and muscular layers can lead to stricture formation (Fig. 49-6). Flattening and rigidity of the mesenteric border combined with pleating of the antimesenteric margin produce the radiographic appearance of multiple sacculations or pseudodiverticula. Progressive fibrosis causes tubular narrowing and a smooth stricture. Stricture of the rectum rarely occurs because of the excellent collateral blood supply to this segment. Ischemic strictures are generally shorter than the original length of ischemic involvement seen on radiographs obtained during the acute stage of the disease, implying that some of the ischemic bowel has retained sufficient blood supply to permit complete healing. Luminal narrowing due to ischemia can present as an annular constricting lesion. If the history is not typical and no prior radiographs

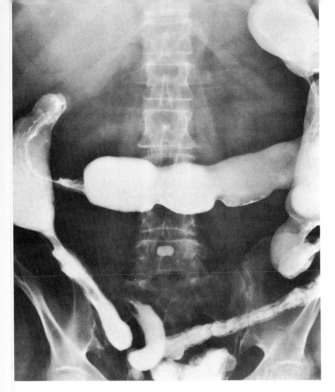

Fig. 49-14. Cathartic colon. Bizarre contractions with irregular areas of narrowing primarily involve the right colon. Although the ileocecal valve is gaping, simulating ulcerative colitis, no ulcerations are identified.

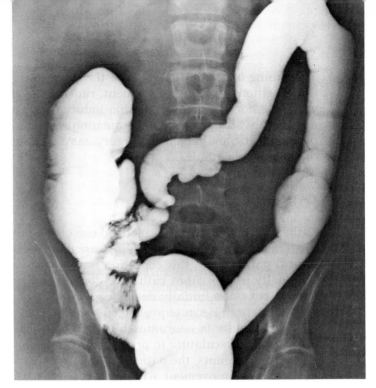

Fig. 49-15. Caustic colitis. Two months after a detergent enema, there is stenosis with irregular sacculations in the midtransverse colon. (Kim SK, Cho C, Levinsohn EM: Caustic colitis due to detergent enema. AJR 134:397–398, 1980. Copyright 1980. Reproduced by permission)

Fig. 49-16. Nonspecific ulcer of the cecum. Fibrotic healing has produced an irregular area of narrowing, without visible ulceration, simulating carcinoma.

Fig. 49-17. Nonspecific ulcer of the transverse colon causing irregular narrowing that simulates annular carcinoma. (Gardiner GA, Bird CR: Nonspecific ulcers of the colon resembling annular carcinoma. Radiology 137:331–334, 1980)

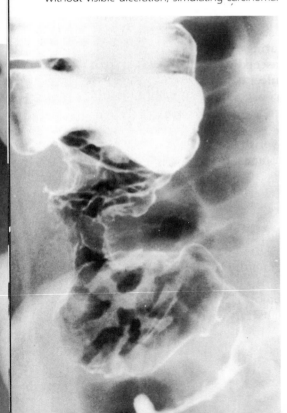

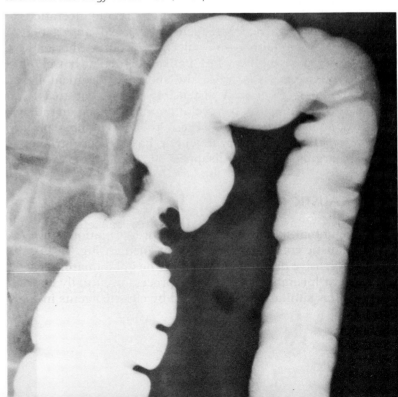

SOLITARY RECTAL ULCER SYNDROME

Stricture formation in the final stage of the solitary rectal ulcer syndrome reflects progressive fibrosis due to long-standing ulceration. If there are no previous barium enema examinations demonstrating mucosal nodularity or ulceration, it can be difficult to differentiate a stricture due to the solitary rectal ulcer syndrome from inflammatory bowel disease, lymphogranuloma venereum, or rectal malignancy.

NONSPECIFIC BENIGN ULCER

Fibrotic strictures are a complication of nonspecific benign ulcers of the colon. Most frequently found in the cecum (Fig. 49-16), nonspecific ulcers can be complicated by perforation or hemorrhage. Fibrotic healing can cause smooth or irregular areas of narrowing, often with no visible ulceration, that can be radiographically indistinguishable from carcinoma (Fig. 49-17).

MALIGNANT LESIONS

ANNULAR CARCINOMA

Annular carcinoma ("apple-core," "napkin-ring") is one of the most typical forms of primary malignancy of the colon (Fig. 49-18). The characteristic combination of narrowing of the bowel lumen and abrupt change from tumor to normal bowel ("tumor shelf," "overhanging margins") is caused by extensive tumor infiltration and rigidity of the bowel wall (Fig. 49-19).

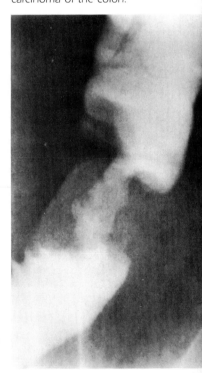

Fig. 49-18. Annular primary carcinoma of the colon.

Among malignant tumors in the United States, the incidence of carcinoma of the colon is second only to that of skin cancer. This malignancy kills more persons than any malignant tumor other than cancer of the lung in men and breast cancer in women. Even with some improvement in lesion detection and medical and surgical therapy, the 5-year survival rate remains about 40%, having changed little in the last several decades.

Adenocarcinoma of the colon and rectum is primarily a disease of elderly persons, the peak incidence being in the 50- to 70-year range. Nevertheless, the disease occasionally develops in younger persons, in whom it tends to be far more aggressive and is associated with a low survival rate.

The etiology of carcinoma of the colon is unknown. There is considerable evidence to suggest that many, if not most, carcinomas of the colon arise in pre-existing villous or adenomatous polyps. It is unclear and controversial whether cancers arise *de novo* in normal colonic mucosa. Several of the hereditary intestinal polyposis syndromes, as well as ulcerative colitis, are known to have a predilection for secondary development of colon cancer. Because the incidence of the disease is far lower in underdeveloped countries than in the West,

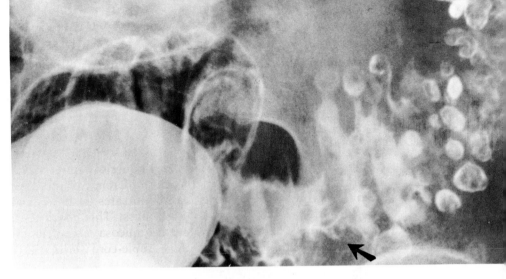

Fig. 49-25. Carcinoma of the sigmoid colon simulating diverticulitis in a patient with multiple diverticula. The lesion **(arrow)** is sharply defined and well demarcated from the adjacent diverticula-laden bowel.

Annular carcinoma can be simulated by an area of transient, localized spasm. This phenomenon can occur anywhere in the colon but is found particularly in the transverse, descending, and sigmoid portions, in which the so-called colonic sphincters are found (Fig. 49-26). These sphincters are areas of spasm that are not due to organic disease but probably reflect localized nerve and muscle imbalance. Unlike the narrowing seen in annular carcinoma, that associated with colon sphincters tends to have tapering margins, changes on sequential films, and is usually relieved by intravenous glucagon. The mucosa running through an area of benign spasm is intact and without ulceration, in contrast to annular carcinoma, in which normal mucosal architecture is destroyed.

SCIRRHOUS CARCINOMA OF THE COLON

Scirrhous carcinoma is a rare variant of annular carcinoma of the colon in which an intense desmoplastic reaction infiltrates the bowel wall with dense fibrous tissue (Fig. 49-27). As the tumor grows, it spreads circumferentially and longitudinally, producing a long segment of bowel (up to 12 cm) with a luminal diameter of only 1 cm to 3 cm. In scirrhous carcinoma, in contrast to the more common annular form of colon cancer, the mucosa can be partially preserved, and the margins of the lesion tend to taper and fade gradually into normal bowel.

Scirrhous carcinoma is a particularly virulent form of colonic malignancy with a poor prognosis. The clinical presentation is insidious, and the relative lack of mucosal destruction makes bleeding an uncommon symptom. Because the tumor grows slowly and only gradually narrows the bowel lumen, the intermittent constipation and progressive decrease in the caliber of the stool may not be readily appreciated by the patient.

Primary scirrhous carcinoma of the colon can be indistinguishable from segmental colonic encasement due either to contiguous spread of carcinoma of the stomach or ovary or to hematogenous metastases from carcinoma of the breast (Fig. 49-28). Patients who develop carci-

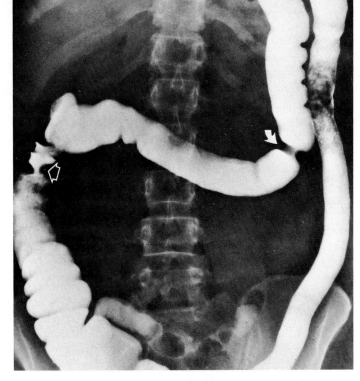

Fig. 49-26. Colonic sphincter (Cannon's point). There is an area of transient, localized spasm in the distal transverse colon **(solid arrow).** A second area of spasm is seen in the hepatic flexure **(open arrow).**

Fig. 49-27. Scirrhous carcinoma of the colon. There is severe circumferential narrowing of a long segment of descending colon.

Fig. 49-28. Scirrhous carcinoma of the colon. The long, circumferentially narrowed area **(arrow)** simulates segmental colonic encasement due to metastatic disease.

Fig. 49-27

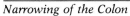

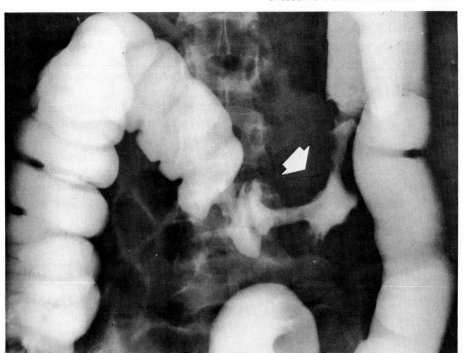

noma of the colon as a late complication of chronic ulcerative colitis often have a scirrhous type of tumor. This can present a diagnostic dilemma, because the appearance of the tumor often closely simulates a benign stricture or the long, stiff, featureless narrowing that is characteristic of the colon in "burned out" ulcerative colitis. Because of this difficulty, the development of scirrhous carcinoma in patients with chronic ulcerative colitis is often not recognized until metastasis or invasion of other organs has occurred.

METASTASES

Metastases to the colon can arise from direct invasion, intraperitoneal seeding, or hematogenous or lymphangitic spread. Rather than a random occurrence, metastases from various primary lesions reflect patterns of spread that are predictable on the basis of anatomic considerations. This is of particular importance, since the site and radiographic appearance of a metastasis can be the foundation for a rational approach to identification of the primary lesion.

Direct Invasion

Direct invasion of the colon from a contiguous primary tumor indicates a locally aggressive lesion that has broken through fascial planes. In men, the most common primary tumor is advanced carcinoma of the prostate gland, which spreads posteriorly across the rectogenital septum (Denonvilliers' fascia) to invade the rectum anteriorly or circumferentially. Because rectal spread of tumor is not infrequent, is often clinically unsuspected, and somewhat alters the therapeutic approach, a barium enema examination is indicated in patients with carcinoma of the prostate.

Spread of carcinoma of the prostate to the rectum can produce one of several radiographic patterns. It can cause a large, smooth, concave pressure defect on the anterior aspect of the rectosigmoid (Fig. 49-29) that is occasionally severe enough to obstruct the colon. Invasion of the anterior rectal wall produces a fungating, ulcerated mass that closely simulates primary rectal carcinoma. The most frequent presentation of prostatic carcinoma metastatic to the colon is a long, asymmetric annular stricture of the proximal rectum or rectosigmoid. The margins of this stricture show irregular scalloping caused either by intramural tumor nodules or by edema infiltrating the bowel wall (Fig. 49-30). Concomitant widening of the retrorectal space is usually seen.

Differentiation between direct extension of prostatic carcinoma and a primary rectal tumor can be difficult. Primary carcinoma of the colon is usually a less extensive lesion that demonstrates a tumor shelf with overhanging margins (Fig. 49-31), in contrast to a metastatic lesion, which has more tapered edges (Fig. 49-32). Elevated serum acid phosphatase activity indicates extension of prostatic carcinoma beyond its fascia but does not indicate whether such extension represents spread to the rectum or to more remote areas, such as liver or bone.

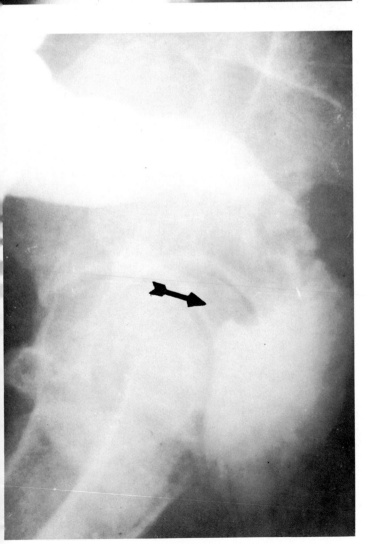

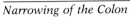

Fig. 49-29. Carcinoma of the prostate involving the colon. The lateral view demonstrates marked anterior compression of the rectosigmoid. (Gengler L, Baer J, Finby N: Rectal and sigmoid involvement secondary to carcinoma of the prostate. AJR 125:910–917, 1975. Copyright 1975. Reproduced by permission)

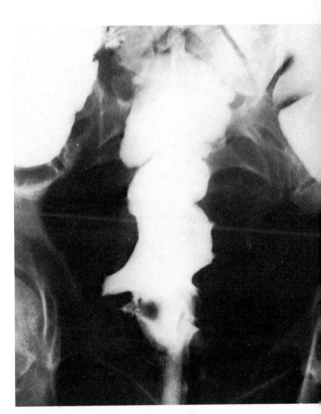

Fig. 49-30. Carcinoma of the prostate involving the colon. The rectum, which has scalloped margins, shows lack of distention and extrinsic infiltration of the bowel wall. (Gengler L, Baer J, Finby N: Rectal and sigmoid involvement secondary to carcinoma of the prostate. AJR 125:910–917, 1975. Copyright 1975. Reproduced by permission)

Fig. 49-31. Primary adenocarcinoma of the rectum. Note the tumor shelf at the inferior aspect of the mass **(arrow).** Such a shelf is not present in secondary prostatic cancer. (Gengler L, Baer J, Finby N: Rectal and sigmoid involvement secondary to carcinoma of the prostate. AJR 125:910–917, 1975. Copyright 1975. Reproduced by permission)

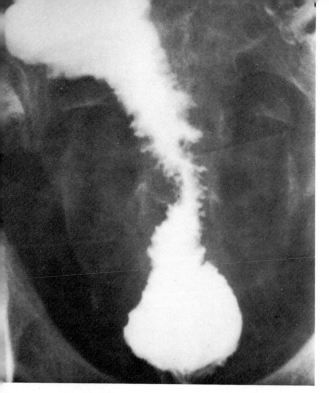

Fig. 49-32. Carcinoma of the prostate involving the rectum. Circumferential involvement causes diffuse rectal narrowing and ulceration. Note the tapered margins of the lesion. There is no evidence of a tumor shelf.

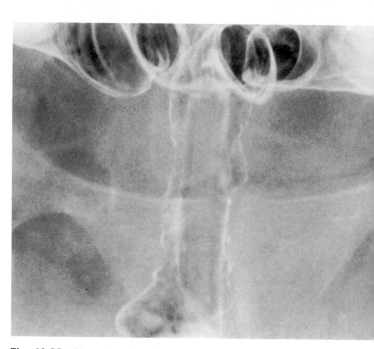

Fig. 49-33. Direct invasion from carcinoma of the cervix concentrically narrowing the rectum.

Fig. 49-34. Extrinsic mass effect on the sigmoid colon due to cystadenocarcinoma of the ovary.

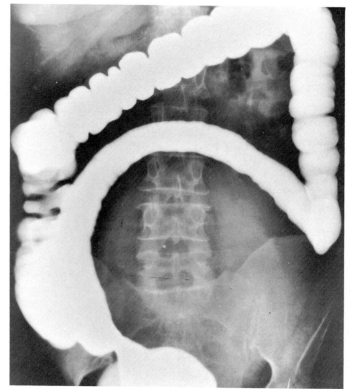

In women, direct invasion from a noncontiguous primary tumor is usually related to a pelvic tumor arising in the ovary or uterus (Fig. 49-33). Invasion of the bowel wall produces a mass effect that is often of great length and does not demonstrate overhanging margins (Fig. 49-34). An associated desmoplastic reaction causes angulation and tethering of mucosal folds and can even lead to the development of an annular stricture (Fig. 49-35).

Primary renal neoplasms can directly invade adjacent segments of the colon, often resulting in large intraluminal masses with no desmoplastic response or significant obstruction. On the left side, direct spread from a renal primary most commonly involves the distal transverse colon or proximal descending colon.

Carcinomas of the stomach and pancreas are noncontiguous primary tumors that can spread to the colon along mesenteric reflections. Primary carcinoma of the stomach (usually scirrhous) extends down the gastrocolic ligament to involve the transverse colon along its superior haustral border (Fig. 49-36). The tumor incites a desmoplastic reaction that causes the colon wall to become thickened, straightened, and irregular. The mucosal folds become tethered and angulated. The inferior border of the transverse colon is initially uninvolved, so that its haustral contours retain their pliability and produce pseudosacculations. Progressive distortion and fixation of the mucosal pattern eventually cause irregular stenoses and an appearance of cobblestoning that simulates Crohn's disease (Fig. 49-37). However, metastases to the transverse colon can usually be distinguished from inflammatory bowel disease by demonstration of the tethering of mucosal folds and the extent of radiographic abnormality, which is localized specifically to the superior border of the transverse colon and tends to end abruptly at the level of the phrenicocolic ligament (extending from the anatomic splenic flexure to the diaphragm), where the mesenteric transverse colon continues as the extraperitoneal descending colon.

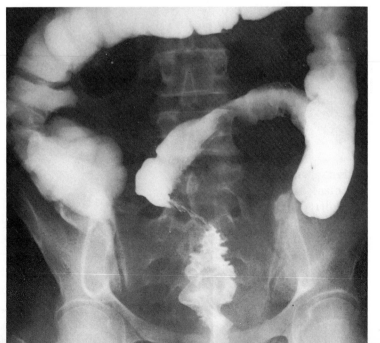

Fig. 49-35. Metastatic cystadenocarcinoma of the ovary. In addition to the mass effect, an associated desmoplastic reaction causes tethering of mucosal folds and an annular stricture.

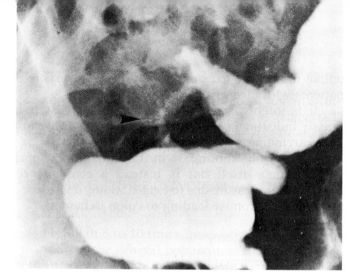

Fig. 49-47. Adenocarcinoma of the colon as a delayed complication of ureterosigmoidostomy. A typical "apple-core" lesion of the sigmoid colon **(arrow)** may be seen. (Parsons CD, Thomas MH, Garrett RA: Colonic adenocarcinoma: A delayed complication of ureterosigmoidostomy. J Urol 118:31–34, 1977)

Fig. 49-46. Ulcerating colitis **(open arrows)** proximal to a high-grade stenosis **(solid arrow)** caused by carcinoma of the sigmoid.

Fig. 49-48. Primary lymphoma of the descending colon. Segmental colonic narrowing **(open arrow)** is complicated by perforation and abscess formation **(solid arrows)** within the tumor mass.

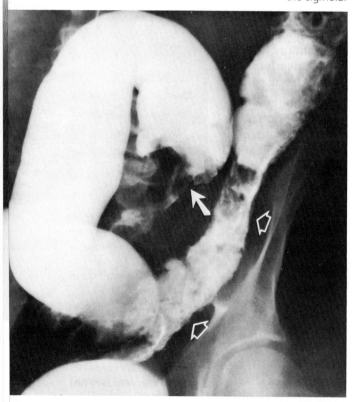

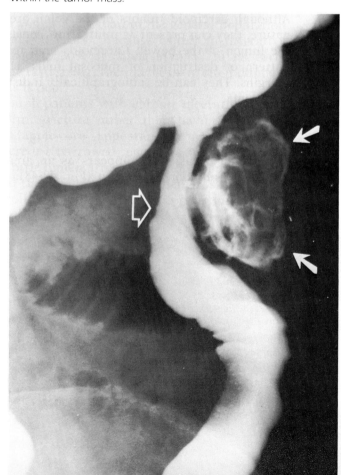

phoma can also present as an aneurysmal dilatation of a short segment of colon. This dilatation is due both to the absence of a desmoplastic response, which permits a malignant ulcer to greatly increase in size, and to destruction of the musucular layer and nerve plexuses. Both of these manifestations of lymphoma, nevertheless, are much less common than the polypoid or diffuse forms of the disease.

A few patients have been described who had a clinical, proctoscopic, and radiographic picture closely simulating ulcerative colitis but in whom malignant lymphoma was diagnosed at surgery. Because these patients had an average of 13 years of symptoms diagnosed as ulcerative colitis, and in view of the poor survival rate in gastrointestinal lymphoma, it is most likely that the lymphoma developed by malignant transformation, possibly by a process similar to the development of adenocarcinoma in patients with chronic inflammatory bowel disease.

DIVERTICULAR DISEASE

Colonic diverticula are acquired herniations of mucosa and submucosa through the muscular layers of the bowel wall (Fig. 49-49). The incidence of colonic diverticulosis increases with age. Rare in persons below the age of 30, diverticula can be demonstrated in up to half of people over 60. In about 95% of patients with diverticular disease, the sigmoid is the major segment of colon affected. Proximal colon involvement is much less frequent and is almost always associated with contiguous disease distally. Diverticula usually develop between the mesenteric and lateral tenia at sites of weakness in the colon wall, where the longitudinal arteries penetrate the inner circular muscle layer to form the submucosal capillary plexus.

Although the precise pathogenesis of diverticulosis is unclear, increased muscular thickening of the colon wall and abnormally exaggerated intraluminal pressure are thought to be major contributing factors. In response to food, emotional stimuli, or cholinergic drugs, the sigmoid colon in patients predisposed to diverticular disease tends to become segmented, and intraluminal pressure becomes elevated. This exaggerated pressure, combined with prominent muscular thickening, causes herniation of mucosal outpouchings at weak points in the colon wall. The reason for the sigmoid colon being the usual site of diverticulosis can be explained by the law of Laplace, which states that, in a cylindrical structure with a given tension, the pressure is inversely related to the radius. Because the sigmoid has the most narrow caliber of any portion of the colon, the tension generated by circular muscle bundles produces far higher pressures in this region than in more proximal parts of the colon, where the lumen diameter is larger. The elevated pressure causes the mucosa and submucosa to herniate through anatomic weak points in the sigmoid musculature and form diverticula.

Epidemiologic data suggest that diet may play a major role in the development of diverticular disease. Diverticulosis is extremely rare in underdeveloped areas in Africa and Asia. It is postulated that the high

Fig. 49-49. Multiple colonic diverticula.

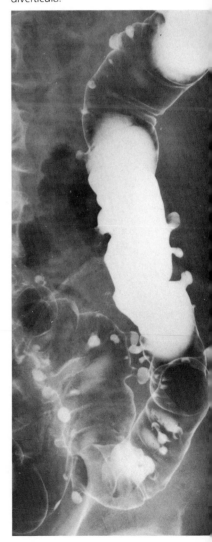

fiber content of native diets results in large volumes of semisolid stool, a large-caliber colonic lumen, and a rapid fecal transit time. In contrast, in the United States and Western Europe, the diet is highly refined and low in roughage. This diet tends to cause a small fecal stream, which leads to excessive segmentation of the sigmoid, increased intraluminal pressure, and smooth muscle hypertrophy, all of which combine to produce diverticulosis.

DIVERTICULOSIS

Clinical Symptoms

The majority of patients with diverticulosis have no symptoms. A substantial number, however, have chronic or intermittent lower abdominal pain frequently precipitated by, or related to, meals and emotional stress. Alternating bouts of diarrhea and constipation are common, and a tender, palpable mass may be present in the left lower quadrant. This symptom complex probably represents the altered motor activity of the thickened colonic musculature rather than diverticular inflammation. Evidence for this hypothesis may be seen in the finding that young patients with "prediverticular" muscle dysfunction may have identical symptoms, even when no true diverticula are radiographically detectable. Thus, the degree of pain and altered bowel habits appear to relate to the intensity of segmentation and the degree of increased intraluminal pressure rather than to the presence of diverticula *per se*.

Painless bleeding is a common complication of diverticulosis. It can range from mild hematochezia to massive hemorrhage. Bleeding is caused by inflammatory erosion of penetrating branches of the vasa recta at the base of the diverticulum. For reasons that are not clear, diverticula of the right colon cause significant bleeding more often than those of the left.

Radiographic Findings

Colonic diverticula appear radiographically as round or oval outpouchings of barium projecting beyond the confines of the lumen. They vary in size from barely visible dimples to saclike structures 2 cm or more in diameter. Giant sigmoid diverticula of up to 25 cm in diameter have been reported (Fig. 49-50). Thought to reflect slowly progressing chronic diverticular abscesses, they appear as large, well-circumscribed radiolucent cystic structures in the lower abdomen (Fig. 49-51). Rectal diverticula are rare, presumably because the longitudinal muscle coat completely encircles this portion of the bowel.

Diverticula are usually multiple and tend to occur in clusters, though a solitary diverticulum is occasionally found. Small numbers of diverticula do not distort or alter the configuration of the bowel. With multiple diverticula, however, deep criss-crossing ridges of thickened circular muscle can produce a series of sacculations (sawtooth configuration) (Fig. 49-52). The involved portion of colon may be shortened and relatively fixed, with narrowing of the lumen.

If multiple diverticula are present, the introduction of barium can cause severe sigmoid spasm and complete obstruction to retrograde flow. This is particularly common if the hydrostatic pressure is excessive (because the enema bag is too high) or the enema solution is too cold. Antispasmodic drugs, such as glucagon, usually permit a successful examination.

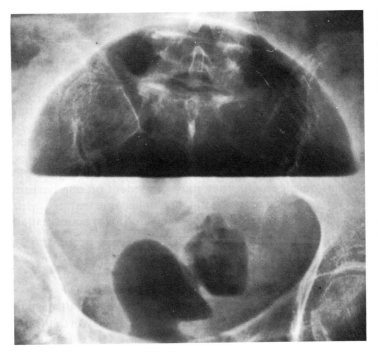

Fig. 49-50. Giant sigmoid diverticulum. A plain abdominal radiograph demonstrates a huge walled-off pelvic abscess with a gas–fluid level.

Fig. 49-51. Giant sigmoid diverticulum. **(A)** A plain abdominal radiograph demonstrates a large, well-circumscribed radiolucent structure **(arrow)** in the lower abdomen. **(B)** A barium enema examination demonstrates filling of the giant sigmoid diverticulum with radiopaque contrast **(arrow)**.

A B

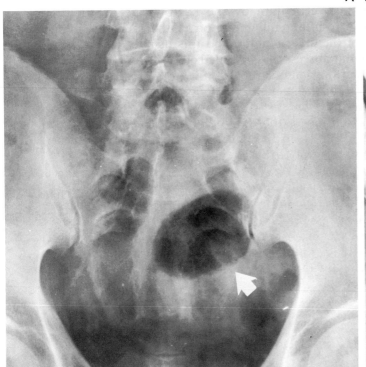

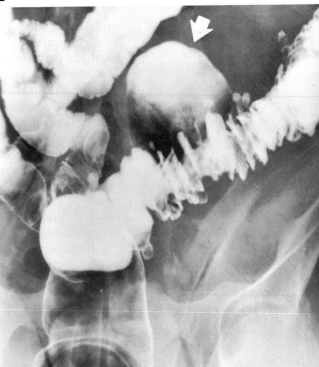

barium or can be dislodged by palpation. Fecal material, however, can be adherent; a repeat examination may be necessary for definite diagnosis. Diverticula seen *en face* rather than in profile can appear to lie within the lumen, rather than projecting beyond it, and may be difficult to distinguish from polyps (Fig. 50-5*A*). Rotation of the patient usually demonstrates that the diverticulum truly extends beyond the colonic lumen (Fig. 50-5*B*). At times, the barium-coated, air-filled diverticulum remains superimposed on the lumen of the bowel on multiple projections. Demonstration of an air–fluid level clearly excludes the diagnosis of a polypoid lesion. Polyps and diverticula can sometimes be differentiated by an evaluation of the quality of the barium coating them. The ring of barium coating a diverticulum has a smooth, well-defined outer border (where it is in contact with the diverticular mucosa) but an irregular inner surface. In contrast, the barium coating a polyp is smooth on its inner border (where it abuts the mucosal surface of the polyp) but is poorly defined on its outer surface (where it is in contact with the fecal stream). Nevertheless, a small adenomatous polyp can easily be hidden in a patient with a large number of diverticula.

There are three major morphologic types of polypoid tumor: sessile, intermediate or protuberant, and pedunculated. The earliest stage is the sessile polyp, a flat lesion attached to the mucosa by a broad base (Fig. 50-6). On *en face* views, the sessile polyp appears rounded. In profile, it may protrude only slightly into the lumen of the colon and may therefore be difficult to differentiate from the normal mucosa of the colon wall. Although the sessile polyp has a central fibrovascular core arising from the submucosa, this potential stalk is not yet detectable radiographically.

Peristaltic waves and the flow of the fecal stream cause traction on a sessile polyp, and this can force the underlying normal mucosa to be drawn out into a pedicle (stalk) (Fig. 50-7). In profile view, the pedicle may appear as a linear lucency in the barium-filled colon (Fig. 50-8*A*) or be thinly coated by barium in an air-contrast examination (Fig. 50-8*B*). When seen *en face* (with the central beam parallel to the long axis of the pedicle), the barium-coated pedicle is seen as a small white

Fig. 50-5. Diverticulum mimicking a colonic polyp. **(A)** On the en face projection, the barium-coated diverticulum simulates a polyp **(arrow)** lying within the lumen. **(B)** A radiograph obtained after rotation of the patient demonstrates that the diverticulum fills with barium **(arrow)** and clearly extends beyond the colonic lumen.

A   B

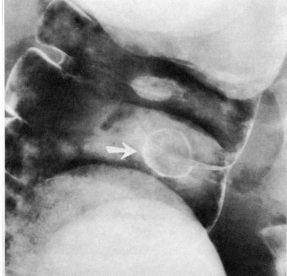
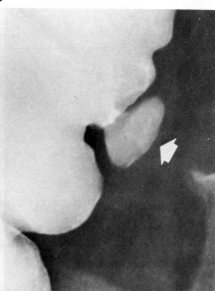

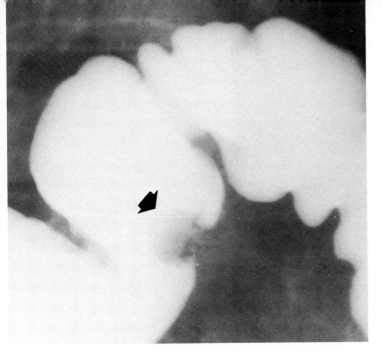

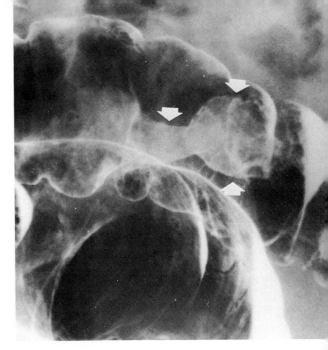

Fig. 50-6. Benign sessile colonic polyp **(arrow).**   **Fig. 50-7.** Pedunculated colonic polyp **(arrows).**

circle within a larger circle of barium covering the body of the polyp (target sign; Fig. 50-9).

The radiographic demonstration of a thin pedicle of 2 cm or more in length is virtually pathognomonic of a benign polyp (see Fig. 50-8). Malignant sessile polyps that have invaded deep into the mucosa will not develop long stalks. When these polypoid carcinomas are pedunculated, the stalks are usually short, thick, and irregular.

Fig. 50-8. Pedunculated colonic polyp. **(A)** On single contrast examination, the stalk appears as a linear lucency in the barium-filled colon **(arrow). (B)** On the double-contrast examination, the stalk of the polyp is thinly coated by barium **(arrow).**

A   B

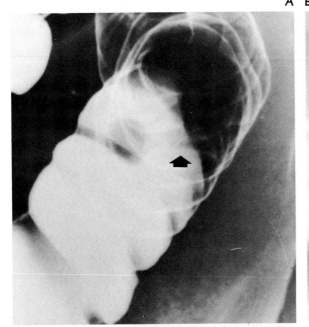

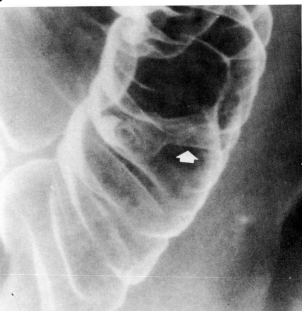

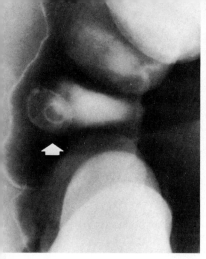
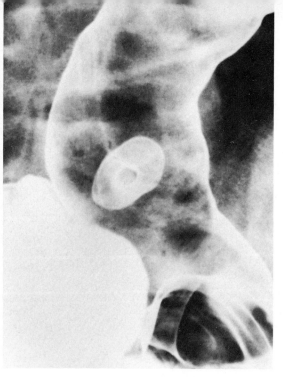

A B

Fig. 50-9. Target sign of pedunculated colonic polyps in two patients. The barium-coated pedicles are seen as small white circles inside the larger circles of barium covering the bodies of the polyps **(arrows)**.

Relationship Between Adenomatous Polyps and Carcinoma

The precise relationship between adenomatous polyps and carcinoma has created considerable controversy. Most authorities believe that the vast majority of adenocarcinomas of the colon arise in pre-existing benign adenomas. Evidence for this theory includes the well-documented coexistence of invasive carcinoma and benign-appearing adenomas, the rare demonstration of *de novo* carcinomas of less than 5 mm in size in otherwise normal colons, and the fact that almost all patients with familial intestinal polyposis who do not have surgery develop colon cancer. It is estimated that the evolution of cancer of the colon from a benign adenomatous polyp requires at least 5 years and may take as many as 20 years. Though it is difficult to establish a true malignancy rate, it is believed that about 5% of adenomatous polyps eventually transform into malignant lesions.

There is a close correlation between the size of adenomatous polyps of the colon and the incidence of invasive carcinoma within them. Adenomas measuring 5 mm to 9 mm in diameter have a 1% probability of containing an invasive malignancy; those under 5 mm have less than a 0.5% incidence. Because more than 90% of colon polyps under 5 mm are hyperplastic (*i.e.*, have no malignant potential) rather than adenomatous, the overall incidence of invasive cancer in such small lesions is less than 0.05%. Adenomatous polyps between 1 cm and 2 cm in size have been reported to have a 4% to 10% incidence of malignancy; those greater than 2 cm in diameter are reported to have a 10% to 46% (average, 25%) malignancy rate (Fig. 50-10).

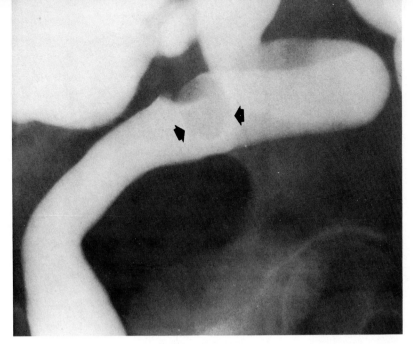

Fig. 50-10. Malignant polyp
(arrows) in the sigmoid colon.
Although the lesion is smooth,
its 4-cm diameter makes
malignancy likely.

Radiographic Differentiation Between Benign and Malignant Polyps

Carcinomatous degeneration of an adenomatous polyp can be suggested by several radiographic criteria: surface characteristics; change in size, shape, or appearance of an associated pedicle; puckering of the base of the tumor; and interval growth on sequential examination.

Benign sessile polyps tend to have a smooth surface and a normal adjacent colon wall. An irregular or lobulated surface suggests malignancy (Fig. 50-11), as does a flat lesion whose base is longer than its height (Fig. 50-12).

Pedunculated polyps with long, thin stalks that move freely on palpation are almost always benign. Carcinomatous transformation in the head of a pedunculated polyp not only enlarges the head but also grows into the stalk. This causes gradual shortening and obliteration of the pedicle and can eventually produce a sessile lesion (Fig. 50-13). It is extremely rare for carcinoma developing in a pedunculated polyp to metastasize to adjacent tissues prior to invading its stalk.

Retraction or indentation (puckering) of the colon wall seen on profile view at the site of origin of a sessile polyp almost invariably indicates that the polyp is malignant (Fig. 50-14). Malignant invasion beneath the mucosal layer, with subsequent retraction of the wall toward the base of the tumor, results in slight concavity of the bowel wall at the base of the lesion. It must be stressed that this description refers only to sessile polyps; benign pedunculated lesions can demonstrate a similar puckered appearance, but, in their case, it is due to tugging of the stalk rather than to malignant invasion of the bowel wall.

Fig. 50-11. Malignant sessile colonic polyp. This large sessile mass has an irregular, lobulated surface.

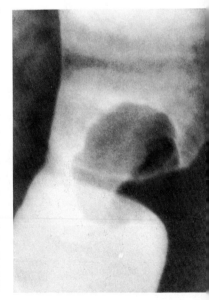

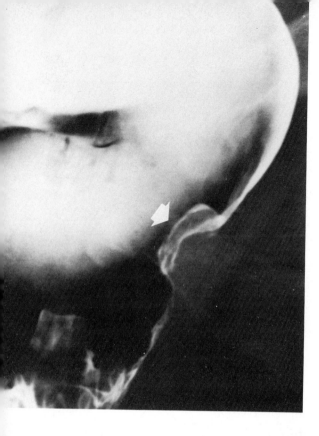

Fig. 50-12. Malignant sessile rectal polyp **(arrow).** Note that the base of this flat lesion is longer than its height.

B   C

Fig. 50-13. Sessile malignant lesion developing from a pedunculated polyp. **(A)** Large pedunculated polyp **(arrows). (B)** Four years later, the mass has become sessile **(arrows). (C)** One year after **(B),** an annular constricting lesion has formed **(arrows).**

A

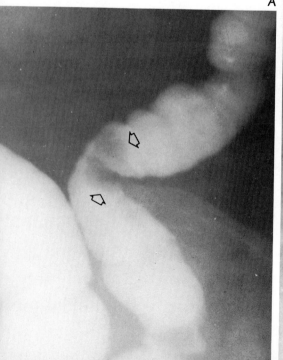

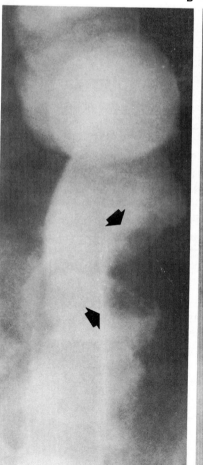

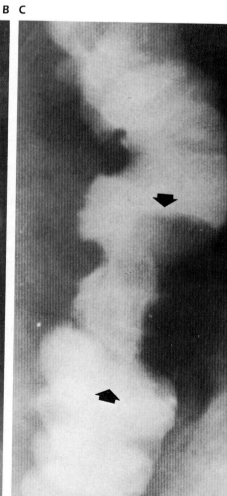

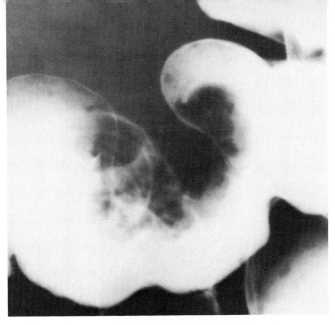

Fig. 50-14. Malignant sessile colonic polyp. Retraction or indentation (puckering) of the colon wall is seen on profile view.

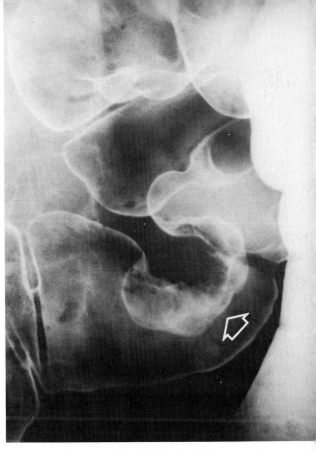

Fig. 50-15. Saddle cancer of the colon. The tumor **(arrow)** appears to sit on the upper margin of the distal transverse colon like a saddle on a horse.

Sudden or steady interval growth of a polyp on sequential examinations strongly suggests malignancy. Although a benign polyp can grow slowly, it tends to maintain its initial configuration. Carcinomatous proliferation alters the growth of a polyp and can change its shape from round or elliptical to a variety of bizarre configurations (*e.g.*, triangular, rectangular, polyhedral).

Another form of carcinoma of the colon is a flat, centrally ulcerated plaque involving a segment of the bowel wall. As the tumor enlarges, it appears to sit on the barium column, much like a saddle on a horse (saddle lesion; Fig. 50-15). Unless they are demonstrated in tangent, saddle carcinomas can be easily overlooked on barium enema examination. These lesions are extremely virulent and grow rapidly, eventually spreading circumferentially about the bowel to become annular carcinomas (Fig. 50-16).

Saddle cancer has been described as analogous to a malignant Carman ulcer of the stomach. Spot-films with compression can demonstrate trapping of barium within a centrally ulcerated lesion with heaped up edges, producing a true Carman meniscus sign.

Because saddle cancers ulcerate at an early stage of development, rectal bleeding is usually the only symptom. Only by meticulous searching for an area of minimal straightening or slight contour defect can these small and subtle, but lethal, lesions be detected.

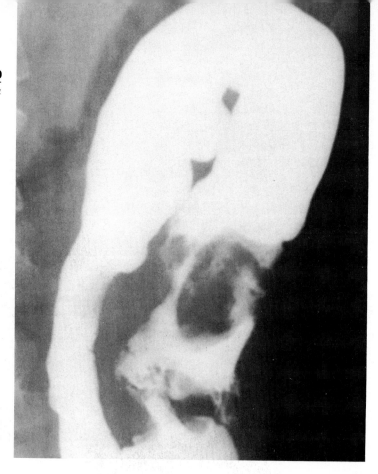

Fig. 50-16. Annular carcinoma of the colon that developed from circumferential spread of a saddle lesion.

VILLOUS ADENOMA

Fig. 50-17. Benign villous adenoma. The bulky descending colon mass has an irregular, corrugated surface **(arrow).**

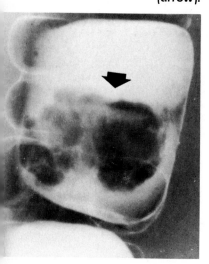

Villous adenomas of the colon are benign exophytic tumors consisting of innumerable villous fronds that give the surface a corrugated appearance (Fig. 50-17). Most are solitary and are located in the rectosigmoid area (Fig. 50-18). However, they can be found anywhere in the colon, particularly in the cecum. Villous adenomas are usually sessile but can be pedunculated (Fig. 50-19). Although they constitute only 10% of all benign neoplastic polyps of the colon, they are of great importance because of their high malignant potential. In contrast to the far more numerous adenomatous polyps, which have a low malignancy rate, about 40% of villous adenomas demonstrate infiltrating carcinoma, usually at the base. Villous adenomas also tend to be much larger than adenomatous polyps; about 75% exceed 2 cm in diameter, whereas only 5% of adenomatous polyps reach this size.

Villous adenomas are often asymptomatic and are frequently an unexpected finding on barium enema examination performed for another purpose. Extremely large tumors (10–15 cm) can produce obstructive symptoms. Large amounts of mucus are occasionally secreted into the lumen across the papillary surface of a villous adenoma. This mucus diarrhea causes severe fluid, protein, and electrolyte (especially potassium) depletion. Rectal bleeding is unusual, since the mucosal surface of a villous adenoma is usually intact and not ulcerated.

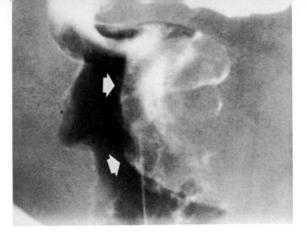

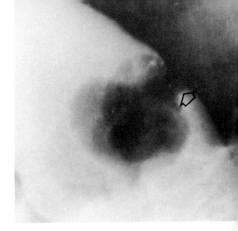

Fig. 50-18. Benign villous adenoma of the rectum **(arrows).** Barium can be seen entering the interstices of the tumor.

Fig. 50-19. Benign villous adenoma of the transverse colon. Note the short stalk **(arrow)** leading to the lobulated mass.

Radiographically, villous adenomas classically present as bulky tumors with a spongelike pattern ("bouquet of flowers") caused by barium filling of deep clefts betwen the multiple fronds (Fig. 50-20). This radiographic feature is best demonstrated on the postevacuation view, in which barium remains within the interstices of the villous tumor. Because the lobular, irregular tumor has a soft consistency, its appearance can change on serial films and with palpation. The adjacent bowel wall is pliable and distensible, since the tumor does not incite a desmoplastic response.

Large size (Fig. 50-21), ulceration, and indentation of the tumor base have been suggested as radiographic signs of malignancy in villous adenomas. Nevertheless, no radiographic finding in villous adenoma is sufficient to exclude malignant degeneration. Because invasive carcinoma in villous adenoma is usually found at the base of a lesion rather than on the surface, biopsies can be unreliable as a result of inadequate tissue sampling. Therefore, even a benign-appearing villous adenoma should be totally excised.

Fig. 50-21. Villous adenocarcinoma. The large size of the mass **(arrows)** suggests malignancy. Barium is seen entering the interstices of the mass, suggesting that the lesion represents a villous tumor.

Fig. 50-20. Benign villous adenoma of the rectum **(arrows).** Barium is seen filling the deep clefts between the multiple fronds.

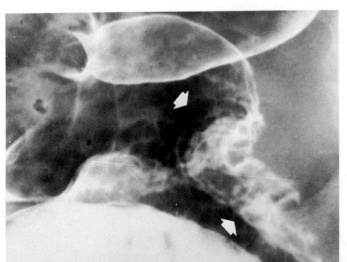

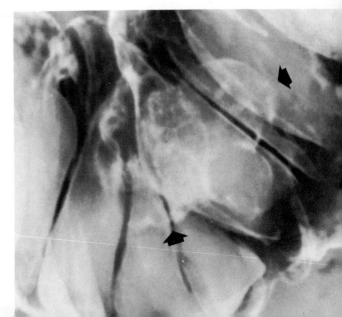

VILLOGLANDULAR POLYP

Villoglandular polyps are composed of mixed adenomatous and villous elements (Fig. 50-22). Although they tend to be pedunculated and grossly simulate adenomatous polyps, villoglandular polyps have an intermediate malignant potential (about 20%) that is higher than that of adenomatous polyps but less than that of villous adenomas.

LIPOMA

Lipomas are the second most common benign tumors of the colon. Submucosal in origin, lipomas grow slowly, rarely cause symptoms, and generally are incidental findings on barium enema examination. The tumors are usually single and occur most commonly in the right colon (Fig. 50-23). Because of the motor activity of the colon and the soft consistency of the tumor, a lipoma tends to protrude into the bowel lumen. The resulting polyp often seems to have a stalk, but this actually represents a thick pseudopedicle of normal mucosa rather than the true pedicle of an adenomatous polyp. Stretching of the epithelium over the lipoma can result in ulceration and continued oozing of blood. Intermittent episodes of intussusception are not uncommon.

On barium studies, lipomas are typically circular or ovoid, sharply defined, smooth filling defects (Fig. 50-24). In comparison with other colon tumors, lipomas have an unusually lucent appearance. This is due both to the fat content of the lesion and to the very smooth surface of the mucosa stretched over the mass, which does not permit as good barium coating as does the more irregular surface of an adenomatous polyp. The adjacent bowel wall is normally distensible, with intact mucosa. If the tumor has an associated pseudopedicle, it generally appears short and thick. The pathognomonic diagnostic feature of lipomas is their changeability in size and shape during the course of

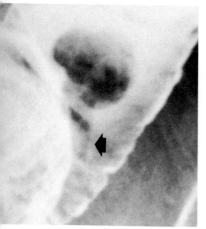

Fig. 50-22. Villoglandular polyp. This benign lesion is composed of mixed adenomatous and villous elements and has a relatively long stalk **(arrow)**.

Fig. 50-23. Lipoma. A large, smooth mass **(arrow)** is visible in the ascending colon.

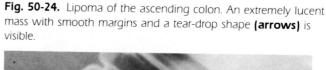

Fig. 50-24. Lipoma of the ascending colon. An extremely lucent mass with smooth margins and a tear-drop shape **(arrows)** is visible.

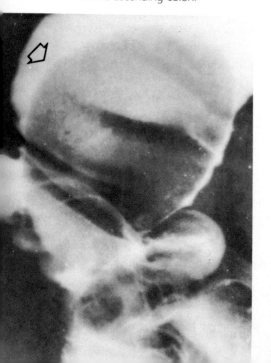

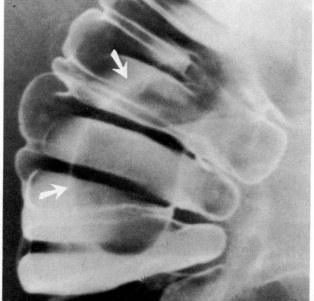

barium enema examination. Because these tumors are extremely soft, their configuration can be altered by palpation and extrinsic pressure. Although a lipoma can appear round or oval on filled films, the malleable tumor characteristically becomes elongated (sausage or banana-shaped) on postevacuation films in which the colon is contracted.

OTHER SPINDLE CELL TUMORS

Other spindle cell tumors (leiomyoma, fibroma, neurofibroma) are rare. They tend to remain more intramural than lipomas (Fig. 50-25), though large lesions can protrude into the lumen and appear as sessile, polypoid tumors mimicking carcinoma (Fig. 50-26). The overlying mucosa tends to be stretched but intact. Unlike lipomas, other spindle cell tumors do not change shape in response to extrinsic pressure or during various phases of filling and emptying of the colon.

Malignant spindle cell tumors are extremely rare (Fig. 50-27). They tend to be much larger and more irregular than their benign counterparts, though differentiation between benign and malignant submucosal tumors can be extremely difficult.

TUMORS WITH INTERMEDIATE MALIGNANT POTENTIAL

CARCINOID TUMOR

Almost all nonappendiceal carcinoid tumors of the colon arise in the rectum (Fig. 50-28). The vast majority are small (under 1 cm in size), solitary, and asymptomatic. Most are found only incidentally on barium

Fig. 50-25. Hemangioma of the sigmoid colon. A large, smooth intramural mass **(arrow)** may be seen.

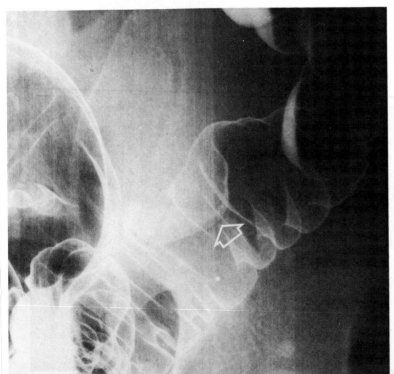

Fig. 50-26. Leiomyoma of the transverse colon. A large mass protrudes into the lumen and appears as a sessile, polypoid filling defect **(arrows)**.

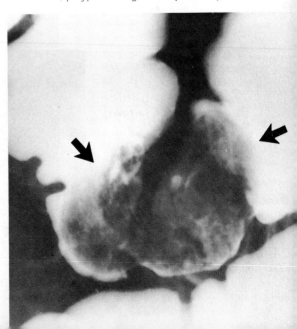

AMEBOMA

An ameboma is a focal hyperplastic granuloma caused by secondary bacterial infection of an amebic abscess in the bowel wall. The lesion has a core of acute and chronic inflammation and necrosis surrounded by a peripheral rim of dense fibrosis.

Amebomas have been reported in 1.5% to 8.5% of patients with amebic colitis. Almost half are multiple; most are associated with evidence of disease elsewhere in the colon. Amebomas are most common in the cecum and ascending colon but can be found anywhere in the large bowel. Most patients with amebomas present with acute or chronic amebic dysentery. Abdominal or rectal examination occasionally demonstrates a large, firm mass that is relatively fixed and tender to palpation.

Radiographically, amebomas are characterized by eccentric or concentric thickening of the entire circumference of the bowel wall. They can appear as discrete luminal masses or as annular, nondistensible lesions with irregular mucosa that simulate colonic carcinoma (Fig. 50-35A).

The differential diagnosis between ameboma and carcinoma can be extremely difficult. The most reliable features of ameboma are multiplicity of lesions, lack of a shelving deformity, and rapid improvement with antiamebic therapy (Fig. 50-35B). Less important findings suggesting ameboma are long length of the lesion, tapered ends, and concentricity of the narrowing. Evidence of mucosal ulcerations elsewhere in the colon, especially in the cecum, strongly suggests amebiasis as the underlying etiology. If a colonic filling defect or annular lesion is suspected to represent an ameboma (especially in a young patient with a history of having lived in or traveled through an endemic area), a trial with antiamebic therapy is essential. Shrinkage of an ameboma in response to antiamebic therapy is often achieved in less than 1 month. In addition, there is a high rate of postoperative morbidity and mortality (over 50% in one series) if a colostomy or other surgical procedure is performed without adequate antiamebic therapy beforehand.

INFLAMMATORY MASSES

Single or multiple small (1–1.5 cm) localized eccentric contour defects have been reported to be an early manifestation of Crohn's disease of the colon. These focal lesions may occur as the only abnormal radiographic finding or may appear in association with more obvious segmental disease elsewhere in the colon. Surface irregularity of the contour defects can suggest the presence of ulceration. These focal lesions seen on barium enema examination correspond pathologically

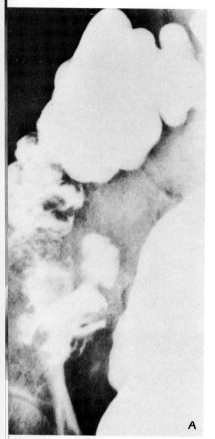

A

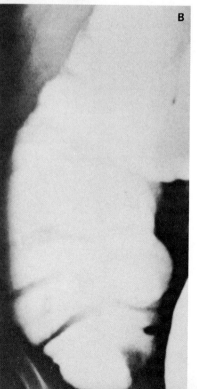

B

Fig. 50-35. Ameboma. **(A)** *Irregular mass in the cecum and ascending colon.* **(B)** *Rapid regression of the lesion following antiamebic therapy. (Cardosa JM, Kimura K, Stoopen M et al: Radiology of invasive amebiasis of the colon. AJR 128:935–941, 1977. Copyright 1977. Reproduced by permission)*

to sharply localized ulcers of variable depth that are associated with pronounced edema and inflammation of the adjacent mucosa and submucosa.

Individual inflammatory pseudopolyps usually measure less than 1.5 cm in diameter and appear as discrete masses scattered throughout involved segments of the colon (Fig. 50-36). A localized giant cluster of pseudopolyps occasionally develops in patients with ulcerative or Crohn's colitis (Fig. 50-37). Adherence and retention of fecal particles within the hyperplastic mass further contribute to the bulk of the lesion. The resultant localized giant pseudopolyp can obliterate the lumen of the colon and simulate a malignant tumor or colonic intussusception.

Although polypoid granulomas caused by schistosomiasis usually present as multiple filling defects in the rectosigmoid, they can occur singly and simulate adenocarcinoma. These masses sometimes become so large that obstruction or intussusception results. A primary submucosal epithelioid tubercule can present radiographically as a sharply outlined contour defect mimicking an intramural tumor; however,

Fig. 50-37. Localized giant pseudopolyposis in ulcerative colitis. Barium enema examination shows obstruction of the splenic flexure by a bulky mass with a nodular surface. Superficial mucosal ulcerations are present in the descending colon. (Bernstein JR, Ghahremani GG, Paige ML et al: Localized giant pseudopolyposis of the colon in ulcerative and granulomatous colitis. Gastrointest Radiol 3:431–435, 1978)

Fig. 50-36. Inflammatory pseudopolyps in Crohn's disease. Multiple nodular filling defects, each less than 1 cm in diameter, are scattered throughout the colon.

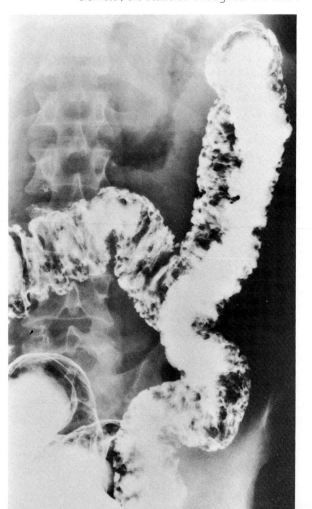

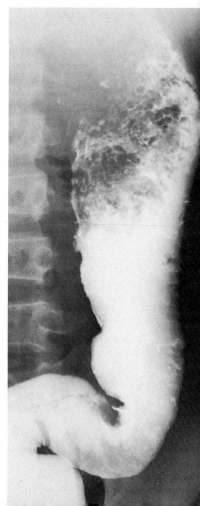

because lesions at this stage of development are asymptomatic, this radiographic pattern is rarely seen. Tuberculosis can also cause an intraluminal mass simulating carcinoma. Rarely, large numbers of *Ascaris lumbricoides* organisms clump together to form a bolus of worms that appears as a polypoid filling defect in the colon. Whenever an intramural or extrinsic filling defect is seen in the cecum (even if on the lateral margin), the possibility of rupture of the appendix and formation of a periappendiceal abscess must be considered (Fig. 50-38). Diverticulitis can appear as a broad intramural or extrinsic colonic filling defect almost always involving the sigmoid (Fig. 50-39). The presence of multiple diverticula intimately associated with the mass, especially if they are deformed, suggests a diverticular abscess. Nonspecific benign ulceration of the colon, which predominantly occurs in the cecum, can present as a large filling defect with or without radiographically demonstrable ulceration (Fig. 50-40). Foreign body perforation with abscess formation, most commonly due to a chicken bone, can also appear as a colonic mass.

MISCELLANEOUS DISORDERS

FECAL IMPACTION

Fecal impactions are large, firm, immovable masses of stool in the rectum that produce filling defects on barium enema examination. They develop whenever there is incomplete evacuation of feces over an extended period. Fecal impactions occur in elderly, debilitated, or

Fig. 50-38. Periappendiceal abscess. Perforation of a retrocecal appendix has produced an inflammatory mass that has caused an extrinsic impression on the lateral margin of the proximal ascending colon **(arrows)**.

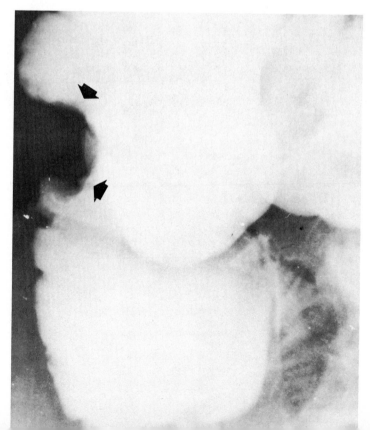

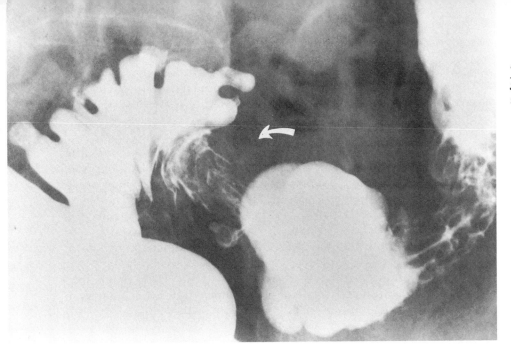

Fig. 50-39. Diverticulitis. The resulting pericolic abscess has caused a large extrinsic filling defect on the sigmoid colon **(arrow).**

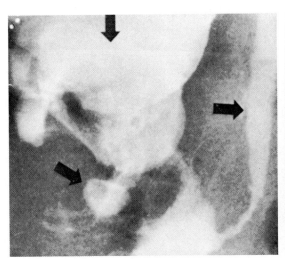 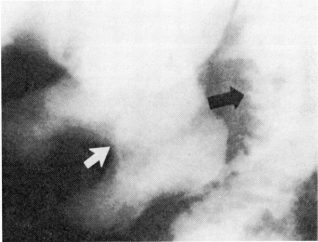

A B

Fig. 50-40. Benign ulceration of the cecum. **(A)** This distorted and incompletely distended cecum is not fixed in appearance, despite its masslike effect [see **(B)**]. The **upper arrow** points to the superior surface of the inflammatory mass. The **slanted arrow** points to the persistent collection of barium representing an ulcer. The **horizontal arrow** points to the partially filled appendix, the base of which is narrowed and irregular. **(B)** The cecum is more distended than in **(A)**, indicating that the distortion is not fixed. The **white arrow** points to the same collection of barium in the ulcer as in **(A)**. The **black arrow** points to the normal terminal ileum with no adjacent mass effect. (Brodey PA, Hill RP, Baron S: Benign ulceration of the cecum. Radiology 122:323–327, 1977)

sedentary persons, in narcotic addicts and patients receiving large doses of tranquilizers, and in children who have undiagnosed megacolon or psychogenic problems. Institutionalized patients, especially those of geriatric age, are prone to the development of fecal impactions.

The symptoms of fecal impaction usually consist of vague rectal fullness and nonspecific abdominal discomfort. A common complaint is overflow diarrhea, the uncontrolled passage of small amounts of watery and semiformed stool around a large obstructing impaction. In elderly, bedridden patients, it is essential that this overflow phenomenon be recognized as secondary to fecal impaction rather than perceived as true diarrhea.

Plain radiographs of the pelvis are usually diagnostic of fecal impaction (Fig. 50-41). Typically, there is a soft-tissue density in the rectum containing multiple small, irregular lucent areas that reflect pockets of gas within the fecal mass. Barium studies demonstrate a large, irregular intraluminal mass.

Fig. 50-41. Fecal impaction. This large rectal mass has multiple irregular lucent areas reflecting pockets of gas within the fecal mass.

ENDOMETRIOSIS

Endometriosis is the presence of heterotopic foci of endometrium in an extrauterine location. Although tissues in proximity to the uterus

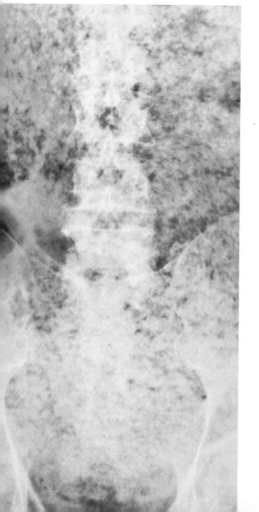

Fig. 50-42. Endometriosis. A polypoid filling defect demonstrated in the proximal sigmoid colon **(arrow)** illustrates the intact mucosa and submucosal appearance characteristic of endometroisis. (Spjut HJ, Perkins DE: Endometroisis of the sigmoid colon and rectum. AJR 82:1070–1075, 1959. Copyright 1959. Reproduced by permission)

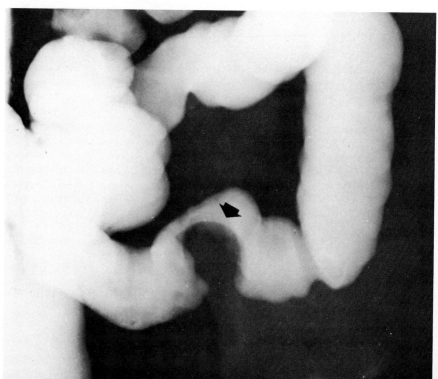

(ovaries, uterine ligaments, rectovaginal septum, pelvic peritoneum) are most frequently involved in endometriosis, the colon and even the small bowel can be affected.

Endometriosis primarily involves those parts of the bowel that are situated in the pelvis (Fig. 50-42). In most instances, the rectosigmoid colon is affected, though endometrial implants can be found in the appendix, cecum, ileum, and even jejunum. The heterotopic endometrium initially invades the subserosal layer of the bowel. Under hormonal influence, the surface epithelium matures and finally sloughs, resulting in bleeding similar to that which occurs in endometriosis in the uterine cavity. If bleeding occurs in an enclosed cystic area, expansion of the lesion can cause necrosis of adjacent tissues. Cyclic repetition of this process causes dissection through the subserosal and muscular layers to the submucosa. Because the spread of endometriosis rarely involves the mucosa, cyclic bleeding into the intestinal lumen is uncommon.

Endometriosis is usually clinically apparent only when ovarian function is active. Although symptoms have been reported in teenagers and even in postmenopausal females, most women who are symptomatic from endometriosis are between 20 and 45 years of age. The typical gastrointestinal complaint is abdominal cramps and diarrhea during the menstrual period. Each exacerbation of disease provokes hyperplasia of smooth muscle and fibrous stroma, which, if sufficiently extensive, can narrow the lumen and cause symptoms of partial colonic or small bowel obstruction. On rare occasions, hemoperitoneum arising from eroded or ruptured endometrial implants can cause acute, intense abdominal pain.

An isolated endometrioma typically presents as an intramural defect involving the sigmoid colon (Fig. 50-43). There can be pleating of the adjacent mucosa due to secondary fibrosis. The sharply defined, eccentric defect simulates a flat saddle cancer. In contrast to the mucosa in primary colonic malignancy, the mucosal pattern underlying and adjacent to an endometrioma usually remains intact.

Endometriosis can also present as a constricting lesion simulating annular carcinoma. Radiographic findings favoring endometriosis are an intact mucosa, a long lesion with tapered margins, and the absence of ulceration within the mass. Repeated shedding of endometrial tissue and blood into the peritoneal cavity can lead to the development of dense adhesive bands causing extrinsic obstruction of the bowel.

INTUSSUSCEPTION

Intussusception, the telescoping of a segment of bowel into the lumen of a contiguous distal portion, produces an intraluminal filling defect that is often associated with intestinal obstruction and vascular compromise. Most intussusceptions occur in children under the age of 2 and consist of invagination of the ileum into the colon (ileocolic intussusception). Colocolic intussusceptions are much less common. In children, a specific cause of intussusception is infrequently demonstrated; the process is most likely a functional disturbance of bowel

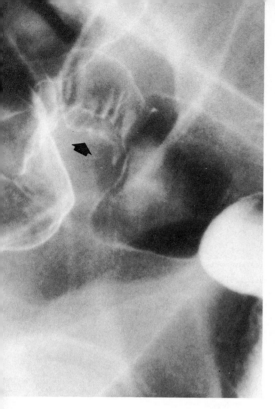

Fig. 50-43. Endometriosis. There is an intramural mass in the proximal sigmoid near the rectosigmoid junction **(arrow)**. The sharply defined, eccentric defect simulates a flat saddle cancer. Pleating of the adjacent mucosa is due to secondary fibrosis.

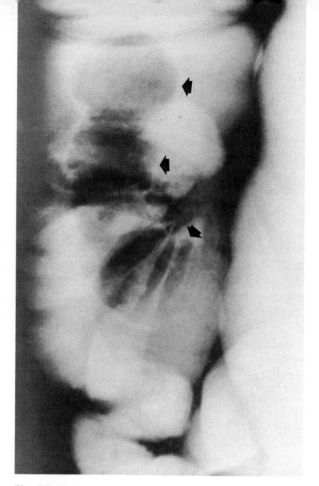

Fig. 50-44. Large polypoid carcinoma intussuscepting into the ascending colon **(arrows)**.

motility resulting from an increased deposition of fat and lymphoid tissue within the bowel. In older children and adults, however, a specific causative lesion can be demonstrated in more than half of all intussusceptions. Common leading points of intussusception are Meckel's diverticula, Peyer's patches, lymphoma, large mesenteric nodes, duplications, and polyps (Fig. 50-44).

Patients with intussusception typically present with recurrent crampy abdominal pain and vomiting. A palpable mass and thick, bloody stools ("currant-jelly" stools) are not uncommon.

Plain abdominal radiographs can reveal a soft-tissue mass with gas in the distal colon outlining the intussuscepting bowel (Fig. 50-45A). A proximal obstructive pattern can often be demonstrated. On barium enema examination, contrast flows in a retrograde fashion through the colon until it reaches the leading point of the intussusception, where it may stop abruptly and produce a concave configuration about the edge of the mass (Fig. 50-45B). Streaks of barium can extend around the mass in a spiral, ringlike fashion to produce a characteristic coiled-spring appearance (Fig. 50-46A). Many intussusceptions can be reduced

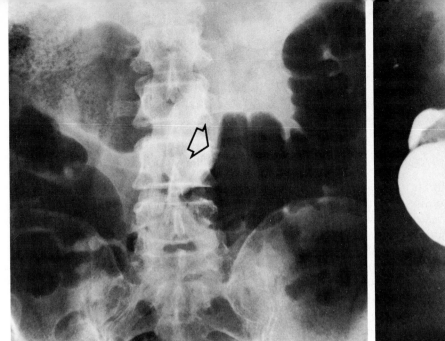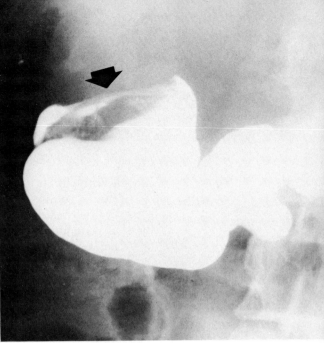

A B

Fig. 50-45. Intussusception. **(A)** A plain abdominal radiograph demonstrates a soft-tissue mass **(arrow)** with gas in the distal colon outlining the intussuscepted bowel. **(B)** Barium enema examination demonstrates obstruction at the level of the intussusception **(arrow)**.

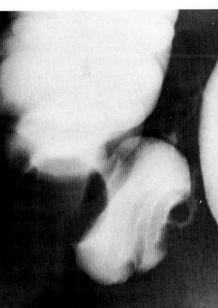

Fig. 50-46. Intussusception. **(A)** Obstruction of the colon at the hepatic flexure. The intussuscepted bowel has a characteristic coiled-spring appearance. **(B)** Partial and **(C)** complete reduction of the intussusception by careful barium enema examination.

B
A C

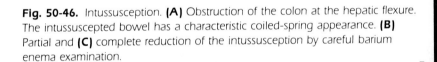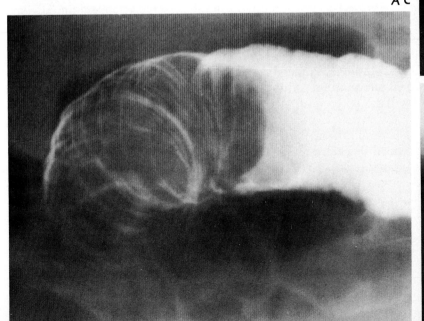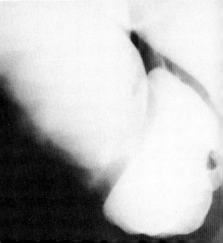

by increased hydrostatic pressure of a barium enema examination (Fig. 50-46*B, C*). In older children and adults, it is recommended that the radiologist carry out a repeat barium enema after reduction to search for a specific etiology for the intussusception.

FOREIGN BODY

Rarely, foreign bodies produce intraluminal filling defects in the colon. Round, undigestable material that reaches the colon from above generally passes without difficulty. Sharp objects (pins, needles, nails) occasionally perforate the rectum at sites of vigorous perstalsis and narrowed lumen caliber. However, even these foreign bodies usually pass without difficulty, presumably because they are coated by semisolid stool and thus are unable to lacerate the bowel wall.

A varied array of foreign bodies have been inserted into the colon from below, usually in homosexuals seeking sexual gratification. These foreign bodies are generally radiopaque and present no diagnostic difficulty (Fig. 50-47). However, foreign bodies inserted into the rectum from below have a higher likelihood of causing perforation or obstruction.

GALLSTONE

On rare occasions, gallstones that have entered the bowel by way of cholecystoduodenal fistulas pass through the terminal ileum and become trapped within the distal sigmoid colon, where they must be differentiated from polypoid filling defects. Rare cases of gallstones lodged in the colon have been reported in patients with fistulas between the gallbladder and the colon and in patients with fistulas between the proximal small bowel and colon that bypass the ileocecal valve.

Fig. 50-47. Vibrator in the rectum.

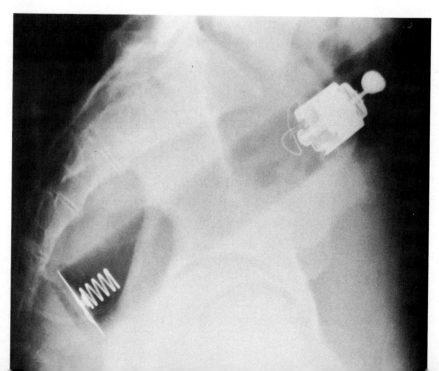

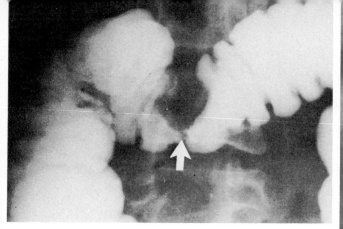

A B

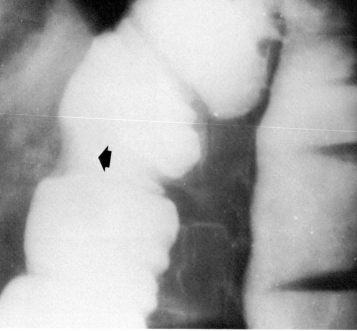

Fig. 50-48. Colonic pseudotumors due to adhesions. Examples of filling defects **(arrows)** in the **(A)** proximal and **(B)** distal portions of the transverse colon. (Kyaw MM, Koehler PR: Pseudotumors of the colon due to adhesions. Radiology 103:597–599, 1972)

PSEUDOTUMORS

Intraluminal or intramural polypoid masses in the colon that closely simulate primary or metastatic tumors can be due to pseudotumors caused by adhesions or fibrous bands (Fig. 50-48). In most patients, these fibrous bands are secondary to previous abdominal surgery. Less frequently, they are the result of changes in the appendices epiploicae secondary to ischemia or to an inflammatory process arising in the bowel wall or adjacent organs. Pseudotumors are usually located in the transverse or sigmoid colon (the distribution of appendices epiploicae) and have an intact mucosa overlying the intraluminal or intramural mass. Nevertheless, these tumorlike lesions may be indistinguishable from colonic neoplasms and require surgical intervention. Another pseudotumor that can be mistaken for a true colonic filling defect is the fortuitous superimposition of a sacral foramen over the rectosigmoid lumen (Fig. 50-49).

OTHER CAUSES OF FILLING DEFECTS

Rarely, a localized collection of amyloid appears as a filling defect in the rectum (Fig. 50-50). Edematous granulation tissue can develop following surgery and present as a distinct mass at the anastomotic site (Fig. 50-51). However, unlike a true neoplastic process, these suture granulomas eventually resolve and disappear. Although usually multiple, colitis cystica profunda can present as a single filling defect mimicking a neoplasm (Fig. 50-52).

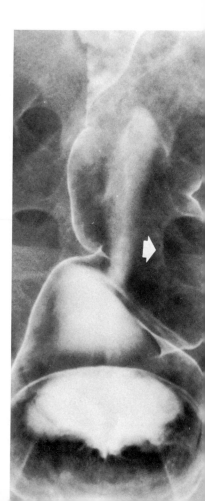

Fig. 50-49. Colonic pseudotumor **(arrow)** due to fortuitous superimposition of a sacral foramen over the rectosigmoid lumen.

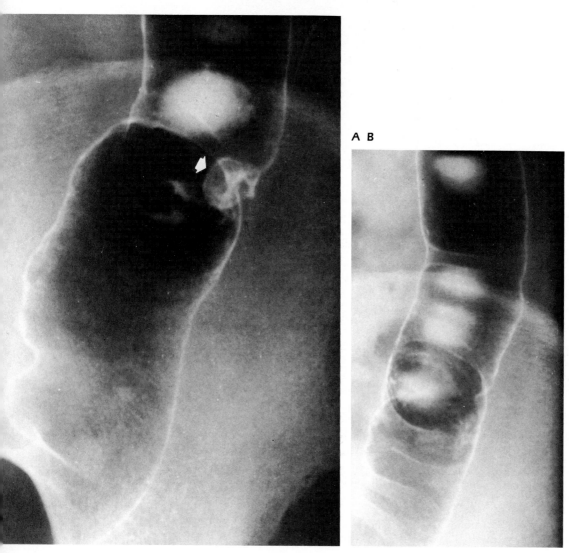

Fig. 50-50. Rectal amyloid presenting as a localized filling defect **(arrow)**.

A B

Fig. 50-51. Suture granuloma simulating recurrent carcinoma. **(A)** Barium enema examination 5 months after resection of a well-differentiated adenocarcinoma clearly shows the mass **(arrow)** at the anastomotic site. **(B)** Repeat examination 2½ years after surgery shows an entirely normal colon. (Shauffer IA, Sequeira J: Suture granuloma simulating recurrent carcinoma. AJR 128:856–857, 1977. Copyright 1977. Reproduced by permission)

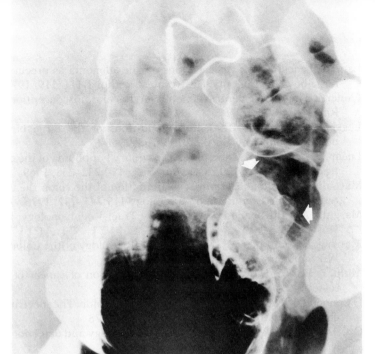

Fig. 50-52. Colitis cystica profunda. A single filling defect **(arrows)** simulates a neoplasm.

BIBLIOGRAPHY

Balthazar EJ, Bryk D: Segmental tuberculosis of the distal colon: Radiographic features in seven cases. Gastrointest Radiol 5:75–80, 1980

Berk RN, Lasser EC: Radiology of the Ileocecal Area. Philadelphia, WB Saunders, 1975

Bernstein JR, Ghahremani GG, Paige ML et al: Localized giant pseudopolyposis of the colon in ulcerative and granulomatous colitis. Gastrointest Radiol 3:431–435, 1978

Brodey PA, Hill RP, Baron S: Benign ulceration of the cecum. Radiology 122:323–327, 1977

Delamarre J, Descombes P, Marti R et al: Villous tumors of the colon and rectum: Double-contrast study of 47 cases. Gastrointest Radiol 5:69–73, 1980

Dreyfuss JR, Benacerraf B: Saddle cancers of the colon and their progression to annular carcinomas. Radiology 129:289–293, 1978

Dreyfuss JR, Janower ML: Radiology of the Colon. Baltimore, Williams & Wilkins, 1980

Grinnel RS, Lane N: Benign and malignant adenomatous polyps and papillary adenomas of the colon and rectum. An analysis of 1,856 tumors in 1,335 patients. Int Abstr Surg 106:519–538, 1958

Joffe N, Antonioli DA, Bettmann MA et al: Focal granulomatous (Crohn's) colitis. Radiologic–pathologic correlation. Gastrointest Radiol 3:73–80, 1978

Jones B, Abbruzzese AA: Obstructing giant pseudopolyps in granulomatous colitis. Gastrointest Radiol 3:437–438, 1978

Kyaw MM, Koehler PR: Pseudotumors of colon due to adhesions. Radiology 103:597–599, 1972

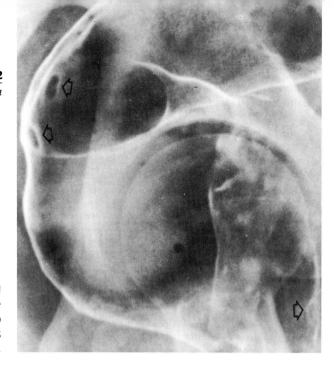

Fig. 51-1. Multiple small adenomatous polyps of the colon **(arrows).** There was no recognized polyposis syndrome.

MULTIPLE ADENOMATOUS POLYPS

Multiple adenomatous polyps of the colon can occur as an isolated event without a recognized polyposis syndrome (Fig. 51-1). In the Malmo series of more than 3000 double-contrast enemas, 12.5% of patients had radiographically demonstrated polyps in the colon. Among those patients with polyps, 24% had multiple polyps (17% had 2 polyps [Fig. 51-2], and 7% had 3 or more polyps [Fig. 51-3]). According to these statistics, therefore, multiple polyps should be expected in about 3% of barium enema examinations.

INTESTINAL POLYPOSIS SYNDROMES

The intestinal polyposis syndromes are a diverse group of conditions that differ widely in the histology of the polyps, the incidence of extracolonic polyps, extra-abdominal manifestations, and the potential for developing malignant disease. An intestinal polyposis disorder should be suspected when a polyp is demonstrated in a young person, when multiple polyps are found in any person, or when carcinoma of the colon is found in a patient under 40 years of age. In these situations, extraintestinal manifestations of the polyposis syndromes should be carefully sought. If one of the hereditary forms of intestinal polyposis is diagnosed, the patient's immediate family should be studied so that a potentially fatal disease is not missed in its premalignant stage.

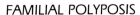

FAMILIAL POLYPOSIS

Familial polyposis is an inherited disease (autosomal dominant) with multiple adenomatous polyps almost exclusively limited to the colon and rectum (Fig. 51-4). Scattered cases of associated adenomas of the stomach and duodenum have also been reported. Small polypoid lesions similar to colonic polyps can be present in the terminal ileum, but these are histologically lymphoid hyperplasia rather than true polyps.

The colonic polyps in this syndrome are not present at birth and tend to arise around puberty. Clinical symptoms, which usually do not

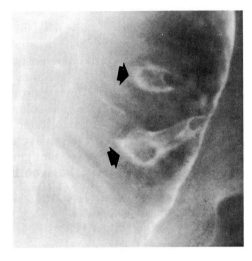

Fig. 51-2. Two benign adenomatous polyps **(arrows).**

Fig. 51-3. Three benign adenomatous polyps **(arrows).**

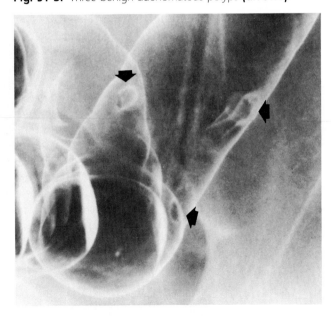

Fi
pc

subt
assu
prod
the
cole
min
to n

GAf

Gard
whic
and
deve
bari

defo
pror
the
the
inclu
towa

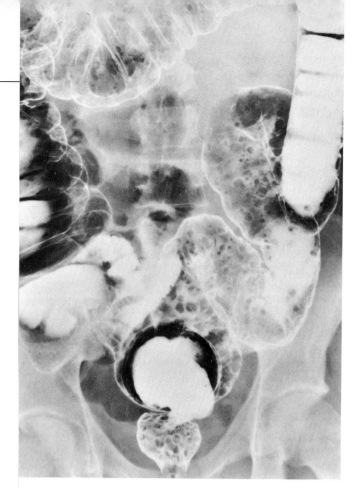

Fig. 51-8. Gardner's syndrome. Innumerable adenomatous polyps throughout the colon present a radiographic appearance indistinguishable from familial polyposis.

Fig. 51-9. Gardner's syndrome. An osteoma **(arrow)** is present in the frontal sinus.

Fig. 51-

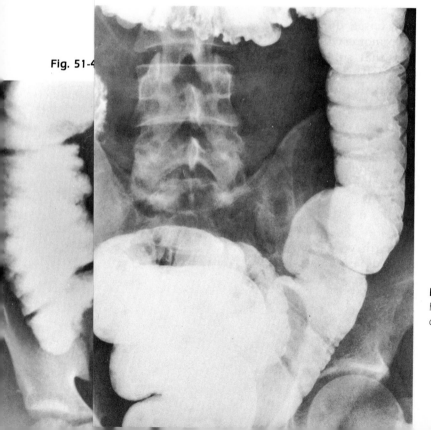

Fig. 51-10. Peutz–Jeghers syndrome. Multiple colonic hamartomas are evident in this patient, who also demonstrated abnormal mucocutaneous pigmentation.

Soft-tissue lesions associated with Gardner's syndrome include sebaceous cysts of the face, scalp, and back, as well as subcutaneous fibromas, leiomyomas, and lipomas. These fibrous tumors tend to progress in number and size regardless of whether colonic polyps are present or the colon has been resected. The fibrous tissue in patients with Gardner's syndrome also has a marked tendency to proliferate, resulting in dense scars or keloids after surgery. In the abdomen, this excessive fibrosis can produce adhesions that may even cause small bowel obstruction.

The distribution and appearance of the adenomatous polyps in Gardner's syndrome are indistinguishable from the pattern in familial polyposis. The polyps are almost always limited to the colon and rectum; extracolonic polyps occasionally occur in the small bowel and stomach. Like patients with familial polyposis, patients with Gardner's syndrome have almost a 100% risk of developing carcinoma of the colon or rectum. Therefore, total colectomy is recommended. In addition, patients with Gardner's syndrome appear to have a predilection toward small bowel malignancies, particularly in the pancreaticoduodenal region.

PEUTZ–JEGHERS SYNDROME

Peutz–Jeghers syndrome is an inherited disorder (autosomal dominant) in which multiple gastrointestinal polyposis is associated with mucocutaneous pigmentation (Fig. 51-10). The syndrome usually develops during childhood or adolescence. The excessive melanin deposits characteristic of Peutz–Jeghers syndrome are flat and small (1–5 mm in size) and occur predominantly on the lips and buccal mucosa. They can also be seen on the face, abdomen, genitalia, hands, and feet. The most common clinical symptom is intermittent colicky pain caused by small bowel intussusception led by one of the polyps. Rectal bleeding or melena is not infrequent, though massive gastrointestinal bleeding is rare.

The polyps in Peutz–Jeghers syndrome are hamartomas, masses of cell types normally present in the bowel, but mixed in abnormal proportions. The polyps are primarily found in the small bowel (especially the jejunum and ileum) but can also occur in the stomach, colon, and rectum. The polypoid lesions in Peutz–Jeghers syndrome are benign and apparently do not undergo malignant transformation. However, about 2% to 3% of patients with the disease develop adenocarcinomas of the intestinal tract (most commonly in the stomach, duodenum, and colon), and 5% of women with the syndrome have ovarian cysts or tumors.

DISSEMINATED GASTROINTESTINAL POLYPOSIS

Disseminated gastrointestinal polyposis refers to a condition in which multiple adenomatous polyps involve the stomach or small bowel as well as the colon, but in which the extraintestinal stigmata of the Gardner's or Peutz–Jeghers syndrome are absent. This very rare condition, which has an extremely high risk of gastrointestinal carcinoma, may be a variant of familial polyposis rather than a discrete clinical entity.

TURCOT SYNDROME

Turcot syndrome (glioma–polyposis syndrome) is the association of multiple colonic adenomatous polyps with malignant tumors of the central nervous system (Fig. 51-11). Patients with this extremely rare syndrome usually present in the second decade of life with neurologic complaints caused by a brain tumor (usually supratentorial glioblastoma) or diarrhea due to colonic polyposis. Because neither brain tumors nor colonic polyps have been noted in the parents of afflicted patients, it seems likely that the disorder is inherited as an autosomal recessive. An increased incidence of colorectal carcinoma has been reported in patients with Turcot syndrome. However, the precise malignant potential of the colonic polyps is unknown, since most patients with this syndrome have died of central nervous system tumors at a very young age.

JUVENILE POLYPOSIS SYNDROMES

There are three rare, but distinct, syndromes associated with juvenile polyps of the colon. These polyps are hamartomatous lesions that are sometimes referred to as retention or inflammatory polyps. Although almost always found in children, juvenile polyps are occasionally first detected in adults. *Juvenile polyposis coli* is probably an inherited disorder in which multiple hamartomatous polypoid lesions can be associated with a variety of congenital anomalies. Juvenile polyps can involve the stomach and small bowel as well as the colon, and if this occurs without any extraintestinal manifestations, it is termed *generalized gastrointestinal juvenile polyposis*. If there is associated hyperpigmentation, alopecia, and atrophy and subsequent loss of fingernails and toenails, the condition is called the *Cronkhite–Canada syndrome*

Fig. 51-11. Turcot syndrome. Multiple colonic adenomatous polyps were found in this young patient, who died of a malignant glioma.

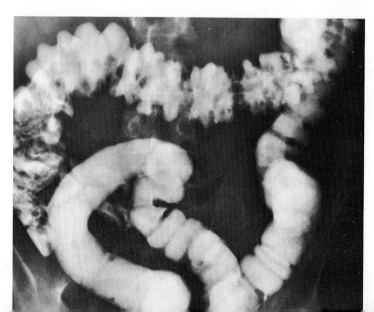

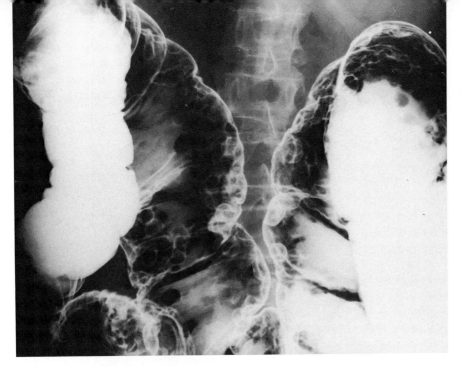

Fig. 51-12. Cronkhite–Canada syndrome. Multiple polypoid lesions simulate familial polyposis. (Dodds WJ: Clinical and roentgen features of the intestinal polyposis syndromes. Gastrointest Radiol 1:127–142, 1976)

(Fig. 51-12). The latter disorder presents much later in life than other intestinal polyposis syndromes (average age of onset, over 50) and may be accompanied by malabsorption and severe diarrhea resulting in substantial electrolyte and protein loss (Fig. 51-13). Although spontaneous remissions occur, the disease is usually relentlessly progressive (especially in women) and leads to death within 1 year of diagnosis.

The hamartomatous (inflammatory) juvenile polyps are not premalignant in any of these three diseases. Several instances of gastrointestinal carcinoma have been described in patients with generalized gastrointestinal juvenile polyposis and the Cronkhite–Canada syndrome, but these may represent merely chance occurrences.

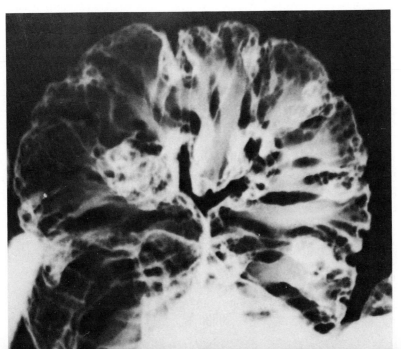

Fig. 51-13. Cronkhite–Canada syndrome. This coned view of the sigmoid colon demonstrates multiple small polyps in a 55-year-old man. (Koehler PR, Kyaw MM, Fenlon JW: Diffuse gastrointestinal polyposis with ectodermal changes: Cronkhite–Canada syndrome. Radiology 103:589–594, 1972)

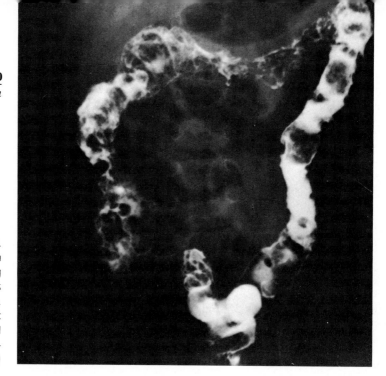

Fig. 51-14. *Juvenile polyposis. A postevacuation radiograph demonstrates many filling defects of various sizes throughout the colon. (Schwartz AM, McCauley RGK: Juvenile gastrointestinal polyposis. Radiology 121:441–444, 1976)*

MULTIPLE JUVENILE POLYPS

The presence of one or more juvenile polyps in the colon of a young child (2–5 years of age) is not uncommon without an inherited disorder and with no evidence of extraintestinal manifestations or associated intestinal malignancy (Fig. 51-14). These juvenile polyps have a smooth, round contour and contain multiple mucin-filled cysts and an abundant connective tissue stroma. Hemorrhage and ulceration are common, leading to symptoms of rectal bleeding, mucus discharge, diarrhea, and, occasionally, abdominal pain. Juvenile polyps are almost always

Fig. 51-15. *Multiple synchronous carcinomas of the colon.* **(A)** *Carcinomas of the ascending and transverse portions of the colon* **(arrows). (B)** *Carcinoma* **(arrows)** *within a tortuous descending colon.*

A B

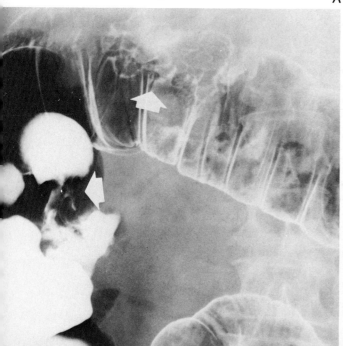

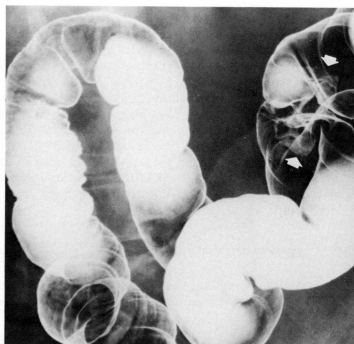

solitary, though multiple polyps (rarely more than a few) do occur. The polyps are benign, have no malignant potential, and tend to autoamputate or regress. Therefore, surgical removal of juvenile polyps is indicated only if there are significant or repeated episodes of rectal bleeding or intussusception.

MULTIPLE ADENOCARCINOMAS

A patient with carcinoma of the colon has a 1% risk of having multiple synchronous colon cancers, which can produce the radiographic pattern of multiple filling defects in the colon (Fig. 51-15). In addition, such a patient has a 3% risk of developing additional metachronous cancers at a later date. Colon carcinomas can also coexist with benign adenomatous polyps (of which there was a 20% incidence in the Malmo series), again presenting the radiographic appearance of multiple colonic filling defects.

METASTASES

Hematogenous metastases to the colon can produce multiple filling defects. Major primary sites include the breast, lung, stomach, ovary, pancreas, and uterus, as well as other primary locations in the colon. Although the colon is the least common site for gastrointestinal metastases from melanoma, single or multiple colonic metastases can represent the initial manifestation of malignant melanoma and can occur without a clinically obvious primary lesion (Fig. 51-16). In addition to discrete masses that mimic intramural, extramucosal tumors, metastases to the colon can also produce thickening of the colon wall, diffuse nodularity, and mesenteric involvement leading to a fibrotic reaction with fixation and acute angulation of the bowel.

LYMPHOMA

Although the gastrointestinal tract is the most common location of primary extranodal lymphoma, the colon is the segment of gut that is least often affected. Lymphoma of the colon can appear as a single (rarely multiple), relatively large lesion or as an extensive infiltrating tumor that extends over long segments of bowel. Diffuse thickening of folds can present as multiple irregular filling defects (Fig. 51-17) that are either scattered throughout the colon or limited to a short segment. Even in one patient, these nodular lesions can vary widely in size and shape in different parts of the colon. Simultaneous extensive involvement of the ileum is not uncommon in lymphoma, in contrast to familial polyposis.

LEUKEMIC INFILTRATION

Leukemic infiltration of the gastrointestinal tract, even when extensive, is usually asymptomatic. Reported clinical complaints range from

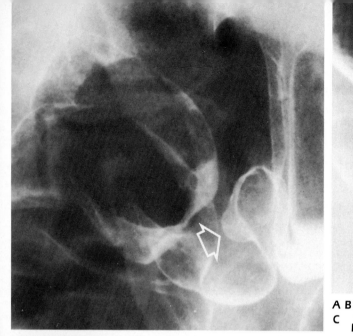

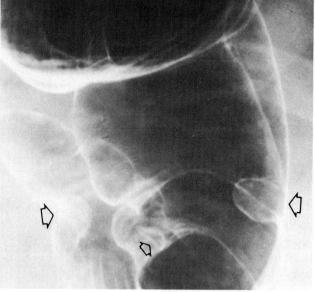

A B
C

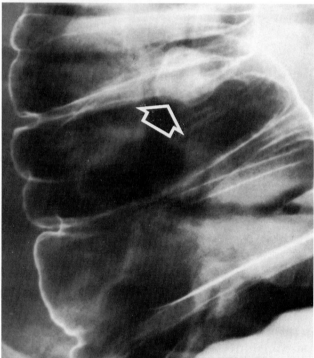

Fig. 51-16. Melanoma metastatic to the colon. **(A)** Double-contrast view of the hepatic flexure showing a single sessile polyp **(arrow)**. **(B)** View of the splenic flexure showing at least three sessile polyps **(arrows)**. **(C)** View of the ascending colon showing a sessile polyp **(arrow)**. (Sacks, BA, Jaffe N, Antonioli DA: Metastatic melanoma presenting clinically as multiple colonic polyps. AJR 129:511–513, 1977. Copyright 1977. Reproduced by permission)

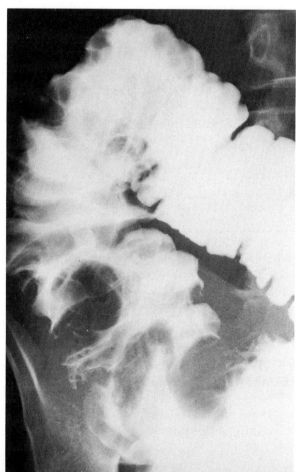

Fig. 51-17. Lymphoma of the colon presenting as multiple irregular nodular filling defects.

nonspecific nausea, mild abdominal pain, and diarrhea to severe necrotizing enterocolitis, bowel hemorrhage, and perforation. In lymphocytic lymphoma, involvement is usually confined to the mucosa and submucosa and can produce a radiographic pattern of diffuse interlacing filling defects in the colon. In myelogenous leukemia, the infiltrate can cause localized or diffuse plaques, nodules, or masses. In addition to colonic lesions, leukemic infiltration can present as intraluminal defects in the esophagus or as an infiltrative process in the stomach that may be indistinguishable from carcinoma.

MULTIPLE SPINDLE CELL TUMORS

Colonic neurofibromatosis associated with von Recklinghausen's disease can produce multiple diffuse intraluminal and intramural defects. These masses, which tend to be larger than the defects seen in the hereditary intestinal polyposis syndromes, are usually detected in patients with characteristic skin lesions.

Colonic lipomatosis can present as multiple filling defects in the colon (Fig. 51-18). This rare lesion can be segmental or diffuse and tends to primarily involve the right colon.

Hemangiomas are a rare cause of multiple intraluminal and intramural filling defects in the colon. The correct diagnosis requires demonstration of characteristic phleboliths associated with the lesions.

MULTIPLE HAMARTOMA SYNDROME (COWDEN'S DISEASE)

The multiple hamartoma syndrome (Cowden's disease) is a rare hereditary disorder associated with multiple malformations, tumors, and various involvement of different organs. The most characteristic clinical features are circumoral papillomatosis and nodular gingival hyperplasia. Several patients with this disorder have demonstrated single or multiple polyps of varied morphology along the gastrointestinal tract (Fig. 51-19). Although there is no convincing evidence of a predisposition to colonic malignancy, the multiple hamartoma syndrome does appear to be associated with an increased incidence of malignant tumors of the thyroid and breast.

INFLAMMATORY PSEUDOPOLYPOSIS

ULCERATIVE AND CROHN'S COLITIS

Pseudopolyps are islands of hyperplastic, inflamed mucosa that remain between areas of ulceration in inflammatory bowel disease (Fig. 51-20). They vary in size, shape, and pattern in relation to the degree and position of the ulceration and the inflammatory response of the bowel. In contrast to the otherwise normal appearance of the bowel in familial polyposis, pseudopolyps in ulcerative and Crohn's colitis are usually associated with radiographic evidence of an inflammatory process

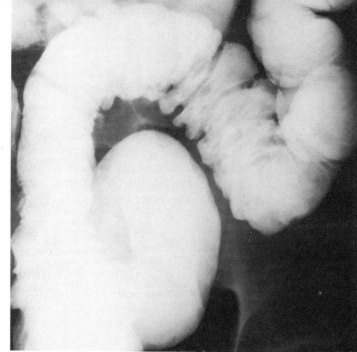

Fig. 51-18. Segmental polypoid lipomatosis presenting as multiple filling defects in the sigmoid colon. (Danoff DM, Nisenbaum HL, Stewart WB et al: Segmental polypoid lipomatosis of the colon. AJR 128:858–860, 1977. Copyright 1977. Reproduced by permission)

Fig. 51-19. Cowden's disease (multiple hamartoma syndrome). Numerous round, sessile polyps are spread over the entire rectum. (Hauser H, Ody B, Plojoux O et al: Radiological findings in multiple hamartoma syndrome (Cowden's disease). Radiology 137:317–323, 1980)

Fig. 51-20. Pseudopolyposis in chronic ulcerative colitis. There was no evidence of acute ulceration.

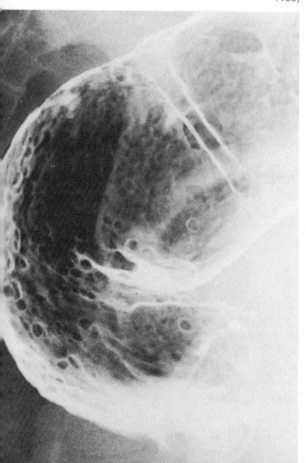

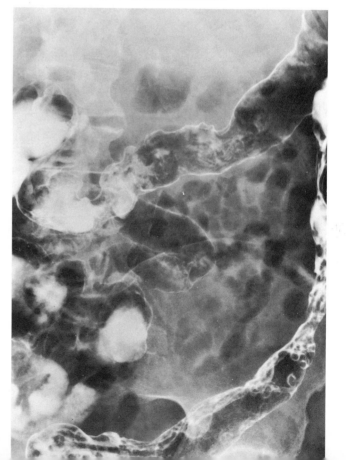

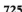
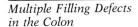

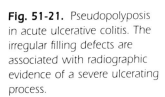

Fig. 51-21. Pseudopolyposis in acute ulcerative colitis. The irregular filling defects are associated with radiographic evidence of a severe ulcerating process.

Fig. 51-23. Pseudopolyposis in Crohn's colitis. The swollen and edematous mucosa surrounded by long, deep, linear ulcers and transverse fissures produces a coarsely nodular cobblestoning appearance.

(ulceration, absence or irregularity of haustral folds, narrowing of the lumen) and a history of chronic diarrhea (Fig. 51-21). However, in an occasional case of ulcerative colitis in which the inflammatory process has healed and the only residual radiographic abnormality is a large number of pseudopolyps, it can be impossible to distinguish this appearance from familial polyposis (Fig. 51-22).

The inflammatory pseudopolyps in ulcerative colitis are usually small and uniform in appearance, producing a somewhat nodular

Fig. 51-22. Pseudopolyposis in chronic ulcerative colitis. If there is no radiographic evidence of inflammatory disease, the pattern is indistinguishable from familial polyposis.

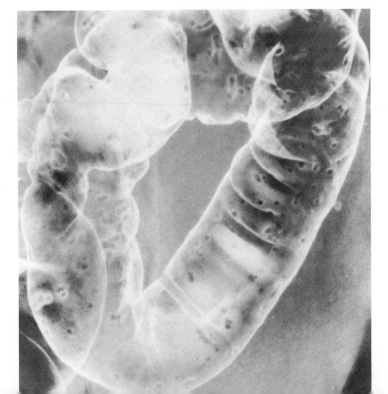

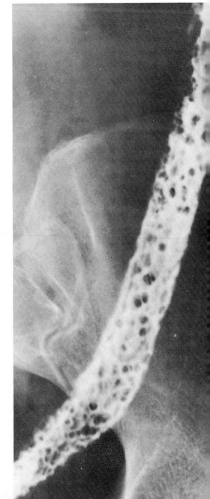

pattern. On rare occasions, however, the mucosa can undergo such extreme hyperplasia that the pseudopolyps appear as large masses simulating fungating polypoid tumors.

When Crohn's disease involves the colon, long, deep linear ulcers and transverse fissures surrounding swollen and edematous mucosa result in a coarsely nodular appearance (cobblestoning) (Fig. 51-23). These irregular pseudopolyps can produce the radiographic appearance of multiple filling defects, simulating the intestinal polyposis syndromes (Fig. 51-24). Patients with pseudopolyposis of the colon due to Crohn's disease usually have concomitant disease of the terminal ileum, unlike patients with ulcerative colitis, in whom ileal involvement is absent or minimal.

Filiform polyposis is a benign, nonspecific sequela of diffuse, severe mucosal inflammation that is seen in both ulcerative and Crohn's colitis. Filiform polyps usually appear as thin, straight filling defects resembling the stalks of polyps without the heads. In some cases, a radiating pattern of filling defects can be seen; in others, there is a branching pattern, particularly at the tip of the polyp (Fig. 51-25). These small lesions can be easily hidden if the barium column is underpenetrated; they can also be mistaken for mucus threads. In most cases, there is no radiologic evidence of acute colitis when filiform polyps are discovered; indeed, the finding of filiform polyposis may be the first clue to the presence of inflammatory bowel disease. Filiform polyps are not associated with the development of carcinoma and therefore should not be mistaken for a neoplastic polyposis syndrome.

Fig. 51-25. Filiform polyposis with a characteristic branching pattern.

Fig. 51-24. Pseudopolyposis in chronic Crohn's colitis. Multiple filling defects without radiographic evidence of inflammatory changes simulate familial polyposis.

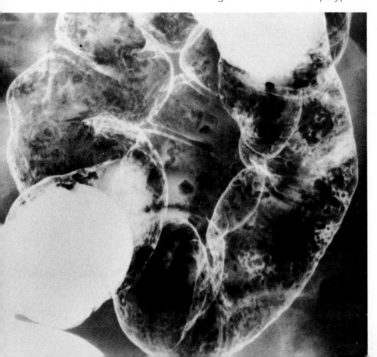

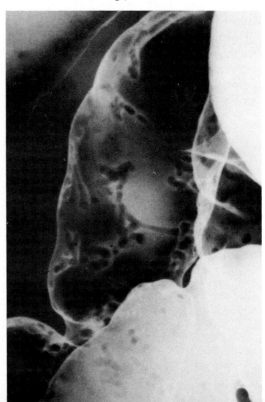

ISCHEMIC COLITIS

In an elderly patient with an acute onset of severe abdominal pain and rectal bleeding and no history of inflammatory bowel disease, diffuse pseudopolyposis should suggest the possibility of ischemic colitis (Fig. 51-26). The radiographic appearance can be indistinguishable from ulcerative or Crohn's colitis; often, only the clinical picture permits differentiation.

AMEBIASIS

The granulomatous reaction that occurs in areas of amebic infestation can produce large, hard masses (amebomas) that are fixed and tender to palpation and can appear as filling defects within the lumen of the bowel. Amebomas can occur anywhere in the colon, though they are most common in the cecum and, to a lesser degree, in the rectosigmoid. They are usually solitary but can be multiple. Amebic infection can also result in a pattern of pseudopolyposis simulating ulcerative colitis or Crohn's disease, giving the radiographic appearance of multiple filling defects in the colon (Fig. 51-27).

SCHISTOSOMIASIS

Schistosomiasis is an infectious disease caused by a blood fluke that inhabits the portal venous system in humans and certain animals. More than 100 million people are infected worldwide, especially in tropical and subtropical countries. After partially maturing in the body of a suitable snail host, the schistosoma organism emerges into the water and enters its human host by penetrating the unbroken skin or buccal membrane. Those larvae that make their way to the liver develop into adult worms, which can reside within the portal venous bed for 20 to 30 years. The mature worms then migrate against the flow of portal venous blood into the smaller venules of the inferior mesenteric vein, where the females deposit their eggs. Those ova that penetrate into the lumen of the bowel are passed from the body and continue the life cycle.

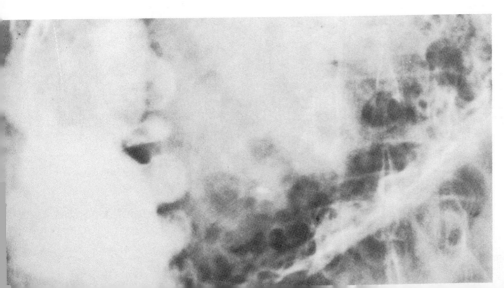

Fig. 51-26. Pseudopolyposis in ischemic colitis. Multiple filling defects are visible along the lower margin of the transverse colon. The diagnosis was suggested by the clinical presentation of acute, severe abdominal pain and rectal bleeding in a patient with no history of inflammatory bowel disease.

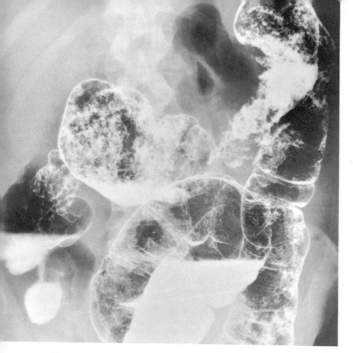

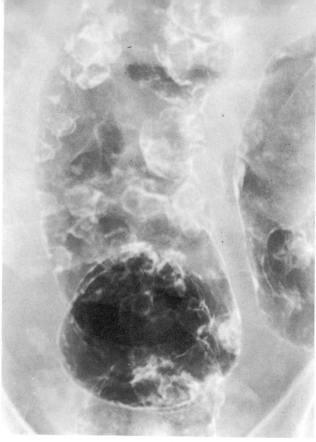

Fig. 51-27. Amebic colitis. Multiple pseudopolyps produce a pattern identical to ulcerative or Crohn's colitis.

Fig. 51-28. Schistosomiasis. Multiple filling defects represent polypoid granulomas.

The irritative effect of the ova that pass through or lodge in the bowel wall stimulates an inflammatory response with granuloma formation and progressive fibrosis. Because the adult worm has a predilection for entering the inferior mesenteric vein, the sigmoid colon is most commonly involved. In severe infestation, the proximal colon can also be affected. The most characteristic radiographic appearance in schistosomiasis is multiple filling defects (usually 1–2 cm large) due to the development of polypoid granulomas (Fig. 51-28). These masses are friable and vascular, and they bleed easily with the passage of feces, which explains the frequently bloody stools associated with severe infestation. Other radiographic findings include ragged ulcerations and edema of the mucosa, as well as narrowing and areas of stricture formation due to reactive fibrosis.

STRONGYLOIDIASIS

Although strongyloidiasis primarily involves the duodenum and jejunum, diffuse colonic ulceration and pseudopolyposis simulating ulcerative or Crohn's colitis occasionally occur (Fig. 51-29). Pseudomembranous colitis can also produce a pattern of extensive hyperplastic pseudopolyposis (Fig. 51-30).

TRICHURIASIS

Trichuris trichiura (whipworm) is a ubiquitous parasite that is primarily found in warm, moist tropics. Humans become infested by ingesting whipworm ova from contaminated soil or vegetables. The ova hatch into larvae that migrate down to the cecum, where they develop into adult worms. Whipworms become attached to the colon and lie embedded between intestinal villi, coiled upon themselves with their blunt caudal portions projecting into the bowel lumen. Mild infections are usually asymptomatic, but heavy infestation, especially in children, can result in chronic diarrhea, abdominal pain, dehydration, weight loss, rectal prolapse, eosinophilia, and anemia.

The radiographic findings in trichuriasis are similar to the appearance in mucoviscidosis (cystic fibrosis) of the colon (Fig. 51-31). There is a diffuse granular mucosal pattern throughout the colon with considerable flocculation of barium due to abundant mucus secretions surrounding the tiny whipworms. In addition, multiple filling defects are produced by the individual outlines of the innumerable worms, which are attached to the mucosa with their posterior portions either tightly coiled or unfurled in a whiplike configuration.

ARTIFACTS

Although the material most commonly confused with polypoid tumors on barium enema examination is feces, the radiographic features of retained fecal material are usually distinctive and should pose no diagnostic problems (Fig. 51-32). A "fecaloma" is generally freely movable, though it occasionally adheres so firmly to the bowel mucosa that it resembles a broad-based polyp. Fecal material tends to be

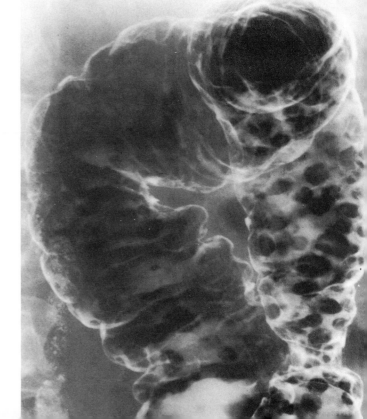

Fig. 51-30. Pseudomembranous colitis. Extensive hyperplastic pseudopolyposis produces a pattern of multiple colonic filling defects.

Fig. 51-29. Strongyloidiasis. Multiple hyperplastic pseudopolyps simulate ulcerative or Crohn's colitis.

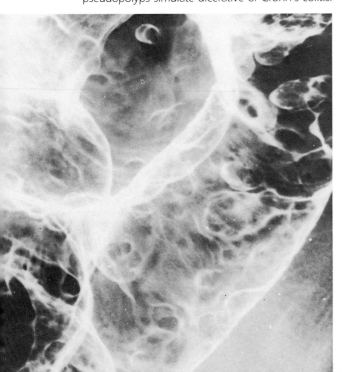

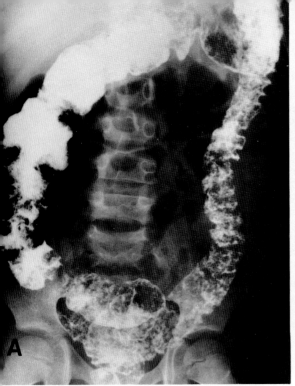

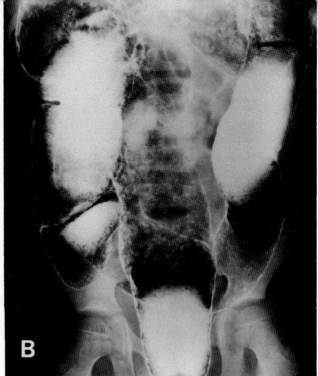

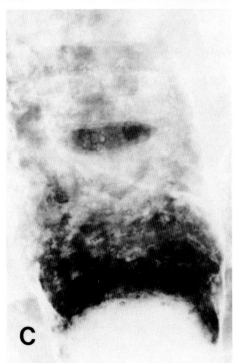

Fig. 51-31. Trichuriasis. **(A)** A postevacuation film from a routine barium enema examination shows flocculation of barium and poor mucosal coating, probably the result of excessive mucus secretions surrounding the numerous whipworms. **(B)** An air-contrast study demonstrates the radiolucent outlines of many small trichurids as they cling to the colon mucosa by their slender anterior ends. **(C)** A magnified view of the rectosigmoid colon from the same air-contrast barium enema shows the outline of many small whipworms attached to the mucosa, their posterior portions either tightly coiled (males) or unfurled in a semilunar or whiplike configuration (females). The composite picture suggests a target or pinwheel appearance of mucosal pattern. (Reeder MM, Palmer PES: The Radiology of Tropical Diseases. Baltimore, Williams & Wilkins, 1981)

irregular in shape, with an uneven barium coating; barium can usually be seen interposed between the fecal mass and the mucosa. The inability to demonstrate the point of attachment of a "polypoid mass" to the wall of the colon should suggest an intraluminal fecal mass rather than a discrete colonic lesion. Complications of fecalomas include ulceration, perforation, and obstruction.

Radiolucent air bubbles surrounded by thin, gradually fading barium margins can simulate multiple colonic filling defects. They frequently appear as several very small air bubbles clustered around a larger one. Oil bubbles from excessive castor oil or mineral oil used as a laxative in preparation for barium enema examination can produce a similar radiographic pattern.

Long, slender lucent strands within the barium column usually represent mucus. They are generally irregular branching defects, are often seen in association with retained fecal material, and are easily differentiated from pathologic lesions.

FOREIGN BODIES

Ingested foreign bodies, especially kernels of corn, can simulate multiple polyposis in the colon (Fig. 51-33). Intact corn kernels have thin outer coverings composed of cellulose that are not digested in the human gastrointestinal tract. These cellulose coverings are normally disrupted by mastication, which permits digestion of the corn by enzymes in the stomach and duodenum. However, in edentulous patients who chew poorly, corn kernels can be swallowed whole, remain undigested, and appear intact in the colon, where they mimic polyps.

MISCELLANEOUS DISORDERS

HEMORRHOIDS

Internal hemorrhoids can produce multiple rectal filling defects that simulate polyps (Fig. 51-34). In most cases, however, hemorrhoids are associated with the linear shadows of the veins from which they arise.

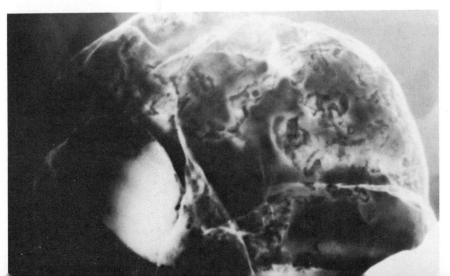

Fig. 51-32. Retained fecal material. There are multiple freely moving colonic filling defects.

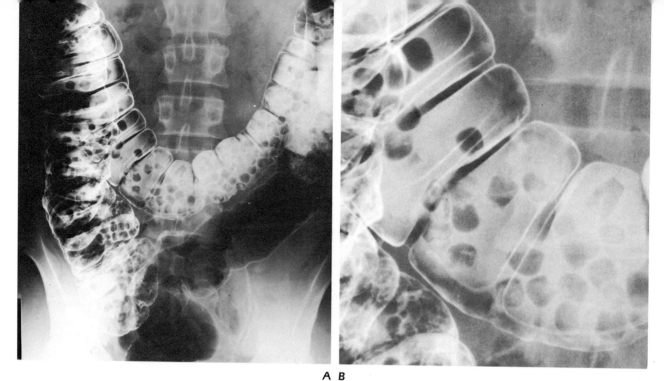

A B

Fig. 51-33. Ingested corn kernels simulating multiple polyposis in the colon. **(A)** Full and **(B)** coned views. (Press HC, Davis TW: Ingested foreign bodies simulating polyposis: Report of six cases. AJR 127:1040–1042, 1976. Copyright 1976. Reproduced by permission)

Fig. 51-34. Internal hemorrhoids. Multiple rectal filling defects **(arrows)** simulate polyps.

Fig. 51-35. Diverticula simulating colonic filling defects. Multiple barium-coated, air-filled diverticula superimposed on the lumen of the bowel mimic discrete colonic filling defects.

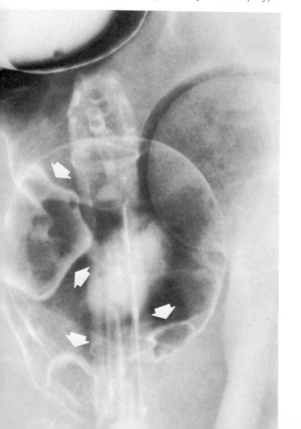

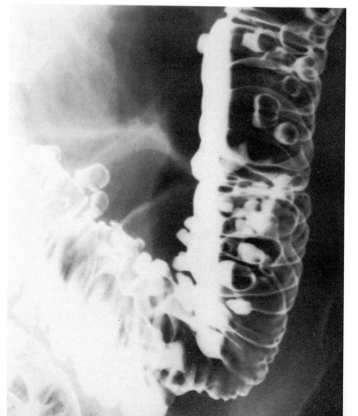

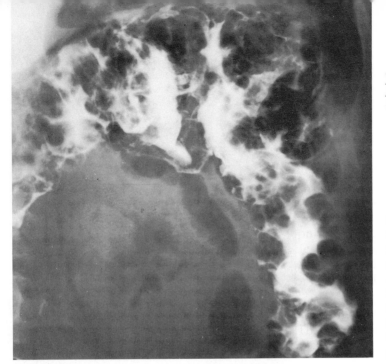

Fig. 51-36. Pneumatosis intestinalis in an asymptomatic person. The intramural collections of gas simulate multiple colonic filling defects. Note that the filling defects in this condition appear to be more radiolucent than the soft-tissue masses in the intestinal polyposis syndromes.

DIVERTICULA

Barium-coated, air-filled diverticula superimposed on the lumen of the bowel sometimes mimic multiple colonic filling defects (Fig. 51-35). However, close attention to the inner and outer borders of the filling defects may permit the distinction to be made between diverticula and polypoid tumors. The ring of barium coating a diverticulum has a smooth, well-defined outer border and a blurred, irregular inner border. Conversely, barium coating a polyp tends to be smooth on its inner border and poorly defined on its outer margin. It is usually necessary, however, to carefully evaluate multiple films in various obliquities to be certain that all of the "filling defects" can be projected clear of the colonic lumen and thus be seen to represent multiple diverticula.

PNEUMATOSIS INTESTINALIS

Intramural collections of gas can simulate multiple colonic filling defects. In contrast to true colonic polyps, the filling defects in pneumatosis intestinalis appear to be more radiolucent and to have broader bases (Fig. 51-36). When the abdomen is palpated, cysts of pneumatosis intestinalis are compressed, and the radiographic defects change shape.

COLITIS CYSTICA PROFUNDA

In colitis cystica profunda, large mucus epithelium-lined cysts up to 2 cm in diameter form in the submucosal layer of the colon. These submucosal cysts are most commonly seen in the pelvic colon and rectum. The disorder almost always involves a short segment of bowel; infrequently, the colon is diffusely affected. Although the pathogenesis of the disease is obscure, its frequent association with proctitis or colitis

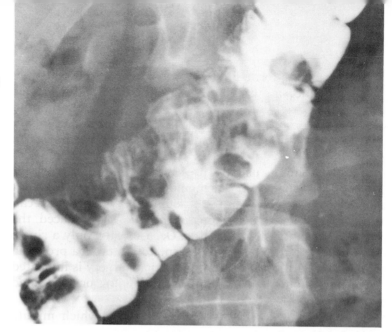

Fig. 51-40. Lymphoma presenting as multiple colonic filling defects. The nodules vary in size and are far larger than those seen in nodular lymphoid hyperplasia.

Fig. 51-41. Cystic fibrosis. These multiple, poorly defined filling defects are caused by residual thick secretions.

Fig. 51-42. Colonic urticaria. Large polygonal, raised plaques are visible in a dilated cecum and ascending colon.

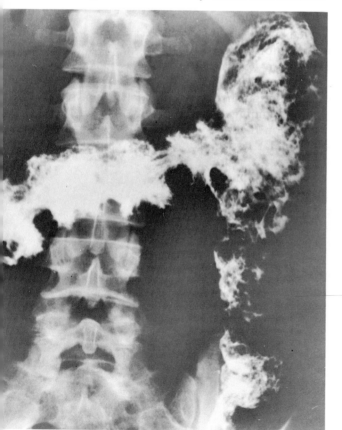

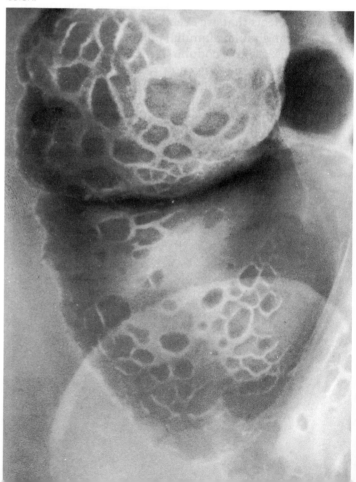

CYSTIC FIBROSIS

Cystic fibrosis in adolescents can produce a striking radiographic appearance of the colon. Because of adherent collections of viscid mucus, adequate cleansing prior to barium enema examination is rarely achieved. The residual thick secretions can cause multiple, poorly defined filling defects that give the colonic mucosa a hyperplastic appearance simulating polyposis (Fig. 51-41).

SUBMUCOSAL EDEMA PATTERN

A characteristic mucosal pattern of large, round or polygonal, raised plaques in a grossly dilated bowel (Fig. 51-42) was first described as an allergic reaction of the colonic mucosa to medication. This "colonic urticaria" predominantly involves the right colon, can be seen without concomitant cutaneous lesions, and regresses once the offending medication is withdrawn. A pattern similar to colonic urticaria has been reported in several other conditions for which the common denominator seems to be submucosal edema. In herpes zoster, an exanthematous neurocutaneous disorder secondary to reactivation or reinfection by a large pox virus, colonic mucosal blebs infrequently appear as multiple small, discrete, polygonal filling defects with sharp angular margins (Fig. 51-43). These blebs correspond morphologically and temporally to the vesicular phase of the cutaneous lesion and are segmentally arrayed in a corresponding or noncorresponding dermatome. A similar radiographic pattern has also been observed in patients with submucosal colonic edema secondary to obstructing carcinoma, cecal volvulus, ischemia, colonic ileus, and benign colonic obstruction.

Fig. 51-43. Herpes zoster. Polygonal filling defects with sharp angular margins are evident in two patients with this disease.

A   B

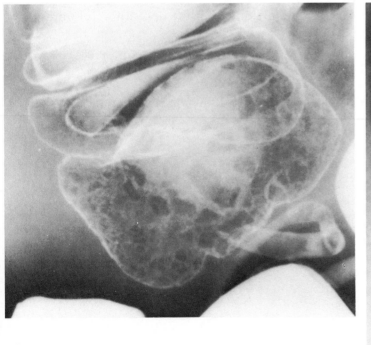

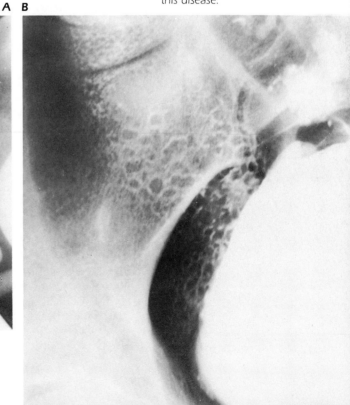

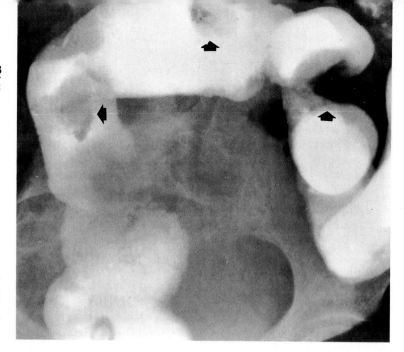

Fig. 51-44. *Amyloidosis. Multiple discrete filling defects* **(arrows)** *represent localized deposition of amyloid in the sigmoid colon.*

ULCERATIVE PSEUDOPOLYPS PROXIMAL TO AN OBSTRUCTION

Ulcerative disease has been described proximal to partial or complete obstruction of the lumen of the esophagus, stomach, small bowel, or colon. In all reported cases, the bowel was normal distal to the point of obstruction. The pathogenesis of ulcerative disease proximal to an obstructing bowel lesion appears to be a function of ischemia caused by distention of the bowel, with decreased blood flow through the vessels extending from the mesenteric border to the bowel wall. In the colon, this process often presents radiographically as prominent nodularity with pseudopolyp formation simulating the appearance of an ulcerating colitis.

AMYLOIDOSIS

Rarely, extensive deposition of amyloid in the colon produces a pattern of multiple discrete filling defects (Fig. 51-44).

BIBLIOGRAPHY

Berk RN, Lasser EC: Radiology of the Ileocecal Area. Philadelphia, WB Saunders, 1975

Berk RN, Millman SJ: Urticaria of the colon. Radiology 99:539–540, 1971

Childress MH, Martel W: Fecaloma simulating colonic neoplasms. Surg Gynecol Obstet 142:664–666, 1976

Denzler TB, Harned RK, Pergam CJ: Gastric polyps in familial polyposis coli. Radiology 130:63–66, 1979

Dodds WJ: Clinical and roentgen features of intestinal polyposis syndromes. Gastrointest Radiol 1:127–142, 1976

Dolan KD, Seibert J, Seibert RW: Gardner's syndrome. AJR 119:359–364, 1973

Dreyfuss JR, Janower ML: Radiology of the Colon. Baltimore, Williams & Wilkins, 1980

El-Afifi S: Intestinal bilharziasis. Dis Colon Rectum 7:1–13, 1964

Godard JE, Dodds WJ, Phillips JC et al: Peutz–Jeghers syndrome: Clinical and roentgenographic features. AJR 113:316–324, 1971

Hauser H, Ody B, Plojoux O et al: Radiological findings in multiple hamartoma syndrome (Cowden disease). Radiology 137:317–323, 1980

Kagan AR, Steckel RJ: Colon polyposis and cancer. AJR 131:1065–1067, 1978

Kelvin FM, Max RJ, Norton GA et al: Lymphoid follicular pattern of the colon in adults. AJR 133:821–825, 1979

Khilnani MT, Marshak RH, Eliasoph J et al: Roentgen features of metastases of the colon. AJR 96:302–310, 1966

Klein MS, Sherlock P: Gastric and colonic metastases from breast cancer. Am J Dig Dis 17:881–886, 1972

Koehler PR, Kyaw MM, Fenlon JW: Diffuse gastrointestinal polyposis with ectodermal changes. Cronkhite–Canada syndrome. Radiology 103:589–594, 1972

Laufer I, de Sa D: Lymphoid follicular pattern: A normal feature of the pediatric colon AJR 130:51–55, 1978

Ledesma–Medina J, Reid BS, Girdany BR: Colitis cystica profunda. AJR 131:529–530, 1978

Margulis AR, Burhenne HJ: Alimentary Tract Roentgenology. St. Louis, C. V. Mosby, 1973

Marshak RH, Lindner AE, Maklansky D: Radiology of the Colon. Philadelphia, WB Saunders, 1980

McCartney WH, Hoffer PB: The value of carcinoembryonic antigen (CEA) as an adjunct to the radiological colon examination in the diagnosis of malignancy. Radiology 110:325–328, 1974

Meyers MA, McSweeny J: Secondary neoplasms of the bowel. Radiology 105:1–11, 1972

Moertel CG, Schutt AJ, Go VLW: Carconoembryonic antigen test for recurrent colorectal carcinoma: Inadequacy for early detection. JAMA 239:1065–1066, 1978

Nebel OT, Masry NA, Castell DO et al: Schistosomal disease of the colon: A reversible form of polyposis. Gastroenterology 67:939–943, 1974

Neitzschman HR, Genet E, Nice CM: Two cases of familial polyposis simulting lymphoid hyperplasia. AJR 119:365–368, 1973

Press HC, Davis TW: Ingested foreign bodies simulating polyposis: Report of six cases. AJR 127:1040–1042, 1976

Pochaczevsky R, Sherman RS: Diffuse lymphomatous disease of the colon: Its roentgen appearance. AJR 87:670–683, 1962

Rabin MS, Bledin AG, Lewis D: Polypoid leukemic infiltration of the large bowel. AJR 131:723–724, 1978

Reeder MM, Hamilton LC: Tropical diseases of the colon. Semin Roentgenol 3:62–80, 1968

Sacks BA, Joffe N, Antonioli DA: Metastatic melanoma presenting clinically as multiple colonic polyps. AJR 129:511–513, 1977

Schwartz AM, McCauley RGK: Juvenile gastrointestinal polyposis. Radiology 121:441–444, 1976

Seaman WB, Clements JL: Urticaria of the colon: A nonspecific pattern of submucosal edema. AJR 138:545–547, 1982

Zegel HG, Laufer I: Filiform polyposis. Radiology 127:615–619, 1978

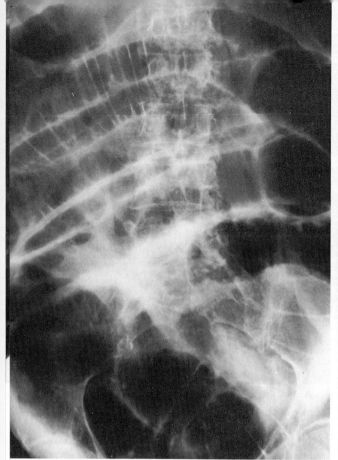
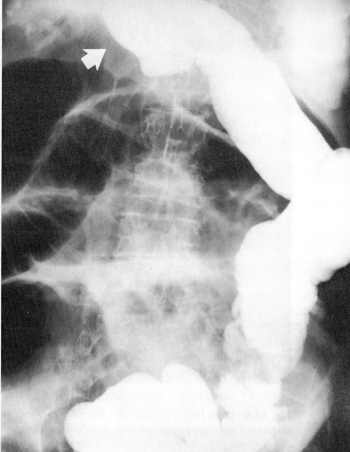

A B

Fig. 52-6. Large bowel obstruction secondary to carcinoma of the colon. **(A)** Plain abdominal radiograph demonstrating massively dilated loops of small and proximal large bowel. **(B)** Complete obstruction to the flow of barium at the site of the malignant lesion **(arrow)**.

INFLAMMATORY STRICTURES

Diverticulitis is the second most common cause of large bowel obstruction. Severe spasm, an adjacent walled off abscess, and fibrous scarring can produce marked narrowing of the lumen of the colon (Fig. 52-7).

Inflammatory bowel disease, such as chronic ulcerative colitis or Crohn's disease, can produce colonic narrowing and obstruction as a result of thickening of the bowel wall by the inflammatory process or of subsequent healing with fibrosis. Infectious granulomatous processes (actinomycosis, tuberculosis, lymphogranuloma venereum) and parasitic diseases (amebiasis, schistosomiasis) can also result in luminal narrowing and colonic obstruction. In Chagas' disease, destruction of the colonic myenteric plexuses by the protozoan *Trypanosoma cruzi* causes striking elongation and dilatation, especially of the rectosigmoid and descending colon (Fig. 52-8). During the healing phase of mesenteric ischemia, intense fibrosis can produce large bowel obstruction.

VOLVULUS

Volvulus of the large bowel is the third most common cause of colonic obstruction. Because torsion of the bowel usually requires a long, movable mesentery, volvulus of the large bowel most frequently involves the cecum and sigmoid colon. The transverse colon, which has a short mesentery, is rarely affected by volvulus.

CECAL VOLVULUS

The ascending colon and cecum may have a long mesentery as a fault of rotation and fixation during development of the gut (Fig. 52-9). This situation predisposes to volvulus, with the cecum twisting on its long axis. It should be stressed, however, that only a few patients with a hypermobile cecum ever develop cecal volvulus. Other factors (colon ileus, distal obstruction as in sigmoid carcinoma, pregnancy, and chronic fecal retention) have been implicated as precipitating causes.

In cecal volvulus, the distended cecum tends to be displaced upward and to the left (Fig. 52-10), though it can be found anywhere within the abdomen. A pathognomonic sign of cecal volvulus is the twisted cecum appearing as a kidney-shaped mass with the torqued and thickened mesentery mimicking the renal pelvis (Fig. 52-11A). A barium enema examination is usually required for definite confirmation of the diagnosis. This study demonstrates obstruction of the contrast column at the level of the stenosis, with the tapered edge of the column pointing toward the site of torsion (Fig. 52-11B).

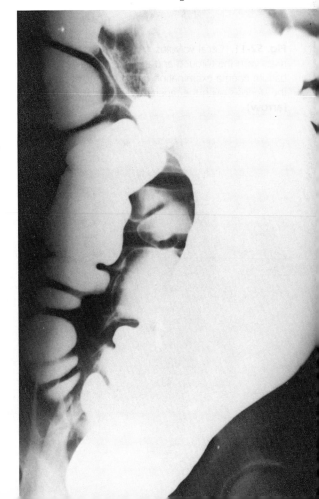

Fig. 52-8. Large bowel obstruction due to Chagas' disease. There is striking elongation and dilatation of the rectosigmoid.

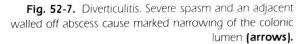

Fig. 52-7. Diverticulitis. Severe spasm and an adjacent walled off abscess cause marked narrowing of the colonic lumen **(arrows).**

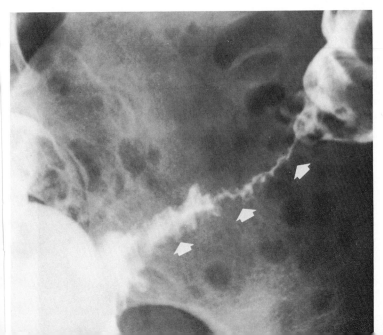

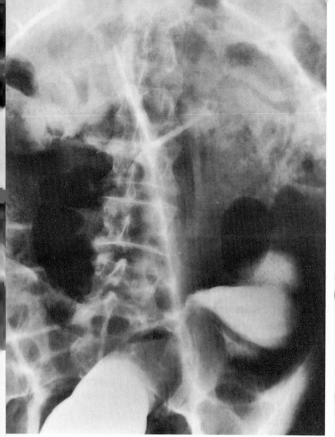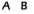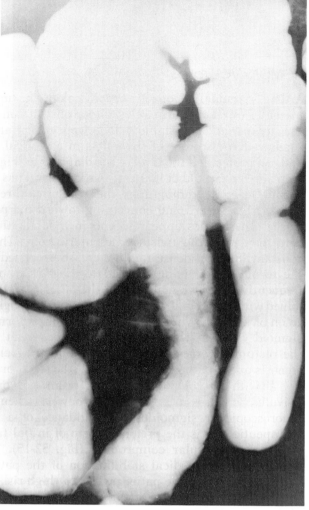

A B

Fig. 52-12. Sigmoid volvulus. **(A)** The massively dilated loop of sigmoid appears as an inverted U-shaped shadow rising out of the pelvis. **(B)** A barium enema examination following reduction of the volvulus demonstrates the severely ectatic sigmoid colon.

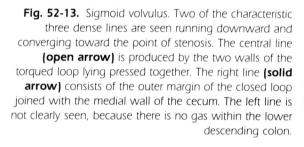

Fig. 52-13. Sigmoid volvulus. Two of the characteristic three dense lines are seen running downward and converging toward the point of stenosis. The central line **(open arrow)** is produced by the two walls of the torqued loop lying pressed together. The right line **(solid arrow)** consists of the outer margin of the closed loop joined with the medial wall of the cecum. The left line is not clearly seen, because there is no gas within the lower descending colon.

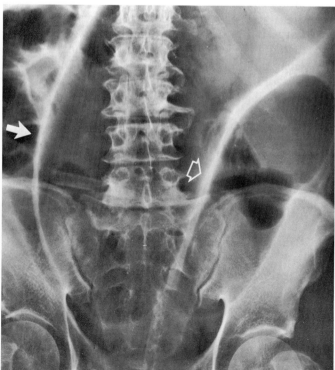

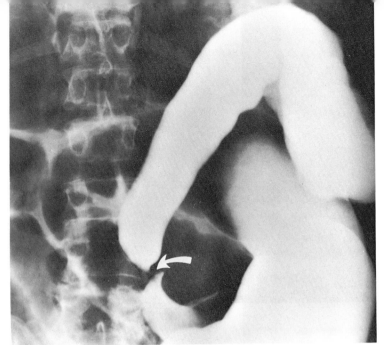

Fig. 52-14. Sigmoid volvulus. A barium enema demonstrates luminal tapering at the site of stenosis producing the characteristic "bird's-beak" configuration.

Fig. 52-15. Sigmoid volvulus with decompression. **(A)** Plain abdominal radiograph demonstrating pronounced dilatation of the sigmoid. **(B)** Following the insertion of a rectal tube, there is resolution of the sigmoid volvulus.

A B

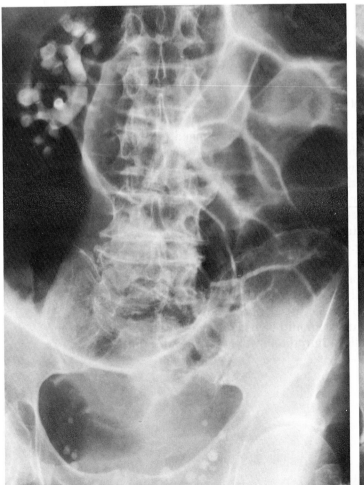
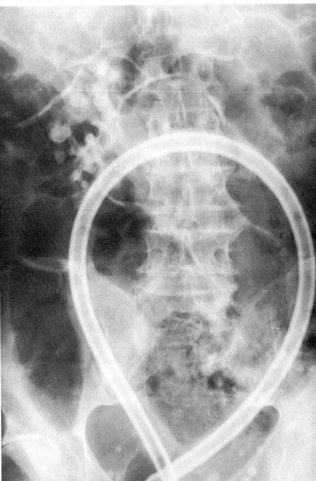

INTUSSUSCEPTION

Colonic obstruction due to intussusception is much more common in infants and children than in adults (Fig. 52-20A). Almost all intussusceptions in children are ileoileal or ileocolic (Fig. 52-21; see also Fig. 52-20); often, no specific cause can be demonstrated. In adults, colocolic intussusceptions are much more common, and the leading edge is frequently shown to be a mucosal or mural colonic lesion (*e.g.* carcinoma, benign polyp, inflammatory disease) (Figs. 52-22, 52-23). Reduction of an intussusception can sometimes be accomplished by barium enema examination, though great care must be exercised to prevent excessive intraluminal pressure and consequent colonic perforation (Figs. 52-20B, 52-21B). If a colonic intussusception is reduced in an adult, a repeat barium enema examination is necessary to determine whether an underlying polyp or tumor is present.

AGANGLIONOSIS (HIRSCHSPRUNG'S DISEASE)

Aganglionosis of the colon (Hirschsprung's disease) can cause massive dilatation of the large bowel and prolonged retention of fecal material within the colon. This congenital form of megacolon, which is most common in males, usually becomes evident in infancy. Clinical symptoms include constipation, abdominal distention and vomiting. The distention can be relieved initially by enemas; eventually, enemas become ineffective. Occasional cases of congenital megacolon are first discovered in late childhood or early adulthood.

The diagnosis of Hirschsprung's disease can often be made from a plain abdominal radiograph. Fecal matter and gas within a severely dilated colon produce the typical mottled shadow of fecal impaction (Fig. 52-24). On lateral view, the rectum or rectosigmoid is not distended

Fig. 52-20. Ileocolic intussusception in a child. **(A)** Characteristic coiled-spring appearance at the point of obstruction. **(B)** Partial reduction of the intussusception by barium enema. **A** **B**

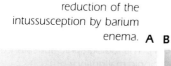

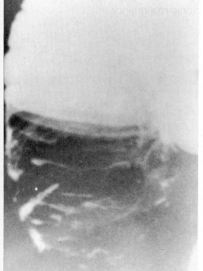

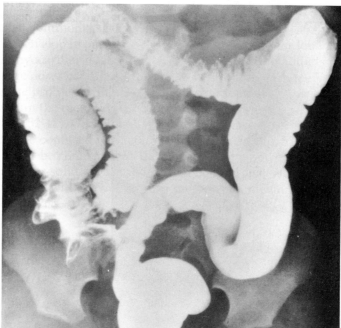

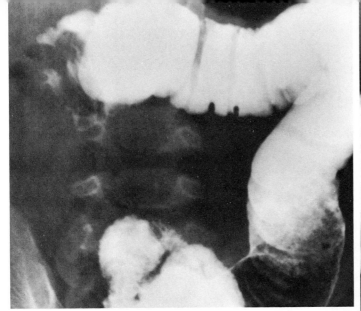

A B

Fig. 52-21. Ileocolic intussusception in a child. **(A)** Complete obstruction in the region of the hepatic flexure. **(B)** A gentle barium enema, which has succeeded in reducing the intussusception, reveals a multilobulated mass in the region of the ileocecal valve.

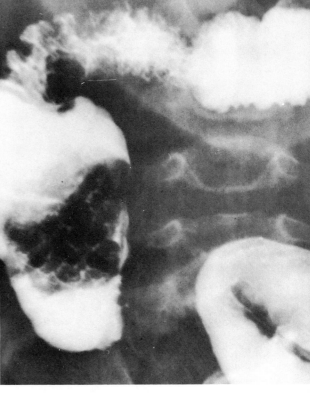

Fig. 52-22. Colocolic intussusception in an adult. Complete obstruction in the region of the hepatic flexure is due to a polypoid carcinoma.

Fig. 52-23. Ileocolic intussusception in an adult caused by intussusception of a pseudolymphomatous mass **(arrow).**

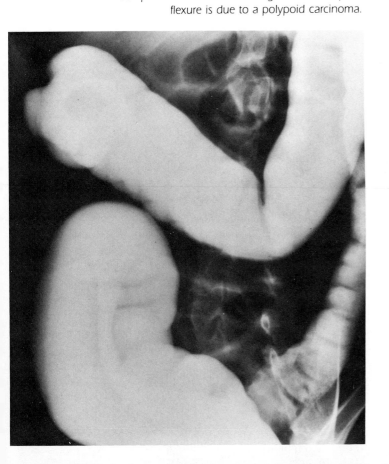

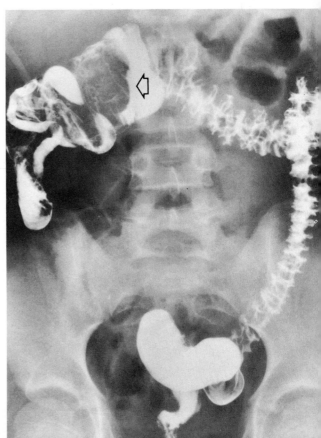

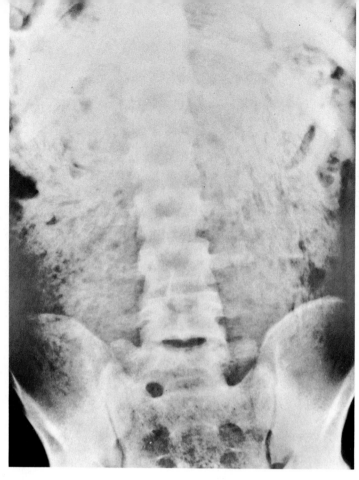

Fig. 52-24. Hirschsprung's disease. A plain abdominal radiograph reveals fecal matter and gas within a severely dilated colon.

Fig. 52-25. Hirschsprung's disease in an adult. **(A)** The abrupt transition between normal caliber and massive dilatation of the bowel is evident. **(B)** A frontal view demonstrates severe dilatation of the descending and transverse portions of the colon.

A B

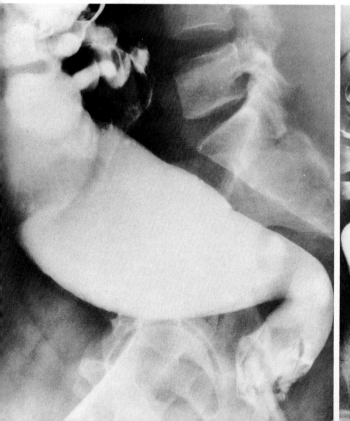

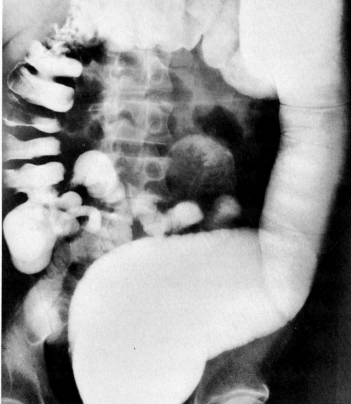

and contains little or no gas or feces. On barium enema examination, the rectum appears to be of essentially normal caliber. At some point in the upper rectum or distal sigmoid, there is an abrupt transition to an area of grossly dilated bowel (Fig. 52-25). It is important to remember that the narrowed, relatively normal-appearing distal colon is actually the abnormal segment in which there is marked diminution or complete absence of ganglion cells in the myenteric plexuses. In contrast, the severely dilated proximal colon has a normal pattern of innervation.

Rarely, aganglionosis involves the entire colon. This condition is associated with a very high mortality rate, possibly because the frequently normal appearance of the colon on barium enema examination makes early diagnosis difficult. In total colonic aganglionosis, the small bowel can be markedly distended, far exceeding the diameter of the colon.

IMPERFORATE ANUS

Imperforate anus refers to the blind ending of the terminal bowel with no opening or fistula to the skin surface. This is one facet of a spectrum of disorders that includes ectopic anus (hindgut opening ectopically at

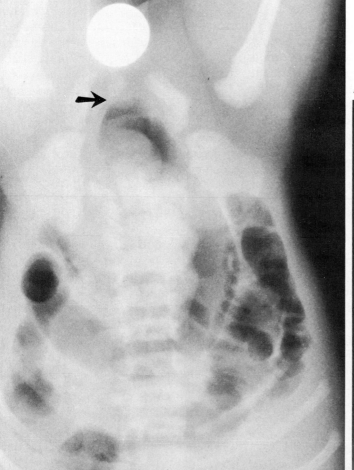

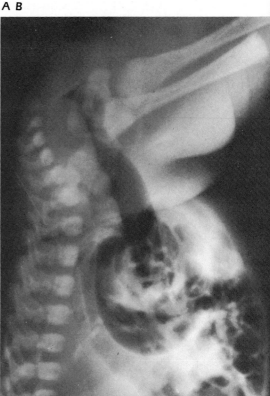

Fig. 52-26. Imperforate anus. **(A)** Frontal and **(B)** lateral views of the abdomen obtained with the infant in an upside-down position demonstrate a wide separation between the end of the gas shadow **(arrow)** and the metallic-density coin placed on the skin.

A B

an abnormally high location, such as the perineum, vestibule, bladder, urethra, vagina, or cloaca), rectal atresia, and anal and rectal stenosis. Plain abdominal radiographs demonstrate a pattern of low colonic obstruction. Upside-down films have traditionally been the major diagnostic study in the assessment of an imperforate anus (Fig. 52-26). If the patient is in this position, gas outlines the distal rectum and thus demonstrates the level of termination of the hindgut. Separation between the end of the gas shadow and a coin placed on the skin in the region of the anal dimple has been considered pathognomic of imperforate anus. However, because the distal colon may not always be filled with gas (because films are taken too early, before gas reaches the distal colon) or because impacted meconium, normal mobility of the hindgut pouch, or distal rectal spasm may produce a false appearance of the distal hindgut, results of the upside-down technique are currently viewed with some skepticism.

MECONIUM PLUG SYNDROME

The term meconium plug syndrome refers to local inspissation of meconium causing a low colonic obstruction during the neonatal period. Plain abdominal radiographs in infants with this condition demonstrate dilatation of the small bowel and proximal colon, mottled and bulky colonic masses, and, rarely, an intracolonic soft-tissue mass of meconium outlined by rectal gas on lateral projection. As soon as the meconium is passed, the obstructive symptoms disappear. This can occur spontaneously or be aided by rectal examination or insertion of a thermometer. If the meconium plug is more persistent, a water-soluble enema can dislodge it, presumably because of the hypertonic nature of the contrast and its stimulation of peristalsis. It must be remembered, however, that the use of such hypertonic contrast tends to draw water into the colon and can lead to severe dehydration. Although the initial radiographic appearance can be difficult to differentiate from aganglionosis of the colon, the clinical course is usually that of a normal, healthy infant once the plug is expelled.

ADHESIONS

Postsurgical, postinflammatory, or congenital adhesions involving the ascending colon can present clinically as acute intestinal obstruction (Fig. 52-27). Such an adhesion causes only partial obstruction, resulting in cecal distention. If there is also an anomaly of mesenteric fixation and therefore a mobile cecum, the distended cecum can become folded anteriorly on the ascending colon over the adhesive band, causing an acute obstruction. This cecal bascule appears radiographically as anterior positioning of the cecum relative to the ascending colon and a folding rather than twisting of the mucosa at the site of obstruction.

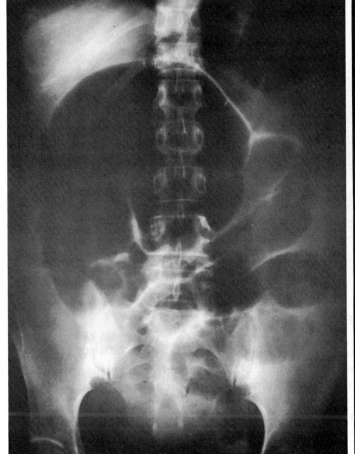
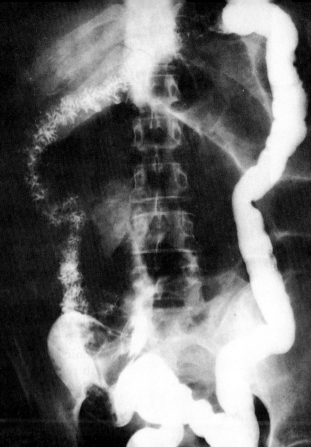
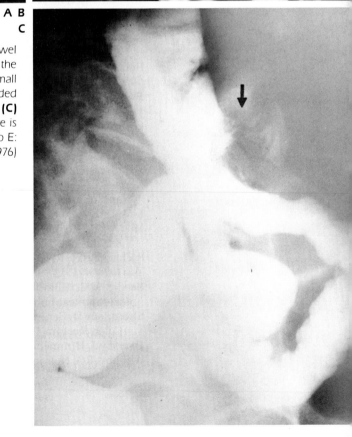

A B
C

Fig. 52-27. Right colonic adhesions causing bowel obstruction. **(A)** A markedly dilated cecum occupies the midabdomen. There is small bowel dilatation. **(B)** A small amount of contrast material has entered the distended cecum. The remainder of the colon is normal in caliber. **(C)** A lateral view reveals the constricted area **(arrow).** There is no twisting of mucosal folds. (Twersky J, Himmelfarb E: Right colonic adhesions. Radiology 120:37–40, 1976)

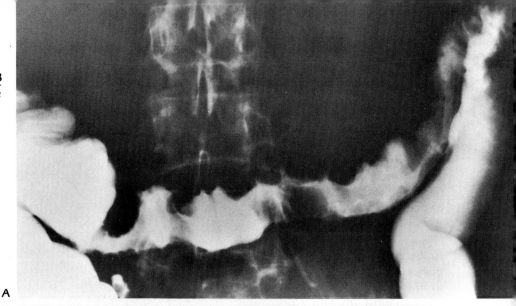

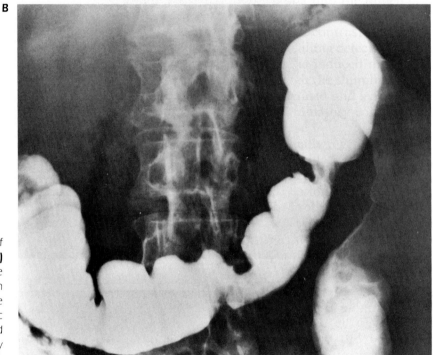

Fig. 54-4. Reversibility of ischemic colitis. **(A)** Thumbprinting involves the transverse colon during an acute ischemic attack. **(B)** One week later, the ischemic changes have reversed, and the patient has clinically recovered.

polymorphonuclear leukocytosis, shock) in response to supportive measures, surgery may become necessary to avoid a fatal outcome.

It must be remembered that ischemic colitis can develop proximal to a colonic carcinoma. Although the mechanism is unclear, malignant obstruction of the colon appears to interfere with the transmural blood supply to the bowel proximal to the lesion. It is therefore essential that the possibility of malignancy be excluded once the acute ischemic episode has subsided.

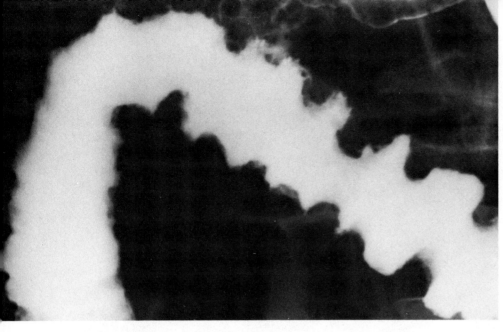

Fig. 54-5. Ulcerative colitis. Multiple filling defects indent the barium-filled transverse colon.

ULCERATIVE AND CROHN'S COLITIS

The intense mucosal inflammation and edema in patients with ulcerative (Fig. 54-5) and Crohn's colitis can produce multiple symmetric contour defects closely resembling the characteristic thumbprinting of ischemic disease. Ulcerative colitis usually involves the rectum, unlike ischemic colitis, in which rectal involvement is infrequent. Demonstration of transverse linear ulcerations, skip areas, and concomitant disease of the small bowel favors the diagnosis of Crohn's colitis.

INFECTIOUS COLITIS

Thumbprinting is an unusual manifestation of acute amebiasis (Fig. 54-6). In this disease, the pattern is caused by extensive necrosis and segmental thickening of the bowel wall due to submucosal and mucosal edema. Thumbprinting can be segmental or generalized but is most frequently seen in the transverse colon. Although the appearance can be similar to that of ischemic colitis, deep ulcerations and a long segment of bowel involvement favors amebiasis or another inflammatory etiology. A similar pattern has been reported in a patient infested by schistosomiasis and strongyloidiasis and in renal transplant patients on immunosuppressive therapy who have a reactivation of latent cytomegalovirus.

PSEUDOMEMBRANOUS COLITIS

A radiographic pattern similar to thumbprinting is a manifestation of pseudomembranous colitis (Fig. 54-7). Although most prominent in the

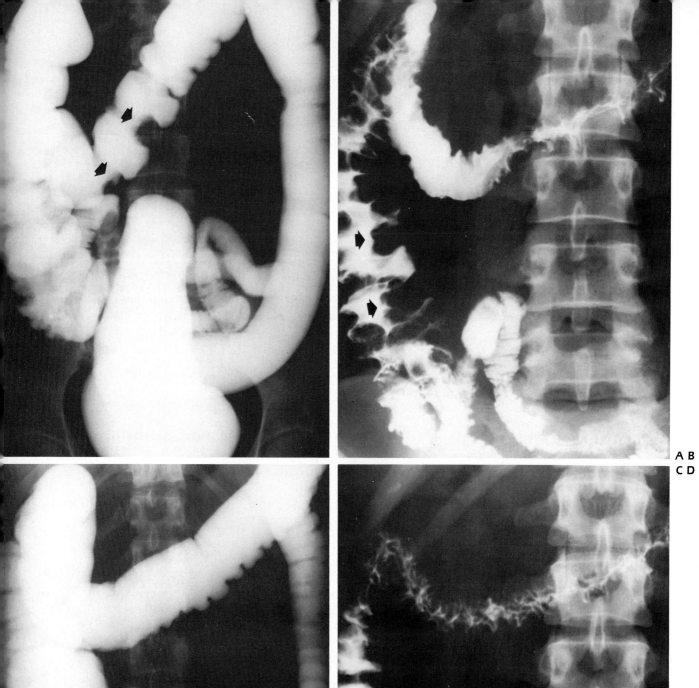

Fig. 54-6. Amebic colitis. **(A)** Filled and **(B)** postevacuation films demonstrate marginal filling defects **(arrows)** and overlying mucosal abnormalities. **(C)** Post-treatment filled and **(D)** postevacuation films illustrate return of the colon to normal. (Hardy R, Scullin DR: Thumbprinting in a case of amebiasis. Radiology 98:147–148, 1971)

Fig. 54-7. Pseudomembranous colitis. **(A)** Polypoid projections into the lumen of the transverse colon simulating the thumbprinting seen in ischemic disease. **(B)** Wide transverse bands of thickened colonic wall **(arrows)**. **(C)** Film from a barium enema demonstrates wide transverse bands of mural thickening identical to the zones of mural thickening visible on plain abdominal radiographs. (Stanley RJ, Nelson GL, Tedesco FJ et al: Plain-film findings in severe pseudomembranous colitis. Radiology 118:7–11, 1976)

A
B C

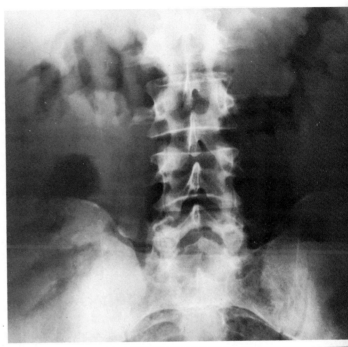

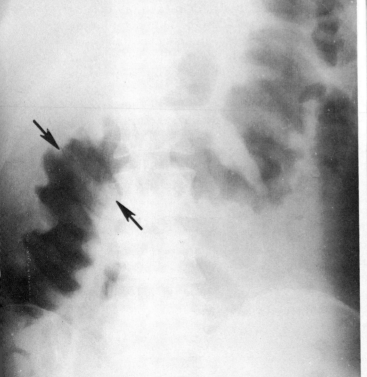

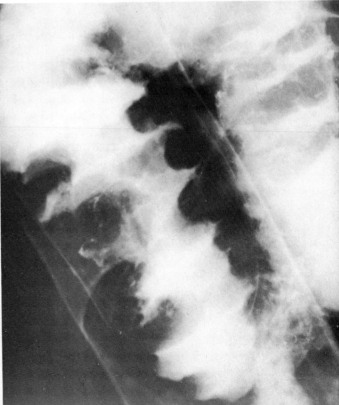

transverse colon, the "thumbprinting" in pseudomembranous colitis is usually generalized rather than segmental, as it is in ischemic disease. In contrast to ischemic colitis, in which thumbprinting reflects submucosal collections of blood or edema fluid, the radiographic pattern in pseudomembranous colitis is due to marked thickening of the bowel wall, which can be so severe that the lumen of the colon is nearly obliterated by the touching surfaces of the haustra on opposite walls of the colon. Wide transverse bands of thickened colonic wall are usually seen. Unlike ischemic colitis, pseudomembranous colitis generally develops after a course of antibiotic therapy and is rarely associated with significant rectal bleeding.

MALIGNANT LESIONS

Localized primary lymphoma of the colon can cause a submucosal cellular infiltrate that produces the radiographic pattern of thumbprinting (Fig. 54-8). A similar appearance can be secondary to hematogenous metastases. In these conditions, the thumbprinting is usually not as symmetric or regular as in ischemic colitis. The clinical onset of colonic lymphoma and metastases to the colon is insidious, unlike the presentation of ischemic colitis, which is acute. In addition, the reversibility of thumbprinting, which is frequently demonstrated in patients with ischemic colitis, does not occur with malignant disease.

OTHER CAUSES

Nonmalignant infiltrative processes can produce a radiographic appearance of thumbprinting that simulates ischemic disease. In women of child-bearing age, the detection of multiple intramural defects suggests endometriosis. Deposition of amyloid in the submucosal layer can present a similar pattern. Pneumatosis intestinalis can be diagnosed as the cause of thumbprinting by the demonstration that the polypoid masses indenting the barium column are composed of air rather than soft-tissue density (Fig. 54-9).

The extensive muscle hypertrophy of the bowel wall that accompanies diverticulosis can cause accentuation of haustral markings and shortening of the colon. This produces an accordionlike effect that can simulate the radiographic pattern of thumbprinting. Although the muscular thickening and spasm in diverticulosis can in some cases be more striking than the actual presence of diverticula, it is generally easy to distinguish this appearance from true thumbprinting due to intramural hemorrhage or an infiltrative process. Walled off abscesses secondary to diverticulitis can also produce discrete masses that indent the barium column and mimic thumbprinting.

Patients with hereditary angioneurotic edema may demonstrate thumbprinting on barium enema examinations performed during acute attacks (Fig. 54-10). The radiographic appearance of the colon rapidly reverts to normal once the acute episode subsides.

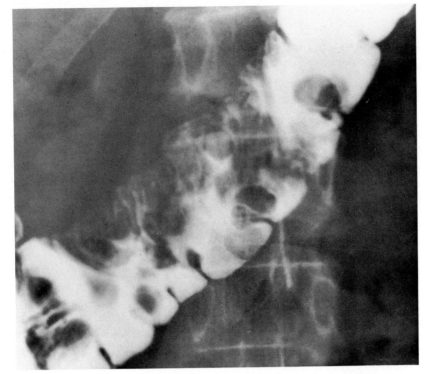

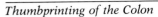

Fig. 54-8. Lymphoma. Submucosal cellular infiltrate produces the radiographic pattern of thumbprinting.

Fig. 54-9. Pneumatosis intestinalis. The polypoid masses indenting the barium column are composed of air rather than soft-tissue density.

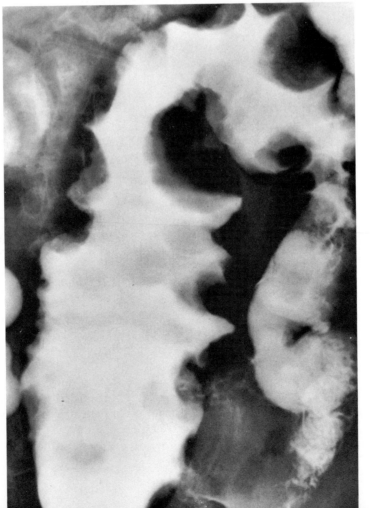

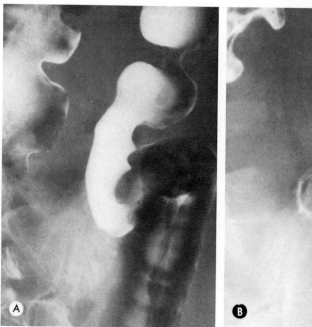 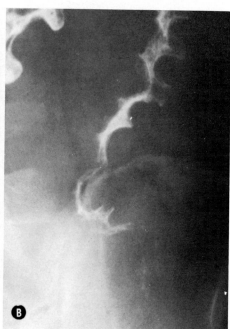

Fig. 54-10. *Hereditary angioneurotic edema. Persistent, localized thumbprinting is demonstrated in the descending colon. The remainder of the colon appears within normal limits. (Pearson KD, Buchignani JS, Shimkin PM et al: Hereditary angioneurotic edema of the gastrointestinal tract. AJR 116:256–261, 1972. Copyright 1972. Reproduced by permission)*

BIBLIOGRAPHY

Boley SJ, Schwartz S, Lash J et al: Reversible vascular occlusion of the colon. Surg Gynecol Obstet 116:53–60, 1963

Cardoso JM, Kimura K, Stoopen M et al: Radiology of invasive amebiasis of the colon. AJR 128:935–941, 1977

Cho SR, Tisnado J, Liu CI: Bleeding cytomegalovirus ulcers of the colon: Barium enema and angiography. AJR 136:1213–1215, 1981

Hardy R, Scullin DR: Thumbprinting in a case of amebiasis. Radiology 98:147–148, 1971

Hyson EA, Burrell M, Toffler R: Drug-induced gastrointestinal disease. Gastrointest Radiol 2:183–212, 1977

Pearson KD, Buchignani JS, Shimkin PM et al: Hereditary angioneurotic edema of the gastrointestinal tract. AJR 116:256–261, 1972

Schwartz S, Boley S, Lash J et al: Roentgenologic aspects of reversible vascular occlusion of the colon and its relationship to ulcerative colitis. Radiology 80:625–635, 1963

Stanley RJ, Melson GL, Tedesco FJ et al: Plain-film findings in severe pseudomembranous colitis. Radiology 118:7–11, 1976

Williams LF, Bosniak MA, Wittenberg J et al: Ischemic colitis. Am J Surg 117:254–264, 1969

DOUBLE TRACKING IN THE SIGMOID COLON 55

Double tracking is the presence of longitudinal extraluminal tracts of barium paralleling the lumen of the sigmoid colon.

Disease Entities

Diverticulitis
Crohn's colitis
Carcinoma of the colon

In diverticulitis, double tracking reflects focal mucosal perforation of the extramural portion of a diverticulum producing a dissecting sinus tract that extends through paracolonic tissues along the axis of the bowel (Fig. 55-1). Multiple communications to the bowel lumen by way of additional perforated diverticula are often seen (Fig. 55-2). Although these may represent independent, coincidental diverticular perforations, the fistulous communications at multiple sites are probably due to a paracolic abscess arising from a single diverticulum that then dissects longitudinally and serially involves adjacent diverticula (Fig. 55-3).

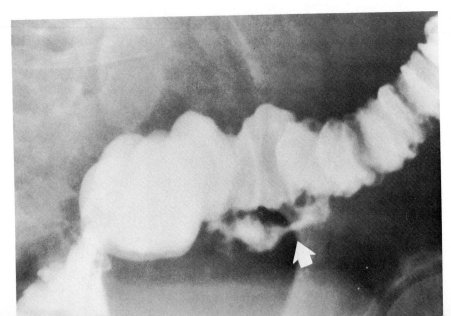

Fig. 55-1. Dissecting peridiverticulitis. There is a short extraluminal track **(arrow)** along the antimesocolic border of the sigmoid colon. Note the apparent absence of other demonstrable diverticula.

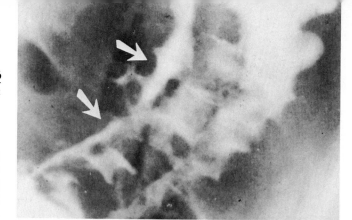

Fig. 55-2. Dissecting peridiverticulitis. The extraluminal tract **(arrows)** extends along the mesocolic border of the sigmoid colon.

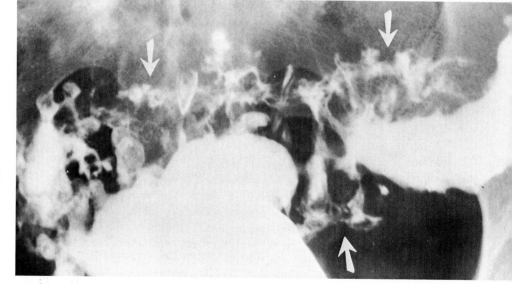

Fig. 55-3. Dissecting peridiverticulitis. There is diffuse sigmoid involvement with extraluminal tracks extending along both the mesocolic **(upper arrows)** and antimesocolic **(lower arrow)** borders.

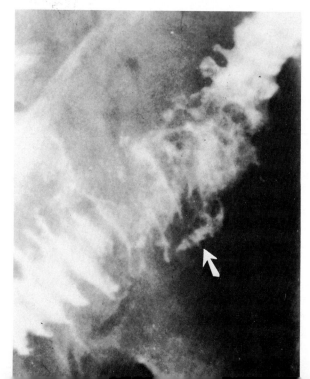

Fig. 55-4. Crohn's colitis grafted on diverticulosis. A short (1.5-cm) track of barium **(arrow)** is visible along the antimesocolic border of the sigmoid. The mucosal fold pattern appears granular and ulcerated, and multiple diverticula are apparent. (Ferrucci JT, Ragsdale BD, Barrett PJ, et al: Double tracking in the sigmoid colon. Radiology 120:307–312, 1976)

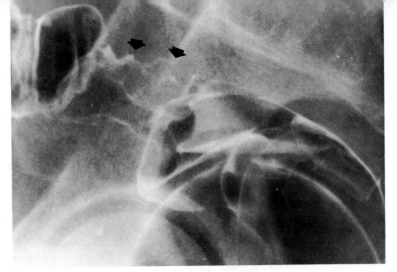

Fig. 55-5. Primary carcinoma
of the rectosigmoid associated
with the radiographic
appearance of double tracking
(arrows).

Extraluminal longitudinal sinus tracts of 10 cm or more in length
have been considered pathognomonic of Crohn's disease of the colon,
in contrast to the shorter tracts (3–6 cm) seen in patients with diverticulitis. However, several examples of double tracking of longer than
10 cm have been reported with diverticulitis.

Differentiation between diverticulitis and Crohn's disease can be
difficult. Not only can the two conditions coexist, but diverticulitis can
be a complication of Crohn's colitis (Fig. 55-4). The characteristic deep
fissuring of Crohn's disease can communicate with one or several
diverticula, leading to peridiverticulitis or abscess formation. The
resulting abscess can then penetrate through the domes of adjacent
diverticula, thereby extending the extraluminal longitudinal sinus tract.

Clinically, both diverticulitis and Crohn's disease can present with
pain, partial obstruction, a lower abdominal mass, rectal bleeding,
fever, and leukocytosis. Radiographically, they can be indistinguishable.
However, the demonstration of ulceration, edematous and distorted
folds, and other sites of colon involvement should suggest the diagnosis
of Crohn's disease.

The radiographic pattern of double tracking can also be demonstrated in patients with primary carcinoma of the sigmoid colon (Fig.
55-5). Transmural ulceration can lead to perforation with abscess
formation in the pericolic fat (Fig. 55-6). A superimposed inflammatory
reaction simulating diverticulitis (thickened mucosal folds, colonic
muscle spasm) can be seen. Although the sinus tracts in carcinoma
have been reported to be wider and more irregular in caliber than
those in diverticulitis, it can be extremely difficult to distinguish these
two entities by their radiographic appearances alone. Regardless of
whether diverticula are visible, the demonstration of double tracking
in the sigmoid colon without clear radiographic evidence of inflammatory bowel disease may require surgical intervention to exclude the
possibility of primary colon carcinoma and allow a definitive diagnosis
to be made.

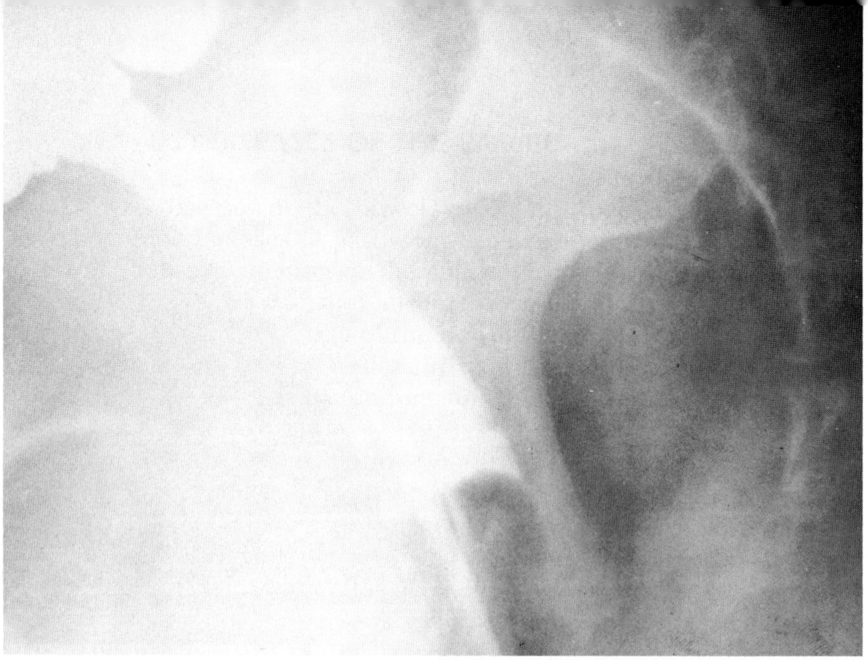

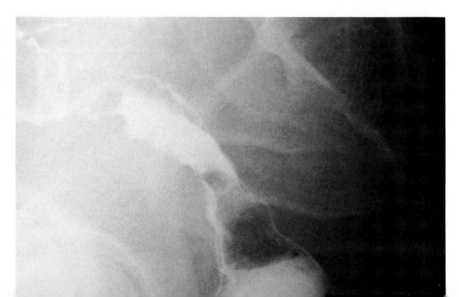

Fig. 56-7. Lymphogranuloma venereum. There is characteristic smooth narrowing of the rectum with widening of the retrorectal space.

granuloma venereum [Fig. 56-7]), radiation (Fig. 56-8), or ischemia. Retrorectal abscesses causing widening of the retrorectal space can be secondary to infected developmental cysts. Such a lesion can present with a draining sinus opening onto the perianal skin between the anus and coccyx or as a communication by way of a fistulous tract between the cyst and the anus, rectum or, very rarely, the vagina. Injection of contrast material into the sinus tract can outline a cystic cavity lying anterior to the coccyx or demonstrate a fistulous connection between the cyst and the rectum or anus. Other causes of retrorectal abscess producing widening of the retrorectal space include diverticulitis (Fig. 56-9), perforated appendix, and perforation due to carcinoma.

BENIGN RETRORECTAL TUMORS

Benign retrorectal tumors that widen the retrorectal space are frequently asymptomatic and are discovered incidentally during routine

Fig. 56-8. Radiation changes. Widening of the retrorectal space is evident 1 year following radiation for carcinoma of the cervix.

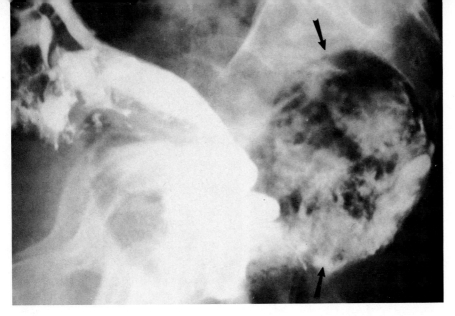

Fig. 56-9. Diverticulitis with a presacral abscess. There is marked widening of the retrorectal space with a large collection of barium in an abscess **(arrows).** The site of perforation was clearly demonstrated on other projections. (Teplick SK, Stark P, Clark RE et al: The retrorectal space. Clin Radiol 29:177–184, 1978)

physical examination or childbirth. In some patients, enlargement of the tumor causes pressure symptoms, such as a feeling of fullness in the pelvis, constipation, and difficulty in urinating. Low back pain is common, and pressure on nerves can lead to pain and numbness in the perineum and legs, as well as to fecal and urinary incontinence.

The most common benign tumors of the retrorectal space are developmental cysts. Most of these are dermoid cysts that are lined by stratified squamous epithelium and contain dermal appendages (hair follicles, sebaceous glands, sweat glands). Less common congenital developmental cysts are enteric cysts (duplications) or postanal (tail gut) cysts. Enteric cysts are lined by squamous or glandular epithelium of the intestinal type; they contain one or more layers of smooth muscle in their wall. Postanal cysts appear to originate from persistent remnants of the embryonic postanal or tail gut. They are lined by squamous or columnar epithelium and contain mucin-secreting goblet cells.

Uncomplicated developmental cysts appear as soft-tissue masses in the retrorectal space. They produce a smooth, extrinsic pressure indentation on the posterior wall of the barium-filled rectum. The overlying rectal mucosa remains intact. The sacrum is usually normal, though smooth, bony erosions due to pressure have been described. Retrorectal developmental cysts often become infected and can present as recurrent retrorectal abscesses with draining sinuses and fistulas to adjacent organs. Sacral osteomyelitis occasionally occurs.

Rare benign retrorectal tumors include lipomas (large, soft, palpable masses) and hemangioendotheliomas.

PRIMARY AND METASTATIC MALIGNANCIES

Primary malignant tumors of the rectum that widen the retrorectal space can be readily diagnosed on barium enema examination. Although most are adenocarcinomas (Fig. 56-10), lymphoma (Fig. 56-11), sarcoma, and cloacogenic carcinoma can produce a similar radiographic pattern.

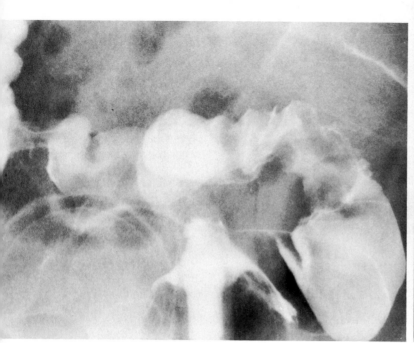 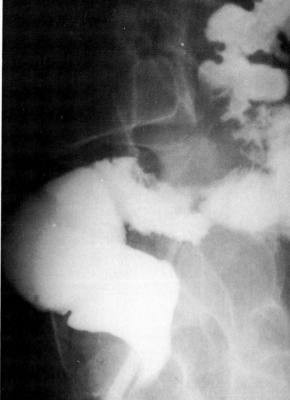

A B

Fig. 56-10. Adenocarcinoma of the rectum causing irregular narrowing of the rectum and widening of the retrorectal space in two patients. (**B** is from Craig JOMC, Highman JH, Palmer FJ: The lateral view in the radiology of the rectum and rectosigmoid. Br J Surg 58:908–912, 1971)

Fig. 56-11. Lymphoma. There is marked widening of the retrorectal space with narrowing of a long segment of the rectosigmoid.

Fig. 56-12. Carcinoma of the prostate. Posterior extension causes an extrinsic mass with spiculation and widening of the retrorectal space.

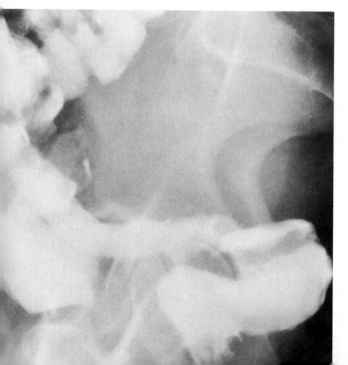 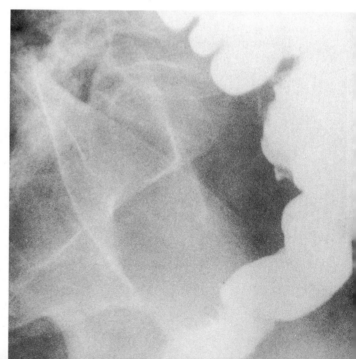

Carcinoma of the prostate can extend posteriorly to involve the rectum and widen the retrorectal space (Fig. 56-12). The tumor tends to encircle the rectum, causing narrowing and, occasionally, obstruction (Fig. 56-13). At times, carcinoma of the prostate simulates primary rectal carcinoma with mucosal destruction and shelf formation. Because of the presence of bone metastases and urinary tract involvement by the time spread to the rectum has occurred, the correct diagnosis of carcinoma of the prostate can usually be made. Direct infiltration of perirectal tissue causing widening of the retrorectal space can be secondary to tumors of the bladder, cervix (Fig. 56-14), or ovary. Following radiation therapy for pelvic carcinoma, it can be difficult to distinguish between a widened retrorectal space caused by radiation effects (Fig. 56-15) and that due to recurrence of tumor (Fig. 56-16). Metastases to lymph nodes in the presacral region can also increase the distance between the rectum and the sacrum.

NEUROGENIC / SACRAL TUMORS

Neurogenic tumors tend to displace the rectum anteriorly without invading the bowel wall. Chordomas arising in the sacrococcygeal region are slow-growing tumors that originate from remnants of the primitive notochord. The lesions commonly cause expansion and destruction of the sacrum and can extend anteriorly to produce a soft-tissue mass that displaces the rectum. Amorphous calcifications are present in about 50% of sacrococcygeal chordomas. Neurofibromas arising in a sacral foramen can enlarge and distort the foramen in addition to causing widening of the retrorectal space.

Primary and secondary malignancies of the sacrum can widen the retrorectal space. These lesions are associated with bone destruction and can usually be diagnosed on the basis of clinical findings and plain radiographs of the sacrum and coccyx.

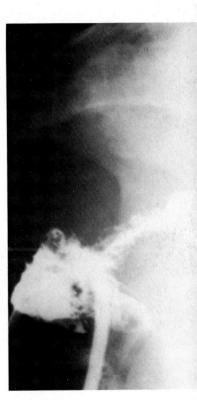

Fig. 56-13. Carcinoma of the prostate. The tumor is encircling the rectosigmoid and extending into the presacral area. The rectal mucosa is normal. The bones are dense from skeletal metastasis. (Teplick SK, Stark P, Clark RE et al: The retrorectal space. Clin Radiol 29:177–184, 1978)

Fig. 56-14. Carcinoma of the cervix. Direct infiltration of the perirectal tissues causes irregular narrowing of the rectosigmoid and widening of the retrorectal space.

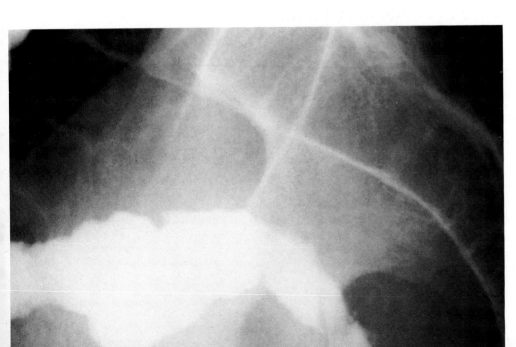

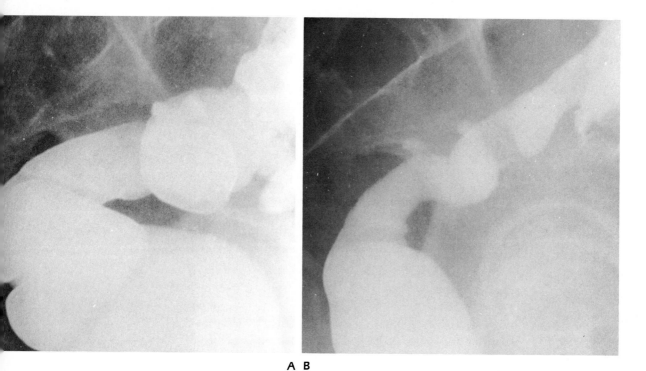

A B

Fig. 56-15. Moderate radiation effect. **(A)** Pretreatment barium examination. **(B)** Ten months after radiation treatments for stage II carcinoma of the cervix, mild rectal bleeding prompted re-examination. An increase in the retrorectal space and moderate foreshortening of the rectosigmoid are evident. Bleeding subsided after stool softeners and a low-roughage diet were instituted. (Meyer JE: Radiography of the distal colon and rectum after irradiation of carcinoma of the cervix. AJR 136:691–699, 1981. Copyright 1981. Reproduced by permission)

Fig. 56-16

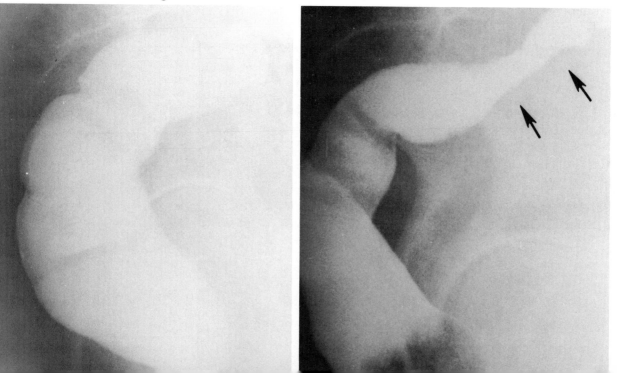

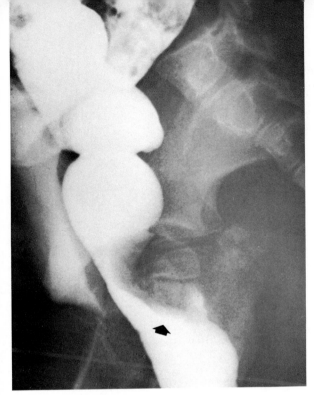

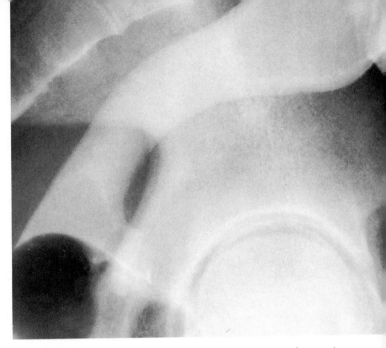

Fig. 56-18. Pelvic lipomatosis. Widening of the retrorectal space is due to massive deposition of fat in the pelvis.

Fig. 56-17. Sacrococcygeal teratoma. There has been contrast filling of rectum and bladder. The large intrapelvically growing tumor mass widens the retrorectal space and compresses the rectal lumen. The **(arrow)** indicates calcifications within the tumor. (Eklof O: Roentgenologic findings in sacrococcygeal teratoma. Acta Radiol [Diagn] (Stockh), 3:41–48, 1965)

Sacrococcygeal teratomas (Fig. 56-17) and anterior sacral meningoceles are causes of widening of the retrorectal space in the pediatric age group. Teratomas frequently contain calcification; anterior sacral meningoceles are readily diagnosed by myelography and can be suspected on the basis of an anomalous sacrum.

◀ **Fig. 56-16.** Recurrent carcinoma of the cervix and mild radiation effect. **(A)** Pretreatment barium examination. **(B)** Fifteen months after radiotherapy for a stage II carcinoma of the cervix, diarrhea and weight loss developed. A loss of volume and increase in the retrorectal space secondary to radiation are evident. The sigmoid is irregularly narrowed and elevated by an adjacent mass, suggesting tumor involvement **(arrows)**. Extensive tumor recurrence was documented at surgical exploration. (Meyer JE: Radiography of the distal colon and rectum after irradiation of carcinoma of the cervix. AJR 136:691–699, 1981. Copyright 1981. Reproduced by permission)

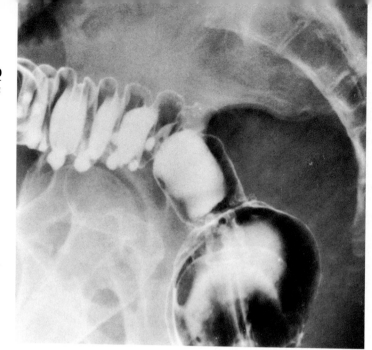

Fig. 56-19. Sigmoid resection for carcinoma. Widening of the retrorectal space is due to operative trauma altering the normal anatomic relationships in the pelvis.

OTHER CAUSES

A widened retrorectal space can sometimes be demonstrated in patients with inguinal hernias containing a segment of colon. Constant pulling on the rectum by a portion of the sigmoid within left-sided hernia sacs may be the cause of enlargement of the retrorectal space; the widening associated with right-sided hernias is probably coincidental. Extensive deposition of amyloid in rectal and perirectal tissues can also widen the retrorectal space. In patients with pelvic lipomatosis (Fig. 56-18) or Cushing's disease, massive deposition of fat in the pelvis can widen the retrorectal space; the surrounding soft tissues often demonstrate excessive lucency. Because the major constituent of the retrorectal space is fatty areolar tissue that can be swollen by edema, widespread

Fig. 56-20. Previous sacral fracture **(arrow).** Bleeding into the presacral soft tissues causes widening of the retrorectal space.

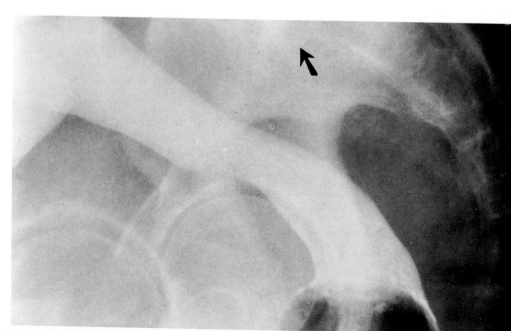

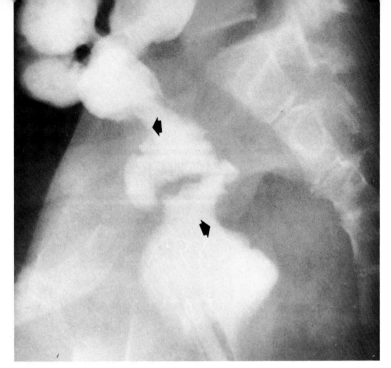

Fig. 56-21. Colitis cystica profunda. Widening of the retrorectal space accompanies multiple intraluminal filling defects **(arrows)** in the rectum. (Ledesma–Medina J, Reid BS, Girdany BR: Colitis cystica profunda. AJR 131:529–530, 1978. Copyright 1978. Reproduced by permission)

venous thrombosis or inferior vena cava obstruction can lead to widening of the space. In patients who have undergone partial sigmoid resection, operative trauma can alter the normal anatomic relationships in the pelvis and produce the radiographic pattern of enlargement of the retrorectal space (Fig. 56-19). A previous sacral fracture (Fig. 56-20) can cause bleeding into the presacral soft tissues and widening of the retrorectal space. Finally, in colitis cystica profunda, cystic dilatation of the mucous glands of the colon can cause widening of the retrorectal space (Fig. 56-21) in addition to multiple intraluminal filling defects.

BIBLIOGRAPHY

Becker JA: Prostatic carcinoma involving the rectum and sigmoid colon. AJR 94:421–428, 1965

Campbell WL, Wolff M: Retrorectal cysts of developmental origin. AJR 117:307–313, 1973

Crispin AR, Fry IK: The presacral space shown by barium enema. Br J Radiol 36:319–322, 1963

Craig JOMC, Higham JH, Palmer FJ: The lateral view in the radiology of the rectum and rectosigmoid. Br J Surg 58:908–912, 1971

Eklof O: Roentgenologic findings in sacrococcygeal teratoma. Acta Radiol [Diagn] (Stockh) 3:41–48, 1965

Jackman RJ, Clark RLM, Smith ND: Retrorectal tumors. JAMA 145:956–961, 1951

Kattan KR, King AY: Presacral space revisited. AJR 132:437–439, 1979

Mather BS: Presacral dermoid cyst. Br J Surg 52:198–200, 1965

Old WL, Stokes TL: Pelvic lipomatosis. Surgery 83:173–180, 1978

Seliger G, Krassner RL, Beranbaum ER et al: The spectrum of roentgen appearance in amyloidosis of the small and large bowel: Radiologic pathologic correlation. Radiology 100:63–70, 1971

Teplick SK, Stark P, Clark RE et al: The retrorectal space. Clin Radiol 29:177–184, 1978

57

NONVISUALIZATION OF THE GALLBLADDER

Disease Entities

Extrabiliary causes of nonvisualization
  Failure of patient to ingest contrast material
  Fasting
  Failure of contrast material to reach
      absorptive surface of small bowel
    Vomiting
    Nasogastric suction
    Diarrhea
    Obstruction
      Esophageal
      Gastric outlet
    Diverticula
      Zenker's diverticulum
      Epiphrenic diverticulum
      Gastric diverticulum
      Duodenal diverticulum
      Multiple jejunal diverticulosis
    Hernias
      Hiatal
      Umbilical
      Inguinal
    Gastric ulcer crater
    Gastric bezoar
    Gastrocolic fistulas (inflammatory,
      neoplastic, surgical)
    Malabsorption diseases

Postoperative ileus
Severe trauma
Inflammatory disease of the abdomen
  Acute pancreatitis
  Acute peritonitis
    Peptic ulcer disease
    Appendicitis
    Diverticulitis
Deficiency of bile salts
  Crohn's disease
  Surgical resection of a large portion of
    terminal ileum
  Cholestyramine therapy
Age of patient under 6 months
Pregnancy
Pernicious anemia
Liver disease
Abnormal communication between biliary
    system and gastrointestinal tract
Intrinsic gallbladder disease
  Previous cholecystectomy
  Anomalous position of gallbladder
    (apparent nonvisualization)
  Obstruction of cystic duct or neck
    of gallbladder
  Chronic cholecystitis

ABSORPTION AND EXCRETION OF ORAL CHOLECYSTOGRAPHIC CONTRAST AGENTS

Oral cholecystographic contrast agents are absorbed from the proximal small intestine. With fat-soluble media (*e.g.*, Telapaque [iopanoic acid]), the presence of bile salts in the intestinal lumen promotes the formation of micelles, which increase the water solubility of the contrast. The bile salts are excreted by the liver, stored in the gallbladder, and emptied into the small bowel under the influence of cholecystokinin, a hormone that is secreted by the duodenal and jejunal mucosa in response to the presence of fat and peptides in the intestinal lumen. The bile salts are then reabsorbed in the terminal ileum and returned to the liver. Water-soluble contrast agents (*e.g.*, Bilopaque [tyropanoate]) dissolve more rapidly in the intestinal lumen. Once they are in aqueous solution, however, they are not absorbed across the mucosa as rapidly as fat-soluble contrast media.

The oral cholecystographic contrast next enters the portal circulation and flows to the liver, where it passes through the hepatic sinusoids and is taken up by the hepatocytes across the sinusoidal hepatic cell membrane. Within the liver, oral contrast media are conjugated with glucuronic acid and converted into more water-soluble substances. The conjugated contrast is then excreted into the bile by a process mediated by active transport involving liver enzymes. With fat-soluble media, an increased rate of excretion of bile salts into bile directly influences the biliary excretion rate, possibly by enhancing bile flow.

Bile normally flows from the liver down the hepatic and common bile ducts into the ampulla of Vater. If the sphincter of Oddi is closed, bile backs up to the level of the opening of the cystic duct. When the cystic duct is patent, most of the contrast enters the gallbladder, and only a small amount is lost in the bile that flows to the duodenum. Once in the gallbladder, reabsorption of water by the gallbladder mucosa concentrates the contrast material. Because the contrast-laden bile entering the gallbladder is diluted by the nonopaque bile already present in the organ, there is a time delay before sufficient radiographic opacification is achieved. With fat-soluble contrast agents, peak opacification of the gallbladder does not occur until 14 hr to 21 hr after ingestion. It should therefore be expected that radiographs obtained 12 hr or less after the ingestion of contrast (as is frequently the case) often result in poor visualization of the gallbladder, even without any gallbladder pathology. In contrast, with water-soluble agents, maximum radiographic opacification occurs 10 hr after ingestion; radiographs should therefore be obtained at about that time.

EXTRABILIARY CAUSES OF NONVISUALIZATION OF THE GALLBLADDER

Probably the most frequent extrabiliary cause of nonvisualization of the gallbladder is simply that the patient either received no contrast material or failed to properly ingest the contrast that was given. A full

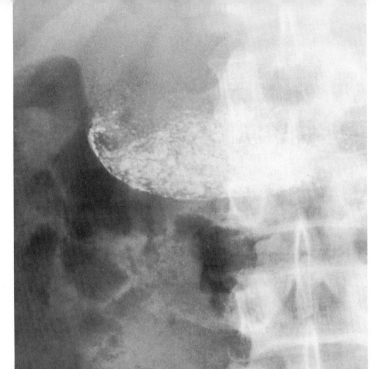

Fig. 57-1. Gastric outlet obstruction. The Telepaque has been trapped in the stomach proximal to the obstruction and therefore has not reached the absorptive surfaces in the small bowel.

abdominal radiograph should be obtained in the patient with a non-visualized gallbladder. This will usually reveal scattered traces of unabsorbed Telapaque in the intestine. The absence of these bits of amorphous density within the bowel suggests that no contrast agent was taken.

In patients who have been fasting, stagnation of concentrated nonopaque bile in the gallbladder due to the lack of fat stimulation can prevent filling of the gallbladder with contrast-laden bile. In addition, patients who are fasting or on a low-fat, low-protein diet tend to sequester their bile salt pool in the gallbladder, resulting in a reduction in biliary excretion of bile salts and consequently decreased absorption and biliary excretion of oral cholecystographic contrast media. Feeding the patient a high-fat lunch the day before the examination (to rid the gallbladder of residual bile) may alleviate this problem.

Any cause of contrast material not reaching the absorptive surface of the proximal small bowel can ultimately result in nonvisualization of the gallbladder. Because Telapaque is an irritant to the gastrointestinal tract, it often provokes vomiting and diarrhea, which decrease the amount of contrast that is absorbed from the small bowel. This most commonly occurs when more than the recommended dose of Telapaque is given. Obstruction of the esophagus (due to malignancy, achalasia, stricture) or gastric outlet obstruction (Fig. 57-1) can prevent contrast material from reaching the small bowel. Similarly, oral cholecystographic contrast can be retained in large diverticula (Zenker's, epiphrenic, gastric, duodenal diverticula [Fig. 57-2], multiple jejunal diverticulosis) or within a hernia sac (hiatal, umbilical, inguinal). Contrast can also be trapped within a gastric ulcer crater (Fig. 57-3) or coat a large gastric bezoar (Fig. 57-4). In patients with gastrocolic fistulas (inflammatory, neoplastic, surgical), oral cholecystographic

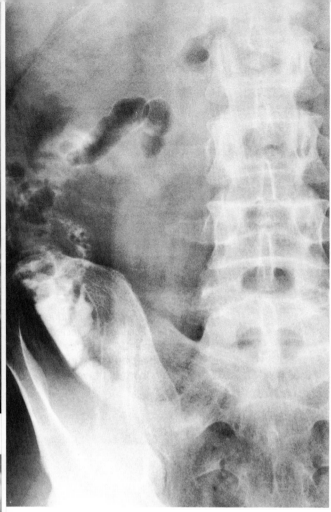

Fig. 57-6. Conjugated Telepaque appearing as a homogeneous, uniform density.

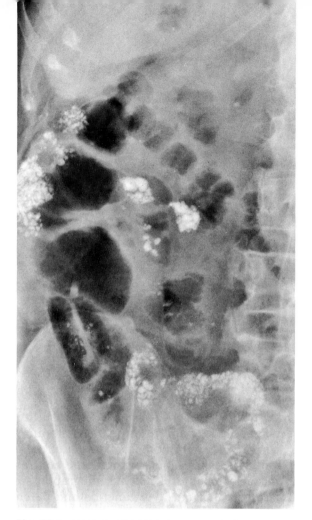

Fig. 57-7. Unconjugated Telepaque producing a dense, granular, particulate pattern.

Mujahed Z: Nonopacification of the gallbladder and bile ducts: A previously unreported cause. Radiology 112:297–298, 1974

Mujahed Z: Factors interfering with the opacification of a normal gallbladder. Gastrointest Radiol 1:183–185, 1976

Mujahed Z, Evans JA, Whalen JP: The nonopacified gallbladder on oral cholecystography. Radiology 112:1–3, 1974

Nathan MH, Newman A: Conjugated iopanoic acid (Telepaque) in the small bowel: An aid in the diagnosis of gallbladder disease. Radiology 109:545–548, 1973

Ochsner SF, Buchtel BC: Nonvisualization of the gallbladder caused by hiatus hernia. AJR 101:589–591, 1967

Sanchez-Ubeda R, Ruzicka FF, Rousselot LM: Effect of peritonitis of nonbiliary origin on the function of the gallbladder as measured by cholecystography, its frequency and its duration. N Engl J Med 257:389–394, 1957

Shehadi WH: Radiologic examination of the biliary tract: Oral cholecystography. Radiol Clin North Am 4:463–482, 1966

Sparkman RF, Jernigan CR: Visualization of gallbladder and bile ducts following trauma. Surgery 41:595–604, 1957

Teplick JG, Adelman BP: Retention of the opaque medium during cholecystography. AJR 74:256–261, 1955

58

ALTERATIONS IN GALLBLADDER SIZE

Disease Entities

Enlarged gallbladder
   Courvoisier phenomenon
   Hydrops
   Empyema
   Vagotomy
   Diabetes mellitus
Small gallbladder
   Chronic cholecystitis
   Cystic fibrosis
   Multiseptate gallbladder
   Hypoplasia

ENLARGED GALLBLADDER

COURVOISIER PHENOMENON

The gallbladder is generally considered to be enlarged when the body of the organ measures 5 cm or more in width. In the presence of jaundice, enlargement of the gallbladder usually indicates the Courvoisier phenomenon secondary to extrahepatic neoplastic disease arising in the head of the pancreas, duodenal papilla, ampulla of Vater, or lower common bile duct (Fig. 58-1). The law of Courvoisier is based on the fact that most patients with malignant biliary obstruction have intrinsically normal gallbladders that can be distended; in contrast, persons with jaundice due to an impacted common duct stone usually have chronically inflamed, scarred, shrunken gallbladders. Gallbladder enlargement is seen in about 90% of patients undergoing surgery for carcinoma of the head of the pancreas, though it is an uncommon finding in patients with common duct stones.

803

It should be stressed that, although the presence of a nontender, palpable gallbladder is a highly reliable indicator of a malignant cause of obstructive jaundice, the converse is certainly not true. Enlargement of the gallbladder may be undetectable on physical examination because hepatomegaly prevents palpation. Simultaneous cystic duct obstruction, even without gallstones, can prevent the gallbladder from distending with bile. In addition, obstructive jaundice caused by a tumor located in the common hepatic duct proximal to the entrance of the cystic duct into the common bile duct is not associated with gallbladder enlargement.

HYDROPS / EMPYEMA

If the gallbladder is enlarged but jaundice is not present, hydrops and empyema are the most likely diagnoses. Hydrops is distention of the gallbladder with clear mucoid fluid secondary to persistent cystic duct obstruction after the inflammation of acute cholecystitis has subsided. Empyema of the gallbladder, also a complication of acute cholecystitis, is accompanied by severe pain and tenderness, fever, chills, leukocytosis, and the finding of pus in the gallbladder. Because these conditions are associated with nonvisualization of the gallbladder, they can be identified radiographically only by the demonstration of a large soft-tissue mass in the right upper quadrant or an impression on adjacent barium-filled loops of bowel (Fig. 58-2).

Fig. 58-1. Courvoisier phenomenon. Huge gallbladder **(arrows)** injected by error at percutaneous transhepatic cholangiography. The patient had carcinoma of the pancreas and presented with painless jaundice.

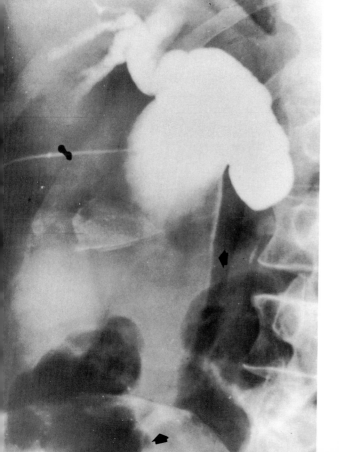

Fig. 58-2. Hydrops of the gallbladder. Marked enlargement of the gallbladder causes an extrinsic impression **(arrow)** on the adjacent barium-filled colon.

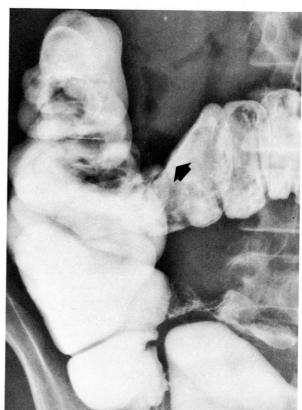

VAGOTOMY

Enlargement of the gallbladder without obstruction of the biliary tract can be seen after vagotomy. The size of the gallbladder in the resting state is reported to approximately double after truncal vagotomy. However, if the patient undergoes a selective vagotomy with sparing of the hepatic vagal branch, no gallbladder enlargement is noted. Emptying of the gallbladder in response to a fatty meal is decreased after vagotomy (especially the truncal type). Although gallbladder enlargement following vagotomy should theoretically lead to stasis of bile and an increased likelihood of gallstone formation, the relationship of gallstones to vagotomy is still very controversial.

DIABETES MELLITUS

Up to 20% of patients with diabetes mellitus have enlarged gallbladders. Gallbladder enlargement in this condition is most likely related to an autonomic neuropathy, possibly due to interference with the vagus nerve. Other suggested mechanisms for gallbladder enlargement in diabetes are an abnormality of gallbladder musculature, a change in the physical and chemical characteristics of bile, and an alteration in function of the valves of Heister. There is no correlation between the degree of gallbladder enlargement and other manifestations of diabetes, the severity of the disease, or the mode of therapy. The impaired function of the gallbladder in diabetics leads to stasis of bile and an increased incidence of gallstones.

RADIOGRAPHIC FINDINGS WITH ENLARGED GALLBLADDERS

In most patients with gallbladder enlargement secondary to obstruction, there is nonvisualization of the gallbladder following the administration of oral cholecystographic contrast media. However, gallbladders enlarged because of vagotomy or diabetes generally may be visualized to some extent. Gallbladder enlargement after vagotomy is usually associated with enlargement of the biliary tree; in diabetics, concomitant common bile duct dilatation does not occur.

SMALL GALLBLADDER
CHRONIC CHOLECYSTITIS

The most common cause for a small, shrunken gallbladder is chronic cholecystitis (Fig. 58-3). After repeated attacks of biliary colic and acute cholecystitis, the gallbladder wall can become greatly thickened and undergo fibrous constriction, resulting in decreased gallbladder size on oral cholecystography.

CYSTIC FIBROSIS

A small, contracted, poorly functioning gallbladder can be seen in 30% to 50% of patients with cystic fibrosis of the pancreas (Fig. 58-4). The

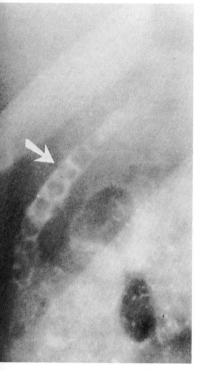

Fig. 58-3. Chronic cholecystitis. Multiple radiolucent stones **(arrow)** fill the small, shrunken gallbladder.

Fig. 58-4. Cystic fibrosis. Diminutive microgallbladder in a 10-year-old boy. (L'Heureux PR, Isenberg JN, Sharp HL et al: Gallbladder disease in cystic fibrosis. AJR 128:953–956, 1977. Copyright 1977. Reproduced by permission)

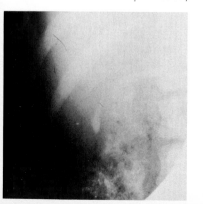

microgallbladders in children and young adults with this disorder have marginal irregularities and multiple weblike trabeculations and are filled with thick, tenacious, colorless bile and mucus. Gallstones are frequently seen in these patients. In view of the high incidence of cholecystographic abnormalities in asymptomatic patients with cystic fibrosis, it is unclear to what extent gallbladder disease is responsible for the frequent attacks of abdominal pain experienced by patients with this condition.

CONGENITAL ANOMALIES

Congenital multiseptate gallbladder is a hyperplastic structure with multiple intercommunicating septa dividing the lumen of the gallbladder. This rare anomaly generally appears on oral cholecystography as a small gallbladder with a honeycomb pattern. The stasis of bile in a multiseptate gallbladder predisposes to infection and gallstone formation.

Infants and children occasionally demonstrate hypoplasia of the gallbladder, which appears as little more than a small, rudimentary pouch at the end of the cystic duct.

BIBLIOGRAPHY

Amberg JR, Jones RS, Mass A et al: Effect of vagotomy on gallbladder size and contractility in the dog. Invest Radiol 8:371–376, 1973

Berk RN, Clemett AR: Radiology of the Gallbladder and Bile Ducts. Philadelphia, WB Saunders, 1977

Bloom AA, Stachenfeld R: Diabetic cholecystomegaly. JAMA 208:357–359, 1969

Bouchier IAD: The vagus, the bile, and gallstones. Gut 11:799–803, 1970

Eaton SB, Ferrucci JT, Margulis AR et al: Unfamiliar roentgen findings in pancreatic disease. AJR 116:396–405, 1972

Fagerberg S, Grevsten S, Johansson H et al: Vagotomy and gallbladder function. Gut 11:789–793, 1970

Harris RC, Caffey J: Cholecystography in infants. JAMA 153:1333–1337, 1953

Hopton DS: The influence of the vagus nerves on the biliary system. Br J Surg 60:216–218, 1973

L'Heureux PR, Isenberg JN, Sharp HL et al: Gallbladder disease in cystic fibrosis. AJR 138:953–956, 1977

Rovsing H, Sloth K: Micro-gallbladder and biliary calculi in mucoviscidosis. Acta Radiol [Diagn] (Stockh) 14:588–592, 1973

DISPLACEMENT OR DEFORMITY OF THE GALLBLADDER

59

Disease Entities

Normal structures
  Duodenum
  Colon
Liver masses
  Hepatoma
  Hemangioma
  Regenerating nodule
  Metastases
  Polycystic liver
  Hydatid cyst
  Hepar lobatum (tertiary syphilis)
  Granuloma
  Abscess
Extrahepatic masses
  Retroperitoneal tumors (renal, adrenal)
  Polycystic kidney
  Lymphoma/metastases to lymph nodes of the porta hepatis
  Pancreatic pseudocyst

The gallbladder normally lies in a fossa on the inferior surface of the liver and is covered to some extent with peritoneum. It has a smooth contour and a generally pear-shaped configuration. The gallbladder can lie as high as the level of the first lumbar vertebra in a hypersthenic patient and as low as the fourth lumbar vertebra in an asthenic person.

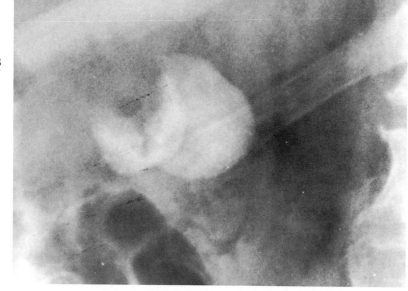

Fig. 59-1. *Hepatoma invading the gallbladder and causing a fixed impression on the superolateral aspect.*

Mass lesions in the right upper quadrant (primarily in the liver or in the region of the porta hepatis; Fig. 59-1), as well as dilatation of adjacent structures (duodenum [Fig. 59-2], colon [Fig. 59-3]), can displace or deform the soft, compressible gallbladder. At times, a contour deformity of the contrast-filled gallbladder on an abdominal radiograph can be the first sign of the presence of a lesion in a nearby organ.

Deformity of the gallbladder secondary to distention of the gas-filled duodenum or the gas- and feces-filled colon is generally variable and inconstant in appearance, changing with the position of the patient. In contrast, mass lesions in the liver produce discrete, localized extrinsic impressions on the gallbladder that are persistent and reproducible and tend not to vary when the patient assumes a different position (Fig. 59-4). Deformities due to hepatic masses also remain constant in radiographs obtained before and after the administration of a fatty meal. Enlarging hepatic masses generally displace the gallbladder downward in relation to the bile ducts or the usual skeletal levels (Fig. 59-5). Depending on its position in the liver, the mass can push the gallbladder laterally or medially as well as downward.

Fig. 59-2. *Indentation of the gallbladder by the gas-filled duodenum.*

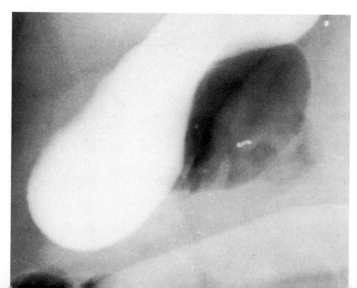

Localized pressure defects of the gallbladder caused by hepatic masses can usually be easily differentiated from intrinsic gallbladder lesions. An exception is the sharply circumscribed impression of a hepatic mass on the fundus of the gallbladder, which simulates an adenomyoma (adenomyomas almost invariably occur at this site).

Radionuclide scanning of the liver provides a simple method for identifying the presence of a hepatic mass. A normal scan, however, does not entirely exclude a hepatic cause for gallbladder deformity, especially when the lesion arises from the inferior aspect of the liver surface. Ultrasound and computed tomography can better characterize a hepatic lesion compressing the gallbladder.

Fig. 59-3. Indentation and compression of the lateral aspect of the gallbladder by the colon, which is distended with feces. (Ochsner SF: Extrinsic abnormalities affecting the biliary system. Semin Roentgenol 11:283–287, 1976. Reproduced by permission)

Fig. 59-4. Polycystic liver causing persistent round filling defects on the lateral aspect of the gallbladder. (Hedgcock MW, Shanser JD, Eisenberg RL et al: Polycystic liver and other hepatic masses mimicking gall-bladder disease. Br J Radiol 52:897–899, 1979)

Fig. 59-5. Massively enlarged liver causing extrinsic compression and downward displacement of the gallbladder.

Fig. 59-4

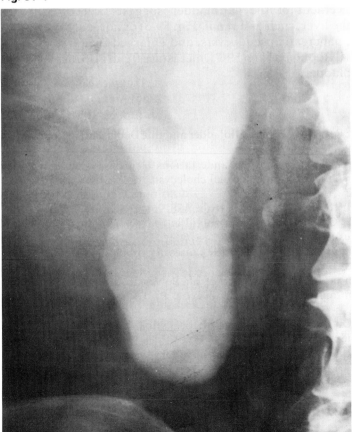

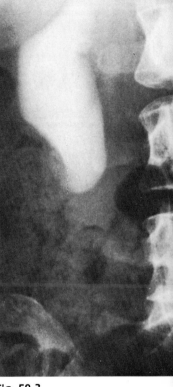

Fig. 59-3

Fig. 59-5

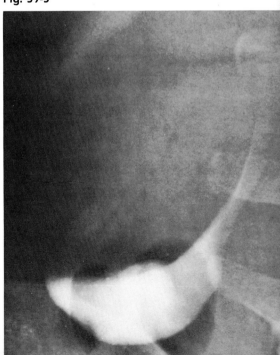

The large majority of filling defects in an opacified gallbladder represent gallstones. Gallstones can develop whenever bile contains insufficient bile salts and lecithin in proportion to cholesterol to maintain the cholesterol in solution. This situation can result from a decrease in the amount of bile salts present (because of decreased reabsorption in the terminal ileum secondary to inflammatory disease or surgical resection) or can be caused by increased hepatic synthesis of cholesterol. Because cholesterol is not radiopaque, most gallstones are radiolucent and visible only on contrast examination. In up to 20% of patients, however, gallstones are composed of calcium bilirubinate or are of mixed composition and contain sufficient calcium to be radiographically detectable. Bilirubin stones are less common and occur in patients with excessive red blood cell destruction (*e.g.*, in persons with hemolytic anemias, such as sickle cell disease or congenital spherocytosis).

Because gallstones are seen with increased frequency in certain disease states, additional signs on plain radiographs should be sought. These include the characteristic thickened trabeculae and "fish-mouth" vertebrae in sickle cell disease, ascites in patients with cirrhosis, abnormal gas-filled loops of bowel in persons with Crohn's disease, severe vascular calcification in patients with diabetes mellitus, and pancreatic calcification in persons with pancreatic disease or hyperparathyroidism. Other conditions apparently associated with a higher than normal incidence of gallstones include prolonged use of estrogen or progesterone, hypothyroidism, hypercholesterolemia, hepatitis, muscular dystrophy, parasitic infestation, and obesity.

RADIOGRAPHIC FINDINGS

The size, shape, number, and degree of calcification of gallstones are extremely varied. Gallstones can be lucent (Fig. 60-1), contain a central nidus of calcification (Fig. 60-2), be laminated (Fig. 60-3), or have calcification around the periphery (Fig. 60-4). They can be as large as 4 cm to 5 cm, or as small as 1 mm to 2 mm. Large numbers of stones can have a sand- or gravel-like consistency and be visible only on radiographs taken with a horizontal beam (upright or lateral decubitus) (Fig. 60-5). Gallstones are almost always freely movable and fall by gravity to the dependent portion of the gallbladder. They frequently layer out at a level that depends on the relation of the specific gravity of the stone to that of the surrounding bile (Fig. 60-6). Occasionally, gallstones of different densities can be seen to lie at separate levels on upright views (Fig. 60-7). Infrequently, a gallstone is coated with tenacious mucus and adheres to the gallbladder wall (Fig. 60-8); this appearance can be impossible to differentiate from the extensive differential diagnosis of fixed filling defects in the opacified gallbladder. Stones can also become trapped in the neck of the gallbladder (Fig. 60-9) or cystic duct (Fig. 60-10).

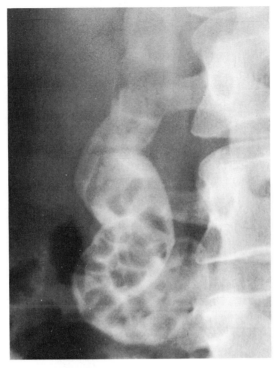

Fig. 60-1. Multiple lucent gallstones.

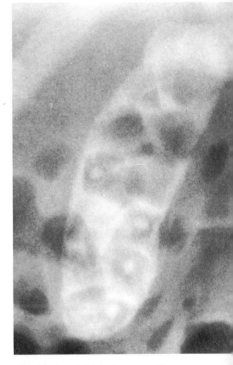

Fig. 60-2. Multiple lucent gallstones, many of which contain a central nidus of calcification.

Fig. 60-3. Laminated gallstone with alternating lucent and opaque layers.

Fig. 60-4. Gallstone with peripheral rim of calcification.

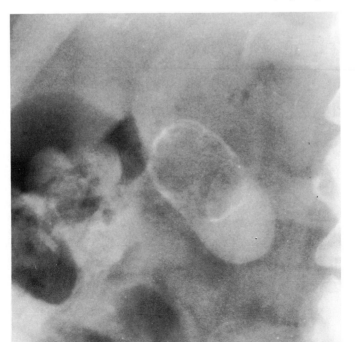

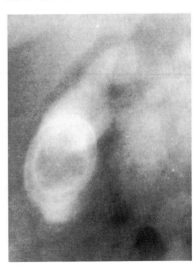

and adenomyomatosis. Radiographically, cholesterolosis and adenomyomatosis are associated with functional abnormalities of the gallbladder, such as hyperconcentration, hypercontractility, and hyperexcretion. In response to a fatty meal, gallbladder contraction in patients with these conditions tends to be hyperactive, with rapid evacuation of the contrast-laden bile.

CHOLESTEROLOSIS

Cholesterolosis ("strawberry" gallbladder) is characterized by abnormal deposits of cholesterol esters in fat-laden macrophages in the lamina propria layer of the gallbladder wall. This fatty material causes coarse, yellow, speckled masses on the surface of a reddened, hyperemic gallbladder mucosa, an appearance resembling strawberry seeds.

Cholesterolosis can produce single or multiple small polypoid filling defects in the opacified gallbladder (Fig. 60-12). These lesions can occur in any portion of the gallbladder and have no malignant potential. The filling defects in cholesterolosis (as well as in adenomyomatosis) are best seen on radiographs made after partial emptying of the gallbladder. Compression or a fatty meal can also be employed to demonstrate the lesions to better advantage. The filling defect of cholesterolosis or adenomyomatosis is fixed in position with respect to the gallbladder wall, in contrast to gallstones, which move freely in response to gravity with changes in patient position. Cholesterol polyps are often attached to the gallbladder wall by delicate stalks. Spontaneous detachment of a cholesterol polyp can provide a nidus for gallstone formation.

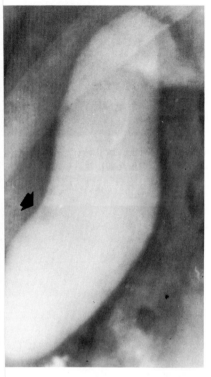

Fig. 60-12. Cholesterol polyp **(arrow).**

Fig. 60-13. Adenomyomatosis. Rokitansky–Aschoff sinuses are limited to the neck and upper body of the gallbladder **(arrow).**

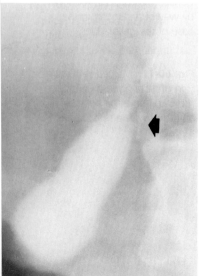

ADENOMYOMATOSIS

Adenomyomatosis is a proliferation of surface epithelium with glandlike formations and outpouchings of the mucosa into or through the thickened muscular layer. The sinuses (Rokitansky–Aschoff) associated with this form of intramural diverticulosis can be limited to a single segment (Fig. 60-13) or be scattered diffusely throughout the gallbladder (Fig. 60-14).

Radiographically, the Rokitansky–Aschoff sinuses appear as single or multiple oval collections of contrast material projected just outside the lumen of the gallbladder (Fig. 60-15). These opaque dots range in diameter from pinpoint size to 10 mm. When multiple and viewed tangentially, they resemble a string of beads closely applied to the circumference of the opacified gallbladder lumen. The clear line separating the opaque sacs from the gallbladder cavity represents the thickness of the mucosa and muscularis. In the annular form of this condition, there is an hourglass-like narrowing surrounded by radiopaque intramural diverticula. Annular thickening can result in a pattern of multiple septal folds. Gallstones are often present in patients with adenomyomatosis; they can be seen in a diverticular sinus or in the fundal portion of a septated gallbladder.

An adenomyoma is a single filling defect in the gallbladder that reflects a localized form of adenomyomatosis rather than a true neoplasm (Fig. 60-16). It is almost invariably situated in the tip of the fundus (Fig. 60-17). Radiographically, an adenomyoma is seen as an intramural mass projecting into the gallbladder (Fig. 60-18), often with an opaque central speck of contrast medium representing umbilication of the mound. Opaque dots representing intramural diverticula can often be seen at the periphery of the nodule. Overdistention of the gallbladder can camouflage the mass so that only the central area of umbilication is seen. When compression is applied, both the mass of the adenomyoma and the surrounding contrast-filled intramural diverticula can be visualized.

In patients with cholesterolosis or adenomyomatosis, the presence of symptoms consistent with gallbladder disease is usually an indication for cholecystectomy, even if there are no demonstrable gallstones. Most of these patients have complete relief from symptoms of vomiting, pain, and specific food intolerance after surgical removal of their gallbladders.

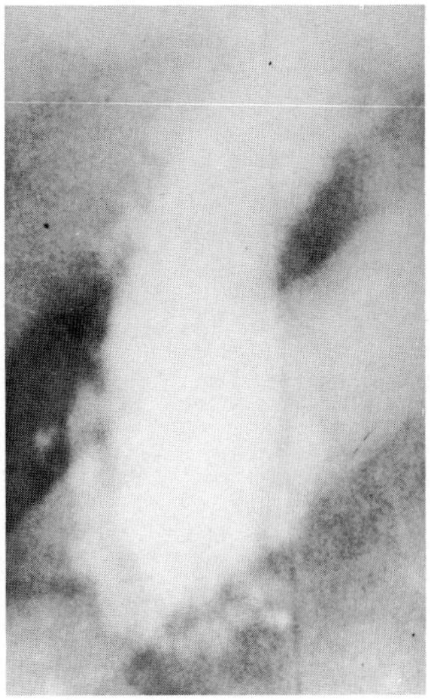

INFLAMMATORY POLYP

Inflammatory polyps are single or multiple localized projections of inflammatory tissue that occasionally develop during the course of chronic cholecystitis. In this condition, hyperplastic mucosa is associated with glandular proliferation, inflammatory cellular infiltrate, thickening of the wall of the gallbladder, prominence of Rokitansky–Aschoff sinuses, and intramural or luminal calculi. Chronic cholecystitis is clearly evident in the adjacent gallbladder mucosa.

BENIGN TUMORS

True benign neoplasms of the gallbladder are rare. Adenomatous polyps are composed primarily of glandular structures with a vascular stroma and minimal inflammatory change (Fig. 60-19). Papillary adenomas (papillomas) have fine villous processes and a loose connective tissue stroma covered by columnar epithelium similar to that of the normal gallbladder (Fig. 60-20). Adenomatous polyps occur throughout the gallbladder, most commonly in or near the fundus. They are generally small and are often best seen on compression films or after a fatty meal. Adenomas are usually pedunculated and often multiple, and they are commonly associated with gallstones and chronic cholecystitis. On oral cholecystography, an adenoma can present on tangential view as a notch in the contour of the gallbladder. The tumor appears as a round, fixed radiolucent filling defect on the *en face* projection.

An adenoma can produce symptoms if a small portion breaks off into the gallbladder and causes intermittent cystic duct obstruction. The tumor can also intussuscept and block the cystic duct; spontaneous reduction usually follows.

The report of several cases of carcinoma, usually *in situ*, arising in adenomas of the gallbladder has raised the possibility that these lesions are premalignant. This has created a controversy as to the proper

Fig. 60-14. Adenomyomatosis. Rokitansky–Aschoff sinuses are scattered diffusely throughout the gallbladder.

Fig. 60-15. Rokitansky–Aschoff sinuses in adenomyomatosis. Collections of intramural contrast appear to parallel the opacified gallbladder lumen, from which they are separated by a lucent space representing the thickness of the mucosa and muscularis.

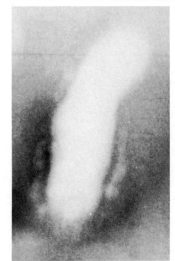

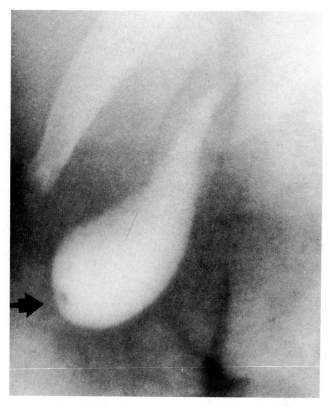

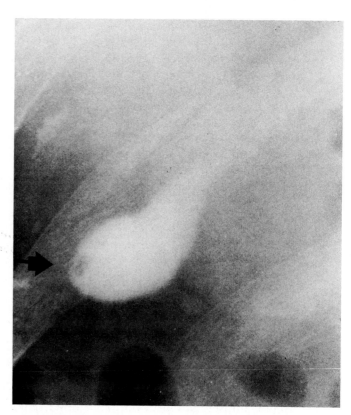

Fig. 60-16. Solitary adenomyoma **(arrow).** (Ochsner SF: Solitary polypoid lesions of the gallbladder. Radiol Clin North Am 4:501–510, 1966)

Fig. 60-17. Solitary adenomyoma of the fundus of the gallbladder **(arrow).** (Ochsner SF: Solitary polypoid lesions of the gallbladder. Radiol Clin North Am 4:501–510, 1966)

Fig. 60-18. Solitary adenomyoma. A broad mass **(arrow)** is evident at the tip of the fundus of the gallbladder.

Fig. 60-19. Glandular adenomatous polyp **(arrow).** (Ochsner SF: Solitary polypoid lesions of the gallbladder. Radiol Clin North Am 4:501–510, 1966)

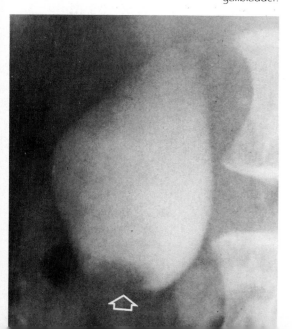

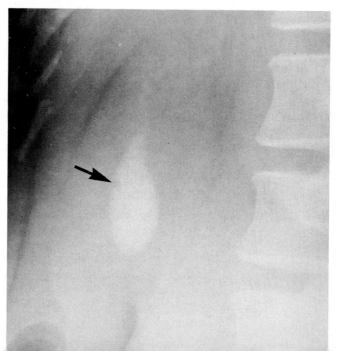

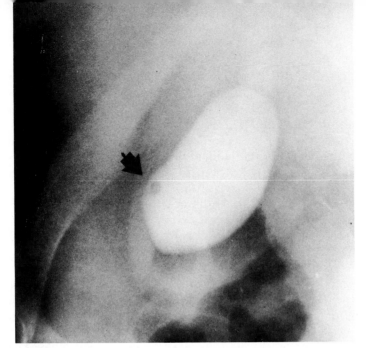

Fig. 60-20. Papillary adenoma **(arrow)**. (Ochsner SF: Solitary polypoid lesions of the gallbladder. Radiol Clin North Am 4:501–510, 1966)

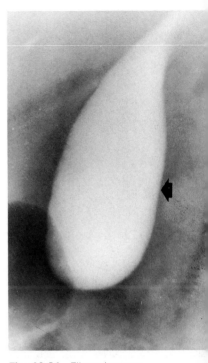

Fig. 60-21. Fibroadenoma **(arrow)**.

Fig. 60-22. Benign gallbladder polyp **(arrow)** composed of mixed cellular elements.

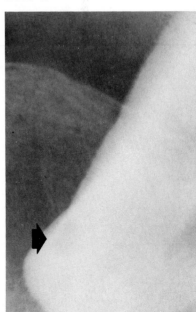

approach to patients with fixed radiolucent filling defects in the gallbladder. Because the risk of carcinoma in a patient with a gallbladder tumor but no calculi is extremely small, the majority opinion holds that, if there are no significant symptoms, there is no indication for cholecystectomy.

Other rarely reported benign tumors of the gallbladder include fibroadenoma (Fig. 60-21), cystadenoma, neurinoma, carcinoid, hemangioma, and tumors of mixed cellular elements (Fig. 60-22).

MALIGNANT TUMORS

CARCINOMA OF THE GALLBLADDER

Carcinoma of the gallbladder usually causes nonvisualization of the organ on oral cholecystography. This is due to obstruction of the cystic duct by an invasive tumor or to the presence of associated chronic cholecystitis or cholelithiasis, which almost invariably accompanies gallbladder cancer. On rare occasions, noninvasive carcinoma appears as a solitary, fixed polyp (Fig. 60-23) or an irregular mural filling defect in a well-opacified gallbladder (Fig. 60-24).

Carcinoma of the gallbladder primarily affects the elderly. Like cholelithiasis, it has a high predominance in women. Cholelithiasis is present in about 80% to 90% of patients with gallbladder carcinoma and is widely considered to be an important predisposing condition.

Most primary carcinomas of the gallbladder are adenocarcinomas; squamous tumors also occur occasionally. In its early stages, carcinoma of the gallbladder is nearly always asymptomatic; if symptoms do occur, they are secondary to coexisting cholecystitis or cholelithiasis. More severe symptoms, such as obstructive jaundice, right upper quadrant pain, anorexia, weight loss, and fatigue, do not appear until the tumor is well advanced and has spread beyond the gallbladder. Carcinoma of the gallbladder is usually rapidly progressive and almost invariably fatal. Death occurs within 1 year of diagnosis in 80% of patients; the 5-year survival rate is a dismal 1% to 5%.

Carcinomas of the gallbladder tend to arise in the body of the organ. The tumor can appear as a bulky mass within or around the gallbladder; scirrhous reaction resulting in thickening and rigidity of the wall can produce a contracted, fibrotic gallbladder. Carcinoma occasionally arises in the cystic duct. Regardless of the site of origin, obstruction of the cystic duct is common and is due either to direct extension of the tumor or to extrinsic compression by spread to adjacent lymph nodes. Local metastases to the porta hepatis and liver are frequent.

The detection of extensive calcification in the wall of the gallbladder ("porcelain gallbladder") should suggest the possibility of carcinoma (Fig. 60-25). Although porcelain gallbladder is uncommon in cases of carcinoma of the gallbladder, the incidence of carcinoma in porcelain gallbladders (up to 60% of cases) is striking. It is generally agreed that carcinoma occurs in the porcelain gallbladder with sufficient frequency to warrant prophylactic cholecystectomy in patients with this condition, even when the disease is asymptomatic.

If a carcinoma of the gallbladder contains mucinous elements, plain abdominal radiographs occasionally demonstrate fine punctate calcifications in the right upper quadrant similar to the calcifications caused by tumors of the same cell type in the colon. Another plain radiographic sign of carcinoma of the gallbladder is the presence of a local, irregular accumulation of gas in the center of the tumor mass (not in the biliary tree). Such gas accumulation is due to a fistulous connection between the gallbladder and the intestinal tract (usually transverse colon or duodenum) and has been considered almost diagnostic of carcinoma of the gallbladder.

Other malignant neoplasms of the gallbladder (carcinoid, leiomyosarcoma) very rarely occur. They have no distinctive clinical or radiographic features.

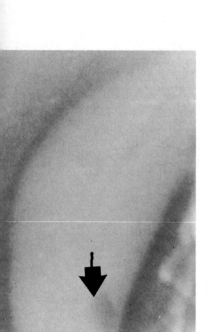

Fig. 60-23. Carcinoma of the gallbladder appearing as a discrete filling defect **(arrow)** in a well-opacified gallbladder. (Cimmino CV: Carcinoma in a well-functioning gallbladder. Radiology 71:563–564, 1958)

Fig. 60-24. Carcinoma of the gallbladder. There is an irregular mural mass **(arrow)** with tumor growth extending into the cystic duct.

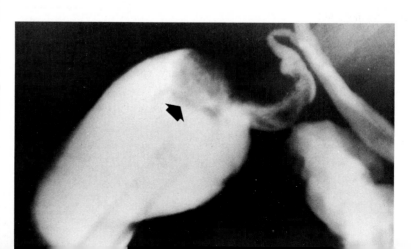

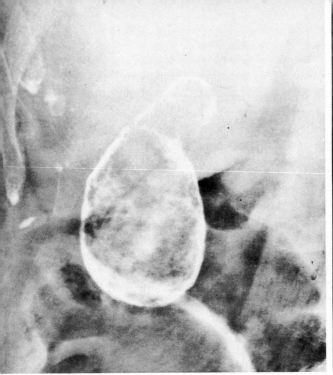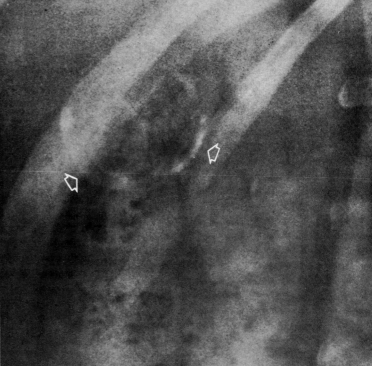

A B

METASTASES

Radiographically apparent hematogenous metastases to the gallbladder are rare and are almost always secondary to metastatic melanoma. Metastases to the gallbladder, however, are not rare in melanoma, occurring in about 15% of patients with the disease (Fig. 60-26). These lesions are usually flat subepithelial nodules that can become polypoid and even pedunculated in the gallbladder lumen. On oral cholecystography, they can occasionally be identified as single or multiple fixed filling defects in an opacified gallbladder. The largest defect is frequently more than 10 mm in diameter, in contrast to most benign lesions, which seldom exceed 7 mm. The "bull's-eye" appearance (large central ulceration) that is characteristic of metastatic melanoma to the bowel is rarely seen when this tumor involves the gallbladder. At times, a large, bulky filling defect in the gallbladder is the first clinical manifestation of melanoma. Metastases to the gallbladder from carcinomas of the lung, kidney, and esophagus have been reported.

Fig. 60-26. Melanoma metastatic to the gallbladder. A sessile lesion appears as a single fixed filling defect **(arrow)** within the opacified gallbladder.

OTHER DISORDERS

PARASITE GRANULOMA

Parasitic infestations of the gallbladder very rarely form tumorlike nodules. In patients with *Ascaris lumbricoides* and *Paragonimus westermanii*, eggs deposited in the wall of the gallbladder incite an intense inflammatory cell infiltration (parasite granuloma) that can appear as a filling defect in an opacified gallbladder.

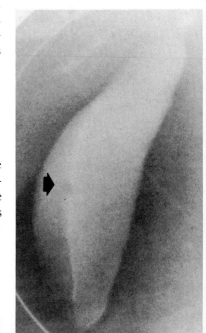

METACHROMATIC LEUKODYSTROPHY

In patients with metachromatic leukodystrophy, a deficiency of the enzyme arylsulfatase-A permits metachromatic sulfatides to deposit in various organs, especially in the central nervous system. Deposition of this substance in macrophages in the mucosa of the gallbladder leads to a progressive inability of the gallbladder to concentrate bile and, rarely, to the formation of single or multiple filling defects.

FIBROXANTHOGRANULOMATOUS INFLAMMATION

Tumorlike nodules of gray-yellow, fat-containing tissue with ulceration of the overlying gallbladder mucosa can be seen in fibroxanthogranulomatous inflammation. This diffuse inflammatory reaction of the gallbladder is very rare and is always associated with acute or chronic cholecystitis, usually with cholelithiasis.

INTRAMURAL EPITHELIAL CYST

Intramural epithelial cysts of the gallbladder are extremely rare. They are reported to present on oral cholecystography as large, smooth intramural defects (Fig. 60-27).

PSEUDOPOLYPS

A variety of pseudopolyps can appear on oral cholecystography as fixed filling defects that simulate true tumors of the gallbladder. A projectional artifact due to folding or coiling of the junction between the neck of the gallbladder and the cystic duct can produce a pseudodefect. A similar defect is occasionally seen when the cystic duct is viewed *en face*, superimposed on the neck of the gallbladder. The cystic duct orifice appears radiolucent because it is not distended at the time the radiograph is made, thereby creating a summation artifact. Placing the patient in a variety of positions will cause this false filling defect to disappear, thereby differentiating it from a true lesion.

Congenital folds or septa within the gallbladder can simulate the appearance of polypoid lesions. The Phyrgian cap is a developmental anomaly in which an incomplete septum extends across the fundus of the gallbladder, partially separating it from the body (Fig. 60-28). Although of no clinical significance, this congenital deformity must be differentiated from localized adenomyomatosis. In a multiseptate gallbladder, the organ is divided into a variable number of intercommunicating chambers. These are lined by mucosa with an underlying muscular coat that may contain Rokitansky–Aschoff sinuses. This anomaly appears to arise during the embryonic stage from persistence of a folding mechanism in the formation of the gallbladder. The gallbladder is usually shrunken and has a characteristic multicystic, honeycomb appearance. The mechanically obstructive features of this anomaly predispose to bile stasis and stone formation.

A rare cause of filling defects in the gallbladder is heterotopic gastric or pancreatic tissue implanted in the gallbladder wall. This

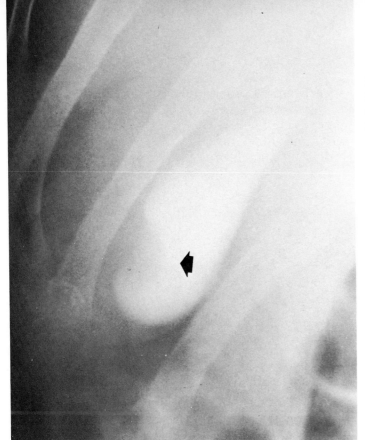

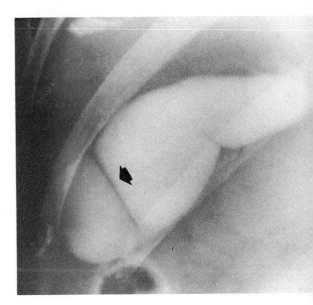

Fig. 60-27. Epithelial cyst of the gallbladder appearing as a large marginal filling defect **(arrow)** on cholecystography. (Ochsner SF, Blalock JB: Epithelial cyst of the gallbladder. Am J Surg 108:419–420, 1964)

Fig. 60-28. Phyrgian cap. An incomplete septum **(arrow)** extends across the fundus of the gallbladder, partially separating it from the body.

condition is usually associated with nonvisualization of the gallbladder on oral cholecystography. Intermittent obstruction due to a ball–valve action of the polyp of heterotopic tissue presumably allows mucus secretions to pass out of the gallbladder but does not permit contrast-laden bile to enter. This partial or intermittent obstruction accounts for the typical symptoms of episodic right upper quadrant pain, nausea, vomiting, and fatty food intolerance that simulate acute cholecystitis. When the gallbladder is opacified, heterotopic gastric or pancreatic tissue can appear as single or multiple mural nodules, most frequently in the neck of the gallbladder or cystic duct (Fig. 60-29).

BIBLIOGRAPHY

Balthazar EJ, Javors B: Malignant melanoma of the gallbladder. Am J Gastroenterol 64:332–335, 1975

Bentivegna S, Hirschl S: Heterotopic gastric mucosa in the gallbladder presenting as a symptom-producing tumor. Am J Gastroenterol 57:423–428, 1972

Berk RN, Armbuster TG, Saltzstein SL: Carcinoma in the porcelain gallbladder. Radiology 106:29–31, 1973

Berk RN, Clemett AR: Radiology of the Gallbladder and Bile Ducts. Philadelphia, WB Saunders, 1977

Christensen AH, Ishak KG: Benign tumors and pseudotumors of the gallbladder: Report of 180 cases. Arch Pathol 90:423–432, 1970

Cimmino CV: Carcinoma in a well-functioning gallbladder. Radiology 71:563–564, 1958

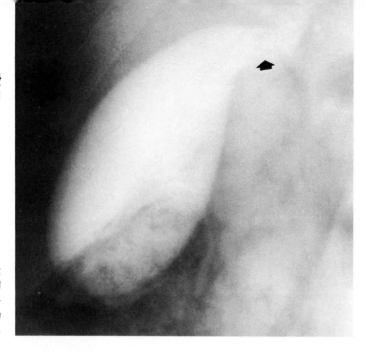

Fig. 60-29. Heterotopic pancreatic tissue implanted intramurally appearing as ill-defined lucencies **(arrow)** in the neck of the gallbladder.

Croce EJ: The multiseptate gallbladder. Arch Surg 107:104–105, 1973

Cynn WS, Forbes T, Schreiber M: Unusual radiographic manifestations of adenomyomatosis of the gallbladder. Radiology 113:577–579, 1974

Evans RC, Kaude JV, Steinberg W: Spontaneous disappearance of large stones from the common bile duct. Gastrointest Radiol 5:47–48, 1980

Harned RK, Babbitt DP: Cholelithiasis in children. Radiology 117:391–393, 1975

Jacobs LA, Demeester TR, Eggleston JC et al: Hyperplastic cholecystoses. Arch Surg 104:193–194, 1972

Jutras JA: Hyperplastic cholecystoses. AJR 83:795–827, 1960

Jutras JA, Levesque HP: Adenomyoma and adenomyomatosis of the gallbladder: Radiologic and pathologic correlations. Radiol Clin North Am 4:483–500, 1966

Khilnani MT, Wolf BS, Finkel M: Roentgen features of carcinoma of the gallbladder on barium-meal examination. Radiology 79:264–273, 1962

Kleinman P, Winchester P, Volberg F: Sulfatide cholecystosis. Gastrointest Radiol 1:99–100, 1976

Laufer I, Gledhill L: The value of the fatty meal in oral cholecystography. Radiology 114:525–527, 1975

McConnell F: Malignant neoplasm of the gallbladder: Roentgenological diagnosis. Radiology 69:720–725, 1957

McGregor JC, Cordiner JW: Papilloma of the gallbladder. Br J Surg 61:356–358, 1974

Melson GL, Reiter F, Evens RG: Tumerous conditions of the gallbladder. Semin Roentgenol 11:269–282, 1976

Meyers MA, O'Donohue N: The Mercedes-Benz sign: Insight into the dynamics of formation and disappearance of gallstones. AJR 119:63–70, 1973

Ochsner SF: Solitary polypoid lesions of the gallbladder. Radiol Clin North Am 14:501–510, 1966

Ochsner SF: Intramural lesions of the gallbladder. AJR 113:1–9, 1971

Ochsner SF, Blalock JB: Epithelial cyst of the gallbladder. Am J Surg 108:419–420, 1964

Shimkin PM, Soloway MS, Jaffe E: Metastatic melanoma of the gallbladder. AJR 116:393–395, 1972

FILLING DEFECTS IN THE BILE DUCTS

61

Disease Entities

Biliary calculi
   Mirizzi syndrome
Artifacts
   Pseudocalculus (contraction of the sphincter of Oddi)
   Air bubble
   Blood clot
Neoplasms
   Malignant tumors
      Cholangiocarcinoma
      Ampullary carcinoma
      Hepatoma
   Benign tumors
      Adenoma
      Papilloma
      Fibroma
      Lipoma
      Neuroma
      Cystadenoma
      Hamartoma
      Carcinoid
  Parasites
   Clonorchis sinensis
   Ascaris lumbricoides
   Fasciola hepatica
   Echinococcus

825

Biliary calculi are the most common filling defects seen in the opacified bile duct (Fig. 61-1). They usually arise in the gallbladder and reach the bile duct either by passage through the cystic duct or by fistulous erosion through the wall of the gallbladder (Fig. 61-2). Calculi rarely originate in either the extrahepatic or the intrahepatic bile ducts, except in patients with congenital or acquired cystic dilatation of bile ducts or strictures due to biliary obstruction (Fig. 61-3). Stones in the extrahepatic bile ducts tend to move freely and change location with alteration in patient position. However, a calculus can beome impacted in the distal common duct and cause obstruction (Fig. 61-4). The impacted stone can usually be diagnosed with confidence because of the characteristic appearance of a smooth, sharply defined meniscus (Fig. 61-5). Occasionally, an irregular stone ("mulberry stone") simulates a polypoid tumor.

MIRIZZI SYNDROME

The Mirizzi syndrome refers to partial obstruction of the common hepatic duct resulting from inflammation associated with a stone in the cystic duct or neck of the gallbladder. This uncommon condition most frequently occurs in patients who have a cystic duct running a parallel course (up to 3 cm in length) with the common hepatic duct. The lumens of the cystic and common hepatic ducts can share a common outer sheath and be separated by only a thin septum. With chronic inflammation of the gallbladder, progressive foreshortening of the gallbladder neck and cystic duct eventually causes compression and partial obstruction of the adjacent common duct (Fig. 61-6). The impression on the common duct is usually noted on its lateral aspect, though medial impressions and concentric narrowing (Fig. 61-7) have been reported. Continued inflammation and pressure necrosis can permit a stone in the neck of the gallbladder or cystic duct to erode into the common hepatic duct, producing a single cavity with diffuse mural inflammation and some degree of duct obstruction.

The diagnosis of Mirizzi syndrome is difficult to make preoperatively by radiographic studies. The gallbladder is usually not visualized on oral cholecystography in patients with this syndrome and may be only faintly opacified on intravenous cholangiography. The diagnosis of Mirizzi syndrome should be suggested whenever narrowing or a compression defect is seen in the common bile duct at or just above the level at which the cystic duct is thought to insert. On rare occasions, multiple filling defects representing small stones can be radiographically demonstrated in a single large cavity in a patient with the Mirizzi syndrome.

A major complication of the Mirizzi syndrome is the danger that, at operation, the surgeon can be confused by the altered anatomy and consider a single large cavity consisting of the gallbladder or cystic duct and the common hepatic duct to represent the gallbladder itself.

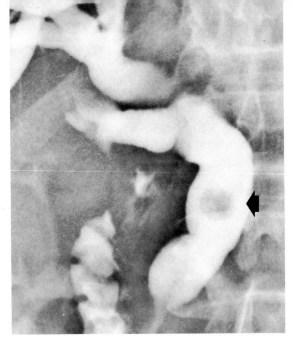
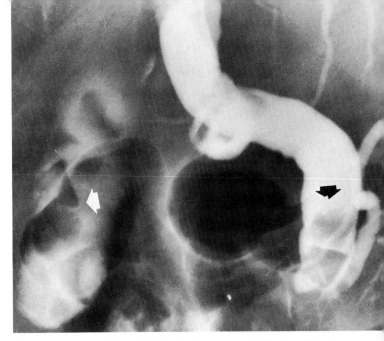

Fig. 61-1. Common bile duct stone **(arrow).**

Fig. 61-2. Calculi seen within both the common bile duct **(black arrow)** and the gallbladder **(white arrow).**

Fig. 61-3. Multiple hepatic duct stones in a patient who developed a stricture at the junction of the left and right hepatic ducts **(arrow).** This juncture was the site of an anastomosis with the jejunum for a previous distal bile duct stricture.

Fig. 61-4. Impacted ampullary stone **(arrow)** with an unusual peanut-shaped configuration.

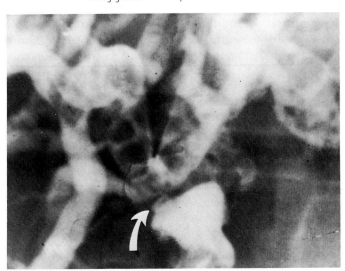

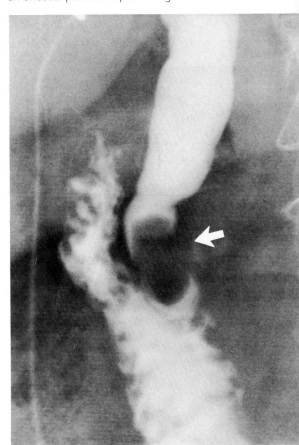

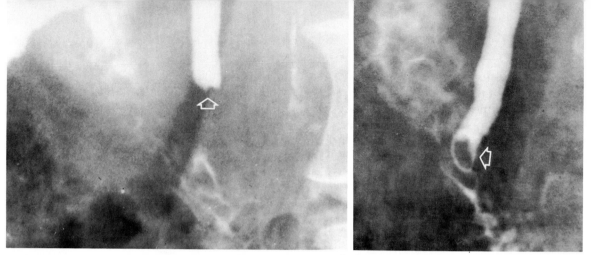

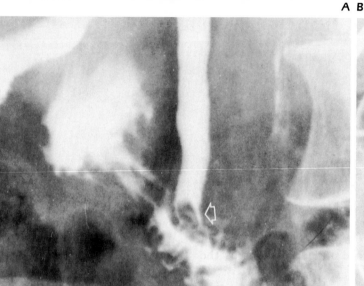

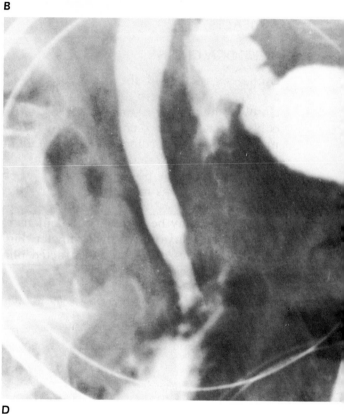

A B

C

D

Fig. 61-9. Pseudocalculus. **(A)** Smooth, slightly lobulated filling defect of the distal common bile duct simulating an impacted stone **(arrow).** Note, however, that some contrast has already flowed into the duodenum. **(B), (C)** Contrast has encircled the stonelike filling defect **(arrows)** in two projections. **(D)** Following relaxation of the sphincter of Oddi, the distal common bile duct appears normal, and contrast flows freely into the duodenum.

AIR BUBBLE

Air bubbles are a particularly vexing cause of artifactual filling defects in the bile duct during T-tube cholangiography. They are smooth, round, and generally multiple, unlike biliary calculi, which are frequently faceted and have a straight border. For an air bubble artifact to be distinguished from a stone in the bile duct, the patient should be raised toward an upright position. Air bubbles are lighter than contrast-laden bile and tend to rise toward the proximal portion of the biliary tree; however, true calculi tend to remain in a stationary position or fall with gravity. If the nature of the lucent filling defect remains in doubt, the examination should be repeated on the following day. Careful prefilling of the injection syringe and tubing should decrease the chance of air bubbles being introduced into the biliary tree during T-tube cholangiography.

BLOOD CLOT

Blood clots are an unusual cause of filling defects in the bile ducts. The margins of blood clots are generally not as smooth as those of biliary calculi. Clots are softer and more easily molded and thus tend to elongate within the duct, rather than having the generally spheroid configuration of stones in the bile ducts.

NEOPLASMS

MALIGNANT TUMORS

Primary malignant lesions of the bile duct (cholangiocarcinoma) occasionally present as filling defects within the common hepatic or bile ducts (Fig. 61-10). However, due to the intense ductal fibrosis that often accompanies the carcinoma, these tumors more typically appear as irregular strictures. A carcinoma of the ampulla that abruptly occludes the common bile duct can be associated with a markedly irregular intraluminal polypoid mass. One manifestation of hepatoma is a bulky intraluminal filling defect in a proximal extrahepatic duct that often causes obstructive jaundice. In the rare villous tumor arising in the common bile duct, contrast enters the interstices of the lesion, as it does also in neoplasms of this cell type elsewhere in the gastrointestinal tract (Fig. 61-11).

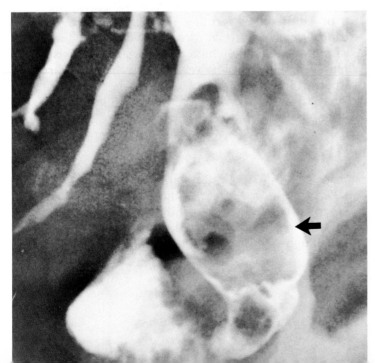

Fig. 61-10. Cholangiocarcinoma presenting as a large filling defect **(arrow)** in the common bile duct.

Fig. 61-11. Villous adenocarcinoma of the common bile duct **(arrow).** Contrast is seen entering the interstices of the lesion.

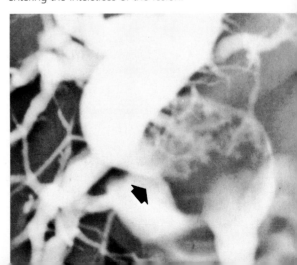

Balthazar EJ: The Mirizzi syndrome. Inflammatory stricture of the common hepatic duct. Am J Gastroenterol 64:144–148, 1975

Belgraier AH: Common bile duct obstruction due to *Fasciola hepatica.* NY State J Med 76:936–937, 1976

Beneventano TC, Schein CJ: The pseudocalculus sign in cholangiography. Arch Surg 98:731–733, 1969

Berk RN, Clemett AR: Radiology of the Gallbladder and Bile Ducts. Philadelphia, WB Saunders, 1977

Clemett AR, Lowman RM: The roentgen features of the Mirizzi syndrome. AJR 94:480–483, 1965

Cremin BJ, Fisher MB: Biliary ascariasis in children. AJR 126:352–357, 1976

Evans JA, Mujahed Z: Percutaneous transhepatic cholangiography. Semin Roentgenol 11:219–222, 1976

Gerlock AJ, Muhletaler CA: Primary common bile duct carcinoid. Gastrointest Radiol 4:263–264, 1979

Goldberg H: Operative and postoperative cholecystocholangiography. Semin Roentgenol 11:203–211, 1976

Harris JD: Rupture of hydatid cysts of the liver into the biliary tracts. Br J Surg 52:210–214, 1965

Koehler RE, Melson GL, Lee JKT et al: Common hepatic duct obstruction by cystic duct stone: Mirizzi syndrome. AJR 132:1007–1009, 1979

Larsen CR, Scholz FJ, Wise RE: Diseases of the biliary ducts. Semin Roentgenol 11:259–267, 1976

Mujahed Z, Evans JA: Pseudocalculus defect in cholangiography. AJR 116:337–341, 1972

Reeder MM, Hamilton LC: Radiologic diagnosis of tropical diseases of the gastrointestinal tract. Radiol Clin North Am 7:57–81, 1969

Tuttle RJ: Cause of recurring obstructive jaundice revealed by percutaneous cholangiography—Hydatid cyst. N Engl J Med 283:805–806, 1970

Van Sonnenberg E, Ferrucci JT: Bile duct obstruction in hepatocellular carcinoma (hepatoma)—Clinical and cholangiographic characteristics. Radiology 130:7–13, 1979

Way LW: Retained common duct stones. Surg Clin North Am 53:1169–1190, 1973

Wright RM, Dorrough RL, Ditmore HB: Ascariasis of the biliary system. Arch Surg 86:402–405, 1963

BILE DUCT NARROWING / OBSTRUCTION

62

Disease Entities

Neoplastic lesions
  Malignant tumors
    Carcinoma of the common bile duct
      (cholangiocarcinoma)
    Ampullary carcinoma
    Carcinoma of the pancreas
    Carcinoma of the duodenum
    Carcinoma of the gallbladder
    Hepatoma
    Metastases to lymph nodes in the
      porta hepatis
    Lymphoma
  Benign tumors
    Papilloma
    Adenoma
    Neurinoma of the cystic duct
    Granular cell myoblastoma
    Fibroma
    Leiomyoma
    Cystadenoma
Inflammatory disorders
  Primary sclerosing cholangitis
  Cholangiolitic hepatitis
  Chronic pancreatitis
  Acute pancreatitis
  Pancreatic pseudocyst
  Duodenal ulcer disease
  Papillary stenosis

Parasites
  Ascaris lumbricoides
  Clonorchis sinensis
  Fasciola hepatica
  Echinococcus granulosis
  Amebiasis
  Shistosomiasis
Granulomatous disease in adjacent
  lymph nodes
  Tuberculosis
  Sarcoidosis
Bile duct calculi
  Impacted stone in ampulla of Vater
  Papillary edema secondary to recent
    passage of biliary stone
  Mirizzi syndrome
Traumatic stricture
Congenital/neonatal anomalies
  Biliary atresia/hypoplasia
  Congenital membranous diaphragm
  Duodenal diverticulum
Vascular impressions
  Calcified portal vein
  Aortic aneurysm
Hepatic cysts (simple, polycystic)
Cirrhosis

Obstruction of the common bile duct by tumor is more commonly caused by an extrinsic malignancy, such as carcinoma of the pancreas, than by a primary carcinoma of the bile duct. However, a distinction between these entities is rarely possible on the basis of radiographic findings. At cholangiography, the duct at the point of obstruction has a nonspecific appearance and can be blunt, rounded, jagged, or tapered or show a "rat-tail" deformity.

MALIGNANT TUMORS

CHOLANGIOCARCINOMA

Primary carcinomas of the bile ducts (cholangiocarcinoma) are almost invariably adenocarcinomas. They have a wide range of histologic appearances, depending on the amount of fibrous stroma present between cells. Because of their strategic location, obstructive jaundice is usually the first clinical manifestation. Pain, weight loss, and other constitutional symptoms are common. In contrast to cancer of the gallbladder, bile duct carcinoma occurs more frequently in men than in women. The peak incidence of cholangiocarcinoma is during the sixth decade of life. Most patients have hepatomegaly; about one-third have a palpable gallbladder (Courvoisier phenomenon). An association between cholangiocarcinoma and chronic ulcerative colitis has been reported. Up to 8% of patients with bile duct carcinoma have chronic ulcerative colitis, and the tumor tends to occur at a much earlier age in patients with this inflammatory bowel disease than in others. The relatively high incidence of biliary carcinoma in the Orient is thought to be related in part to chronic infestation by *Clonorchis sinensis*.

Carcinoma can occur at any site along the bile ducts. The most common locations are in the retroduodenal or supraduodenal segments of the common bile duct and in the common hepatic duct at the carina (Fig. 62-1). Because of their infiltrative nature, most bile duct carcinomas are far advanced at the time of diagnosis, with regional lymph node metastases and extension along the bile ducts. Tumors arising at the junction of the right and left hepatic ducts (Klatskin tumors) behave as distinct clinical entities (Fig. 62-2). They tend to grow slowly and to be late to metastasize.

Cholangiocarcinoma most commonly presents radiographically as a short, well-demarcated segmental constriction (Fig. 62-3). The tumor usually begins as a plaquelike lesion of the wall that infiltrates and spreads along the duct in both directions. An extensive desmoplastic response tends to produce diffuse narrowing of the duct (Fig. 62-4); little intraluminal extension of tumor is seen. An obstructing tumor most often causes abrupt occlusion of the common bile duct with proximal dilatation. Passage of contrast through the lesion can demonstrate the site of occlusion to be smooth or to contain small, irregular polypoid masses protruding into the lumen. Cholangiocarcinoma occasionally appears as a discrete, bulky polypoid tumor with a large intraluminal component. If the mass is relatively smooth, it may

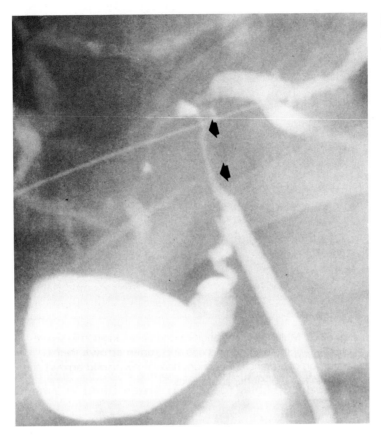

Fig. 62-1. Cholangio-carcinoma presenting as a smooth stricture **(arrows)** extending from the carina to the junction of the cystic duct. Areas of relative narrowing of the right and left hepatic ducts may represent additional sites of tumor involvement.

Fig. 62-2. Klatskin tumor. Sclerosing cholangiocarcinomas **(arrows)** in two patients are visible arising at the junction of the right and left hepatic ducts.

A B

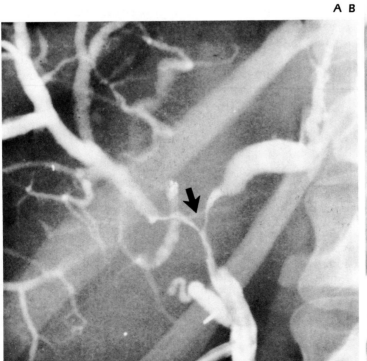

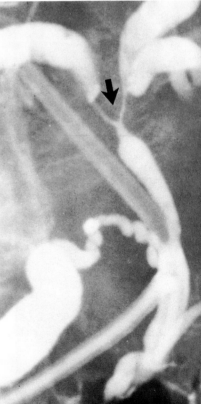

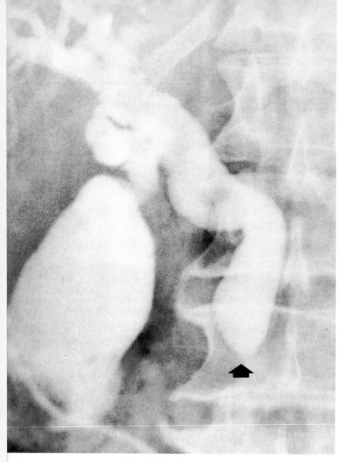

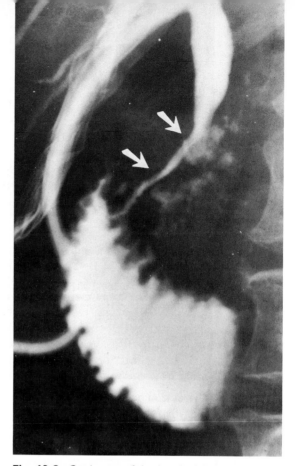

Fig. 62-7. Adenocarcinoma of the ampulla causing an abrupt occlusion **(arrow)** of the distal common bile duct.

Fig. 62-8. Carcinoma of the head of the pancreas. There is irregular narrowing of the common bile duct **(arrows).** The calcifications reflect underlying chronic pancreatitis.

Fig. 62-9. Carcinoma of the pancreas causing complete obstruction of the bile duct **(arrow).**

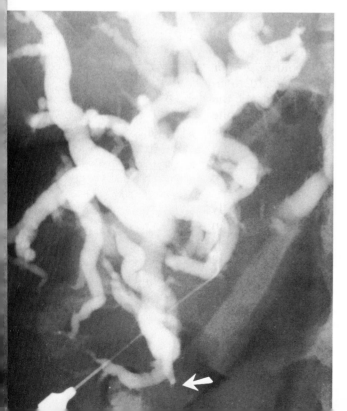

obstructive jaundice (Fig. 62-10). A mass in the gallbladder fossa with simultaneous obstruction of the common hepatic and cystic ducts suggests direct spread of carcinoma of the gallbladder. Extension of a strategically placed hepatoma very rarely produces bile duct obstruction and jaundice. Hepatomas tend to undergo necrosis and degeneration, especially in a large tumor nodule. Necrosis and degeneration of a hepatoma contiguous with a bile duct may conceivably permit a large tumor fragment to enter the biliary tree and flow distally until it becomes lodged in the common bile duct.

METASTASES

Metastases to lymph nodes in the porta hepatis or along the medial margin of the descending duodenum can cause extrinsic obstruction of the main hepatic or common bile ducts (Fig. 62-11). These metastases are usually secondary to primary malignancies of the gastrointestinal tract but can also represent spread from carcinoma of the lung or breast. In these conditions, the diffuse desmoplastic response evoked by the metastasis can simulate the appearance of primary cholangiocarcinoma. It must be remembered that involvement of the extrahepatic biliary tree by metastatic carcinoma is not common. The usual cause of jaundice in these patients is massive liver replacement by metastatic tumor.

LYMPHOMA

Lymphoma involving nodes in the porta hepatis can also produce obstructive jaundice. Whenever the bile duct is deviated as well as obstructed, the possibility of lymph node metastases should be considered.

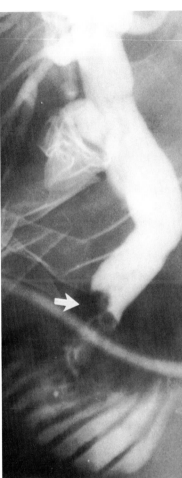

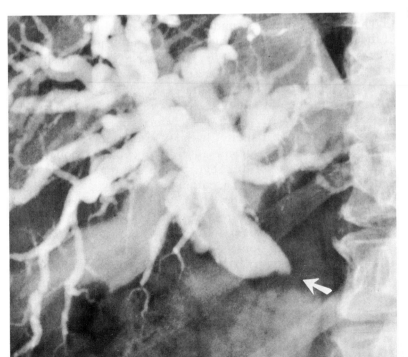

Fig. 62-10. Adenocarcinoma arising in the second portion of the duodenum and causing an irregular mass in the distal common bile duct **(arrow)** with a high-grade biliary stenosis.

Fig. 62-11. Extrinsic obstruction of the common bile duct **(arrow)** due to nodal metastases from carcinoma of the colon.

CHRONIC PANCREATITIS

Because of the intimate relationship of the pancreas to the distal common bile duct, chronic fibrotic changes in the pancreas can lead to inflammatory strictures of the common bile duct (Fig. 62-14). Radiographically, inflammatory and fibrotic changes in the periductal tissues cause smooth, concentric, gradual tapering of the common bile duct with moderate dilatation of the proximal extrahepatic ducts and mild dilatation of intrahepatic ducts. Associated pancreatic calcification is seen not infrequently (Fig. 62-15). Complete common duct obstruction is rare. The stricture involves that portion of the bile duct that lies in the pancreatic tissue. There is often an abrupt transition between the encased "pipestem" segment and the dilated suprapancreatic portion of the duct (Fig. 62-15). Although the strictured bile duct can be tortuous, the smooth margins and relative lack of dilatation of the intrahepatic ducts serve to differentiate this appearance from that of pancreatic carcinoma.

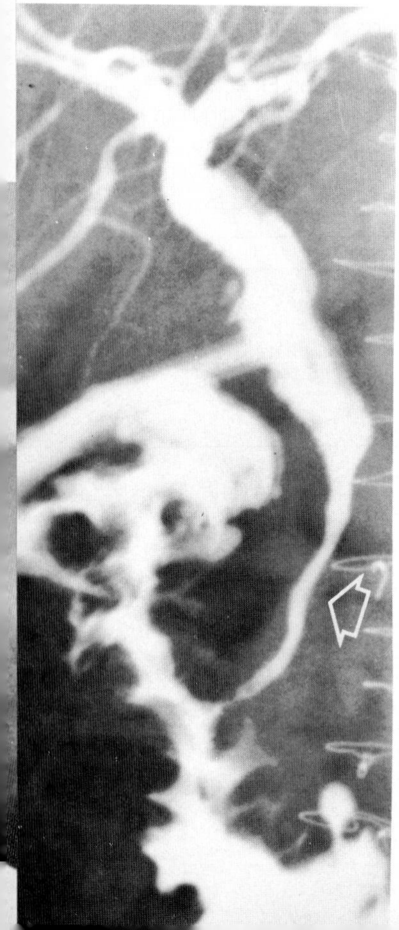

ACUTE PANCREATITIS / ULCER DISEASE

In acute pancreatitis, the enlarged edematous pancreas can circumferentially narrow the common bile duct (Fig. 62-16). This appearance is often reversible when the acute inflammatory process subsides. A strategically located pseudocyst in the head of the pancreas can also displace and narrow the bile duct, producing obstructive jaundice. An unusual cause of benign stricture is a penetrating duodenal ulcer in the region of the bile duct.

Fig. 62-14. Chronic pancreatitis causing smooth narrowing of the intrapancreatic portion of the common bile duct **(arrow)**. Note the associated irregular thickening of folds in the adjacent second portion of the duodenum.

Fig. 62-15. Chronic pancreatitis causing severe narrowing of the common bile duct. Note the abrupt transition between the encased "pipestem" segment and the dilated suprapancreatic portion of the common bile duct **(arrow)**. Calcification suggestive of chronic pancreatitis can also be seen.

Fig. 62-16. Acute pancreatitis. Enlargement of the edematous pancreas circumferentially narrows the common bile duct **(arrows)**.

Fig. 62-15   **Fig. 62-16**

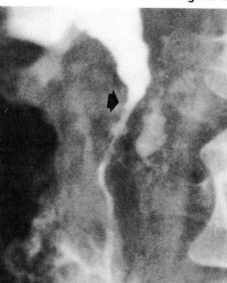
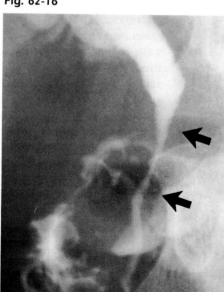

PAPILLARY STENOSIS

Papillary stenosis (stenosis of the sphincter of Oddi) is an ill-defined and controversial entity for which the surgical criterion is failure to pass a dilator larger than a Bakes No. 3 from the common bile duct into the duodenum. Papillary stenosis is associated with chronic inflammatory disease of the biliary tract and pancreas. It appears pathologically as an inflammatory process consisting of mucosal ulceration, granulation tissue, and fibrosis. Papillary stenosis has been suggested as the cause of postcholecystectomy symptoms resembling biliary colic. It can be successfully treated by surgical relief of the obstruction at the choledochoduodenal junction. Radiographically, there is smooth stenosis of the terminal portion of the bile duct with prolonged retention of contrast material in dilated proximal bile ducts.

PARASITIC INFESTATION

Obstructive jaundice can be secondary to parasitic infestation of the biliary tree. The larvae of the liver fluke *Clonorchis sinensis,* ingested by humans who eat uncooked fish in endemic areas in the Orient, enter the biliary tree by passing through the ampulla of Vater. Most of the organisms migrate into the peripheral branches of the bile duct, though some may remain in the larger ducts. The larvae burrow into the duct walls and incite a diffuse inflammatory reaction leading to biliary stricture and stone formation, which, in addition to causing conglomerations of the worms themselves, can result in obstructive jaundice. *Fasciola hepatica* can produce a similar radiographic appearance. In endemic areas of the United States, *Ascaris lumbricoides* infects up to 30% of the population. Although primarily a disease of the bowel, the worms can cross the sphincter of Oddi and cause partial or complete obstruction of bile ducts with resultant cholangitis, cholecystitis, and stone formation.

Many parasites indirectly affect the bile ducts by inhabiting the liver. In patients with *Echinococcus* infestation, large parent cysts can communicate with the biliary tree. Daughter cysts shed into the bile ducts can be trapped in the region of the ampulla and obstruct the common bile duct. Both echinococcal cysts and amebic abscesses can displace and narrow bile ducts. Fibrosis of the periportal connective tissue and contraction of the liver in patients with schistosomiasis can cause irregular narrowing and tortuosity of intrahepatic bile ducts simulating the pattern in cirrhosis.

GRANULOMATOUS DISEASE

Inflammatory processes occurring in lymph nodes adjacent to the common bile duct and porta hepatis can result in biliary obstruction (Fig. 62-17). Tuberculosis (Fig. 62-18), sarcoidosis, and other chronic granulomatous diseases involving periductal lymph nodes can cause compression, narrowing, and even secondary invasion of the hepatic or common bile ducts.

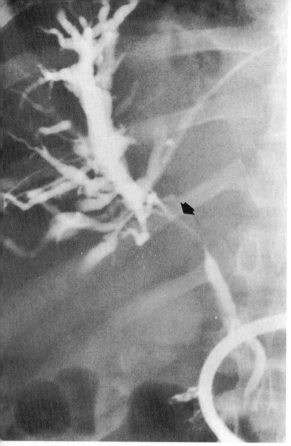

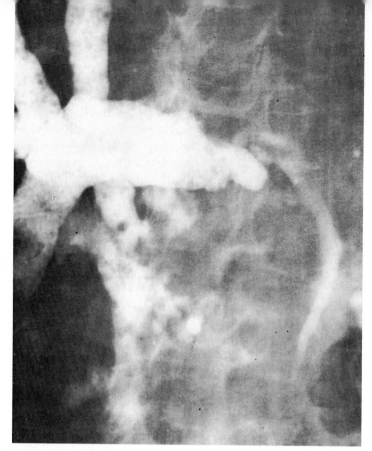

Fig. 62-17. Nonspecific inflammatory mass in the porta hepatis causing narrowing of the common bile duct **(arrow).**

Fig. 62-18. Tuberculous involvement of the biliary ductal system. There is severe stenosis near the junction of the right and common hepatic ducts with innumerable calculi in the intrahepatic ducts.

BILIARY CALCULI

A common duct stone impacted in the ampulla or edema of the papilla secondary to a recently passed stone is a relatively common cause of bile duct obstruction. On cholangiography, an impacted stone in the ampulla appears as a characteristic smooth, concave intraluminal filling defect (Fig. 62-19). In some instances, other radiolucent stones can be identified in proximal segments of the dilated ductal system. An impacted stone or edema following passage of a stone can cause swelling of the papilla that is detectable on an upper gastrointestinal series.

Calculi in the biliary ducts are almost always secondary to gallstones that enter the common bile duct by way of the cystic duct or by erosion. True primary common duct stones arising in the intrahepatic or extrahepatic biliary tree are unusual and tend to occur proximal to a pre-existing stricture or narrowing of the common bile duct. "Common duct stones" in patients who have had their gallbladders removed usually represent retained intrahepatic or extrahepatic duct stones that were not identified at the time of cholecystectomy. After cholecystec-

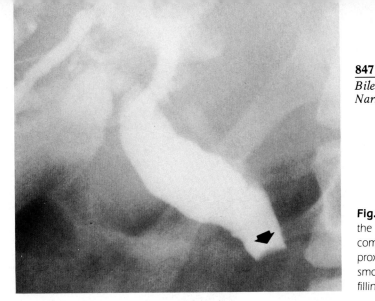

Fig. 62-19. Impacted stone in the ampulla producing common duct obstruction proximal to a characteristic smooth, concave intraluminal filling defect **(arrow)**.

tomy, stones can develop secondary to stasis in a large cystic duct remnant.

In the Mirizzi syndrome, a stone impacted in the cystic duct or neck of the gallbladder erodes into the adjacent common hepatic duct and can result in inflammatory or machanical obstruction of the biliary tree. This characteristically produces narrowing of the ductal lumen as a result of a broad extrinsic impression on the lateral aspect of the common hepatic duct.

SURGICAL / TRAUMATIC STRICTURES

The overwhelming majority of benign strictures of the common bile duct are related to previous biliary tract surgery (Fig. 62-20). They can be caused by severing, clamping, or excessive probing of the common bile duct during the operative procedure. In many cases, the operation is completed without the surgeon being aware that an accident to a major bile duct has occurred. Postoperatively, stricture of the bile duct can be secondary to a suture, biliary leakage, or prolonged T-tube placement. Tearing of a major bile duct can cause a biliary fistula. If the common bile duct or common hepatic duct has been ligated, the patient becomes obviously jaundiced within a few days of surgery. There is often considerable drainage of bile from the T-tube; the volume varies inversely with the degree of jaundice. Infrequently, biliary strictures can be secondary to blunt abdominal trauma with torsion injuries to the common bile duct (Fig. 62-21).

Radiographically, the postoperative stricture is generally smooth and concentric, with the obstructed end appearing funnel-shaped or convex distally, in contrast to the concave margin produced by an obstructing calculus. Unlike malignant lesions, benign strictures tend to involve long segments of the bile duct without total obstruction; there is usually a gradual transition to normal segments of the duct.

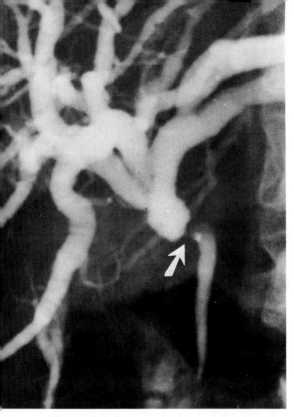

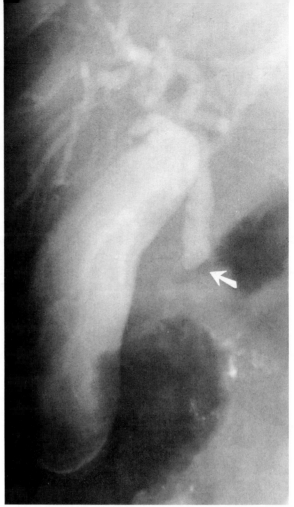

Fig. 62-20. Benign stricture of the common bile duct **(arrow)** related to previous biliary tract surgery.

Fig. 62-21. Benign stricture of the common bile duct **(arrow)** following blunt abdominal trauma.

CONGENITAL / NEONATAL ANOMALIES

BILIARY ATRESIA

The most common cause of persistent neonatal jaundice is biliary atresia. Rather than representing a congenital defect, biliary atresia probably develops postpartum as a complication of a chronic inflammatory process that causes ductal lumen obliteration, which is often segmental and irregular in distribution. Indeed, this condition and neonatal hepatitis may represent opposite extremes of the same disease, with biliary atresia reflecting hepatitis with a component of sclerosing cholangitis of the extrahepatic ducts. The entire extrahepatic biliary ductal system usually is atretic, though the common hepatic duct or common bile duct may be individually involved. Children with this anomaly generally have an unfavorable prognosis. However, in patients with some types of extrahepatic atresia and in persons with biliary hypoplasia, biliary–intestinal anastomosis can result in a cure rate of up to 30% if the diagnosis is made before liver damage progresses to an advanced stage.

MEMBRANOUS DIAPHRAGM

Congenital membranous diaphragm of the common bile or hepatic duct is an extremely rare lesion that is usually not diagnosed until early adult life (Fig. 62-22). The diaphragm can cause chronic partial biliary obstruction resulting in bile stasis, stone formation, and recurring cholangitis.

DUODENAL DIVERTICULUM

Most duodenal diverticula arise within 1 cm to 2 cm of the ampulla. Infrequently, the common duct empties directly into a duodenal diverticulum. When this occurs, the duodenal diverticulum may obstruct the common duct because of anatomic distortion of its entry into the duodenum, diverticulitis, or the presence of an enterolith (of bile acids) within the sac.

OTHER CAUSES OF BILE DUCT NARROWING / OBSTRUCTION

VASCULAR IMPRESSIONS

An extremely rare cause of obstructive jaundice is benign vascular compression of the common bile duct. This mechanism has been reported in two patients, one with a calcified portal vein and another with an aortic aneurysm compressing and occluding the common bile duct.

HEPATIC CYSTS

Rarely, obstructive jaundice is produced by nonparasitic cysts of the liver. Strategically positioned simple cysts or cysts in a polycystic liver can cause a mass effect in the porta hepatitis that narrows the common or hepatic ducts. Decompression of the liver cysts at surgery or under ultrasound guidance results in rapid clearing of jaundice.

CIRRHOSIS

Cirrhosis of any etiology is characterized by progressive destruction of liver cells associated with regeneration of liver substance and fibrosis. During its early stages, the disease usually has little or no effect on the biliary ductal system. Fatty infiltration can cause straightening, elongation with separation, and occasional dilatation of the intrahepatic ducts. As the disease progresses, extrinsic pressure of the regenerating nodules can displace ductal structures. As the liver shrinks with increasing fibrosis, the intrahepatic ducts become crowded together and often assume an irregular tortuous or corkscrew appearance, with of without changes in caliber, that simulates the pattern seen on angiography.

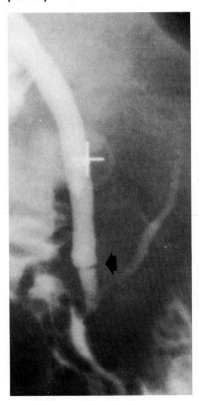

Fig. 62-22. Congenital membranous diaphragm (web) of the common bile duct **(arrow).**

Ameres JP, Levine MP, DeBlasi HP: Acalculous clonorchiasis obstructing the common bile duct. Am Surg 42:170–172, 1976

Balthazar EJ: The Mirizzi syndrome: Inflammatory stricture of the common hepatic duct. Am J Gastroenterol 64:144–148, 1975

Berk RN, Clemett AR: Radiology of the Gallbladder and Bile Ducts. Philadelphia, WB Saunders, 1977

Buonocore E: Transhepatic percutaneous cholangiography. Radiol Clin North Am 14:527–542, 1976

Chang SF, Burrell MI, Brand MH et al: The protean gastrointestinal manifestations of metastatic breast carcinoma. Radiology 126:611–617, 1978

Ergun H, Wolf BH, Hissong SL: Obstructive jaundice caused by polycystic liver disease. Radiology 136:435–436, 1980

Geisse G, Melson GL, Tedesco FJ et al: Stenosing lesions of the biliary tree. Evaluation with endoscopic retrograde cholangiopancreatography (ERC) and percutaneous transhepatic cholangiography (PTC). AJR 123:378–385, 1975

Gerson PD, Schinella RA: Hepatoma presenting as extrahepatic biliary obstruction. Am J Dig Dis 14:42–47, 1969

Ho CS, Wesson DE: Recurrent pyogenic cholangitis in Chinese immigrants. AJR 122:368–374, 1974

Klatskin G: Adenocarcinoma of the hepatic duct at its bifurcation within the porta hepatis: An unusual tumor with distinctive clinical and pathological features. Am J Med 38:241–256, 1965

Krieger J, Seaman WB, Porter MR: The roentgenologic appearance of sclerosing cholangitis. Radiology 94:369–374, 1970

Lang EK: Percutaneous transhepatic cholangiography. Radiology 112:283–290, 1974

Larsen CR, Scholz FJ, Wise RE: Diseases of the biliary ducts. Semin Roentgenol 11:259–267, 1976

Legge DA, Carlson HC: Cholangiographic appearance of primary carcinoma of the bile ducts. Radiology 102:259–266, 1972

Legge DA, Carlson HC, Dickson ER et al: Cholangiographic findings in cholangiolitic hepatitis. AJR 113:16–20, 1971

Menuck L, Amberg J: The bile ducts. Radiol Clin North Am 14:499–523, 1976

Mujahed Z, Evans JA: Pseudocalculus defect in cholangiography. AJR 116:337–341, 1972

Ritchie JK, Allan RN, Macarthney J et al: Biliary tract carcinoma associated with ulcerative colitis. Q J Med 43:263–279, 1974

Rohrmann CA, Ansel HJ, Freeny PC et al: Cholangiographic abnormalities in patients with inflammatory bowel disease. Radiology 127:635–641, 1978

Shingleton WW, Gamburg D: Stenosis of the sphincter of Oddi. Am J Surg 119:35–37, 1970

Tuttle RJ: Cause of recurring obstructive jaundice revealed by percutaneous cholangiography—Hydatid cysts. N Engl J Med 283:805–806, 1970

Warren KW, Mountain JC, Lloyd–Jones W: Malignant tumors of the bile ducts. Br J Surg 59:501–502, 1972

Wastie ML, Cunningham IGE: Roentgenologic findings in recurrent pyogenic cholangitis. AJR 119:71–77, 1973

CYSTIC DILATATION OF THE BILE DUCTS

63

Disease Entities

General bile duct dilatation (see Chap. 62)
Dilatation of extrahepatic bile ducts
  Choledochal cyst
  Choledochocele
  Hepatic duct diverticulum
Dilatation of intrahepatic bile ducts
  Congenital anomalies
    Caroli's disease
    Congenital hepatic fibrosis
  Neoplastic disease
    Papillomatosis
    Epithelioma
  Choledocholithiasis
    Western type
    Oriental type
  Cholangitis
  Cholangiohepatitis (recurrent pyogenic cholangitis)
  Secondary involvement
    Benign tumors
    Malignant tumors
    Parasites (hydatid cysts, *Clonorchis sinensis*, *Ascaris lumbri-coides*)
    Liver infarcts after transcatheter embolization of hepatic artery branches

851

The diameter of the common bile duct on cholangiography should measure 11 mm or less. General dilatation of the bile ducts is usually secondary to an obstructing lesion in the distal common duct. This may be due to an inflammatory or neoplastic process or to an impacted or recently passed biliary calculus (see Chap. 62). It is controversial whether the common bile duct dilates after cholecystectomy because it must assume a reservoir function. It is generally agreed that, unless bile duct pathology (*e.g.*, stenosis, stones, cancer) develops, an extrahepatic system that is normal before gallbladder removal will remain normal in most cholecystectomized patients. In most cases, the finding of an enlarged common bile duct after cholecystectomy merely reflects dilatation that was already present, but possibly not appreciated, before surgery. This interpretation is supported by the fact that the common bile duct frequently does not return to a normal caliber after the operative relief of biliary obstruction.

CHOLEDOCHAL CYST

Fig. 63-1. Choledochal cyst. There is fusiform dilatation of the common bile duct and adjacent portions of the common hepatic and cystic ducts.

A choledochal cyst is a cystic or fusiform dilatation of the common bile duct and adjacent portions of the common hepatic and cystic ducts (Fig. 63-1) that is typically associated with localized constriction of the distal common bile duct (Fig. 63-2). Concomitant dilatation of intra-

Fig. 63-2. Choledochal cyst. Note the localized constriction **(arrow)** separating the cyst from the normal-caliber distal duct.

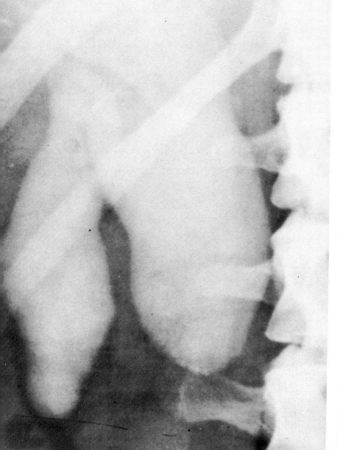

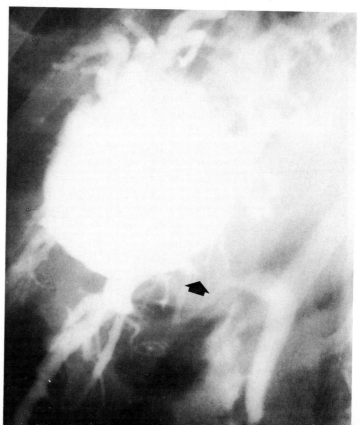

hepatic bile ducts has recently been recognized with increasing frequency (Fig. 63-3). Although usually considered to be a congenital, developmental abnormality, many choledochal cysts are probably acquired lesions caused by regurgitation of pancreatic secretions into the distal common bile duct. This regurgitation, which causes cholangitis, gradual stricture formation, and ductal dilatation over a long period of time, is apparently due to a minor variation in the anatomic development of the confluence of the common bile and pancreatic ducts.

Choledochal cysts are classically described as presenting with a triad of upper abdominal pain, mass, and jaundice. Although the presence of all three is relatively unusual, most patients have at least one of these clinical manifestations. Jaundice is the most common presenting symptom, seen in about 70% of patients. Cholangitis is a frequent complication. Very large cysts can compress neighboring organs, such as the duodenal sweep and head of the pancreas. Rarely, choledochal cysts perforate and cause biliary peritonitis.

A soft-tissue mass representing the markedly dilated bile duct is often seen on plain abdominal radiographs (Fig. 63-4). Upper gastrointestinal examination can demonstrate displacement of the duodenum anteriorly, inferiorly, and to the left. Oral cholecystography and intravenous cholangiography can opacify the choledochal cyst if they are performed between attacks of hepatic dysfunction, but are usually unsuccessful when there is jaundice or distal obstruction. Ultrasound and radionuclide scanning permit specific preoperative diagnosis of a choledochal cyst.

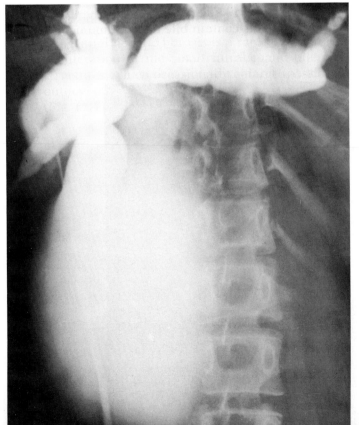

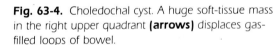

Fig. 63-3. Choledochal cyst. The intrahepatic bile ducts are also involved in the generalized dilatation of the biliary system.

Fig. 63-4. Choledochal cyst. A huge soft-tissue mass in the right upper quadrant **(arrows)** displaces gas-filled loops of bowel.

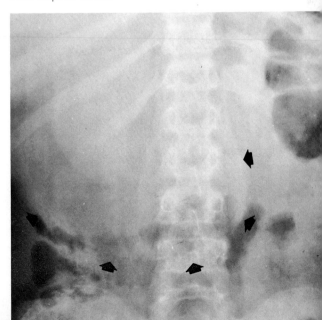

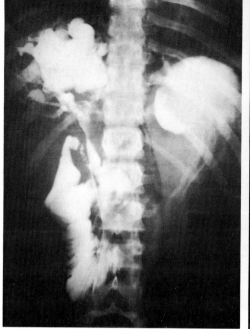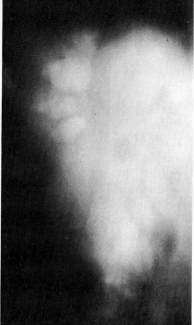

A B

hepatic fibrosis is usually seen in children and is complicated by massive periportal fibrosis leading to portal hypertension, liver decompensation, and gastrointestinal bleeding. Death occurs at an early age as a result of liver failure and portal hypertension.

RADIOGRAPHIC FINDINGS

In both Caroli's disease and congenital hepatic fibrosis, T-tube or operative cholangiography demonstrates large or small cystic spaces communicating with the intrahepatic bile ducts. This produces a "lollipop-tree" appearance of the biliary system (Fig. 63-8A). On intravenous cholangiography, careful evaluation can sometimes demonstrate multiple patchy collections of contrast material in the liver reflecting pools of contrast in dilated, often stone-filled biliary spaces (Fig. 63-8B).

BENIGN TUMORS

Papillomas are fairly common neoplasms of the extrahepatic biliary tract that are most frequently found at the ampulla, where the tumor represents only hypertrophy of a normal anatomic structure. Papillomatosis of the intrahepatic biliary ducts is a rare disease that has been associated with similar tumors in the extrahepatic biliary system and has been described to occur after resection of the ampulla for a papilloma. Colicky right upper abdominal pain and intermittent jaundice, often dating from childhood, is caused by biliary obstruction due to thick mucus material produced by the villous tumors, by fragmentation of the papillary fronds, or by amputation of entire polyps into the biliary tract. Bleeding into the bile ducts from intrahepatic papillomatosis can present as upper gastrointestinal hemorrhage. Radiographically, multiple rounded filling defects resembling nonopaque calculi are evident in the bile ducts. When intrahepatic or extrahepatic ducts are obstructed by large tumors, proximal bile duct dilatation occurs. A high incidence of carcinoma has been reported in patients with this disorder.

Primary epitheliomas of the intrahepatic bile duct are rare. Secondary epitheliomas, also uncommon, can be caused by hepatomatous nodules, which are often large and extend into the biliary ducts, where they obliterate the lumen and cause proximal cystic dilatation.

CHOLEDOCHOLITHIASIS

In Western countries, intrahepatic calculi are almost invariably associated with either extrahepatic calculi or an obstruction in the hilum of the liver. In Oriental countries, intrahepatic lithiasis and cystic dilatation of bile ducts are frequently complications of parasitic infestation. Ascariasis and the liver fluke *Clonorchis sinensis* can cause large, round filling defects in a dilated intrahepatic ductal system. *Clonorchis* infestation is associated with an increased frequency of intrahepatic bile duct carcinoma.

CHOLANGITIS

Cholangitis of any etiology causes diffuse periductal inflammatory fibrosis leading to strictures of varying length and areas of cystic dilatation of the bile ducts. In patients with severe acute suppurative cholangitis, single or multiple small liver abscesses can communicate with the biliary tree and enhance the radiographic appearance of cystic dilatation of intrahepatic bile ducts (Fig. 63-9).

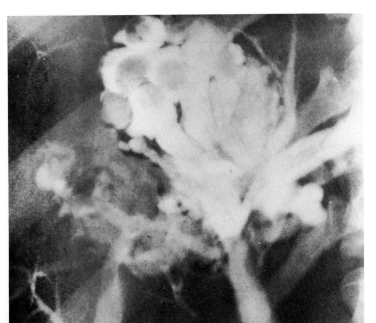

Fig. 63-9. Communicating hepatic abscess simulating localized cystic dilatation of an intrahepatic bile duct.

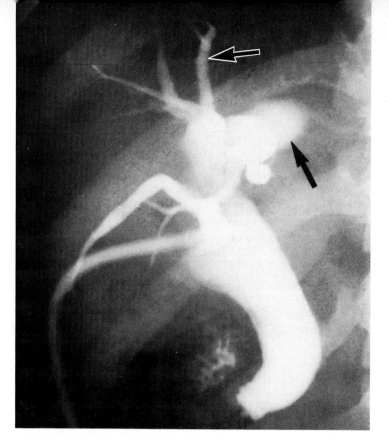

Fig. 63-10. Cholangiohepatitis (recurrent pyogenic cholangitis). A T-tube cholangiogram demonstrates that the common bile duct and intrahepatic duct **(lower arrow)** are dilated. The **upper arrow** shows a moderately dilated bile duct with short branches arising at right angles to the duct. (Ho CS, Wesson DE: Recurrent pyogenic cholangitis in Chinese immigrants. AJR 122:368–374, 1974. Copyright 1974. Reproduced by permission)

CHOLANGIOHEPATITIS

Cholangiohepatitis (recurrent pyogenic hepatitis) is a major cause of an acute abdomen in the Far East and is occasionally seen in Asian immigrants in the United States (Fig. 63-10). It is unclear whether the disease is secondary to *Clonorchis sinensis* infestation causing stone formation, biliary obstruction, stasis, and superimposed infection or whether it is related to portal septicemia resulting from poor eating habits. Cholangiohepatitis is characterized clinically by episodic attacks of right upper quadrant pain, fever, chills, and jaundice; patients may develop severe septicemia and obstructive jaundice requiring immediate surgical drainage of the common bile duct. Radiographic findings include a decreased and abnormal arborization pattern of intrahepatic radicles and segmental dilatation of bile ducts along with areas of rapid peripheral tapering (arrowhead sign). Radiolucent calculi and dilatation of the common bile duct (up to 3–4 cm in diameter) are usually present.

SECONDARY INVOLVEMENT OF THE BILIARY SYSTEM

If large enough, any intrahepatic growth (benign or malignant tumor, parasitic infestation) will distort the segmental biliary ducts of the affected lobe, causing partial obstruction and cystic dilatation of portions of the intrahepatic biliary tree. In patients with hydatid cysts,

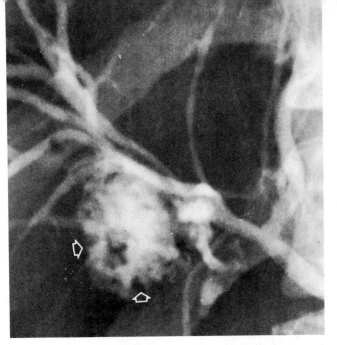

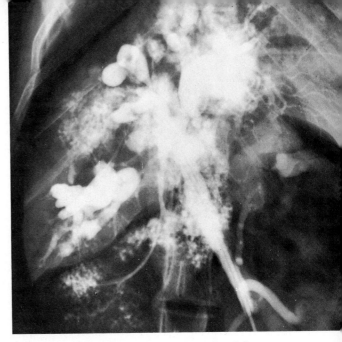

Fig. 63-11. Hydatid disease (echinococcosis). Fistulous communications between the cysts and the bile ducts mimic intrahepatic bile duct dilatation.

Fig. 63-12. Bile duct cysts secondary to liver infarcts. (Doppman JL, Dunnick NR, Girton M et al: Bile duct cysts secondary to liver infarcts: Report of a case and experimental production by small vessel hepatic artery occlusion. Radiology 130:1–5, 1979)

fistulous communications between the cysts and the bile ducts can mimic intrahepatic bile duct dilatation (Fig. 63-11).

Improvements in transcatheter embolization techniques have permitted superselective occlusion of hepatic artery branches for control of hepatic bleeding and for palliative treatment of liver tumors. Rarely, this procedure leads to irreversible ischemia, infarction, and the development of bile cysts that communicate with the biliary tree (Fig. 63-12).

BIBLIOGRAPHY

Babbitt DP, Starshak RJ, Clemett AR: Choledochal cyst: A concept of etiology. AJR 119:57–62, 1973

Belamaric J: Intrahepatic bile duct carcinoma and *C. sinensis* infection in Hong Kong. Cancer 31:468–473, 1973

Berk RN, Clemett AR: Radiology of the Gallbladder and Bile Ducts. Philadelphia, WB Saunders, 1977

Caroli J: Diseases of the intrahepatic biliary tree. Clin Gastroenterol 2:147–161, 1973

Doppman JL, Dunnick NR, Girton M et al: Bile duct cysts secondary to liver infarcts. Report of a case and experimental production by small vessel hepatic artery occlusion. Radiology 130:1–5, 1979

Han BK, Babcock DS, Gelfand MH: Choledochal cyst with bile duct dilatation: Sonography and [99mTc] IDA cholescintigraphy. AJR 136:1075–1079, 1981

Hatfield PM, Scholtz FJ, Wise RE: Congenital disease of the gallbladder and bile ducts. Semin Roentgenol 11:235–243, 1976

Ho CS, Wesson DE: Recurrent pyogenic cholangitis in Chinese immigrants. AJR 122:368–374, 1974

Mall JC, Ghahremani GG, Boyer JL: Caroli's disease associated with congenital hepatic fibrosis and renal tubular ectasia. Gastroenterology 66:1029–1035, 1974

Mueller PR, Ferrucci JT, Simeone JF et al: Postcholecystectomy bile duct dilatation. Myth or reality? AJR 136:355–358, 1981

Mujahed Z, Glenn F, Evans JA: Communicating cavernous ectasia of the intrahepatic ducts (Caroli's disease). AJR 113:21–26, 1971

Reeder MM, Hamilton LC: Radiologic diagnosis of tropical diseases of the gastrointestinal tract. Radiol Clin North Am 7:57–81, 1969

Rosenfield N, Griscom NT: Choledochal cysts: Roentgenographic techniques. Radiology 114:113–119, 1975

Rosewarne MD: Cystic dilatation of the intrahepatic bile duct. Br J Radiol 45:825–827, 1972

Schey WL, Pinsky SM, Lipschutz HS et al: Hepatic duct diverticulum simulating a choledochal cyst. AJR 128:318–320, 1977

Scholz FJ, Carrera GF, Larsen CR: The choledochocele: Correlation of radiological, clinical and pathological findings. Radiology 118:25–28, 1976

Unite I, Maitem A, Bagnasco FM et al: Congenital hepatic fibrosis associated with renal tubular ectasia: A report of three cases. Radiology 109:565–570, 1973

ENLARGEMENT OF THE PAPILLA OF VATER

64

Disease Entities

Normal variant
Papillary edema
  Impacted common duct stone
  Pancreatitis
  Acute duodenal ulcer
Perivaterian neoplasms
  Carcinoma
  Adenomatous polyp
Papillitis
Lesions simulating enlarged papilla
  Benign spindle cell tumor
  Ectopic pancreas

The papilla of Vater is an elevated mound of tissue which projects into the duodenal lumen and into which opens the common bile duct. It can be identified radiographically in about 60% of barium upper gastrointestinal series. It appears as a small, regular indentation surrounded by normal mucosal folds. The papilla is most frequently situated on the inner border of the second portion of the duodenum at or just below the promontory (Fig. 64-1). In about 8% of patients, it is located in the third portion of the duodenum.

The papilla is generally considered to be enlarged whenever the greatest dimension seen radiographically exceeds 1.5 cm. In about 1% of examinations, however, the papilla appears to be larger than 1.5 cm (up to 3 × 1.2 cm) without there being any disease process (Fig. 64-2). This normal variant is a diagnosis of exclusion; all other causes of an enlarged papilla must be ruled out before a normal variant can be seriously considered.

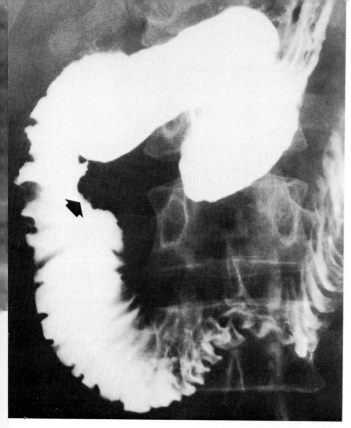

Fig. 64-5. Enlargement of the papilla **(arrow)** in acute pancreatitis.

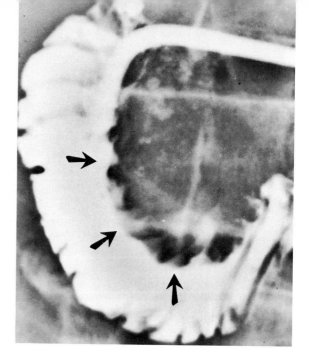

Fig. 64-6. Enlargement of the papilla **(arrows)** in a patient who had chronic pancreatitis and was experiencing an acute exacerbation of the disease.

Fig. 64-7. Enlargement of the papilla in a patient with diffuse peptic ulcer disease **(arrows).** There is generalized thickening of folds throughout the first and second portions of the duodenum.

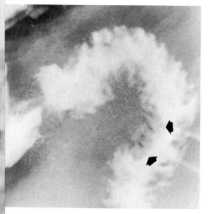

of pancreatitis, it does not exclude the possibility of an impacted biliary stone. However, given that pancreatic calcification develops only infrequently in pancreatitis secondary to gallstones, the presence of such calcification in a patient with an enlarged papilla makes an impacted common duct stone an unlikely diagnosis.

In patients with acute duodenal ulcer disease, diffuse enlargement of the duodenal mucosal folds can occur. When the second portion of the duodenum is involved, maximum fold thickening tends to occur at the apex of the bulb, with the enlarged folds gradually decreasing in size distally. This enlargement of folds extends to and beyond the region of the papilla. The papillary fold can participate in this generalized edema and, because the papilla is larger than other duodenal folds, can become especially prominent (Fig. 64-7). If enlargement of the papilla is due to acute duodenal ulcer disease, a bulbar ulcer crater can almost invariably be demonstrated.

In patients with an impacted common duct stone, the papilla is primarily enlarged; duodenal fold thickening gradually decreases away from the papilla. In pancreatitis, the pattern of papilla enlargement and thickening of duodenal folds can appear identical to that seen in peptic ulcer disease. However, associated pancreatic swelling or calcification is usually also seen.

PERIVATERIAN NEOPLASMS

Perivaterian carcinomas (a collective term for malignancies arising in the duodenum, head of the pancreas, distal common bile duct, and ampulla of Vater) can protrude into the duodenal lumen and give the radiographic appearance of enlargement of the papilla (Fig. 64-8). In addition to the tumor mass, papillary enlargement can reflect malignant lymphatic obstruction with secondary papillary edema. In patients with perivaterian neoplasms, the surface of the papilla is often irregular and can demonstrate local erosion (Fig. 64-9). There is no thickening of surrounding duodenal folds, as may be seen in enlargement of the papilla due to edema. Perivaterian carcinoma occasionally has a smooth surface and appears identical to a benign edematous process.

Adenomatous polyps of the papilla of Vater can have a radiographic appearance simulating enlargement of the papilla. These tumors often have considerable inflammatory hyperplasia. Because evidence of foci of low-grade malignancy is usually histologically detectable, these adenomatous polyps of the papilla are generally considered to be premalignant lesions.

PAPILLITIS

Periductal inflammation and hyperplastic ductal proliferation can result in papillary "polyps." Rather than being a true neoplasm, this process is more likely an inflammatory reaction (papillitis) that eventually produces sphincter stenosis because of the formation of exuberant fibrosis.

Fig. 64-8. Adenocarcinoma of the duodenum giving the radiographic appearance of enlargement of the papilla **(arrows).**

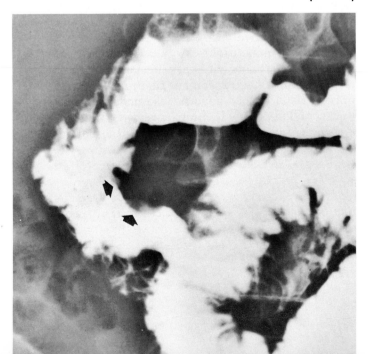

Fig. 64-9. Villous adenocarcinoma of the ampulla producing irregular enlargement of the papilla **(arrows).**

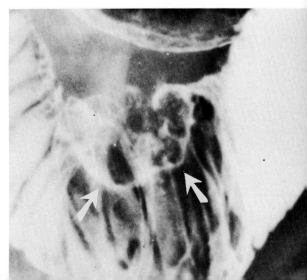

A benign spindle cell tumor situated on the inner aspect of the second portion of the duodenum can mimic an enlarged papilla and, unless the papilla itself is clearly demonstrated, can be difficult to distinguish from papillary enlargement. Similarly, ectopic pancreatic tissue in the descending duodenum can simulate papillary edema. The presence of a central barium collection (ulcer or rudimentary duct) in what appears to be an enlarged papilla should suggest the possibility of a spindle cell tumor (especially leiomyoma) or ectopic pancreas.

DIFFERENTIAL DIAGNOSIS

Because a variety of entities can produce an almost identical radiographic pattern of enlargement of the papilla, clinical and laboratory data are essential to the proper diagnosis. Whenever an enlarged papilla is seen without jaundice, the most likely cause is ectopic pancreas, duodenal leiomyoma, or a large normal papilla. If jaundice, inflammatory manifestations, or clinical signs of malignancy are present, papillary enlargement suggests an impacted common duct stone, pancreatitis, duodenal ulcer disease, or perivaterian carcinoma. Jaundice is usually progressive in patients with malignancy; it can subside or fluctuate in patients with impacted common duct stones and is generally mild in persons with pancreatitis.

Patients with impacted common duct stones frequently have a previous history of cholelithiasis or biliary colic. Persons with pancreatitis causing papillary enlargement report similar episodes of abdominal pain and a history of alcohol abuse. In both of these benign conditions, the abdominal pain usually has an abrupt onset; in contrast, the pain associated with malignancy is generally more insidious. Fever and leukocytosis are frequently noted in patients with impacted common duct stones or acute pancreatitis; weight loss is more likely to reflect a malignant tumor or chronic pancreatitis. Guaiac-positive stools are fairly common in patients with perivaterian malignancy but rare in persons with impacted stones or pancreatitis. A palpable gallbladder can be felt in about one-fourth of patients with perivaterian malignancy but is rare in persons with papillary enlargement due to pancreatitis or an impacted common duct stone. Serum amylase or lipase levels are almost universally elevated in patients with pancreatitis. Transient elevation of these enzymes can be seen in about one-third of patients with impacted common duct stones but is unusual in persons with malignant perivaterian neoplasms.

BIBLIOGRAPHY

Berk RN, Clemett AR: Radiology of the Gallbladder and Bile Ducts. Philadelphia, WB Saunders, 1977

Bree RL, Flynn RE: Hypotonic duodenography in the evaluation of choledocholithiasis and obstructive jaundice. AJR 116:309–319, 1972

Eaton SB, Ferrucci JT, Benedict KT et al: Diagnosis of choledocholithiasis by barium duodenal examination. Radiology 102:267–273, 1972

Eaton SB, Ferrucci JT, Margulis AR et al: Unfamiliar roentgen findings in pancreatic disease. AJR 116:396–405, 1972

Griffen WO, Schaefer JW, Schindler S et al: Ampullary obstruction by benign duodenal polyps. Arch Surg 97:444–449, 1968

Jacobson HG, Shapiro JH, Pisano D et al: The vaterian and peri-vaterian segments in peptic ulcer. AJR 79:793–798, 1958

Oh C, Jemerin EE: Benign adenomatous polyps of the papilla of Vater. Surgery 57:495–503, 1965

Poppel MH: The roentgen manifestations of relapsing pancreatitis. Radiology 62:514–521, 1954

Poppel MH, Jacobson HG, Smith RW: The Roentgen Aspects of the Papilla and Ampulla of Vater. Springfield, IL, Charles C Thomas, 1953

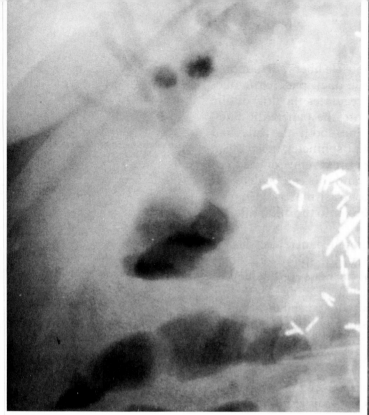

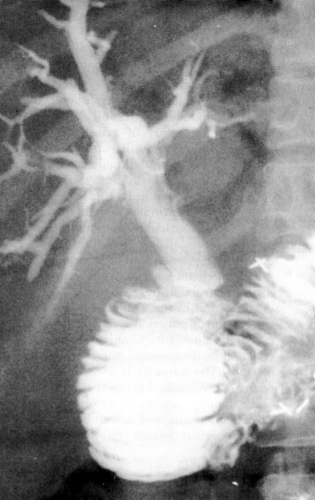

Fig. 65-1. (A) Gas in the biliary tree and **(B)**
pancreaticoduodenal reflux of barium in a patient who had
undergone a surgical procedure to relieve biliary
obstruction.

Fig. 65-2. Gas in the biliary tree following
cholecystoduodenostomy for stricture of the common bile
duct.

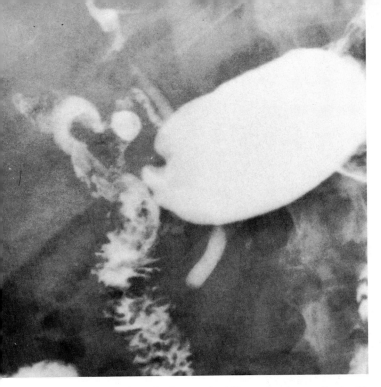

Fig. 65-3. Pancreaticobiliary reflux in a patient with gallstone ileus. Note that barium fills the tract extending from the gallbladder to the duodenal bulb. The distal common bile duct and region of the papilla are normal.

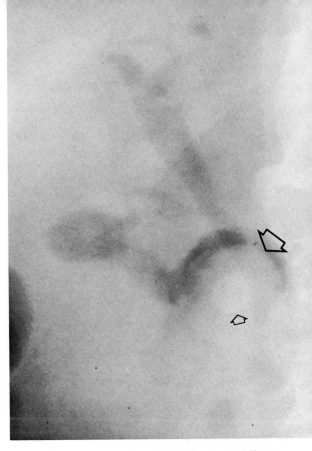

Fig. 65-4. Gas in the biliary tree due to fistulization between the gallbladder and duodenum. Note the central calcification **(small arrow)** within the offending gallstone **(large arrow),** which is situated in the duodenum.

Fistulas between the biliary system and duodenum are occasionally present without gas in the biliary tree. This occurs in the patient with a cholecystoduodenal fistula in whom the cystic duct is obstructed by a stone or tumor. In this situation, gas is unable to enter the biliary tree, though it is often present in the gallbladder.

In patients with severe peptic ulcer disease, fistulas can extend from the duodenum or stomach into the gallbladder or bile duct. Jaundice or cholangitis can develop in these patients, but biliary involvement is often asymptomatic and is usually only incidentally discovered on plain abdominal radiographs or on an upper gastrointestinal series. Acute spasm or fibrous healing of a postbulbar ulcer adjacent to the papilla or acute inflammation of the head of the pancreas can deform the orifice of the ampulla and lead to incompetence of the sphincter of Oddi and pancreaticobiliary reflux (Fig. 65-6).

Rigidity of the duodenal wall, caused by the diffuse cicatrization that is associated with granulomatous disease of the duodenum, can result in gas in the biliary tree and pancreaticobiliary reflux. In Crohn's disease, reflux is postulated to occur either by fistula formation or through a damaged ampulla of Vater. In strongyloidiasis, periampullary scarring and incompetence of the sphincter of Oddi can produce a similar radiographic appearance.

Gas in the biliary tree and pancreaticobiliary reflux can be due to biliary infestation by *Clonorchis sinensis* or *Ascaris lumbricoides. Clon-*

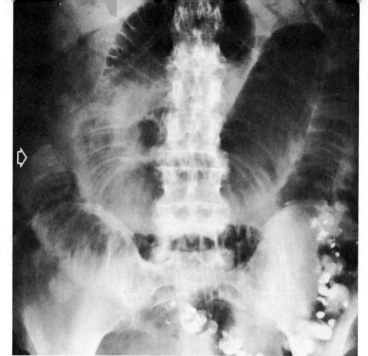

Fig. 65-5. Gallstone ileus. An obstructing stone **(open arrow)** causes dilatation of proximal small bowel loops. Note the gas in the biliary tree **(solid arrow).**

Fig. 65-6. Two patients with pancreaticobiliary reflux associated with postbulbar peptic ulcers **(arrows).**

A B

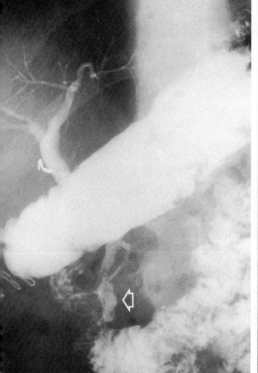 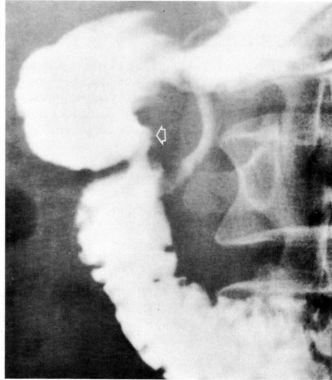

orchis is a parasitic fluke that is acquired by the ingestion of raw freshwater fish. The parasite migrates from the duodenum into the biliary tree, where it may live for many years and incite an inflammatory reaction. This inflammation predisposes to stone formation, obstruction, secondary bacterial infection, and scarring. Recurrent attacks of abdominal pain and cholangitis are common. *Clonorchis* should be considered a possible cause of gas in the biliary tree and pancreaticobiliary reflux in patients with the appropriate clinical symptomatology who have spent a long time in the Orient. *Ascaris* invades the bile ducts by passing through the sphincter of Oddi from the duodenum. Migration of the worms can disrupt the normal sphincter architecture and permit reflux into the common bile duct. Once in the biliary system, the worms or their ova induce an inflammatory response that can lead to progressive cholangitis and bile duct obstruction.

MALIGNANT DISEASES

Gas in the biliary tree and pancreaticobiliary reflux can be seen in patients with primary or metastatic lesions involving the ampulla of Vater or perivaterian region. Indeed, the appearance of biliary reflux in a patient without a history of surgery or known Crohn's disease points to perivaterian malignancy as the most likely etiology.

EMPHYSEMATOUS CHOLECYSTITIS

Gas in the bile ducts is an infrequent occurrence in patients with emphysematous cholecystitis (Fig. 65-7). Its presence suggests that the cystic duct is patent, allowing gas to escape from the gallbladder lumen. If gas is not also identified in the wall of the gallbladder, the diagnosis of emphysematous cholecystitis may not even be considered.

CONGENITAL ANOMALY

Spontaneous reflux from the duodenum into the pancreatic or common bile duct can occur without any duodenal or pancreaticobiliary disease. This is a rare occurrence that is usually associated with the anomalous insertion of one or both of these ducts into a duodenal diverticulum.

PSEUDOPNEUMOBILIA

An appearance simulating gas in the biliary tree (pseudopneumobilia) is occasionally produced by the normal periductal fat that surrounds and parallels the course of the major bile ducts (Fig. 65-8). This lucent band is continuous with the extraperitoneal fat outlining the visceral border of the liver. It is typically wider than a nonobstructed ductal system, is not as radiolucent as gas in the bile ducts, and does not involve the intrahepatic portion of the biliary tree. The true nature of pseudopneumobilia is readily apparent on intravenous cholangiography.

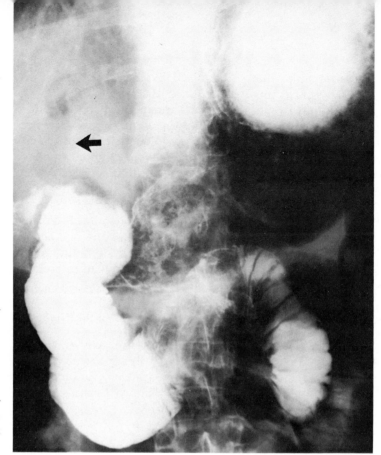

Fig. 65-7. Gas in the biliary tree **(arrow)** in a patient with phlegmonous emphysematous gastritis.

Fig. 65-8. Pseudopneumobilia. **(A)** On a plain abdominal radiograph, the curved tubular radiolucent band **(arrows)** projecting over the upper renal pole (together with the liver shadow) was interpreted as "air in the biliary system." An upper gastrointestinal series showed no fistulous communication. **(B)** An intravenous cholangiogram demonstrates the shape and position of the normal common bile ducts, particularly the sleevelike lucent periductal fat paralleling their contours. Extraperitoneal fat outlining the visceral border of the liver is continuous with the periductal hilar fat. (Govoni AF, Meyers MA: Pseudopneumobilia. Radiology 118:536, 1976)

A B

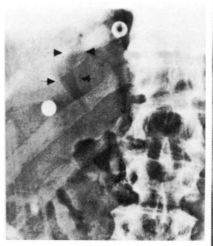
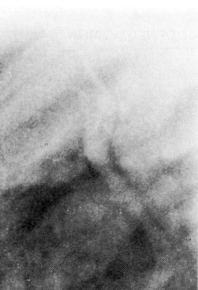

Berk RN, Clemett AR: Radiology of the Gallbladder and Bile Ducts. Philadelphia, WB Saunders, 1977

Eaton SB, Benedict KT, Ferrucci JT et al: Hypotonic duodenography. Radiol Clin North Am 8:125–137, 1970

Eaton SB, Ferrucci JT, Margulis AR et al: Unfamiliar roentgen findings in pancreatic disease. AJR 116:396–405, 1972

Govoni AF, Meyers MA: Pseudopneumobilia. Radiology 118:526, 1976

Haff RC, Wise L, Ballinger WF: Biliary–enteric fistulas. Surg Gynecol Obstet 133:84–88, 1971

Harley WD, Kirkpatrick RH, Ferrucci JT: Gas in the bile ducts (pneumobilia) in emphysematous cholecystitis. AJR 131:661–663, 1978

Hoppenstein JM, Medoza B, Watne AL: Choledochoduodenal fistula due to perforating duodenal ulcer disease. Ann Surg 173:145–147, 1971

Legge DA, Carlson HC, Judd ES: Roentgenologic features of regional enteritis of the upper gastrointestinal tract. AJR 110:355–360, 1970

Poppel MH, Jacobson HG, Smith RW: The Roentgen Aspects of the Papilla and Ampulla of Vater. Springfield, IL, Charles C Thomas, 1953

Shehadi WH: Radiologic examination of the biliary tree. Radiol Clin North Am 4:463–482, 1966

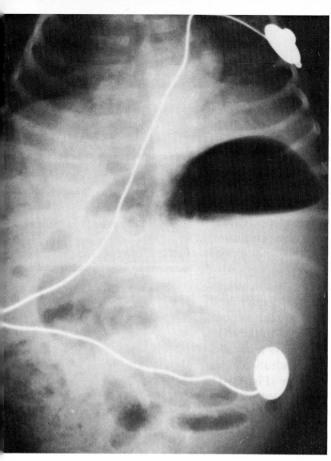

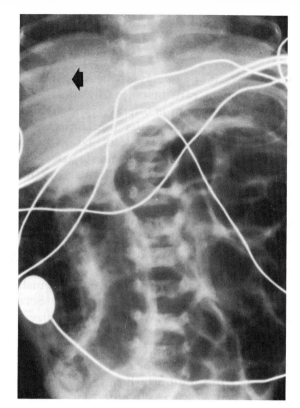

Fig. 66-2. Portal vein gas **(arrow)** in an infant who died of necrotizing enterocolitis.

Fig. 66-1. Portal vein gas. Note the characteristic radiographic appearance of tubular lucencies extending to the edge of the liver. This infant died from acute necrotizing enterocolitis.

where they cause hemolysis of fetal red blood cells. This hemolysis of fetal cells before birth causes jaundice, anemia, edema, splenomegaly, and hepatomegaly in the newborn infant. The presence of gas in the portal veins is a dire prognostic sign.

UMBILICAL VEIN CATHETERIZATION

In relatively asymptomatic infants, the presence of an umbilical vein catheter in association with portal vein gas excludes most serious illnesses (Fig. 66-3). Portal vein gas in these infants is caused by inadvertent injection of air during umbilical venous catheterization or during drug administration through the catheter and does not reflect a potentially fatal disorder. Umbilical venous catheterization offers a simple pathway through which to give fluids and medications to infants with respiratory distress and other medical problems. The tip of the catheter should be positioned in the inferior vena cava, just below the right hemidiaphragm. To reach this point, the catheter must pass through the umbilical vein and cross the ductus venosus before entering the inferior vena cava. If the catheter lodges in the umbilical vein or ductus venosus, or if it reaches the portal sinus, any gas inadvertently administered through it is injected almost directly into the hepatic portal venous system.

ADULT DISORDERS

In adults, most cases of gas in the portal veins are associated with mesenteric arterial occlusion and bowel infarction. Gas in the portal veins has also been described in patients with diabetes, mesenteric vein thrombosis, hemorrhagic pancreatitis, diverticulitis, pelvic abscesses, perforated gastric ulcers, necrotic colon carcinoma, and emphysematous cholecystitis (Fig. 66-4), and after acute necrotizing gastroenteritis following the ingestion of corrosive substances or hydrogen peroxide colon lavage. Portal vein gas has been demonstrated in a few patients with ulcerative or Crohn's colitis after barium enema examination. Unless associated with free perforation, this complication does not cause symptoms or appear to be associated with complications.

PROGNOSIS OF PORTAL VEIN GAS

On rare occasions, the discovery of gas in the portal veins has led to immediate surgery and patient survival. Nevertheless, except in the case of the asymptomatic infant with an umbilical venous catheter or the patient with ulcerative or Crohn's colitis following barium enema examination, gas in the portal veins is generally associated with an extremely dismal prognosis.

Fig. 66-3. Portal vein gas related to umbilical catheterization. **(A)** This newborn male infant was noted to have "grunting respirations." The symptoms rapidly cleared. Note the portal vein gas **(open arrow)** and the tip of the catheter in the umbilical vein **(solid arrow). (B)** This newborn male infant had mild respiratory distress, which cleared rapidly. Note the portal vein gas **(arrow)** and the umbilical catheter, its tip (not identified in this picture) in the umbilical vein. (Swaim TJ, Gerald B: Hepatic portal venous gas in infants without subsequent death. Radiology 94:343–345, 1970)

A B

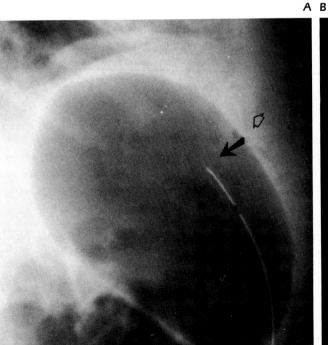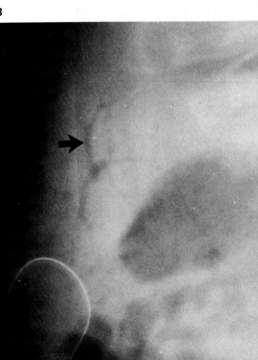

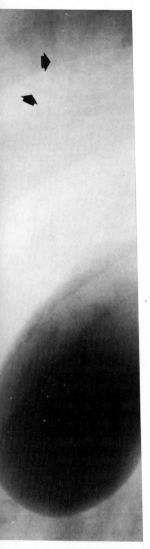

Fig. 66-4. Porta
(arrows) associ
emphysematous cho

BULL'S-EYE LESIONS IN THE GASTROINTESTINAL TRACT

Disease Entities

Metastatic melanoma
Primary neoplasms
   Spindle cell tumor (benign or malignant)
   Lymphoma
   Carcinoid
   Carcinoma
Hematogenous metastases
   Breast cancer
   Lung cancer
   Renal cancer
   Kaposi's sarcoma
Eosinophilic granuloma
Ectopic pancreas

Bull's-eye or target lesions of the gastrointestinal tract reflect ulceration or umbilication of mass lesions. The ulceration can cause gastrointestinal hemorrhage and, if the underlying mass lesion is sufficiently large, can be associated with intestinal obstruction.

METASTATIC MELANOMA

Multiple bull's-eye lesions in the gastrointestinal tract are highly suggestive of metastatic melanoma (Fig. 67-1). This tumor metastasizes widely and frequently involves the gastrointestinal tract, usually sparing the large bowel. Metastases of melanoma can be well-circumscribed round or oval nodules, plaques, or sessile or pedunculated polypoid masses. As the metastasis outgrows its blood supply, central ulceration

883

is common. The borders of the filling defect are sharply defined, and the ulcer is quite large relative to the size of the metastatic mass. Some nodules of metastatic melanoma can be centrally umbilicated without there being actual ulceration. Metastatic melanoma in the form of an enlarging pedunculated mass projecting into the bowel lumen can lead to intussusception. Gastrointestinal metastases can be the first clinical manifestation of metastatic melanoma; at times, it can be impossible to identify the primary tumor site. In a patient with a known primary melanoma, the presence of multiple bull's-eye gastrointestinal lesions is virtually pathognomonic of metastatic melanoma.

PRIMARY NEOPLASMS

Spindle cell tumors of the bowel (especially leiomyoma) can demonstrate central necrosis and ulceration of the overlying mucosal surface, which give rise to gastrointestinal hemorrhage and the radiographic appearance of a single bull's-eye lesion (Fig. 67-2). Central ulceration of a discrete mass (occasionally multiple) is one of the many manifestations of gastrointestinal lymphoma (Fig. 67-3). Infrequently, an ulcerated carcinoid tumor or primary carcinoma of the small bowel can present as an isolated bull's-eye lesion.

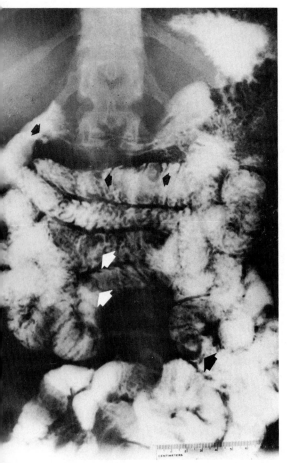

Fig. 67-1. Metastatic melanoma. Multiple nodular filling defects **(arrows)** varying from 6 mm to 2 cm in diameter are present throughout the small bowel. Central ulceration can be identified in most of the lesions; in some, the central ulcer is large in relation to the size of the mass, causing a bull's-eye appearance. At least ten separate discrete nodular lesions could be identified on the complete series of original radiographs. Except for the isolated lesions, the small bowel is normal in appearance. (Cavanagh RC, Buchignani JS, Rulon DB: RPC of the month from the AFIP. Radiology 101:195–200, 1971)

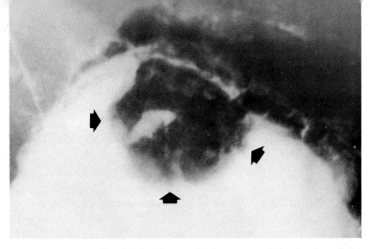

Fig. 67-2. Ulcerated leiomyoma of the fundus of the stomach **(arrows)** causing a bull's-eye appearance.

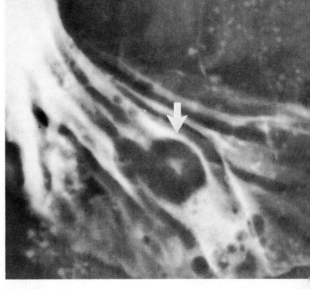

Fig. 67-3. Lymphoma of the stomach **(arrow)** with central ulceration presenting as a bull's-eye lesion.

HEMATOGENOUS METASTASES

Hematogenous metastases can cause multiple ulcerating mass lesions of the bowel (Fig. 67-4). Breast cancer metastasizes to the gastrointestinal tract, especially the stomach and duodenum, in about 15% of cases. Although this tumor does not elicit a desmoplastic response, the highly cellular deposits can narrow and deform the lumen, causing a scirrhous appearance. Metastases to the small bowel usually produce large mesenteric masses, with infiltration of the bowel wall, fixation, and angulation. Occasionally, there are discrete submucosal masses that may have central ulceration (Fig. 67-5).

KAPOSI'S SARCOMA

Kaposi's sarcoma is a systemic disease that characteristically affects the skin and causes an ulcerated hemorrhagic dermatitis. The typical nodules or pigmented patches initially involve the extremities and are frequently associated with intense edema, which causes the limbs to become firm, thick, and heavily pachydermatous. Biopsy and histologic studies show that the Kaposi's lesions are composed of capillaries that sometimes anastomose freely. The space between the blood vessels is filled with spindle-shaped cells and reticulin fibers resembling a well-differentiated fibrosarcoma. The lesions are sensitive to irradiation and have a low-grade malignant course.

Kaposi's sarcoma is most common in middle-aged or elderly men from countries in Eastern Europe and northern Italy. It is also extremely prevalent in parts of Africa, where it makes up 10% of all malignant neoplasms.

Most patients with multiple skin nodules inevitably develop visceral disease as well, though this may not be manifest at the time of the

and delay in transit time can be noted. In the more common left paraduodenal hernia, small bowel loops pass into the paraduodenal fossa posteriorly and into the left mesocolon, producing dilated loops of small bowel clustered in the left upper quadrant of the abdomen lateral to the fourth portion of the duodenum (Fig. 68-2). Paraduodenal hernias occurring on the right side are associated with incomplete intestinal rotation. The junction of the duodenum and jejunum has a low, right paramedian position. The duodenum is dilated, and the jejunal loops are situated on the right side of the abdomen, extending into the right transverse mesocolon. In both types of paraduodenal hernia, the transverse colon tends to be depressed inferiorly by the mass.

Repeated episodes of paraduodenal herniation can increase the size of the defect and lead to adhesions between the intestinal loops or between the trapped bowel and hernia sac. This process can result in obstruction or circulatory compromise. Therefore, even a small paraduodenal hernia is potentially dangerous and is usually considered an operable condition.

LESSER SAC HERNIA

Herniation into the lesser peritoneal sac through the foramen of Winslow is a rare condition that typically presents as an acute abdominal emergency. Unless promptly relieved by surgery, it can rapidly lead to intestinal strangulation and death. The lesser sac is a potential space bounded anteriorly by the caudate lobe of the liver, the lesser omentum, the posterior wall of the stomach, and the anterior layer of the greater omentum. The posterior border includes the left kidney and adrenal gland, pancreas, transverse colon and mesocolon, and posterior layer of the greater omentum. The lateral margin consists of the spleen and the phrenicolienal and gastrolienal ligaments. The free edge of the hepatoduodenal ligament (containing the bile duct, hepatic arteries,

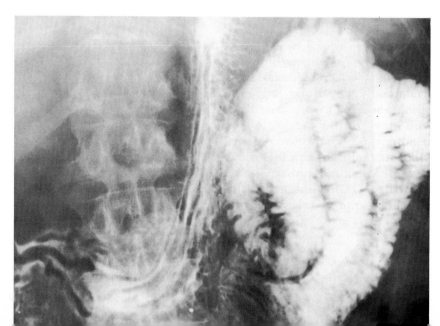

Fig. 68-2. Left paraduodenal hernia. Small bowel loops are clustered in the left upper quadrant lateral to the fourth portion of the duodenum and the stomach.

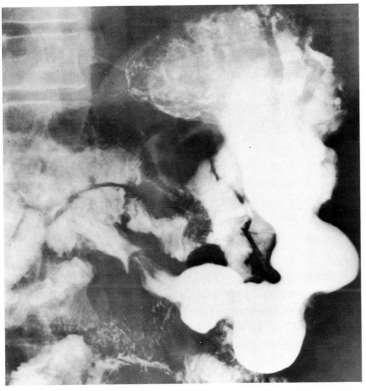

Fig. 68-3. Herniation through the foramen of Winslow into the lesser sac. Loops of small bowel are seen in an abnormal position along the lesser curvature medial and posterior to the stomach.

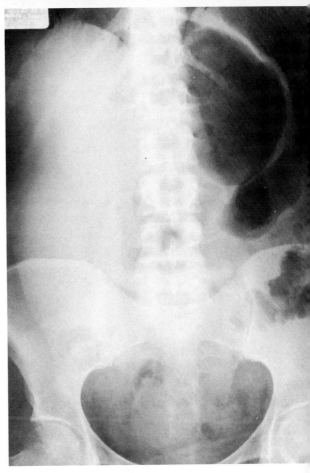

Fig. 68-4. Cecal herniation through the foramen of Winslow. Gas in the cecum is seen medial and posterior to the stomach. There is no gas or fecal material in the right lower quadrant. (Henisz A, Matesanz J, Westcott JL: Cecal herniation through the foramen of Winslow. Radiology 112:575–578, 1974)

and portal vein) forms the right border of the lesser sac and the anterior margin of the foramen of Winslow. The posterior margin of the foramen is the anterior surface of the inferior vena cava.

Lesser sac hernias can contain small bowel, colon, gallbladder, or merely omentum. Radiographically, abnormal gas-filled loops of bowel can be seen along the lesser curvature medial and posterior to the stomach. The herniated bowel and omentum displace the stomach and transverse colon anteriorly, inferiorly, and to the left. Oral contrast reveals bunched and dilated bowel confined, as if in a bag, in the left upper and midabdomen (Fig. 68-3). If incarceration occurs, multiple fluid levels can be seen within the limits of the lesser sac. Dilatation, stretching, and medial displacement of the duodenum are commonly seen. This finding is of value in the differentiation of an intestinal hernia from a lesser sac abscess, which displaces the descending duodenum laterally rather than medially. If large bowel (especially cecum) protrudes into the lesser sac, the presence of gas medial and posterior to the stomach is associated with an absence of gas and fecal material in the right lower quadrant (Fig. 68-4). A barium enema examination in this condition can demonstrate compression of the colon as it passes through the foramen of Winslow, or tapering of a contrast-filled segment pointing to the opening of the lesser peritoneal sac.

OTHER INTERNAL HERNIAS

Very rarely, internal hernias occur in one of the four principal fossae located in the region of the cecum (ileocolic, ileocecal, retro-appendiceal, and retrocecal; Fig. 68-5). Herniation through the small bowel mesentery (Fig. 68-6), sigmoid mesentery, or broad ligament is also extremely rare. Posterolateral herniation of colon or small bowel with bowel gas overlying the posterior portion of the spine (lumbar hernia) is an uncommon lesion that usually follows trauma but occasionally occurs spontaneously.

INGUINAL / FEMORAL HERNIAS

Herniation of loops of bowel into an inguinal or femoral hernia sac is relatively frequent. When this occurs, gas-filled loops of bowel can be seen to extend beyond the normal pelvic contour on plain abdominal radiographs or may be filled with barium during contrast examination. Left-sided hernias tend to involve the sigmoid colon. Right-sided hernia sacs usually contain small bowel (Fig. 68-7); infrequently, the cecum is present in the hernia. A long segment of bowel occasionally extends into a large scrotal hernia (Fig. 68-8). Although inguinal hernias tend to be larger than femoral ones, it is usually difficult to distinguish between them radiographically.

Fig. 68-5. Internal hernia of the ileum. **(A)** A plain abdominal radiograph demonstrates a large soft-tissue mass (pseudotumor) in the right lower quadrant. **(B)** A barium enema examination demonstrates obstruction to flow in the distal ileum **(arrow)** as it enters the internal hernia.

A B

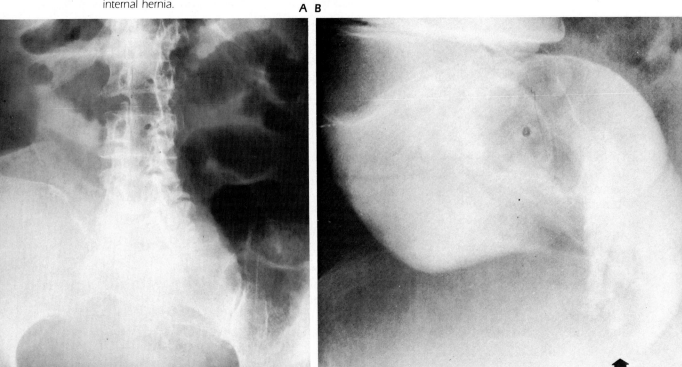

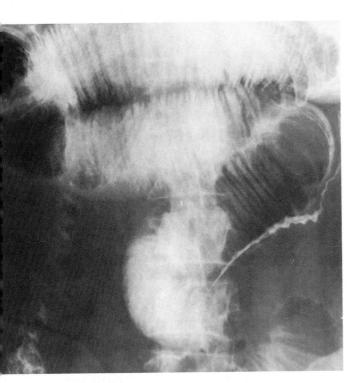

Fig. 68-6. Herniation of small bowel through a hole in the mesentery. Note the marked dilatation of small bowel proximal to the point of obstruction.

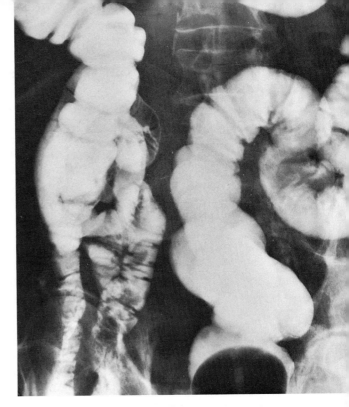

Fig. 68-7. Right inguinal hernia containing distal ileum.

Fig. 68-8. Large scrotal hernia containing sigmoid colon.

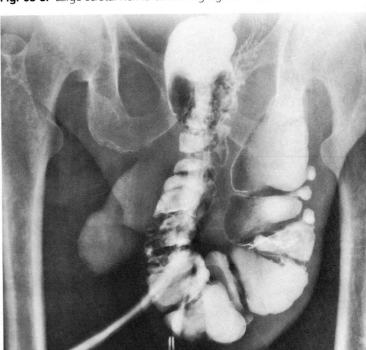

OBTURATOR HERNIA

Obturator hernias are rare lesions that are far more common in females than males and occur most often on the right side (Fig. 68-9). An obturator hernia can contain any or all of the internal female genital organs, urinary bladder, variable segments of small and large bowel, appendix, and omentum. Early diagnosis is imperative, because the signs of small bowel obstruction in an obturator hernia are more apt to become manifest after strangulation or other complication occurs. A positive Howship–Romberg sign, although not always present, is highly indicative of this condition. The sign consists of pain along the inner aspect of the thigh to the knee or below and is due to compression of the obturator nerve by the hernial contents. Although the hernia is infrequently palpable externally, it can often be felt by vaginal or rectal examination. Radiographic examination may demonstrate gas or contrast agent within a herniated segment of bowel confined to the region of the obturator canal.

HERNIATION THROUGH THE ANTERIOR ABDOMINAL WALL

Herniation of bowel occurs not uncommonly through the anterior abdominal wall (umbilical hernia, ventral hernia, postoperative incisional hernia). Because this is essentially a clinical diagnosis, radiographic examination is used only to demonstrate the nature of the

Fig. 68-9. Obturator hernia containing sigmoid colon.

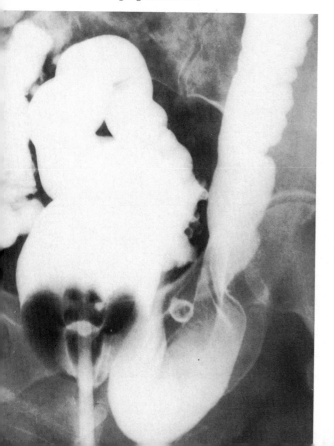

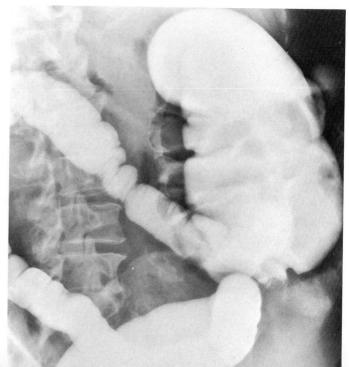

Fig. 68-10. Umbilical hernia. A barium enema examination demonstrates a dilated cecum in the hernia sac.

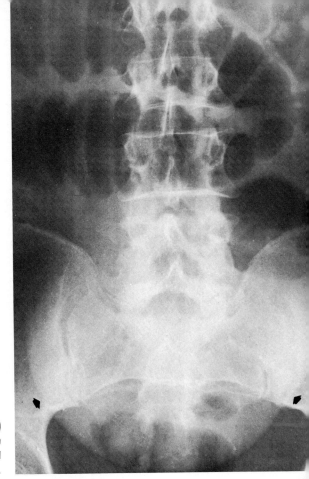

Fig. 68-11. Umbilical hernia. A large soft-tissue mass **(arrows)** in the midabdomen and upper pelvis is clearly demonstrated on a plain abdominal radiograph. The loops of small bowel proximal to the obstruction are dilated.

Fig. 68-12. Umbilical hernia. **(A)** On the frontal view, bowel loops within the hernia sac are superimposed on normal intraperitoneal loops. **(B)** A lateral radiograph clearly shows that the bowel loops are in the hernia sac.

A B

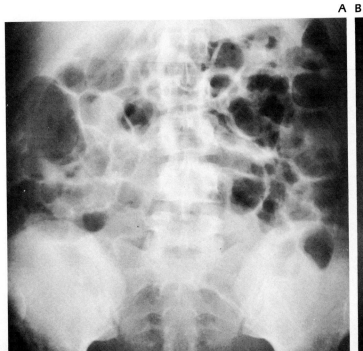 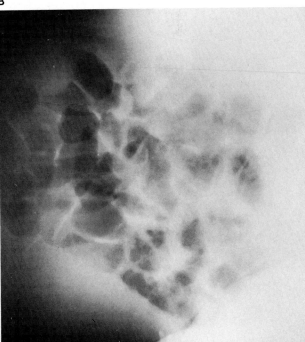

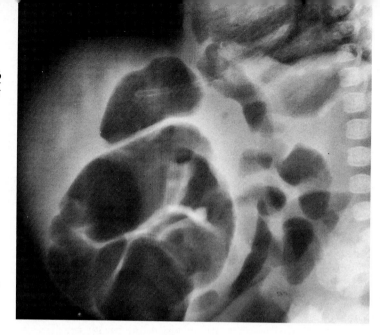

Fig. 68-13. Omphalocele containing loops of gas-filled small bowel.

herniated contents (Fig. 68-10) and to determine whether there is evidence of bowel obstruction (Fig. 68-11). On the anteroposterior view, bowel loops herniated into an anterior abdominal wall sac are super-imposed on normal intraperitoneal loops (Fig. 68-12A). Therefore, oblique or lateral radiographs of the abdomen are required for optimum evaluation (Fig. 68-12B).

OMPHALOCELE

An omphalocele is a protrusion of the abdominal viscera into the base of the umbilical cord with an associated defect in the abdominal wall. It represents persistence of normal fetal herniation with failure of complete withdrawal of the midgut from the umbilical cord during the tenth fetal week. The hernia contains loops of small bowel, which are usually filled with gas and are readily seen on plain abdominal films (Fig. 68-13). Liver, colon, spleen, and pancreas can also be trapped in

Fig. 68-14. Spigelian hernia. Small bowel is trapped in the hernia sac **(arrow)** that arises along the left semilunar line.

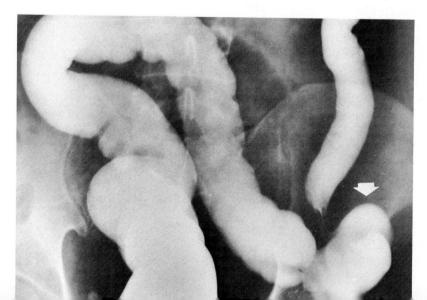

the hernia sac. Complications of an omphalocele include infection, rupture, and obstruction of loops of bowel entering or exiting from the hernia sac.

SPIGELIAN HERNIA

An interesting form of ventral hernia is the lateral spigelian hernia, a spontaneous defect of the abdominal wall that arises along the linea semilunaris (Fig. 68-14). This curved depression runs just lateral to the outer border of the rectus abdominis muscle, extending from the tip of the costal cartilage of the ninth rib to the symphysis pubis. Spigelian hernias pass through the fibers of the transverse and internal oblique muscles but stay beneath the intact external oblique aponeurosis and can therefore be difficult to palpate. Although the precise etiology of spigelian hernias is unclear, they tend to occur more frequently in persons with greater than normal intra-abdominal pressure, such as heavy laborers, and in persons with urinary retention, chronic lung disease, and gastric outlet obstruction. They can also be seen in multiparous women and in patients who have recently lost large amounts of weight.

Intermittent abdominal pain with point tenderness or a mass in the region of the semilunar line should suggest the possibility of spigelian hernia. Small bowel, colon, or omentum can be trapped in the narrow-necked hernia sac. Incarceration of herniated bowel can present with symptoms simulating gallbladder disease, acute appendicitis, or intermittent small bowel obstruction. Radiographically, gas- or contrast-filled bowel can be found laterally, outside the confines of the peritoneal cavity. Bowel loops often appear sharply constricted as they enter and exit from the hernia sac.

BIBLIOGRAPHY

Bartlett JD, Martel W, Lindenauer SM: Right paraduodenal hernia. Surg Gynecol Obstet 132:443–449, 1971

Frimann–Dahl J: Roentgen examinations in acute abdomen diseases. Springfield, IL, Charles C Thomas, 1974

Gibson LD, Gaspar MR: A review of 606 cases of umbilical hernia. Surg Gynecol Obstet 109:313–322, 1959

Goldberger LE, Berk RN: Cecal hernia into the lesser sac. Gastrointest Radiol 5:169–172, 1980

Harper J, Holt J: Obturator hernia. Am J Surg 92:562–565, 1956

Henisz A, Matesanz J, Westcott JL: Cecal herniation through the foramen of Winslow. Radiology 112:575–578, 1974

Holder LE, Schneider HJ: Spigelian hernias: Anatomy and roentgenographic manifestations. Radiology 112:309–313, 1974

Lawler RE, Duncan TR: Retrocecal hernia. Radiology 87:1051–1052, 1966

Meyers MA: Paraduodenal hernias: Radiologic and arteriographic diagnosis. Radiology 95:29–37, 1970

Schaefer C, Waugh D: Mesentericoparietal hernia. Am J Surg 116:847–852, 1968

Williams AJ: Roentgen diagnosis of intra-abdominal hernia. Radiology 59:817–825, 1952

Zausner J, Dumont AE, Ring SM: Obturator hernia. AJR 115:408–410, 1972

69 GAS IN THE BOWEL WALL (PNEUMATOSIS INTESTINALIS)

Gas in the bowel wall (pneumatosis intestinalis) can exist as an isolated entity or in conjunction with a broad spectrum of diseases of the gastrointestinal tract or respiratory system. In primary penumatosis (about 15% of cases), no respiratory or other gastrointestinal abnormality is present. Primary penumatosis usually occurs in adults and mainly involves the colon. Secondary pneumatosis intestinalis (about 85% of cases) more commonly involves the small bowel and is associated with a wide variety of pre-existing disorders. In the primary form, gas collections usually appear cystic; in the secondary type, a linear distribution of gas is generally seen.

Disease Entities

Primary (idiopathic)
Secondary
   Gastrointestinal disease with bowel necrosis
      Necrotizing enterocolitis in infants
      Ischemic necrosis due to mesenteric vascular disease
      Intestinal obstruction (especially if there is strangulation)
      Primary infection of the bowel wall
      Ingestion of corrosive agents
   Gastrointestinal disease without associated necrosis of the bowel wall
      Pyloroduodenal peptic ulcer disease
      Inflammatory bowel diseases (*e.g.*, ulcerative colitis, Crohn's disease, tuberculosis)
      Connective tissue disease
      Gastrointestinal endoscopy/colonoscopy

Jejunoileal bypass surgery
Obstructive lesions of the colon in children (*e.g.*, imperforate anus, Hirschsprung's disease, meconium plug)
Steroid therapy
Perforated jejunal diverticulum
Whipple's disease
Intestinal parasites
Obstructive pulmonary disease
Pulmonary emphysema
Bullous disease of the lung
Chronic bronchitis
Asthma

PRIMARY PNEUMATOSIS INTESTINALIS

Primary pneumatosis intestinalis is a relatively rare benign condition characterized pathologically by multiple thin-walled, noncommunicating, gas-filled cysts in the subserosal or submucosal layer of the bowel. The overlying mucosa is entirely normal, as is the muscularis. The disorder primarily involves the colon (particularly the left side), is usually segmental in distribution, and rarely affects the rectum. Because patients with primary pneumatosis intestinalis have no associated gastrointestinal or respiratory abnormalities, symptoms are infrequent, and gas in the bowel wall is usually an unexpected finding on plain abdominal radiographs or barium studies.

The appearance of radiolucent clusters of cysts along the contours of the bowel is diagnostic of primary pneumatosis intestinalis (Fig. 69-1). On barium examinations, the filling defects are seen to lie between the lumen (outlined by contrast) and the water density of the outer wall of the bowel. The radiographic pattern of pneumatosis can simulate more severe gastrointestinal conditions. Small cysts may be confused with tiny polyps. Larger cysts can produce scalloped defects simulating inflammatory pseudopolyps or the thumbprinting seen with intramural hemorrhage (Fig. 69-2). At times, the cysts of pneumatosis intestinalis concentrically compress the lumen, causing gas shadows that extend on either side of the bowel contour surrounding a thin, irregular stream of barium and mimicking the appearance of an annular carcinoma. To differentiate pneumatosis intestinalis from these other conditions, it is important to note the striking lucency of the gas-filled cysts in contrast to the soft-tissue density of an intraluminal or intramural lesion. In areas of obstruction, the overhanging edges are relatively lucent, in contrast to the soft-tissue density of tumors. Other distinguishing factors are the compressibility of the cysts on palpation and the not infrequent occurrence of asymptomatic pneumoperitoneum. The large amount of extraluminal gas within the peritoneal cavity can present a spectacular radiographic appearance and suggest a perforated viscus. However, the discovery of pneumoperitoneum in an apparently healthy patient with no peritoneal signs should make pneumatosis intestinalis the likely

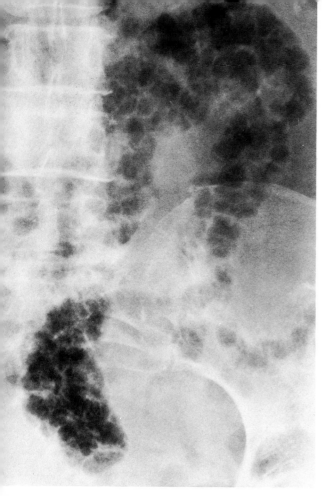

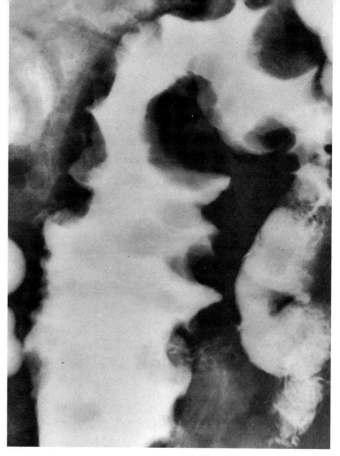

Fig. 69-1. Primary pneumatosis intestinalis in an asymptomatic man. Radiolucent clusters of gas-filled cysts are seen along the contours of the bowel.

Fig. 69-2. Primary pneumatosis intestinalis in an asymptomatic elderly man. The large gas-filled cysts produce scalloped defects in the colon simulating inflammatory pseudopolyps or the thumbprinting seen with intramural hemorrhage.

Fig. 69-3. Pneumatosis intestinalis in a premature infant with underlying necrotizing enterocolitis. Intramural gas **(arrows)** parallels the course of the bowel loops.

Fig. 69-4. Pneumatosis intestinalis in a premature infant with necrotizing enterocolitis. The bubbly appearance of gas in the wall of diseased colon resembles fecal material **(arrows);** although this appearance is normal in adults, it is always abnormal in premature infants.

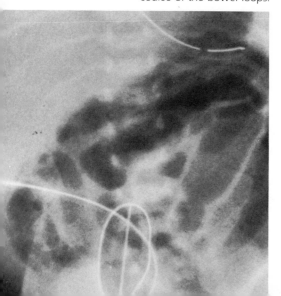

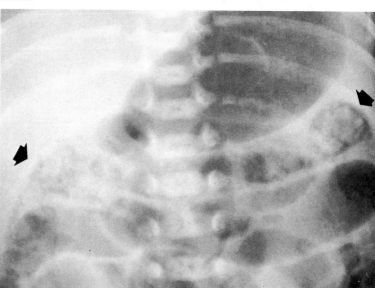

diagnosis. If the amount of gas that is absorbed by the peritoneum (about 100 ml/day) equals the amount that enters daily from ruptured cysts, a "balanced" pneumoperitoneum is the result, and large amounts of free intraperitoneal gas may be continuously present for months or years.

Primary pneumatosis intestinalis usually requires no treatment and resolves spontaneously. Surgery is required only in the very rare case of a patient with hemorrhage, obstruction, or perforation. In some severe cases, oxygen breathing (70% for 6 days) has been reported to be effective in decompressing the gas-filled cysts. Breathing high concentrations of oxygen alters the balance of diffusion of gases between the cysts and venous blood in favor of absorption of gases in the cysts, thereby causing cyst decompression.

GASTROINTESTINAL DISEASE WITH BOWEL NECROSIS

NECROTIZING ENTEROCOLITIS

Pneumatosis intestinalis in infants is usually associated with an underlying necrotizing enterocolitis, for which there is a very low survival rate (Fig. 69-3). The disease primarily occurs in premature or debilitated infants, who apparently have a decreased ability to fight infection. Gas-forming bacteria from the lumen invade the bowel wall through an insufficiently resistant mucosa, leading to a fulminant necrotizing cellulitis and septicemia. Necrotizing enterocolitis most commonly affects the ileum and right colon, though total gut involvement may occur. There is variable mucosal destruction, and a dirty brown pseudomembrane often covers the denuded areas. The bowel wall tends to be thickened and friable; multiple perforations can be present.

Babies who develop necrotizing enterocolitis are usually asymptomatic during the first 48 hr to 72 hr of life. On the third or fourth day, the infant begins to vomit bile-tinged material and develops mild to severe abdominal distention and respiratory distress. About half of the infants with this condition have a few loose blood-streaked stools; severe diarrhea, however, is infrequent. Clinical deterioration is usually progressive and rapid. Unless vigorous therapeutic measures are instituted, the infant can suffer spells of apnea, jaundice, and shock before succumbing.

Radiographic Findings

Pneumatosis intestinalis in infants suffering from necrotizing enterocolitis is characterized by a frothy or bubbly appearance of gas in the wall of diseased bowel loops (Fig. 69-4). The appearance often resembles fecal material in the right colon. However, it must be remembered that, although this feces-like appearance is perfectly normal in adults, it is always abnormal in premature infants. The gas in the wall of the colon in necrotizing enterocolitis is probably related to mucosal necrosis and subsequent passage of intraluminal gas into the bowel wall. This is complicated by the presence of intraluminal gas-forming organisms that also penetrate the diseased mucosa to reach the inner layers of the bowel wall. Gas entering the damaged intestinal capillary bed can spread to the intrahepatic branches of the portal vein. The radiographic detection of this appearance is an ominous sign. Extensive necrosis can result in perforation of the bowel wall and pneumoperitoneum. In contrast to pneumatosis intestinalis in adults, in whom cyst rupture and pneumoperitoneum are usually asymptomatic, bowel perforation in infants with necrotizing enterocolitis results in peritonitis and usually a fatal outcome.

The radiographic appearance of pneumatosis in a child with necrotizing enterocolitis is pathognomonic, especially if it is associated with pneumoperitoneum or portal vein gas. A barium enema examination is rarely needed for diagnosis; indeed, in view of the friable consistency of the colon, this procedure is hazardous.

Several cases have been reported of pneumatosis in neonates with a "benign" form of necrotizing enterocolitis. This relatively mild inflammatory process may be related to transient intestinal hypoxia; it does not progress to significant bowel necrosis.

MESENTERIC VASCULAR DISEASE

Two basic mechanical factors are implicated in the development of most cases of secondary pneumatosis intestinalis in adults. Regardless of the underlying etiology, most patients with gas in the bowel wall have loss of mucosal integrity and/or increased intraluminal pressure in the bowel. In those with ischemic, infectious, or traumatic damage to the mucosa, pneumatosis intestinalis can reflect a potentially fatal bacterial invasion (Fig. 69-5).

Peripheral occlusion of mesenteric vascular branches results in a transient ischemic break in the integrity of the highly sensitive mucosa and intramural extension of bowel gas. Although mesenteric vascular disease most commonly occurs in elderly persons, it occasionally arises in younger patients with conditions predisposing to the premature onset of occlusive disease (*e.g.*, diabetes, hypercholesterolemia, hypothyroidism). Bowel ischemia can be produced by an aneurysm of the abdominal aorta or be a complication of reconstructive surgery of the cardiac valves or the aorta.

Pneumatosis intestinalis secondary to mesenteric arterial (or venous) thrombosis presents as crescentic linear gas collections in the wall of ischemic bowel loops (Fig. 69-6). When gas is present in the bowel wall without intestinal necrosis, signs of severe peritoneal irritation are absent, and pneumatosis typically disappears once blood flow to the affected segment of bowel improves. The concomitant finding of gas in the portal vein, however, is a reliable indicator of irreversible intestinal necrosis and a poor prognostic sign.

Mucosal ischemia can be secondary to strangulating obstructions, such as volvulus or incarcerated hernia. Even if strangulation has not occurred, markedly increased intraluminal pressure proximal to an

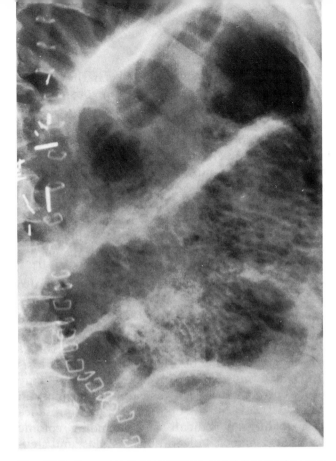

Fig. 69-5. Pneumatosis intestinalis in an adult secondary to a fatal necrotizing enterocolitis that developed following a motor vehicle accident and partial colon resection.

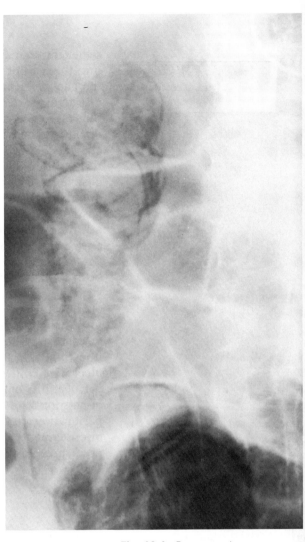

Fig. 69-6. Pneumatosis intestinalis due to mesenteric arterial thrombosis. Crescentic linear gas collections are seen in the wall of ischemic bowel loops.

obstruction can compress the intramural circulation and lead to vascular compromise and ischemic necrosis (Fig. 69-7). Mucosal necrosis can also be caused by infectious organisms that invade the bowel wall or by powerful corrosive agents (*e.g.*, lye, hydrochloric acid, formalin) that have been ingested accidentally or intentionally in a suicide attempt.

GASTROINTESTINAL DISEASE WITHOUT BOWEL NECROSIS

Even if there is no necrosis of the bowel wall, any gastrointestinal tract lesion that results in mucosal ulceration or intestinal obstruction may be associated with gas in the bowel wall. The most common of these conditions is obstructive peptic ulcer disease of the pyloroduodenal region. In severe pyloric stenosis, the increase in intraluminal pressure proximal to the obstructing lesion apparently forces intraluminal gas

the right iliac fossa, and, when large amounts are involved, can be seen along the flank down to the minor pelvis.

When the patient is in the supine position, free intraperitoneal gas accumulates between the intestinal loops and is much more difficult to demonstrate. However, a large quantity of gas can be diagnosed indirectly, because it permits visualization of the outer margins of the intestinal wall (Fig. 70-3). The distinct demonstration of the inner and outer contours of the bowel wall is often the only sign of pneumoperitoneum in patients in such poor condition that they cannot be turned on their side or be examined upright.

In children, pneumoperitoneum can be manifest as a generalized greater than normal radiolucency of the entire abdomen. This radiolucency often assumes an oval configuration ("football" sign) because of the accumulation of large amounts of free gas in the uppermost (anterior) portion of the peritoneal cavity when the child is supine. Another sign of pneumoperitoneum on the supine radiograph is demonstration of the falciform ligament (Fig. 70-4). This curvilinear water-density shadow in the upper abdomen to the right of the spine is outlined only when there is gas on both sides of it, as in a pneumoperitoneum.

PNEUMOPERITONEUM WITH PERITONITIS

PERFORATED VISCUS

The most frequent cause of pneumoperitoneum with peritonitis is perforation of a peptic ulcer, either gastric or duodenal (Fig. 70-5). However, in about 30% of perforated peptic ulcers, no free intraperitoneal gas can be identified. Therefore, failure to demonstrate a pneumoperitoneum is of no value in excluding the possibility of a perforated

Fig. 70-2. Pneumoperitoneum. **(A)** On the semi-erect view, there is no evidence of free intraperitoneal gas beneath the domes of the diaphragm. **(B)** On the lateral decubitus view, the free intraperitoneal gas is clearly seen collecting under the right side of the abdominal wall. Gas can even be seen extending down the flank to the region of the pelvis.

A   B

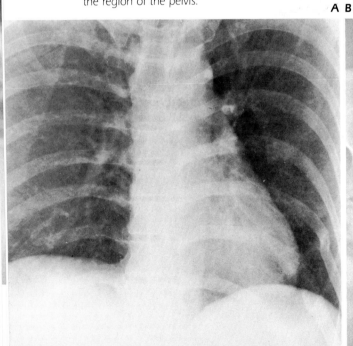 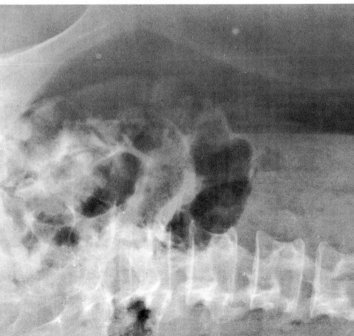

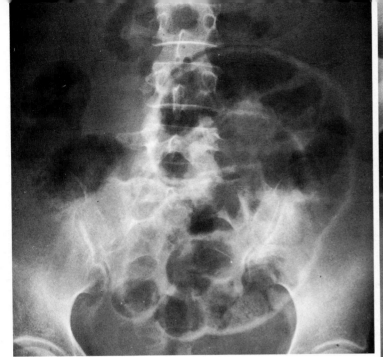

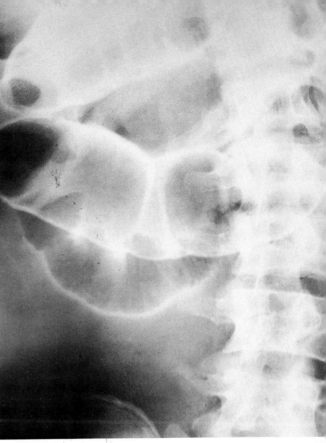

A B

Fig. 70-3. Pneumoperitoneum demonstrated on supine view. Large quantities of free intraperitoneal gas may be diagnosed indirectly in these two patients because the gas permits visualization of the outer margins of the intestinal wall.

Fig. 70-4. Falciform ligament sign of pneumoperitoneum. **(A)** On the supine view, the falciform ligament appears as a curvilinear water density shadow **(arrows)** in the upper abdomen to the right of the spine. This implies that there is a pneumoperitoneum with gas on both sides of the ligament. **(B)** An upright view clearly demonstrates free gas under the right hemidiaphragm.

A B

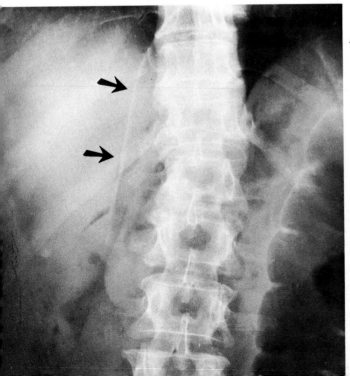

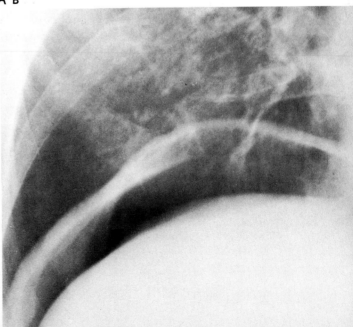

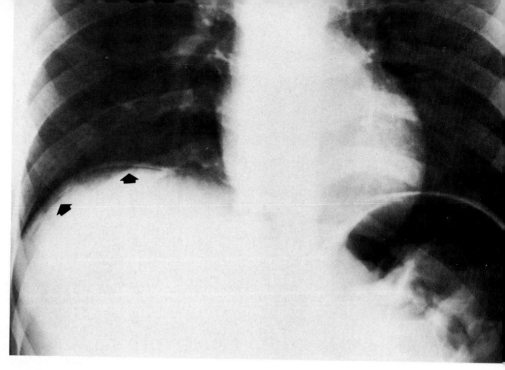

Fig. 70-5. *Pneumoperitoneum caused by a perforated duodenal ulcer.*

ulcer. In general, absence of gas in the stomach and the presence of gas scattered throughout the small and large bowel suggests a gastric perforation as the cause of pneumoperitoneum. Little or no colonic gas in the presence of a gastric gas–fluid level and small bowel distention makes a colonic perforation more likely. However, these radiographic findings can be difficult to discern and misleading, so that a firm diagnosis of the site of perforation often cannot be made on plain film examination and may require a barium study (Fig. 70-6).

Colonic perforations, especially those involving the cecum, give the most abundant quantities of free intraperitoneal gas (Fig. 70-7). Colonic perforations can be due to obstructing malignancy or severe ulcerating colitis leading to toxic megacolon. Perforation due to diverticulitis usually results in a localized pericolic abscess. Occasionally, gas from a diverticular perforation enters the general peritoneal space and produces a pneumoperitoneum, which predominantly collects under the left hemidiaphragm. Pneumoperitoneum rarely occurs in patients with acute appendicitis.

ULCERATIVE BOWEL DISEASE

Inflammatory lesions with ulcerations in the intestinal wall can give rise to pneumoperitoneum. In the small bowel, this is most commonly seen in patients with tuberculosis or typhoid fever. Because the small bowel does not usually contain substantial amounts of gas, perforations of this organ produce relatively small amounts of free intraperitoneal gas. Ulceration within Meckel's diverticula, especially in children, can lead to perforation (Fig. 70-8), as can ulcerations in patients with chronic ulcerative colitis or lymphogranuloma venereum.

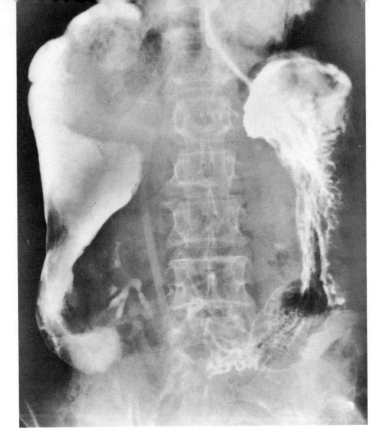

Fig. 70-6. Perforated duodenal ulcer. There is extensive extravasation from the upper gastrointestinal tract following the oral administration of contrast material.

Fig. 70-7. Extensive pneumoperitoneum following colonic perforation.

Fig. 70-8. Pneumoperitoneum following perforation of an ulcerated Meckel's diverticulum in a child.

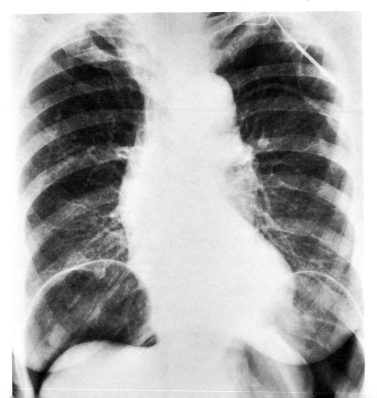

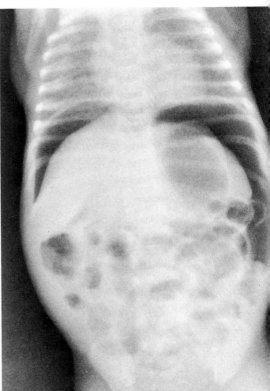

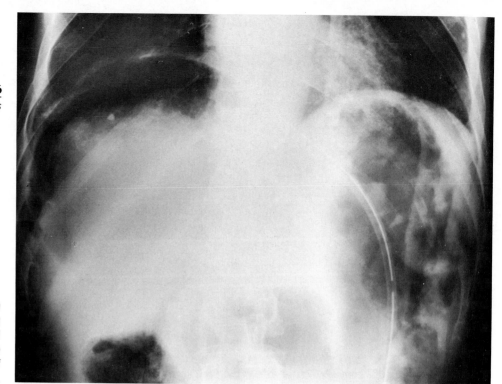

Fig. 70-9. Pneumoperitoneum that developed following trauma. Note the thickened gastric folds due to hemorrhage into the wall of the stomach.

INFECTION / TRAUMA

Septic infection of the peritoneal cavity by gas-forming organisms can result in the production of a substantial amount of gas and the radiographic appearance of pneumoperitoneum. Pneumoperitoneum can also develop following penetrating injuries of the abdominal wall and after blunt trauma causing rupture of a hollow viscus (Fig. 70-9).

DELAYED COMPLICATION OF RENAL TRANSPLANTATION

Spontaneous perforation of the colon is one of the most significant gastrointestinal complications that develop in renal transplant patients on long-term immunosuppressive therapy (Fig. 70-10). Many of these perforations are associated with diverticular disease occurring months or years after successful transplantation and are unrelated to periods of transplant rejection. Free peritoneal perforation is common with diverticular disease in transplant patients; in contrast, diverticular perforations are usually localized in nontransplant patients. Colon necrosis and perforation in transplant patients can also be caused by ischemic colitis or pseudomembranous colitis. In the immediate post-transplant period, perforation can be due to the development of a perinephric abscess. Colon and small bowel perforations outnumber gastroduodenal perforations more than 2 to 1 in post-transplant patients. Upper abdominal pain is the predominant clinical symptom. Clinical signs of an intra-abdominal catastrophe are infrequent or delayed, probably because of steroid or other immunosuppressive therapy. The overall mortality rate of gastrointestinal perforation in renal transplant patients is about 75%.

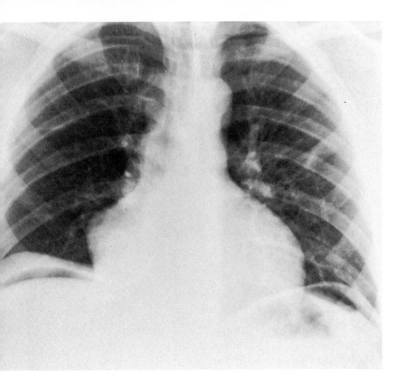

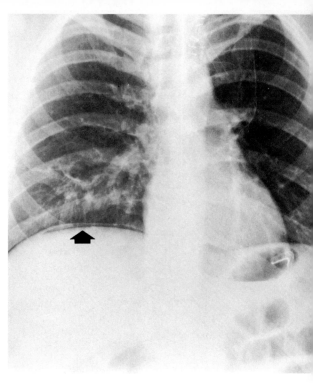

Fig. 70-10. Pneumoperitoneum resulting from spontaneous perforation of the colon in a renal transplant patient on long-term immunosuppressive therapy.

Fig. 70-11. Iatrogenic pneumoperitoneum **(arrow)** following laparotomy.

PNEUMOPERITONEUM WITHOUT PERITONITIS

IATROGENIC CAUSES

Iatrogenic pneumoperitoneum is generally asymptomatic and usually follows laparotomy (Fig. 70-11). In one large study, pneumoperitoneum was demonstrated in almost 60% of cases after abdominal surgery. Pneumoperitoneum usually occurs after operations on the gallbladder, stomach, or intestines, in which relatively large incisions are required. This phenomenon is seen rarely after repairs of inguinal hernias and infrequently after appendectomies. Postoperative pneumoperitoneum can be radiographically detectable for up to 3 weeks after surgery but usually can no longer be demonstrated after the first postoperative week. The time required for absorption of the free intraperitoneal gas depends primarily on the volume of gas originally trapped in the abdomen (as seen on the initial postoperative radiograph). Body habitus of the patient also appears to play a major role in the incidence and rate of absorption of postoperative pneumoperitoneum. In one study, over 80% of asthenic patients showed pneumoperitoneum. Only 25% of obese patients demonstrated this finding, and, in this group, the intraperitoneal gas was nearly always gone by the third postoperative day. Therefore, free intraperitoneal gas is a normal postoperative radiographic finding that, in the event of postoperative abdominal symptoms, should not enter into decisions of diagnosis or management. The major exception is in obese patients and children, in whom the presence of free intraperitoneal gas more than 3 days after surgery suggests, although it certainly does not confirm, the possibility of perforation.

An increasing amount of gas in the peritoneal cavity on serial radiographs strongly suggests a persistent abdominal abnormality and may indicate breakdown of a surgical anastomosis or other rupture of the intestinal tract. For this determination to be made, however, it is essential that all radiographs be obtained with the patient in the same position for the same length of time and without abdominal drains.

Examples of rare iatrogenic causes of pneumoperitoneum include perforation during endoscopic procedures and the old and seldom used technique of pneumoperitoneum for diagnostic purposes. In a diagnostic pneumoperitoneum, gas is introduced into the abdominal cavity to aid in delineating the viscera, particularly the liver and spleen, to outline abdominal masses, and to demonstrate the undersurface of the diaphragm.

ABDOMINAL CAUSES

In unusual instances, free intraperitoneal gas develops without gastrointestinal perforation, infection, trauma, or recent surgery. Patients with this "spontaneous pneumoperitoneum" are only mildly ill or even totally asymptomatic. It is essential that the causes of spontaneous pneumoperitoneum be carefully considered to prevent the patient from being subjected to immediate and unwarranted laparotomy.

Pneumoperitoneum can occur as a complication of pneumatosis intestinalis following rupture of one or several of the multiple gas-filled cysts that are present in the walls of the gastrointestinal tract. Spontaneous pneumoperitoneum without peritonitis can be the result of a *forme fruste* perforation of a peptic ulcer. It is postulated that a tiny perforation, usually missed at operation, may produce a valvelike flap that permits only gas to escape from the lumen. A similar mechanism of leakage of gas from the bowel lumen may result from lesions such as carcinoma of the stomach and Crohn's disease. There also is evidence that gas can traverse the intact wall of a severely distended viscus. Leakage through the stomach by this mechanism can be due to aerophagy, gastroscopy, excessive intake of oral sodium bicarbonate, or a misplaced oxygen tube.

Jejunal diverticulosis is one of the leading gastrointestinal causes of pneumoperitoneum without peritonitis or surgery (Fig. 70-12). In this condition, the distended diverticular mucosa may function as a semipermeable membrane allowing transmural gas equilibration. Intestinal gas enters the peritoneal cavity without gross fecal contamination.

GYNECOLOGIC CAUSES

Infrequently, gynecologic causes of pneumoperitoneum have been reported (Fig. 70-13). Gas injected into the fallopian tubes as part of the Rubin test for tubal patency can escape into the peritoneal cavity in amounts sufficient to be visualized radiographically. Ascent of air

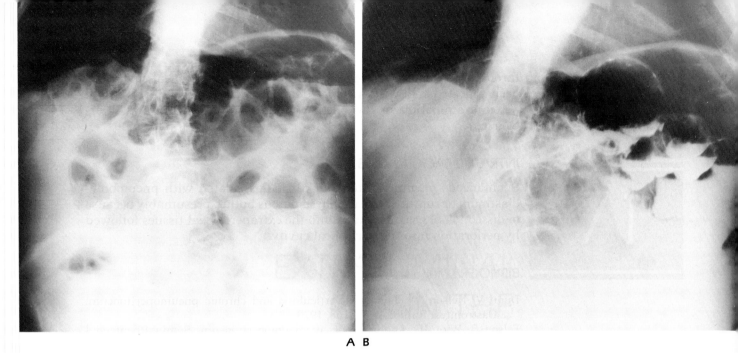

A B

Fig. 70-12. Pneumoperitoneum associated with jejunal diverticulosis. **(A)** An erect abdominal radiograph demonstrates pneumoperitoneum as well as an unusual small bowel gas pattern from gas-filled diverticula. **(B)** An erect film taken during small bowel follow-through shows gas–barium levels in multiple large jejunal diverticula as well as the presence of the pneumoperitoneum. (Dunn V, Nelson JA: Jejunal diverticulosis and chronic pneumoperitoneum. Gastrointest Radiol 4:165–168, 1979)

Fig. 70-13. Pneumoperitoneum following orogenital intercourse. **(A)** Frontal and **(B)** lateral chest radiographs demonstrate a large amount of free intraperitoneal gas. (Gantt CB, Daniel WW, Hallenbeck GA: Nonsurgical pneumoperitoneum. Am J Surg 134:411–414, 1977)

A B

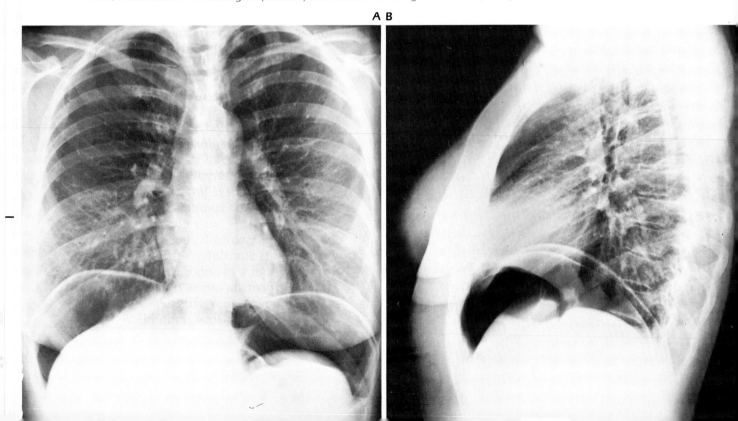

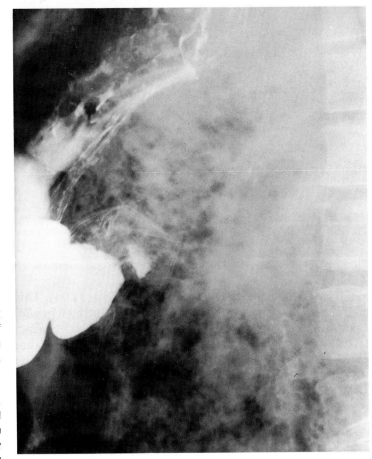

Fig. 71-12. Pancreatic abscess. The characteristic mottled pattern of speckled radiolucencies, with normal fat intermingled with areas of water density, involves much of the retroperitoneal space.

Fig. 71-13. Lesser sac abscess. **(A)** A plain abdominal radiograph and **(B)** a film from a barium study reveal a huge abscess cavity with a prominent gas–fluid level **(arrows).**

A B

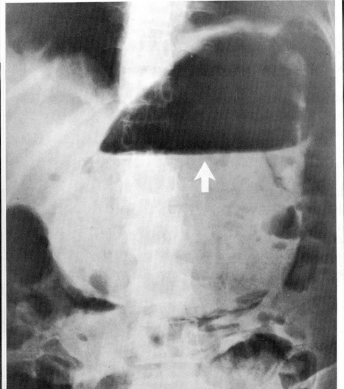

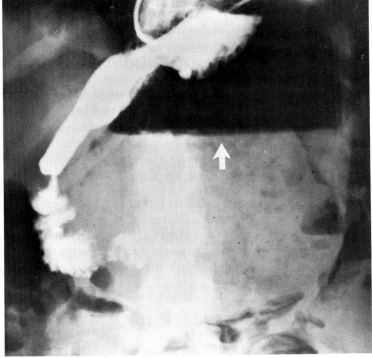

GAS WITHIN THE BOWEL WALL

Gas in the wall of the stomach can be an ominous sign of severe infection associated with phlegmonous gastritis or other necrotizing condition. It can also be a benign complication of endoscopy, gastric pneumatosis, or rupture of a pulmonary bullus into the esophageal wall.

Pneumatosis intestinalis can reflect mesenteric ischemia and necrosis in adults or necrotizing enterocolitis in children. It can also be a benign phenomenon of no clinical significance. This condition is discussed in detail in Chapter 69.

GAS IN THE BILIARY / PORTAL SYSTEM

Gas in the biliary tree is due to fistulization between the gallbladder or bile duct and the stomach or duodenum. This condition can be due to previous surgery (sphincterotomy), cholecystitis, severe peptic ulcer disease, trauma, or a tumor. Gas in the biliary tree is discussed in detail in Chapter 65.

Emphysematous cholecystitis is a rare condition in which gas-forming organisms (*Escherichia coli, Clostridium welchii*) cause collections of gas in the lumen of the gallbladder, within its wall or surrounding tissue, or in both places (Fig. 71-14). Bacterial growth in the gallbladder is facilitated by cystic duct obstruction (most often by stones), which causes stasis and ischemia in the gallbladder. Up to half of reported cases of emphysematous gastritis have been in patients with poorly controlled diabetes.

Abdominal radiographs demonstrate gas in the gallbladder lumen, in the wall of the gallbladder, or in the pericholecystic tissues (Fig. 71-15). It is postulated that gas distention of the gallbladder lumen

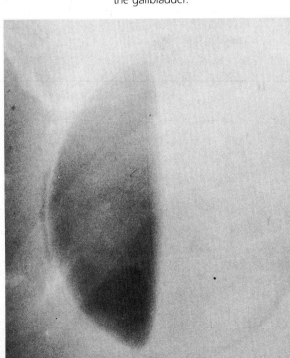

Fig. 71-15. Emphysematous cholecystitis. Gas is evident within the lumen and wall of the gallbladder.

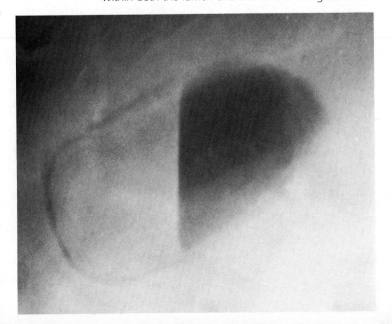

Fig. 71-14. Emphysematous cholecystitis. Gas is found within both the lumen and the wall of the gallbladder.

occurs first. At this stage, the gas filling the lumen of the gallbladder can be mistaken for a normal collection of gas in the stomach or intestine. Extension of gas into the wall of the gallbladder and adjacent tissues produces the pathognomonic appearance of a rim of translucent bubbles or streaks outside and roughly parallel to the gallbladder lumen. Because there is almost always obstruction of the cystic duct in emphysematous gastritis, gas is absent from the biliary ducts in the early stages of disease. If the infection spreads into the biliary tree, gas is seen in the ductal system.

At times, it may be necessary to eliminate the possibility of an internal biliary fistula as the source of the gas in the gallbladder lumen. This can be effectively done if there is no gas in the biliary ductal system.

Gas in the portal veins, discussed in detail in Chapter 66, is usually an ominous prognostic sign. It is generally related to necrotizing enterocolitis in children and mesenteric ischemia and bowel necrosis in adults. In children, a benign form of portal vein gas can be related to placement of an umbilical venous catheter.

CHILAIDITI'S SYNDROME

The transverse colon and the hepatic flexure are occasionally found interposed between the liver and the right hemidiaphragm (Chilaiditi's syndrome) (Fig. 71-16). This type of interposition is common, especially in mentally retarded or psychotic patients with chronic colonic enlargement. It sometimes occurs in association with chronic lung disease, postnecrotic cirrhosis, or pregnancy. This anomalous position of the colon is often transient and generally of little clinical significance. At

Fig. 71-16. Chilaiditi's syndrome. The transverse colon and hepatic flexure are interposed between the liver and the right hemidiaphragm.

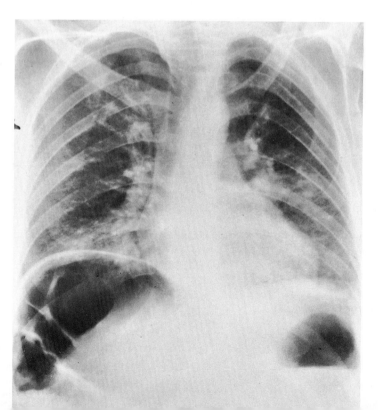

times, however, Chilaiditi's syndrome is characterized by abdominal pain that becomes increasingly worse during the day and is often accentuated by deep breathing. Abdominal radiographs show a striking appearance of gas in the hepatic flexure interposed between the liver and diaphragm. It is essential that this pattern not be confused with free intraperitoneal gas.

PEFORATION DUE TO A FOREIGN BODY

Most ingested foreign bodies pass through the gastrointestinal tract without incident. Less than 1%, especially those that are either sharp or elongated, cause perforation and localized abscess formation. The intentional ingestion of foreign bodies is common in young children and emotionally disturbed persons. Predisposing factors in adults include decreased palatal sensitivity due to dentures, excessive alcohol intake or drug use, ingestion of extremely cold liquids, poor vision, or rapid eating. The radiographic demonstration of the offending foreign body (*e.g.*, a chicken bone) with an associated mass or extraluminal gas collection in a patient with signs of peritonitis, mechanical bowel obstruction, or pneumoperitoneum strongly suggests this diagnosis.

OTHER CAUSES OF EXTRALUMINAL GAS

A ruptured aortic aneurysm with dissection of blood into the retroperitoneal fat can produce a mottled appearance that simulates a retroperitoneal abscess. If there are no clinical signs of infection, a ruptured aortic aneurysm must be considered a possible cause of this radiographic pattern.

Postoperative perirenal hematoma can simulate a perirenal abscess. The apparent etiology of this condition is liquefaction of the hematoma, with gas entering it from the drain site.

Gas is occasionally demonstrated in the abdominal wall after surgery (Fig. 71-17). It may also be related to localized abscess formation.

Rarely, gas gangrene involves intra-abdominal structures other than the liver and gallbladder and causes the radiographic appearance of gas in the soft tissues or in the walls of abdominal organs (Fig. 71-18).

BIBLIOGRAPHY

Berenson JE, Spitz HB, Felson B: The abdominal fat necrosis sign. Radiology 100:567–571, 1971

Connell TR, Stephens DH, Carlson HC et al: Upper abdominal abscess: A continuing and deadly problem. AJR 134:759–765, 1980

Evans JA, Meyers MA, Bosniak MA: Acute renal and perirenal infections. Semin Roentgenol 6:274–290, 1971

Grainger K: Acute emphysematous cholecystitis: Report of a case. Clin Radiol 12:66–69, 1961

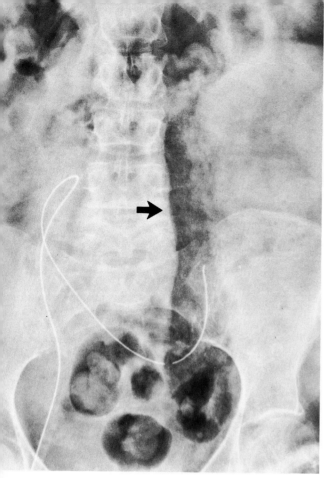

Fig. 71-17. Gas within a wound infection in the rectus sheath **(arrow)** following abdominal surgery.

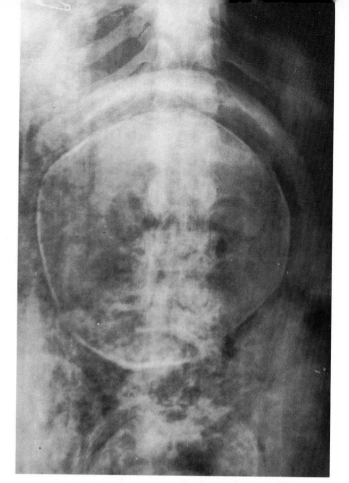

Fig. 71-18. Gas gangrene of the uterus. Gas is evident in the wall of the uterus and the surrounding soft tissues.

Harned RK: Retrocecal appendicitis presenting with air in the subhepatic space. AJR 126:416–418, 1976

Love L, Baker D, Ramsey R: Gas producing perinephric abscess. AJR 119:783–792, 1973

Maglinte DDT, Taylor SD, Ng AC: Gastrointestinal perforation by chicken bones. Radiology 130:597–599, 1979

Mellins HZ: Radiologic signs of disease in lesser peritoneal sac. Radiol Clin North Am 2:107–120, 1964

Miller WT, Talman EA: Subphrenic abscess. AJR 101:961–969, 1967

Nelson SW: Extraluminal gas collections due to diseases of the gastrointestinal tract. AJR 115:225–248, 1972

Woodard S, Kelvin FM, Rice RP et al: Pancreatic abscess: Importance of conventional radiology. AJR 136:871–878, 1981

FISTULAS INVOLVING THE SMALL OR LARGE BOWEL

Gastrointestinal fistulas are abnormal communications between the gastrointestinal tract and another segment of bowel (enteric–enteric fistula), another intra-abdominal organ (internal fistula), or the skin (external fistula).

CAUSES OF ENTERIC–ENTERIC FISTULAS

Crohn's disease
Diverticulitis
Malignant neoplasms (primary, metastatic)
Gastric ulcer
Radiation therapy
Ulcerative colitis
Infectious diseases
  Tuberculosis
  Pelvic inflammatory disease
  Actinomycosis
  Amebiasis
  Shigellosis
Marginal ulcer (after gastric surgery)

Fistula formation is a hallmark of chronic Crohn's disease, found in at least half of all patients with this condition (Fig. 72-1). The diffuse inflammation of the serosa and mesentery in Crohn's disease causes involved loops of bowel to be firmly matted together by fibrous **935**

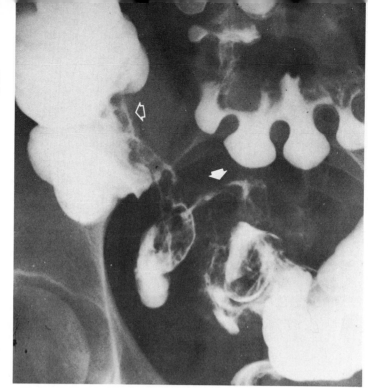

Fig. 72-1. Crohn's disease. There is fistulization between the terminal ileum and sigmoid **(solid arrow)** and double-tracking along the cecum **(open arrow).**

peritoneal and mesenteric bands (Fig. 72-2). Fistulas apparently begin as ulcerations that burrow through the bowel wall into adjacent loops of small bowel and colon (Fig. 73-3). Enteric–enteric fistulas can cause severe nutritional problems if they bypass extensive areas of intestinal absorptive surface (Fig. 72-4); the recirculation of intestinal contents and subsequent stasis can permit bacterial overgrowth and malabsorption. In addition to enteric–enteric fistulas, a characteristic finding in Crohn's disease is the appearance of fistulous tracts ending blindly in

Fig. 72-2. Crohn's disease. There is a fistula between the distal ileum and sigmoid **(arrow).**

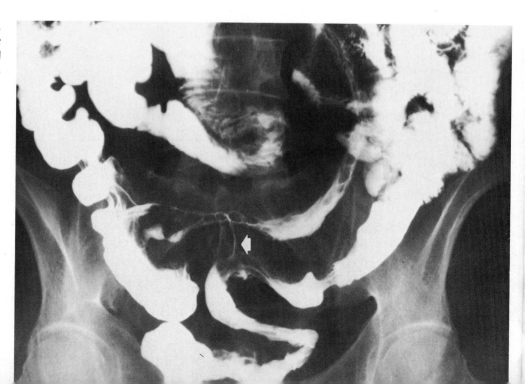

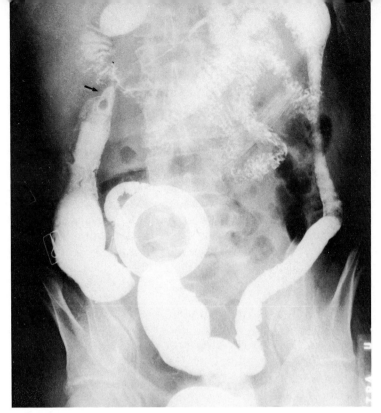

Fig. 72-3. Crohn's disease. A duodenocolic fistula is evident **(arrow).** (Korelitz BI: Colonic–duodenal fistula in Crohn's disease. Dig Dis 22:1040–1048, 1977)

Fig. 72-4. Crohn's disease with development of a duodenocolic fistula. **(A)** A barium enema examination demonstrates retrograde filling of the fistula to the distal descending duodenum **(arrow).** There is marked irregularity of the colon with pseudopolyposis. **(B)** A delayed film from an upper gastrointestinal series demonstrates prominent duodenal folds **(arrow)** resulting from secondary reactive inflammation and not Crohn's disease. (Smith TR, Goldin RR: Radiographic and clinical sequelae of the duodenocolic anatomic relationship: Two cases of Crohn's disease with fistulization of the duodenum. Dis Colon Rectum 20:257–262, 1977)

A B

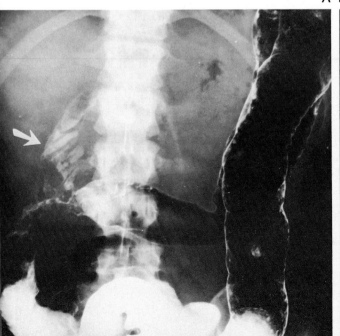
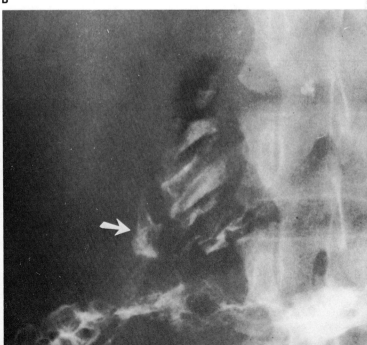

abscess cavities surrounded by dense inflammatory tissue. These abscess cavities are situated intraperitoneally, retroperitoneally, or deep within the mesentery and can produce palpable masses, persistent fever, or pain.

Fistulous communications between the colon and small bowel can be seen in about 10% of patients with diverticulitis (Fig. 72-5). These fistulas are often multiple and, when combined with a colovesical communication, can produce intractable perineal pain and itching, excoriation, or severe fluid and electrolyte imbalance due to loss of small bowel contents by way of the enterovesical fistula. A classic finding in this disease is dissection along the wall of the colon (double tracking; see Chap. 55). Although most commonly seen in diverticulitis and once thought to be pathognomonic of this disorder, double tracking can also develop in patients with Crohn's disease or carcinoma of the colon.

Primary or metastatic malignancy of the small bowel or colon can extend to form mesenteric or serosal deposits that draw bowel loops together toward a central point (Fig. 72-6). This can lead to irregular ulceration and the creation of a fistulous communication between adjacent bowel loops (Fig. 72-7).

Gastrocolic and duodenocolic fistulas can originate from primary carcinomas of the colon (Fig. 72-8) or stomach. These tumors are almost always bulky and infiltrating and are associated with a marked inflammatory reaction. The tumor apparently extends from the serosa of one viscus into the wall of another, followed by lumen-to-lumen necrosis. The presence of growing tumor and fibrous stroma within the wall of a malignant fistula accounts for the length of these tracts and the relative separation of bowel loops. A similar radiographic pattern can be caused by carcinoma of the pancreas spreading to involve both the stomach and colon (Fig. 72-9).

Malignant gastrocolic fistulas are frequently demonstrated during barium enema examination but are rarely detected on upper gastrointestinal series. This phenomenon is probably related to preferential flow from the colon to the stomach or small bowel. The higher than usual intraluminal pressure in the colon at the time of a barium enema examination may overcome resistance in the rigid, nondistensible fistula, allowing passage of barium into the stomach or small bowel. When an upper gastrointestinal series is performed under more physiologic conditions, the intraluminal pressure in the proximal gastrointestinal tract may not be sufficient to overcome this resistance.

Gastrocolic fistulas are a rare complication of benign gastric ulcer disease (Fig. 72-10). Gastric ulcers causing this condition are invariably located along the greater curvature or posterior wall of the antrum. As an ulcer penetrates posteriorly, involvement of the mesocolon permits spread of inflammation to the superior border of the transverse colon, which is almost always the site of the colonic end of the fistula (Fig. 72-11). Benign ulcer-induced gastrocolic fistulas are especially common in patients receiving steroids or aspirin, both of which have well-known ulcerogenic properties. These medications also decrease the inflam-

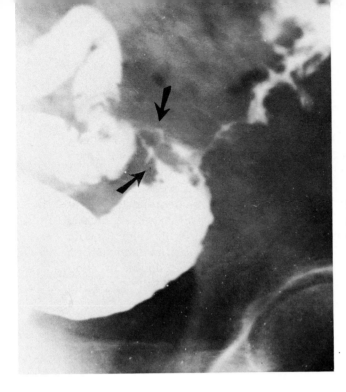

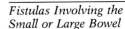

Fig. 72-5. Diverticulitis. Fistulous tracts **(arrows)** connect the sigmoid colon and ileum. (Kroening PM: Sigmoido-ileal fistulas as a complication of diverticulitis. AJR 96:323–325, 1966. Copyright 1966. Reproduced by permission)

Fig. 72-6. Malignant duodenocolic fistula. **(A)** An upper gastrointestinal series demonstrates a lesion in the antrum of the stomach. There is marked deformity of the second portion of the duodenum with a duodenocolic fistula and mass deformity of the proximal transverse colon **(arrows). (B)** A barium enema examination demonstrates the duodenocolic fistula, a lesion of the proximal transverse colon, and deformity of the cecum. (Vieta JO, Blanco R, Valentini GR: Malignant duodenocolic fistula: Report of two cases, each with one or more synchronous gastrointestinal cancers. Dis Colon Rectum 19:542–552, 1976)

A B

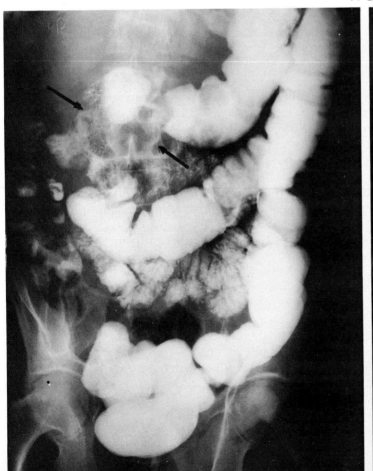

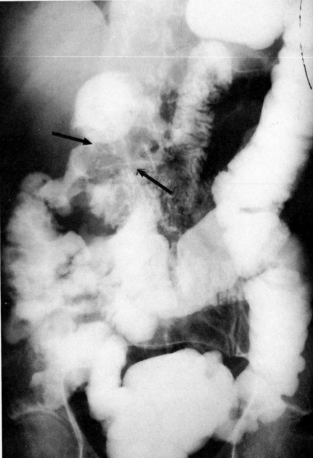

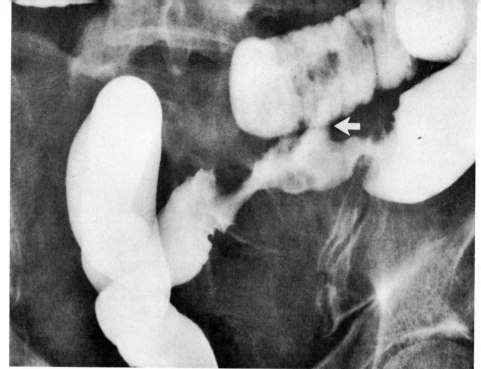

Fig. 72-7. Ileocolic fistula **(arrow)** secondary to carcinoma of the sigmoid colon.

Fig. 72-8. Gastrocolic fistula **(arrow)** caused by adenocarcinoma of the colon.

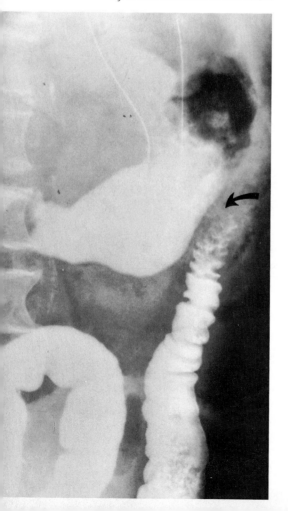

Fig. 72-9. Gastrocolic fistula due to invasive carcinoma of the tail of the pancreas. Contrast **(arrow)** appears in the stomach during a barium enema examination.

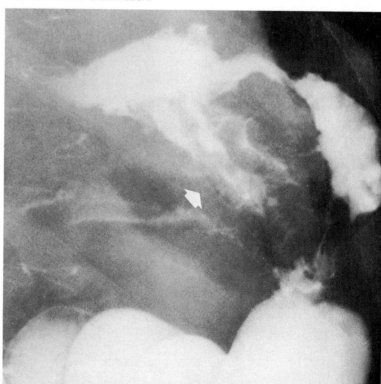

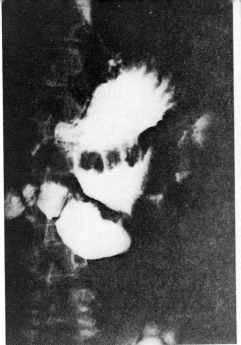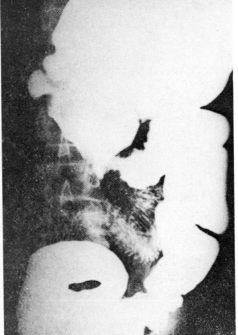

A B

Fig. 72-10. Gastrocolic fistula as a complication of benign gastric ulcer disease. **(A)** An upper gastrointestinal series shows contrast material entering the transverse colon through the gastrocolic fistula. **(B)** A barium enema examination demonstrates reflux of contrast material into the stomach through the gastrocolic fistula. (Smith DL, Comer TP: Gastrocolic fistula, a rare complication of benign gastric ulcer. Dis Colon Rectum 17:769–770, 1974)

Fig. 72-12. Tuberculosis. A colocolic fistula with surrounding abscess formation is evident in the region of the splenic flexure.

Fig. 72-11. Gastrocolic fistula secondary to benign ulcer disease. An upper gastrointestinal series demonstrates the fistula between the greater curvature of the stomach and the superior border of the transverse colon. (Swartz MJ, Paustian FF, Chleborad WJ: Recurrent gastric ulcer with spontaneous gastrojejunal and gastrocolic fistulas. Gastroenterology 44:527–531, 1963)

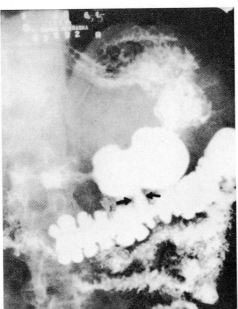

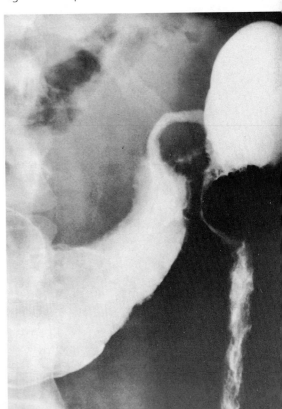

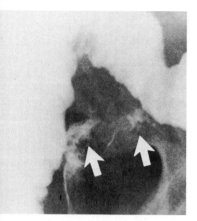

Fig. 72-13. Shigellosis. There is a fistulous tract between the rectum and sigmoid colon **(arrows).**

matory reaction that would ordinarily seal off a penetrating gastric ulcer. In addition, steroids can mask the severe clinical symptoms, thereby permitting a penetrating ulcer to develop into a gastrocolic fistula.

Radiation therapy, especially to the pelvic organs, can cause ischemic and inflammatory changes in the small and large bowel. In addition to mucosal ulceration and stricture formation, radiation enteritis often leads to the development of enteric–enteric fistulas.

Although enteric–enteric fistulas occur in ulcerative colitis, they are found in less than 0.5% of patients with this disease. Fistulas can also develop in other inflammatory bowel diseases, such as tuberculosis (Fig. 72-12), pelvic inflammatory disease, actinomycosis, amebiasis, and shigellosis (Fig. 72-13).

A fistulous communication between the stomach, jejunum, and colon (gastrojejunocolic fistula) or directly between the stomach and colon represents a grave complication of marginal ulceration after gastric surgery (especially gastrojejunostomy) for peptic ulcer disease (Fig. 72-14). Most patients with this condition (there is a heavy predominance in men) have diarrhea and weight loss; pain, vomiting, and bleeding occur in one-third to one-half of cases. The first evidence of the presence of such a fistula is sometimes obtained during a barium enema examination in which contrast is observed to extend directly from the transverse colon into the stomach. These postsurgical fistulas are associated with a high mortality rate, especially if recognized late.

CAUSES OF INTERNAL FISTULAS

Diverticulitis
Ulcerative colitis
Crohn's disease
Malignant neoplasm
Radiation therapy
Pancreatitis
Prosthetic aortic graft
Gallbladder–bowel fistulas
    Acute cholecystitis
    Peptic ulcer disease
    Trauma
    Carcinoma
Duodenum–kidney fistulas
    Pyelonephritis (especially tuberculous)
    Duodenal ulcer
Extravasation of contrast from bowel mimicking fistulas
    Diverticulitis
    Perforated viscus
    Trauma
    Surgery
    Abscess

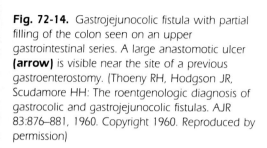

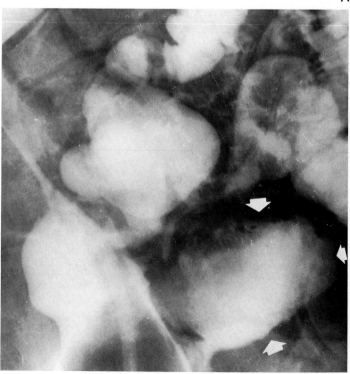

Fig. 72-14. Gastrojejunocolic fistula with partial filling of the colon seen on an upper gastrointestinal series. A large anastomotic ulcer **(arrow)** is visible near the site of a previous gastroenterostomy. (Thoeny RH, Hodgson JR, Scudamore HH: The roentgenologic diagnosis of gastrocolic and gastrojejunocolic fistulas. AJR 83:876–881, 1960. Copyright 1960. Reproduced by permission)

Fig. 72-15. Colovesicoenteric fistula. **(A)** A barium enema examination demonstrates barium entering the bladder **(arrows)** and small intestine by way of the sigmoid colon. **(B)** A radiograph from a cystogram shows filling of the small intestine from the bladder **(arrows.)** The presence of a colovesicoenteric fistula due to acute diverticulitis was confirmed at surgery. (Smith HJ, Berk RN, Janes JO et al: Unusual fistulae due to colonic diverticulitis. Gastrointest Radiol 2:387–392, 1978)

A B

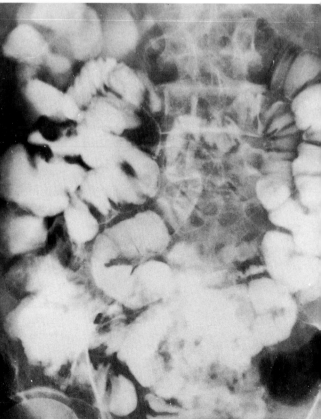

Internal fistula formation is a frequent complication of diverticulitis. Colovesical fistulas (more common in men than women) account for more than 50% of all fistulas in this disease (Fig. 72-15). They can cause recurrent urinary tract infections, chronic cystitis, pneumaturia, or fecaluria. Plain radiographs of the abdomen occasionally demonstrate gas in the bladder; excretory urography, cystography, or barium enema examinations sometime show the presence of a fistula (Fig. 72-16). In women, rectovaginal fistulas can permit passage of feces or gas through the vagina (Fig. 72-17). After surgical treatment of diverticulitis, colo-ureteral, colocutaneous, or multiple internal fistulas can occur.

Rectovaginal fistulas occur in about 2% to 3% of women with ulcerative colitis. These fistulas frequently do not heal after local surgical repair; colectomy with ileostomy or a temporary diverting procedure is often required. Colovesical fistulas can also be seen in ulcerative colitis (Fig. 72-18). Although less common than enteric–enteric fistulas, internal fistulas extending from the bowel to the bladder or vagina can occur in patients with Crohn's disease (Fig. 72-19). Extension of a lower abdominal malignancy can also produce a colovesical or rectovaginal fistula. Radiation therapy to the pelvic organs can cause fibrous inflammatory adhesions between bowel and bladder that permit the development of enteric–vesical fistulas.

Fig. 72-16. Colovesical fistula (diverticulitis). A barium enema examination demonstrates barium in the fistulous tract **(solid arrow)** between the sigmoid colon and the bladder. Barium can also be seen lining the base of the gas-filled bladder **(open arrows)**.

Fig. 72-17. Rectovaginal fistula in diverticulitis. The **open arrow** points to the fistulous tract; the **closed arrows** point to contrast in the vagina.

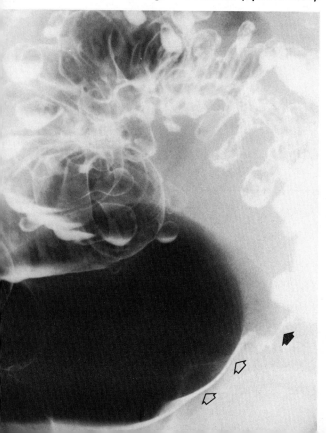

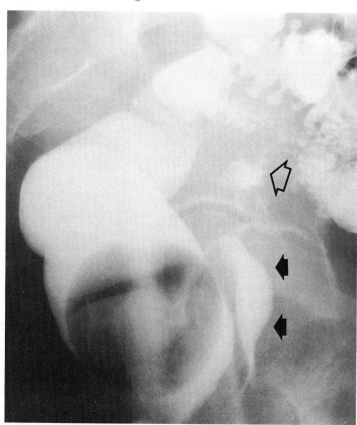

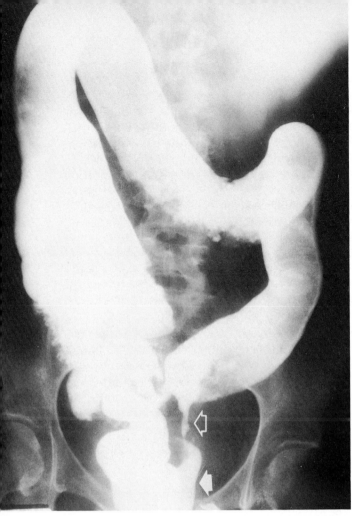

Fig. 72-18. Colovesical fistula in ulcerative colitis. The **open arrow** points to the fistula; the **closed arrow** points to contrast in the bladder.

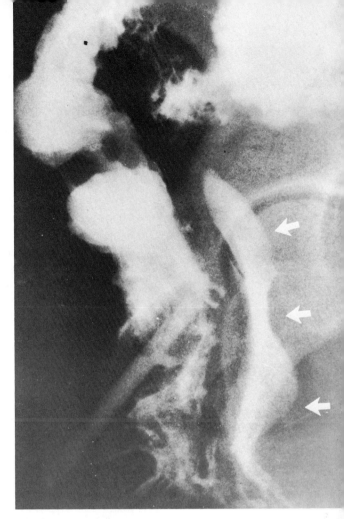

Fig. 72-19. Rectovaginal fistula in a patient with Crohn's disease. The **arrows** point to contrast in the vagina.

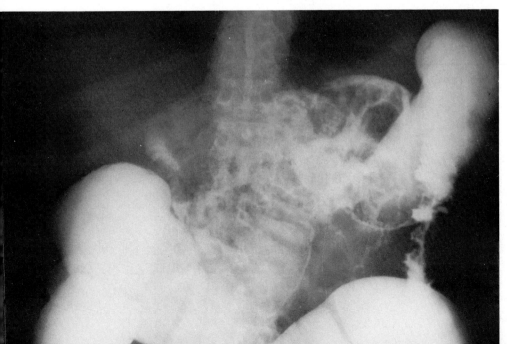

Fig. 72-20. Spontaneous perforation of a pancreatic pseudocyst into the colon and duodenum. (Shatney CH, Sosin H: Spontaneous perforation of a pancreatic pseudocyst into the colon and duodenum. Am J Surg 126:433–438, 1973)

Various types of internal fistula can result from severe pancreatitis or be complications of surgery for pancreatic cancer. About 2.5% of pseudocysts rupture spontaneously into the stomach, duodenum, or colon (Fig. 72-20). Unlike free rupture into the peritoneal cavity, which is generally a catastrophic event, perforation into the gastrointestinal tract can present a variable clinical picture ranging from potentially lethal hemorrhage to substantial improvement in the patient's condition (Fig. 72-21).

Fistulas between the aorta and adjacent bowel (usually the duodenum) develop in up to 2% of patients who have undergone aortic aneurysm resection. In patients with upper or lower intestinal bleeding (often massive) occurring 3 weeks or more after aortic surgery, the possibility of a paraprosthetic–enteric fistula must be excluded. Fistula formation between the colon and venous structures can be a complication of diverticulitis (Fig. 72-22).

Fistulas between the gallbladder and bowel can be secondary to acute cholecystitis (90%) or severe peptic ulcer disease (6%). The remaining cases are the result of trauma or tumor. An acutely inflamed gallbladder can create a cholecystoenteric fistula by perforating into the lumen of an adjacent visceral organ, most commonly the duodenum. Fistulas can extend into the hepatic flexure, stomach, or jejunum. In patients with severe peptic disease, a penetrating duodenal or gastric ulcer can perforate into the gallbladder or bile duct. Regardless of the etiology, plain abdominal radiographs generally demonstrate gas within the biliary tree. On upper gastrointestinal series, barium usually fills the cholecystoenteric fistula.

Fistulas between the duodenum and right kidney are most often secondary to pyelonephritis, often tuberculous in origin. The pathologic mechanism is usually rupture of a perirenal abscess into the duodenum,

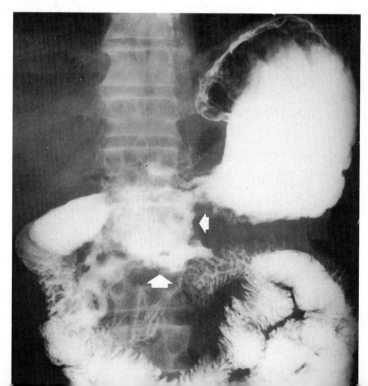

Fig. 72-21. Spontaneous transenteric rupture of a pancreatic pseudocyst. Note the collection of extraluminal barium **(arrows)** in the pseudocyst cavity. Following the perforation, the patient's clinical condition improved. (Bradley EL, Clements JL: Transenteric rupture of pancreatic pseudocysts: Management of pseudocystenteric fistulas. Am J Surg 42:827–837, 1976)

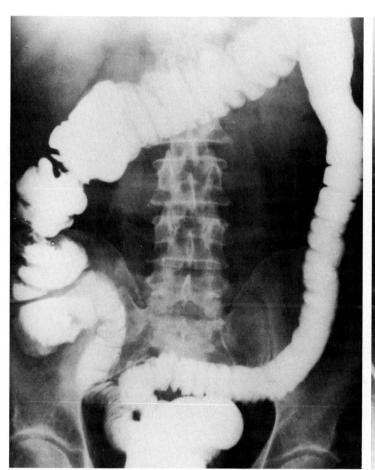

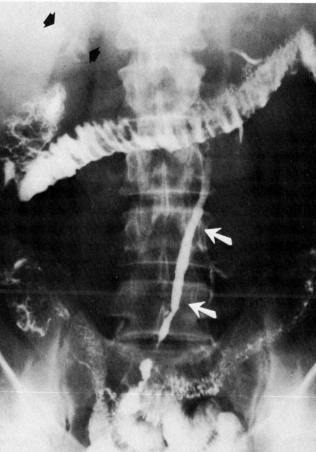

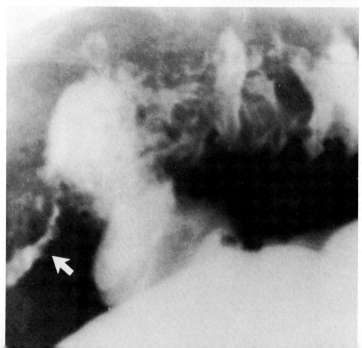

A C
B

Fig. 72-22. Colovenous fistula. **(A)** A barium enema examination shows only minimal changes of spastic colon disease. **(B)** A spot film made during the barium enema examination shows narrowing of the sigmoid colon and a fistulous tract **(arrow).** A few diverticula are present. **(C)** A postevacuation radiograph shows barium in the inferior mesenteric vein **(white arrows).** Barium and gas are visible in a liver abscess **(black arrows).** The barium remained in the vein for 3 days after the examination and was gradually replaced by gas. At surgery, a small abscess was found that was due to peforation of the sigmoid colon. The patient did well for 8 days following the operation but then suddenly developed irreversible shock and died. Autopsy confirmed the presence of barium in the inferior mesenteric vein and showed thrombosis of the portal and splenic veins and multiple liver abscesses. (Smith HJ, Berk RN, Janes JO et al: Unusual fistulae due to colonic diverticulitis. Gastrointest Radiol 2:387–392, 1978)

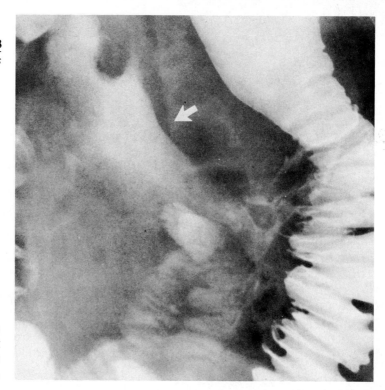

Fig. 72-23. Diverticulitis with extravasation of contrast **(arrow)** into the retroperitoneal space.

which is best demonstrated on retrograde pyelography. On rare occasions, a duodenal ulcer penetrates into the tissues surrounding the kidney and produces a renoduodenal fistula.

An appearance resembling fistulization can be produced by extravasation of contrast from the bowel into the retroperitoneal or peritoneal space. This can be caused by such entities as diverticulitis (Fig. 72-23), a perforated viscus (Fig. 72-24), trauma (Fig. 72-25), surgery (Fig. 72-26), or erosion by an abscess cavity (Fig. 72-27).

Fig. 72-24. Perforated duodenal ulcer. Extravasated contrast is seen surrounding the liver **(arrows).**

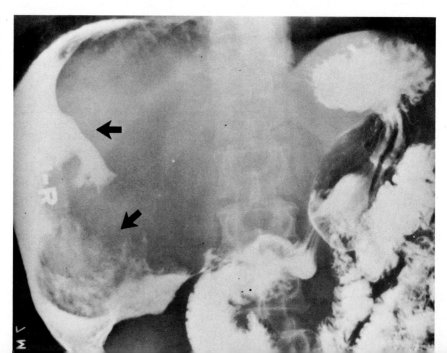

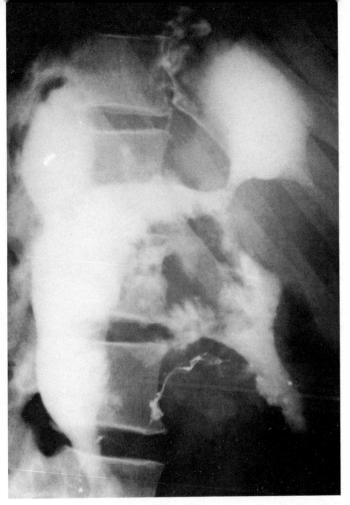

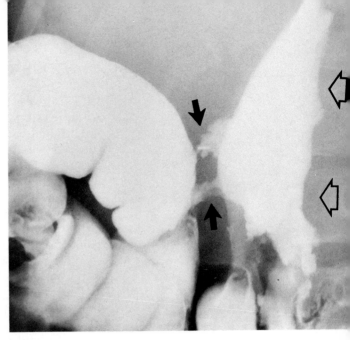

Fig. 72-26. Fistulous communication **(solid arrows)** between the colon and a retroperitoneal abscess **(open arrows)** following nephrectomy.

Fig. 72-25. Diffuse internal fistula formation following a gunshot wound to the abdomen.

Fig. 72-27. Extravasation of contrast from the colon into the huge subphrenic abscess **(arrows)**.

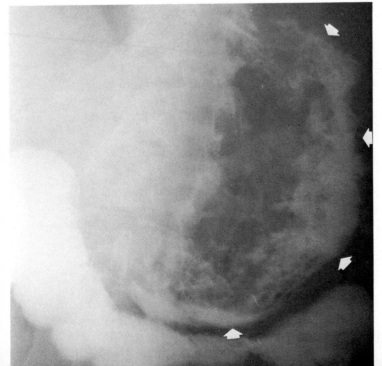

Postoperative fistulas
   Complication of surgery
   Intentional creation (gastrostomy, ileostomy, colostomy)
Pancreatic fistulas
   Trauma
   External drainage of pseudocyst
   Complication of surgery
Fistulas due to underlying gastrointestinal disease
   Crohn's disease
   Anorectal causes
      Malignancy
      Radiation therapy
      Tuberculosis
      Lymphogranuloma venereum
   Diverticulitis
      Colocutaneous
      Colocoxal

The major complication of external gastrointestinal fistulas is the drainage of large amounts of electrolyte-rich fluid through them. External fistulas arising in the proximal portion of the gastrointestinal tract generally produce a large volume of fluid loss; those developing from the distal small bowel and colon are usually low-output fistulas. In addition to dehydration and electrolyte imbalance, external fistulas that bypass a large percentage of the functioning intestine often cause severe weight loss and protein–calorie malnutrition. Because intraperitoneal infections accompany many external fistulas, there are frequently abscesses along the fistulous tracts that wall off and persist if the fistulas are not adequately drained. Injection of water-soluble contrast into an external fistula usually demonstrates the source of the fistula and any communicating abscess cavities (Fig. 72-28).

The morbidity rate for external gastrointestinal fistulas is high. Even though about three-quarters of these fistulas close spontaneously if treated properly, hospitalization is frequently prolonged.

Most external gastrointestinal fistulas are complications of abdominal surgery in which an anastomosis fails to heal properly. Various factors that contribute to this lack of adequate healing include foreign bodies (*e.g.,* rubber drains) close to the suture line, excessive tension on the anastomosis, infection, ischemia, and radiation enteritis. Anastomosis through inadequately resected malignant tissue, surgical injury to the bowel, and intra-abdominal abscesses can also result in postoperative external gastrointestinal fistulas.

External gastrointestinal fistulas arising from the pancreas can occur after trauma, external drainage of a pseudocyst, or surgical procedures on the pancreas. Traumatic fistulas usually result from undetected or inadequately treated injury to the pancreatic duct. Pancreatic pseudocysts fail to obliterate after external surgical drainage in about one-third of cases, often leading to the development of pancreatic fistulas.

External gastrointestinal fistulas are commonly encountered in patients with Crohn's disease. They usually extend to the perianal area and produce chronic indurated rectal fistulas with associated fissures and perirectal abscesses (Fig. 72-29). Involvement of the skin around the umbilicus also occurs.

Anorectal fistulas are granulation-tissue-lined tracts between the anal canal or rectum and one or more openings in the perianal skin. These fistulas can arise from infections in the bowel wall that extend to form an abscess, which then ruptures and forms a fistulous tract to the skin. Anorectal fistulas can be associated with Crohn's disease, malignancy, radiation therapy, trauma, tuberculosis, or lymphogranuloma venereum.

Colocutaneous fistulas occur in approximately 6% of patients who have received surgical treatment for diverticulitis. However, spontaneous colocutaneous fistulas are rare. A colocoxal fistula is an unusual complication of colonic diverticulitis that causes a communication between the colon (usually the sigmoid) and the hip, buttock, or thigh. This condition is characterized by emphysematous cellulitis that presents as gas between muscles and interstitial planes, in contrast to gangrene, which usually produces gas in muscle bundles. The major mechanism involved in this phenomenon is the pressure gradient between the colonic lumen and the surrounding interstitium, which allows intraluminal gas to flow into the relatively low-pressure soft tissues.

Fig. 72-28. External fistula complicating abdominal surgery. Contrast introduced through the fistulous tract fills loops of small bowel.

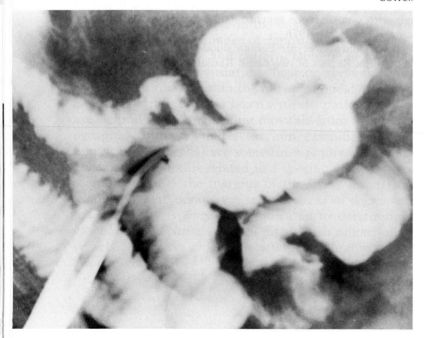

Fig. 72-29. Crohn's disease causing perirectal abscess and fistulization to the prostate.

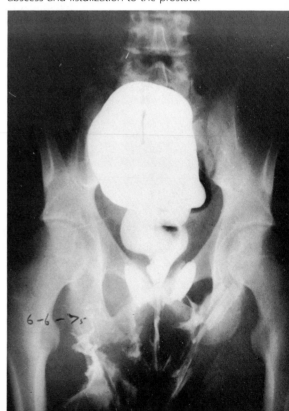

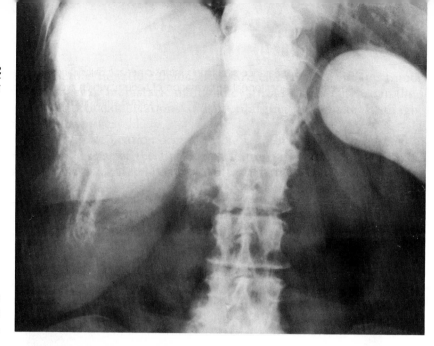

Fig. 73-13. Calcification of the liver and spleen caused by a prior injection of Thorotrast.

CALCIFICATION IN THE SPLEEN

Disseminated calcifications
  Phleboliths
  Granulomatous disease
    Histoplasmosis
    Tuberculosis
    Brucellosis
Cysts
  Congenital
  Post-traumatic
  Echinococcal
  Dermoid
  Epidermoid
Capsular and parenchymal calcification
  Pyogenic or tuberculous abscess
  Infarction
  Hematoma
Vascular calcification
  Splenic artery calcification
  Splenic artery aneurysm
Generalized increased splenic density
  Sickle cell anemia
  Hemochromatosis
  Residual Thorotrast

Multiple small, round or ovoid calcified nodules are frequently distributed throughout the spleen. These can represent phleboliths in the splenic veins or the healed granulomas of a widely disseminated infection. In the past, most of these lesions were thought to represent

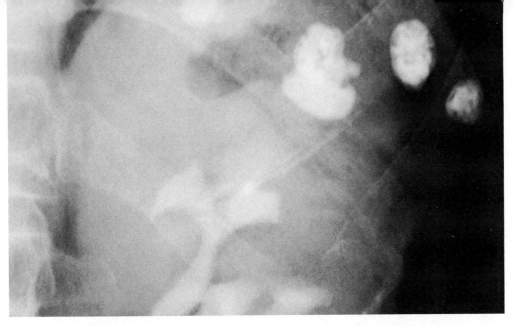

Fig. 73-14. Calcified splenic granulomas in a patient with chronic brucellosis.

calcified tuberculous nodules (see Fig. 73-1). Currently, it is believed that they more likely represent healed foci of histoplasmosis (see Fig. 73-2), especially when they are seen in patients from endemic areas. Similar calcifications are often distributed extensively throughout the lungs; occasionally, they are found in the liver.

Multiple calcified granulomas and chronic abscesses of the spleen can be demonstrated in chronic brucellosis (Fig. 73-14). Unlike the lesions in histoplasmosis and tuberculosis, the lesions in chronic brucellosis tend to be still active and suppurating even in the presence of calcification. The calcified nodules in chronic brucellosis are larger (about 1–3 cm in diameter) and consist of a flocculent calcified center in a radiolucent area that is surrounded by a laminated calcified rim.

Splenic cysts calcify infrequently (Fig. 73-15). In the United States, most are of congenital origin. Occasionally, a post-traumatic hematoma becomes cystic and develops a calcified wall. In endemic areas, splenic cysts are usually due to echinococcal disease (Fig. 73-16). These hydatid cysts are often multiple and tend to have thicker and coarser rims of peripheral calcification than simple splenic cysts. Echinococcal calcification can reflect a hydatid cyst in the spleen or extension of cysts arising from neighboring organs. Dermoid and epidermoid cysts very rarely demonstrate calcification.

Plaques of calcification in a thickened and fibrotic splenic capsule can be found secondary to a pyogenic or tuberculous abscess, infarct, hematoma (Fig. 73-17), or hydatid cyst. Splenic infarcts calcify infrequently. Although they are usually single, multiple calcified infarcts can occur. The calcification in a splenic infarct is often triangular or wedge-shaped, the apex of the density appearing to point toward the center of the organ. Calcified hematomas and abscesses of the spleen are rare.

Calcification within the media of the splenic artery is extremely common and produces a characteristic tortuous, corkscrew appearance

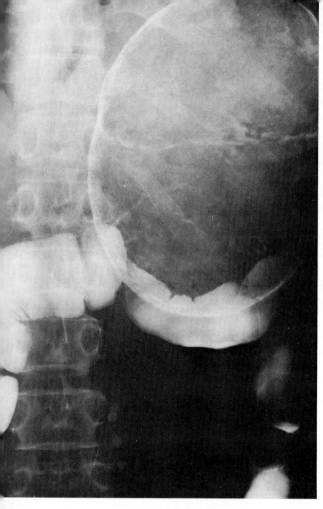

Fig. 73-15. Huge calcified splenic cyst.

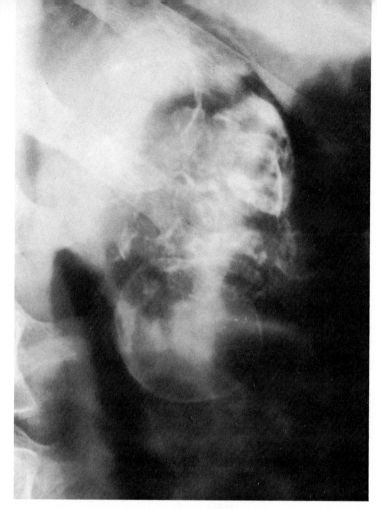

Fig. 73-16. Calcified hydatid cyst of the spleen (echinococcal disease).

Fig. 73-17. Calcified splenic hematoma.

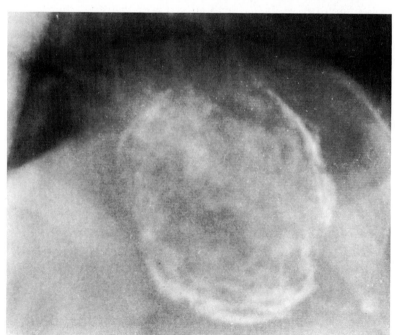

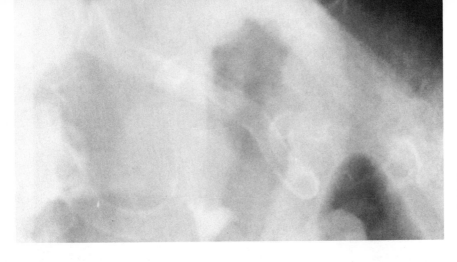

Fig. 73-18. Calcification of the splenic artery in a patient with diabetes. Note the characteristic tortuous, corkscrew appearance.

(Fig. 73-18). When viewed end-on, splenic artery calcification appears as a thin-walled ring. A similar circular pattern (Fig. 73-19) or bizarre configuration (Fig. 73-20) of calcification in the left upper quadrant can be due to a saccular aneurysm of the splenic artery.

A generalized increase in splenic density is seen in up to 5% of patients with sickle cell anemia (Fig. 73-21). Fine miliary shadows are produced by calcification and iron deposits in the fibrotic nodules of siderosis. Contraction and atrophy of the spleen cause these concretions to become confluent, producing irregular areas of calcification and a diffuse increase in density. Generalized opacity of the spleen can also

Fig. 73-19. Splenic artery aneurysm with a calcified rim.

Fig. 73-20. Splenic artery aneurysm. Note the bizarre, lobulated calcification.

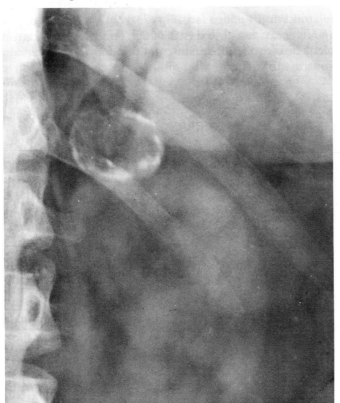

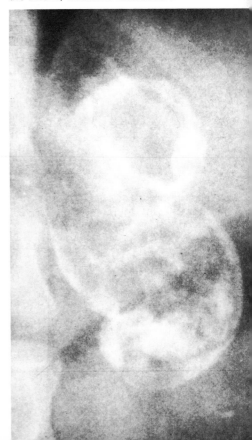

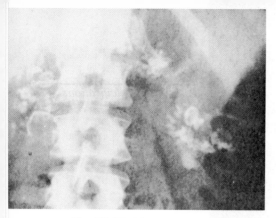

Fig. 73-25. Hereditary pancreatitis. The calcifications are rounder and larger than those usually found in other pancreatic diseases. (Ring EJ, Eaton SB, Ferrucci JT et al: Differential diagnosis of pancreatic calcification. AJR 117:446–452, 1973. Copyright 1973. Reproduced by permission)

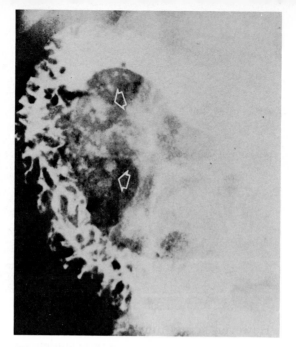

Fig. 73-26. Cystic fibrosis. These finely granular calcifications are primarily found in the head of the pancreas. (Ring EJ, Eaton SB, Ferrucci JT et al: Differential diagnosis of pancreatic calcification. AJR 117:446–452, 1973. Copyright 1973. Reproduced by permission)

cations of pancreatic disease, such as diabetes and steatorrhea, are common and tend to develop at an early age. Abdominal pain is a less prominent feature than would be expected in patients with pancreatic disease in Western countries.

True calcification of the pancreatic parenchyma can occur following intraparenchymal hemorrhage due to trauma or infarction. In patients who bleed from small intrapancreatic aneurysms secondary to pancreatitis, the resulting hematomas can subsequently calcify.

Pancreatic calcification occasionally occurs in patients who have no clinical evidence of pancreatic disease. Although the precise mechanism involved is unclear, these persons usually have nonspecific pancreatic ductal stenosis with formation of calculi upstream from the site of obstruction.

CALCIFICATION IN THE GALLBLADDER / BILE DUCT

Gallstone
Porcelain gallbladder
Milk of calcium bile
Common duct stone
Stone in the cystic duct remnant
Mucinous adenocarcinoma of the gallbladder

About 20% of gallstones contain sufficient calcium to be radiopaque (Fig. 73-27). Stones composed of pure cholesterol or a mixture of cholesterol and bile pigments are nonopaque. Although opaque gall-

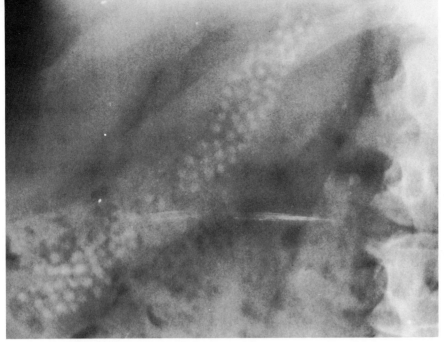

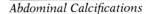

Fig. 73-27. Multiple small radiopaque stones in a large gallbladder.

Fig. 73-28. Calcified gallstone. The radiolucent center is surrounded by a dense outer rim.

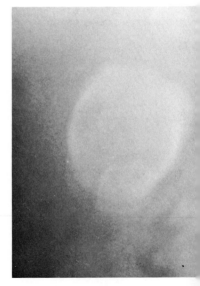

stones vary greatly in radiographic appearance, they generally have a dense outer rim consisting of calcium bilirubinate or carbonate and a more transparent center composed of cholesterol, bile pigment, or both (Fig. 73-28). Gallstones are often laminated, consisting of alternating opaque and lucent rings (Fig. 73-29). Solitary gallbladder stones are usually rounded; multiple stones are generally faceted (Fig. 73-30).

Several opacities in the right upper quadrant can simulate gallstones. A renal calculus can be differentiated from a gallstone overlying the renal shadow by obtaining a film in which the patient is rotated into an oblique position. A stone within a long retrocecal appendix or residual barium within a diverticulum in the hepatic flexure of the colon can mimic a radiopaque gallstone (see Fig. 73-36).

In patients with cholecystoduodenal or other fistulas between the biliary and alimentary tracts, gallstones can be demonstrated at any point in the duodenum, small bowel, or colon (Fig. 73-31). Impaction of a gallstone in the ileum or jejunum can cause small bowel obstruction (gallstone ileus).

"Porcelain gallbladder" refers to extensive mural calcification around the perimeter of the gallbladder forming an oval density that corresponds to the size and shape of the organ (Fig. 73-32). The term reflects the blue discoloration and brittle consistency of the gallbladder wall. The calcification in a porcelain gallbladder can appear as a broad, continuous band in the muscular layers or be multiple and punctate and occur in the glandular spaces of the mucosa. Extensive gallbladder wall thickening is always accompanied by mural thickening and fibrosis secondary to chronic cholecystitis. Although a procelain gallbladder is an uncommon finding in patients with gallbladder carcinoma, there is a very high incidence of carcinoma in patients with extensive calcification of the gallbladder wall. Therefore, even if they are asymptomatic, patients with porcelain gallbladders are usually subjected to prophylactic cholecystectomy.

Enteroliths
   Appendicolith
   Meckel's stone
   Diverticular stone
   Rectal stone
Calcified mucocele of the appendix
Calcified appendices epiploicae
Ingested foreign bodies
   Calcified seeds and pits
   Birdshot (from ingestion of wild game)
Mucinous carcinoma of the stomach and colon
Gastric or esophageal leiomyoma
Mesenteric calcification
   Fat deposit
   Lipoma
   Cyst

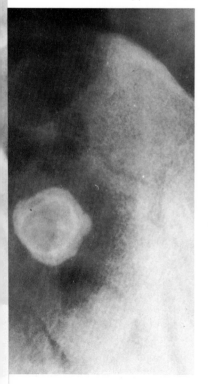

Fig. 73-35. Laminated calcification in an appendicolith.

Enteroliths are smooth, often faceted stones with radiopaque laminated calcifications. They are thought to result from stasis and are usually found proximal to an area of stricture or within diverticula. Enteroliths are not expelled with the fecal stream and can remain in place for years. They can cause mucosal ulcerations and be responsible for lower abdominal pain. Rectal enteroliths can produce fecal impaction and, if sufficiently numerous, bowel obstruction.

The most clinically important enterolith is the appendicolith. Appendicoliths are round or oval laminated stones of varying size that are found in 10% to 15% of cases of acute appendicitis (Fig. 73-35). In patients with fever, leukocytosis, and right lower quadrant pain, the radiographic demonstration of an appendicolith is highly suggestive of acute appendicitis. Surgical experience suggests that the presence of an appendicolith in combination with symptoms of acute appendicitis usually implies that the appendix is gangrenous and likely to perforate. Appendicoliths are generally situated within the lumen of the appendix but in rare instances may penetrate through the wall and lie free in the peritoneal cavity or in a periappendiceal abscess. Most appendicoliths are located in the right lower quadrant. Depending on the length and position of the appendix, an appendicolith can also be seen in the pelvis or in the right upper quadrant (in the case of a retrocecal appendix), where it can simulate a gallstone (Fig. 73-36). An appendicolith located near the midline can mimic a ureteral stone (Fig. 73-37); this is of great clinical significance, since an inflamed appendix in this region can cause hematuria and lead the physican to suspect renal colic rather than appendicitis.

Faceted stones can develop in a Meckel's diverticulum (Fig. 73-38); impaired drainage from the diverticulum leads to stasis and enterolith formation. Complications of Meckel's stones include inflammation with perforation and peritonitis, ulceration, and hemorrhage.

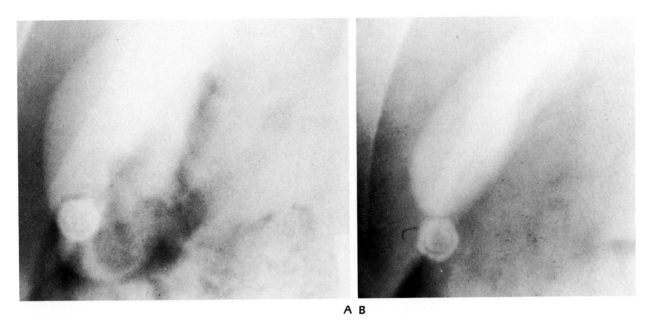

A B

Fig. 73-36. Appendicolith in a retrocecal appendix mimicking a gallstone. **(A)** The calcified appendicolith appears to lie in the opacified gallbladder. **(B)** After a fatty meal, the appendicolith is clearly seen to lie outside the confines of the shrunken gallbladder.

A large cresent-shaped or circular calcification in the right lower quadrant is characteristic of a calcified mucocele of the appendix. A mucocele is a collection of mucinous material in a dilated portion of the appendix (usually the tip). It is caused by fibrotic obstruction of the proximal lumen (*e.g.,* healed appendicitis) and an accumulation of mucus produced by the lining epithelium. A mucocele can vary in size

Fig. 73-37. Appendicolith mimicking a ureteral stone in a patient with hematuria. **(A)** On a plain abdominal radiograph, the appendicolith **(arrow)** is positioned in the region of the lower right ureter. **(B)** At excretory urography, the appendicolith **(arrow)** is seen to be separate from the nonobstructed right ureter.

A B

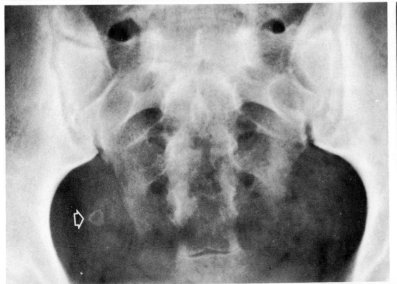
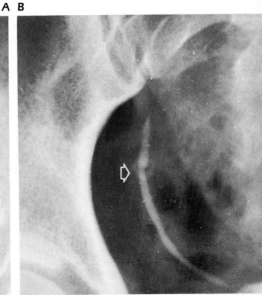

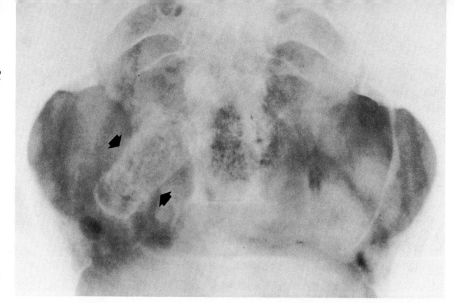

Fig. 73-38. Calcified enterolith **(arrows)** in a Meckel's diverticulum.

Fig. 73-39. Calcified appendix epiploica **(arrow).** The cystlike calcific density was detached from the colon and changed position on serial films.

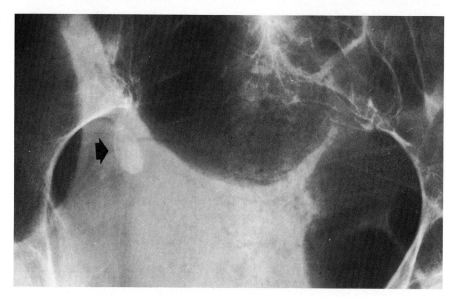

from slight bulbous swelling to a large mass completely replacing the appendix and displacing the cecum.

Appendices epiploicae are small, pedunculated fat pads that are covered by visceral peritoneum and are located along the surface of the colon. Infarction of appendices epiploicae results in cystlike calcific densities adjacent to the gas-filled colon, most commonly the ascending portion (Fig. 73-39). These calcified appendices epiploicae can become detached from the colon and appear radiographically as small, ring-shaped calcifications that lie free in the peritoneal cavity and change position on serial films.

Ingested material (*e.g.*, seeds, pits) can become trapped in the colon within the appendix or diverticula or be found proximal to an area of stricture. The deposition of calcium on these nonopaque foreign bodies results in a characteristic ringlike appearance. In persons who have eaten wild game, ingested birdshot can present as rounded metallic densities trapped in the appendix (Fig. 73-40) or in colonic diverticula.

Some mucinous adenocarcinomas of the stomach and colon contain small mottled or punctate deposits of calcium (Fig. 73-41). Most reported cases have been in patients under 40 years of age. The calcifications can be limited to the tumor mass or involve regional lymph nodes, the adjacent omentum, or metastatic foci in the liver.

About 4% of leiomyomas of the stomach demonstrate some radiographic evidence of calcification. The circumscribed, stippled, or patchy calcification in these tumors simulates the pattern seen in uterine fibroids. Because the actual size of such tumors is clearly reflected by the extent of calcification, a larger, bulky lesion suggesting leiomyosarcoma may be correctly recognized.

Leiomyomas are the only esophageal tumors that have been reported to calcify. The rare calcification in these distal esophageal lesions initially presents as scattered punctate densities. This pattern progresses to the more characteristic appearance of coarse calcium deposits seen in tumors of this cell type in other sites.

Single or multiple mobile opaque nodules can reflect calcified fat deposits in the omentum. Deposition of calcium salts in omental fat can be the result of local interference with blood supply, inflammatory or traumatic pancreatic fat necrosis, or any infectious process causing

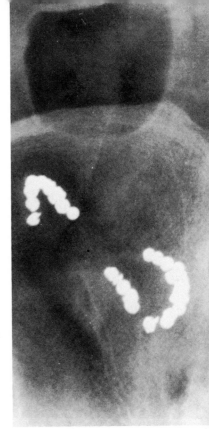

Fig. 73-40. Metallic foreign bodies in the appendix representing ingested birdshot in a patient who ate wild game.

Fig. 73-41. Calcified mucinous adenocarcinoma of the stomach. **(A)** A plain abdominal radiograph demonstrates calcification in the left upper quadrant. **(B)** An upper gastrointestinal series reveals that the calcification is related to a large adenocarcinoma of the stomach.

A   B

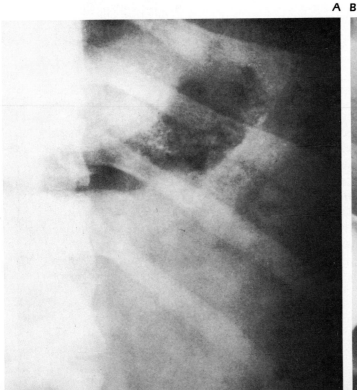
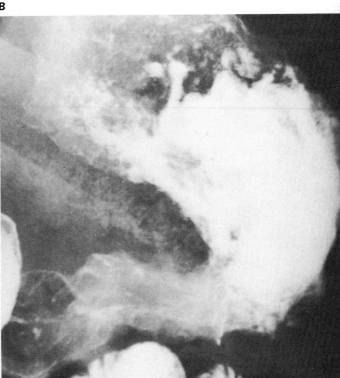

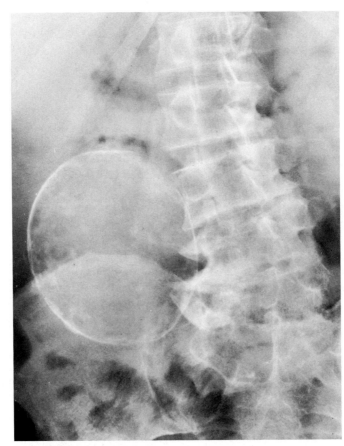

Fig. 73-42. Calcified mesenteric cyst.

Fig. 73-43. Multiple calculi in the renal pelvis. Although the calculi are opaque on the plain abdominal radiograph **(A)**, they appear lucent on the excretory urogram **(B)** because their density is less than that of the iodinated contrast material.

A B

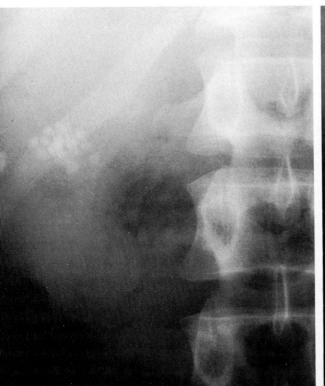

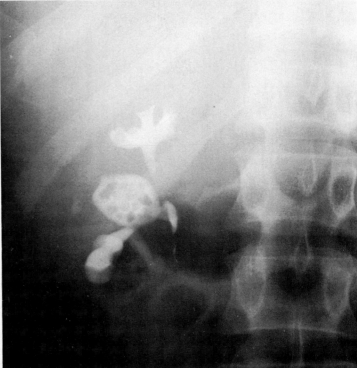

caseating necrosis. More extensive concretions can develop in mesenteric lipomas. Cysts of the mesentery or peritoneum, especially chylous cysts, can demonstrate unilocular or multilocular calcification (Fig. 73-42). Hydatid cysts, presumably forming through rupture of the primary hepatic cyst into the peritoneal cavity, can also calcify.

CALCIFICATION IN THE KIDNEY

    Calculus
    Nephrocalcinosis
        Skeletal deossification
            Hyperparathyroidism
            Metastatic carcinoma to bone
            Primary carcinoma
            Severe osteoporosis
            Cushing's disease
            Steroid therapy
        Increased intestinal absorption of calcium
            Sarcoidosis
            Milk–alkali syndrome
            Hypervitaminosis D
        Renal tubular acidosis
        Medullary sponge kidney
        Hyperoxaluria
        Renal papillary necrosis
        Tuberculosis
        Chronic pyelonephritis
    Cystic disease
        Simple benign cyst
        Polycystic kidney
        Multicystic kidney
        Echinococcal cyst
    Perirenal hematoma/abscess
    Renal cell carcinoma
    Xanthogranulomatous pyelonephritis
    Cortical calcification
        Acute cortical necrosis
        Chronic glomerulonephritis
        Hereditary nephritis
        Dialysis therapy
    Vascular calcification
        Renal artery aneurysm
        Arteriovenous malformation
    Renal milk of calcium
    Residual Pantopaque in a renal cyst

Calculi are frequently demonstrated in the calyces and the renal pelvis (Fig. 73-43). Occasionally, almost the entire pelvocalyceal system is filled with a large staghorn calculus (Fig. 73-44). Urinary stasis and infection are important factors in promoting calculus formation. Calculi composed of calcium phosphate and calcium oxalate usually have uniform dense radiopacity; magnesium ammonium phosphate stones are much less radiopaque. Cystine calculi, though often considered nonopaque, are usually moderately opaque and present a frosted or ground-glass appearance. Completely radiolucent calculi contain no calcium and are composed of pure uric acid or urates, xanthine, or matrix concretions that are a combination of mucoprotein and mucopolysaccharide. These calculi usually form in the presence of *Proteus* infection. Renal calculi can be laminated as a result of deposition of alternate layers of densely radiopaque material (calcium phosphate, calcium oxalate) and material of relatively low radiodensity (magnesium ammonium phosphate, urate).

Nephrocalcinosis refers to radiographically detectable diffuse calcium deposition within the renal parenchyma, chiefly in the medullary pyramids. Histologically, calcium may be deposited in the interstitium, in tubular epithelial cells, or along basement membranes of the collecting ducts, distal convoluted tubules, or ascending limb of the loop of Henle. Calcification can also occur in the tubular lumen. Radiographically, the calcification in nephrocalcinosis varies from a few scattered punctate densities to very dense and extensive calcifications throughout both kidneys.

Nephrocalcinosis occurs in about 25% of patients with hypercalcemia due to primary hyperparathyroidism, which is caused by an adenoma or carcinoma of a single gland or diffuse hyperplasia of all the parathyroid glands. Excess secretion of parathyroid hormone increases osteoclast activity, with resulting deossification of the skeleton and hypercalcemia.

Fig. 73-44. Staghorn calculi. **(A)** Unilateral, and **(B)** bilateral.

A B

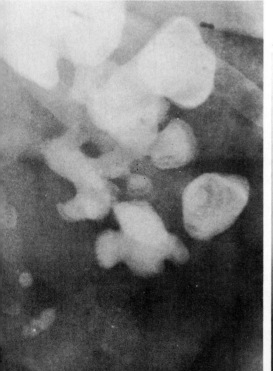
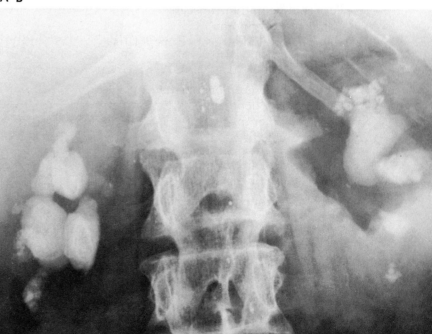

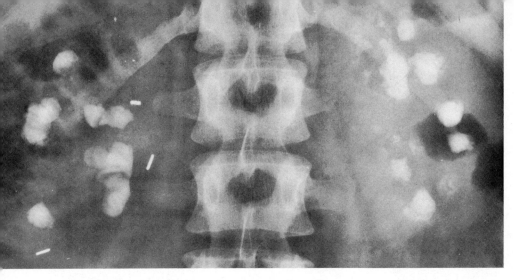

Fig. 73-45. Milk–alkali syndrome causing nephrocalcinosis.

Bone destruction in patients with metastatic carcinoma leads to a release of excess amounts of calcium from osseous structures, and this can result in nephrocalcinosis. Deossification of the skeleton and subsequent nephrocalcinosis can also occur in patients with severe osteoporosis (due to immobilization, menopause, senility) or Cushing's disease and in persons receiving steroid therapy. Patients with primary carcinomas, especially of the lung or kidney, may develop a paraneoplastic syndrome with hypercalcemia and nephrocalcinosis that appears to be related to inappropriate secretion by the tumor of specific humoral factors.

Increased intestinal absorption of calcium can lead to nephrocalcinosis. In patients with sarcoidosis, an increased intestinal sensitivity to vitamin D results in excessive absorption of dietary calcium. A similar mechanism occurs in patients with hypervitaminosis D; an excess of vitamin D also promotes dissolution of calcium salts from bone. Patients with the milk–alkali syndrome have a long history of excessive calcium ingestion, usually in the form of milk and antacids containing calcium carbonate (Fig. 73-45). The large tubular load of calcium and phosphate in the presence of alkaline urine and interstitial fluid causes the development of nephrocalcinosis.

Renal tubular acidosis is a disorder in which the kidney is unable to excrete an acid urine (below pH 5.4) because the distal nephron cannot secrete hydrogen against a concentration gradient. In addition to nephrocalcinosis and nephrolithiasis, patients with renal tubular acidosis frequently suffer from osteomalacia. The parenchymal calcification in renal tubular acidosis is characteristically very dense and extensive, diffusely involving the medullary portion of the renal lobes (Fig. 73-46).

Calcification within cystic dilatations of the distal collecting ducts is a manifestation of medullary sponge kidney (Fig. 73-47). The calculi are usually small and round, tending to cluster around the apices of the pyramids. Many patients with this disease are entirely free of urinary tract symptoms unless stone formation, urinary tract infection, or hematuria supervenes.

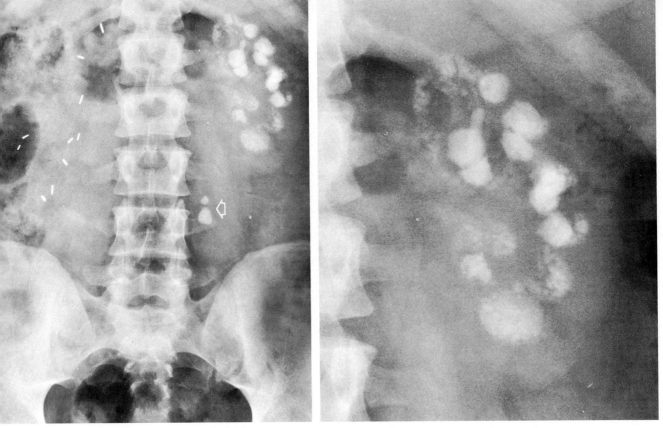

A B

Fig. 73-46. Renal tubular acidosis causing nephrocalcinosis. **(A)** An abdominal radiograph demonstrates diffuse calcification in the medullary pyramids of the left kidney. In addition, two stones (one of which is causing an obstruction) are seen in the midportion of the left ureter **(arrow).** The patient had previously undergone a right nephrectomy. **(B)** A close-up view of the left kidney demonstrates the intrarenal calcification.

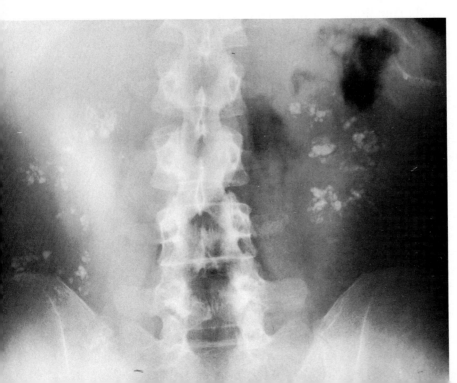

Fig. 73-47. Medullary sponge kidney. Multiple small and large densities in the papillae present a pattern that is indistinguishable from other causes of nephrocalcinosis. (Davidson AJ: Radiologic Diagnosis of Renal Parenchymal Disease. Philadelphia, WB Saunders, 1977)

Hyperoxaluria produces nephrocalcinosis by interstitial deposition of calcium oxalate. The primary form is a rare inherited metabolic disease in which symptoms of urinary tract calculi occur early in childhood (Fig. 73-48). Infection, hypertension, and obstructive uropathy usually cause a fatal outcome before the patient reaches the age of 20. Secondary oxaluria occurs in association with intestinal diseases, especially Crohn's disease (Fig. 73-49), in which increased absorption of dietary oxalate is related to the inflammatory process.

Nephrocalcinosis is a common finding in patients with renal papillary necrosis (Fig. 73-50). This disease is characterized by infarction of renal papillae resulting in necrosis with sloughing of the involved tissue. Renal papillary necrosis can be secondary to analgesic abuse (*e.g.*, phenacetin), diabetes mellitus, obstruction of the urinary tract, pyelonephritis, or sickle cell anemia. The necrotic papilla can remain *in situ* and become calcified or become detached and serve as a nidus for calculus development. A characteristic radiographic finding in papillary necrosis is the "ring shadow," a triangular radiolucency surrounded by a dense opaque band representing calcification of a sloughed papilla.

Fig. 73-48. Primary calcium oxalosis. There are diffuse, mottled renal parenchymal calcifications. Other evidence of the disease includes a "rugger–jersey" spine and sclerotic bands in the iliac crests and acetabuli. (Carsen GM, Radkowski MA: Calcium oxalosis: A case report. Radiology 113:165–166, 1974)

Fig. 73-49. Secondary oxaluria associated with Crohn's disease. Multiple calcifications are evident in both kidneys, both ureters, and the bladder. Calcifications are also present in the gallbladder and cystic duct. (Chikos PM, McDonald GB: Regional enteritis complicated by nephrocalcinosis and nephrolithiasis. Radiology 121:75–76, 1976)

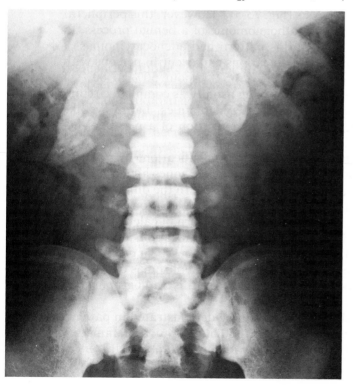

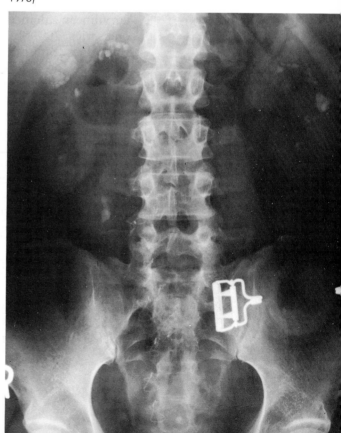

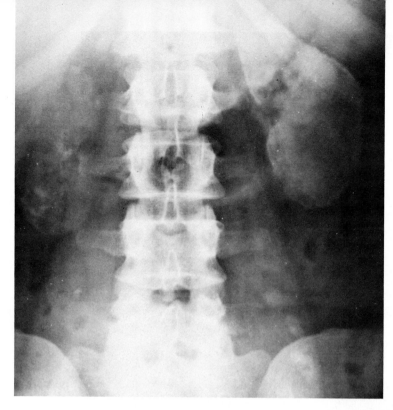

Fig. 73-54. Bilateral renal cortical necrosis.

Fig. 73-55. Calcification in a renal artery aneurysm. **(A)** A plain abdominal radiograph demonstrates circular calcification with a cracked-eggshell appearance at the renal hilus. **(B)** A selective right arteriogram shows contrast filling the saccular aneurysm **(arrow)**.

A B

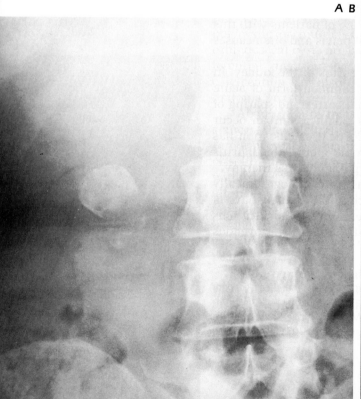

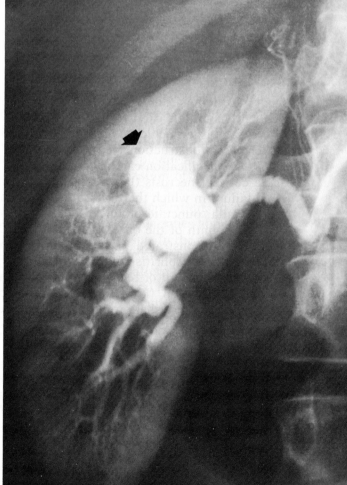

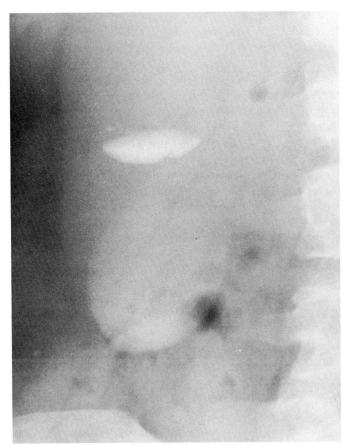

Fig. 73-56. Renal milk of calcium. **(A)** A supine abdominal radiograph demonstrates an oval density suggesting a renal calculus. **(B)** On the upright view, the calcium-containing sediment gravitates to the bottom of the renal cyst, resulting in the characteristic "half-moon" contour. **(C)** An excretory urogram shows that the milk of calcium is situated at the bottom of a large right upper pole renal cyst.

A
B C

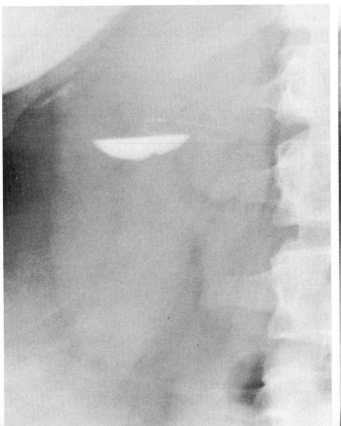

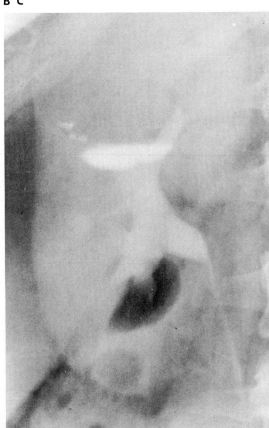

"Renal milk of calcium" refers to a suspension of fine sediment containing calcium that is most commonly found in a cyst or calyceal diverticulum. Less frequently, milk of calcium has been associated with obstruction of the urinary collecting system and hydronephrosis. The precise etiology of this process is unclear, but it may be related to stasis and infection. Renal milk of calcium usually is asymptomatic and an incidental finding. On plain abdominal radiographs in which the patient is supine, the appearance suggests an ordinary round or oval solid calculus (Fig. 73-56A). With the patient upright or sitting, however, the calcific material gravitates to the bottom of the cyst, resulting in a characteristic "half-moon" contour (Fig. 73-56B,C,).

Residual Pantopaque from prior renal cyst puncture can appear as a confusing heavy-metal density that simulates a swallowed coin on abdominal radiographs (Fig. 73-57). Unlike water-soluble contrast, Pantopaque takes several years to be absorbed from a renal cyst and may present a diagnosis dilemma if a history of prior cyst puncture is not available.

URETERAL CALCIFICATION

Calculus
Schistosomiasis
Tuberculosis

Fig. 73-57. Residual Pantopaque from prior renal cyst puncture. **(A)** A plain abdominal radiograph demonstrates two heavy-metal densities, one in the upper pole of the left kidney and the other in the lower pole of the right kidney. **(B)** Nephrotomography demonstrates that the two heavy-metal densities lie within renal cysts. (Eisenberg RL, Mani RL: Residual Pantopaque in renal cysts: An addition to the differential diagnosis of intra-abdominal heavy-metal densities. Clin Radiol 29:227–229, 1978)

A B

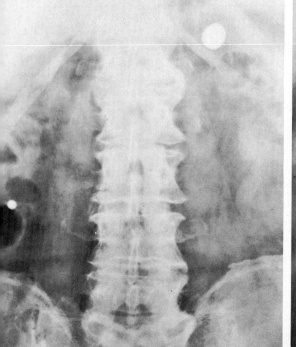
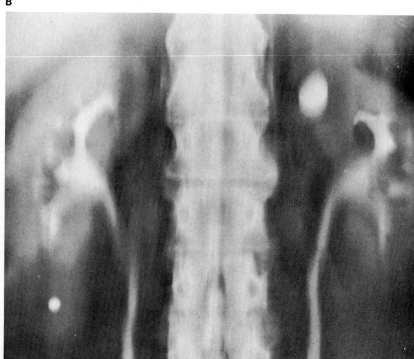

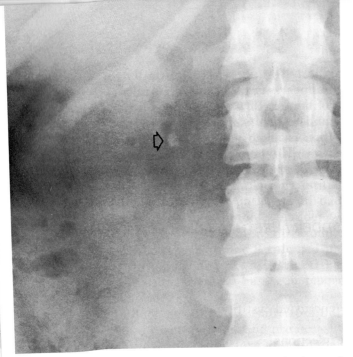

Fig. 73-58. Ureteral calculus **(arrow).**

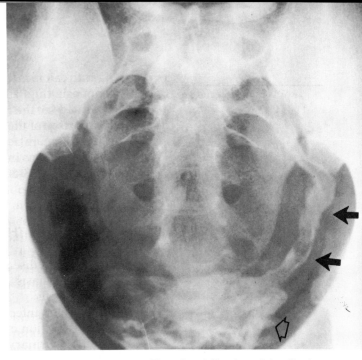

Fig. 73-59. Schistosomiasis. There is calcification of the distal ureter **(solid arrows)** and bladder **(open arrow).**

Ureteral calculi are extremely common, and their detection is clinically important (Fig. 73-58). They are usually small, irregular, and poorly calcified and are therefore easily missed on abdominal radiographs that are not of good quality. Calculi most commonly lodge in the lower portion of the ureter, especially at the ureterovesical junction and at the pelvic brim. Ureteral calculi are often oval in shape, their long axes paralleling the course of the ureter. They must be differentiated from the far more common phleboliths, which are spherical in shape and are located in the lateral portion of the pelvis below a line joining the ischial spines. In contrast, ureteral calculi are situated medially above the interspinous line.

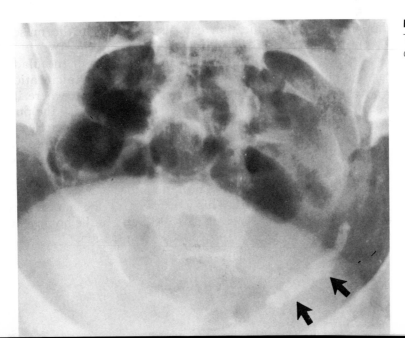

Fig. 73-60. Tuberculosis. There is calcification of the distal ureter **(arrows).**

Curvilinear calcifications may develop in the periphery of the jellylike masses that are secondary to pseudomyxoma peritonei (Fig. 73-79). This condition is a complication of spontaneous or surgical rupture of pseudomucinous carcinoma of the ovary. Deposition of tumor cells throughout the mesentery and serosa of the bowel incites a foreign-body type of peritonitis with thickening, fibrosis, and calcification.

Tuberculous salpingitis can produce a "string-of-pearls" calcification bilaterally within the pelvis. Tuberculous involvement causes the fallopian tubes to have an irregular contour, a small lumen, and multiple strictures.

Placental calcification is a physiological phenomenon associated with involution of the placenta, which usually occurs after the 32nd week of fetal life. The calcification typically has a fine lacelike pattern, best seen in the lateral projection, that outlines the crescentic shape of the placenta and is 15 cm to 20 cm in length and about 3 cm in average thickness. Because the deposition of calcium is greatest at the periphery of the cotyledons, the outer margin of the placenta is delineated.

Although infrequently seen, a lithopedion is easily diagnosed by recognition of fetal skeletal parts in the area of calcification (Fig. 73-80). The lesion can be intrauterine, from an old missed abortion, or extrauterine, from a previous ectopic pregnancy.

Bilateral laminated calcifications that closely approximate the lateral pelvic wall have been reported as a specific complication in patients treated with parametrial injections of ^{198}Au colloid (Fig. 73-81). This radionuclide was formerly used as an adjunct to surgery and radium therapy in the treatment of the lateral parametrium and lymph node drainage of carcinoma of the cervix. Excessive complications and the introduction of supervoltage treatment forced this mode of therapy to be discontinued. The calcification in this condition appears within 5 years of treatment, is gradually progressive, and varies from thin and linear to thick and globular. Multiple short, thin metallic densities can be identified in patients treated with gold seed implants for pelvic malignancy (Fig. 73-82).

Fig. 73-79. Pseudomyxoma peritonei. Curvilinear calcifications develop at the periphery of the jellylike masses, which are a complication of spontaneous rupture of pseudomucinous carcinoma of the ovary.

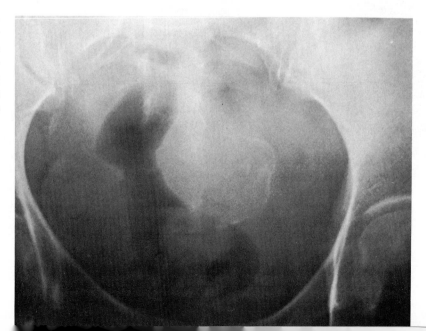

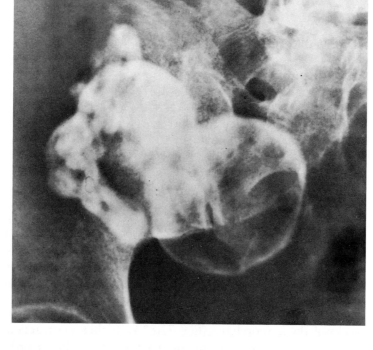

Fig. 73-80. Lithopedion. This calcified fetus was seen in a 78-year-old woman.

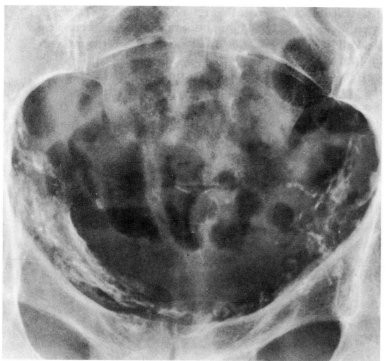

Fig. 73-81. Parametrial calcification in a patient with cervical carcinoma treated with radioactive gold. (Deeths TM, Stanley RJ: Parametrial calcification in cervical carcinoma patients treated with radioactive gold. AJR 127:511–513, 1976. Copyright 1976. Reproduced by permission)

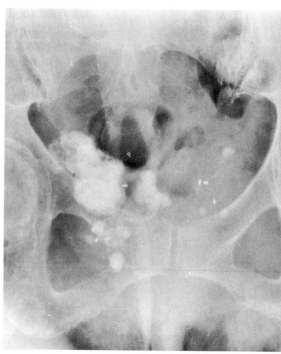

Fig. 73-82. Gold seed implants in a patient treated for transitional carcinoma of the bladder. Note the multiple short, thin metallic densities.

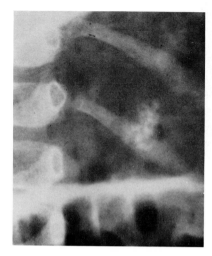

Fig. 73-85. Calcification in a Wilms' tumor.

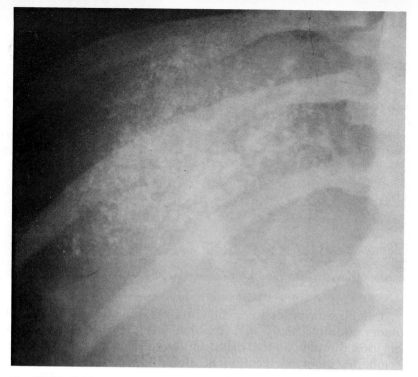

Fig. 73-86. Diffuse amorphous calcification in a large neuroblastoma.

Fig. 73-87. Psammomatous calcification of ovarian cystadenocarcinoma. The granular, sandlike calcifications represent metastatic spread throughout the abdomen.

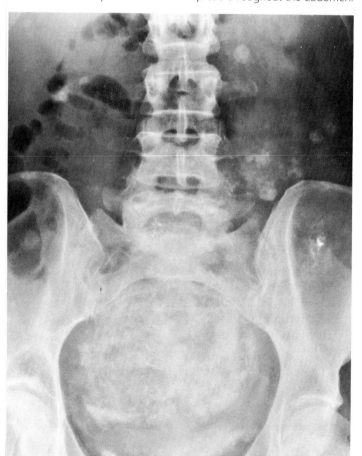

Fig. 73-88. Bizarre masses of calcification not conforming to any organ in a patient with an undifferentiated abdominal malignancy. (Dalinka MK, Lally JF, Azimi F et al: Calcification in undifferentiated abdominal malignancies. Clin Radiol 26:115–119, 1975)

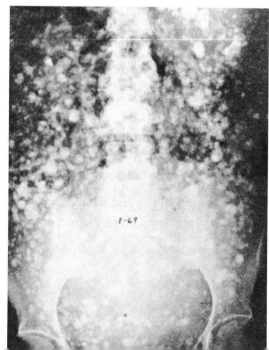

Neuroblastoma, a tumor of adrenal medullary origin, is the second most common malignancy in children. About 10% arise outside of the adrenal gland, primarily in sympathetic ganglia. The tumor is highly malignant and can attain great size before detection. Calcification in a neuroblastoma is common (occurring in about 50% of all cases), in contrast to the relatively infrequent calcification in Wilms' tumor, from which a neuroblastoma must be differentiated. The calcification in a neuroblastoma has a fine granular or stippled appearance (Fig. 73-86); occasionally, there is a single mass of amorphous calcification.

Retroperitoneal teratomas are less common than either Wilms' tumor or neuroblastoma. The tumor is almost always discovered in infancy and is generally located in the upper abdomen near the midline. Most teratomas have visible calcified spicules of cartilage or bone. Teeth inclusions, pseudodigits, or pseudolimbs may be identified. Retroperitoneal cavernous hemangiomas in children can appear as large masses containing multiple phleboliths in unusual locations.

Retroperitoneal hematomas, hydatid cysts, and tuberculous psoas abscesses can calcify. However calcification in retroperitoneal tumors in adults is extremely rare.

GENERALIZED ABDOMINAL CALCIFICATION

> Psammomatous calcification (cystadenocarcinoma of the ovary)
> Pseudomyxoma peritonei
> > Pseudomucinous cystadenoma of the ovary
> > Mucocele of the appendix
> Undifferentiated abdominal malignancy
> Tuberculous peritonitis
> Oil granulomas
> Meconium peritonitis

Several diverse conditions can result in widespread abdominal calcifications. The granular or sandlike psammomatous calcification of ovarian cystadenocarcinoma can be confined to the primary tumor or diffusely involve metastases throughout the abdomen (Fig. 73-87). Pseudomyxoma peritonei, caused by rupture of pseudomucinous cystadenoma of the ovary or mucocele of the appendix, can cause widespread abdominal calcifications that are annular in appearance and tend to be most numerous in the pelvis (see Fig. 73-79).

Bizarre masses of calcification that do not conform to any organ have been described in undifferentiated abdominal malignancies (Fig. 73-88). Patients with this condition have large soft-tissue masses with multiple linear or nodular calcific densities that can coalesce to form distinctive conglomerate masses.

Tuberculous peritonitis of long duration occasionally produces widespread abdominal calcifications. These calcifications are mottled and simulate residual barium in the gastrointestinal tract.

Oil granulomas, which can occur as a late effect of the instillation of liquid petrolatum into the peritoneal cavity to prevent adhesions, occasionally result in widespread annular or plaquelike deposits simulating pseudomyxoma peritonei (Fig. 73-89). The calcifications are located in masses of fibrous tissue surrounding the oil droplets. Clinically, oil granulomas can produce hard palpable masses that simulate carcinomatosis or cause intestinal obstruction.

Multiple small calcific deposits scattered widely throughout the abdomen in the newborn can represent meconium peritonitis (Fig. 73-90). This condition is a chemical inflammation of the peritoneum caused by the escape of sterile meconium into the peritoneal cavity. Meconium peritonitis usually results from perforation *in utero* secondary to a congenital stenosis or atresia of the bowel or to meconium ileus.

CALCIFICATION IN VASCULAR STRUCTURES

Arteries
Veins (pheboliths)
Lymph nodes
   Chronic granulomatous disease
   Residual lymphographic contrast
   Silicosis

Fig. 73-89. Intraperitoneal granulomatosis. The patient was treated with intraperitoneal mineral oil many years previously in an attempt to prevent the formation of abdominal adhesions.

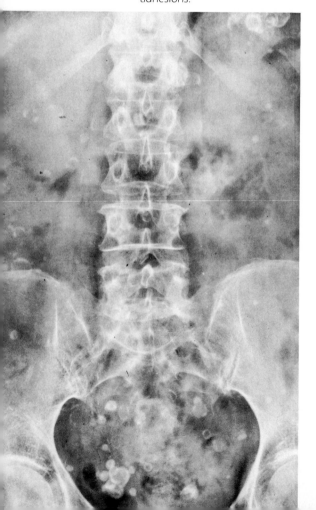

Fig. 73-90. Meconium peritonitis. Multiple small calcific deposits **(arrows)** are scattered throughout the left lower abdomen.

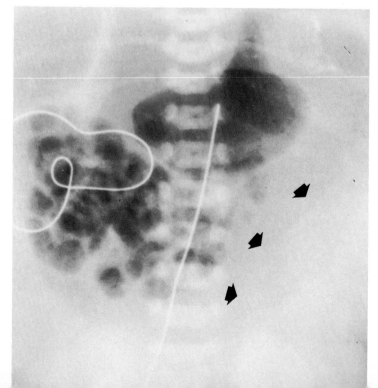

Calcification of atheromatous plaques in the walls of large abdominal arteries is a frequent observation in radiographs of middle-aged and elderly patients (Fig. 73-91). Similar calcification can also be seen in young persons, expecially those suffering from diabetes. The aorta, splenic artery, and iliac artery are most frequently calcified. Arterial calcification is seen as irregular plaquelike areas that vary in size from small flecks to parallel lines several centimeters in length. The amount of visible calcification bears no relationship to the severity of vascular occlusion; complete obstruction can exist with no detectable calcification.

The calcified splenic artery typically is tortuous (see Fig. 73-18) and, when viewed end-on, appears as a thin-walled ring in the left upper quadrant. Fragmentary calcification of the iliac arteries just below the sacroiliac joints can be mistaken for a ureteral calculus.

A phlebolith is a calcified thrombus within a vein. Phleboliths are most frequently found along the lateral aspect of the pelvis; almost all adults have at least a few of them (Fig. 73-92). These calcifications are round or slightly oval in shape and vary in size from very tiny densities to opacifications of 0.5 cm or more in diameter. They can be of homogeneous density, be laminated, or have the characteristic ringlike appearance of a lucent center and dense periphery. The detection of many of these small, rounded rings of calcification in a localized area suggests the possibility of multiple phleboliths in a hemangioma.

In patients with symptoms of ureteral colic, phleboliths can be confused with a calculus in the distal ureter. Unlike a smooth, rounded phlebolith, a ureteral calculus is often irregular in shape and, if elliptical, has its long axis lying parallel to that of the ureter. Ureteral calculi are

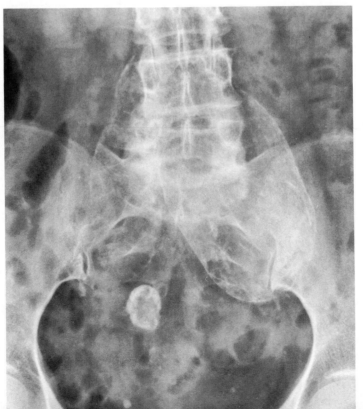

Fig. 73-91. Calcified atheromatous plaques in the walls of aneurysms of the lower abdominal aorta and both common iliac areries.

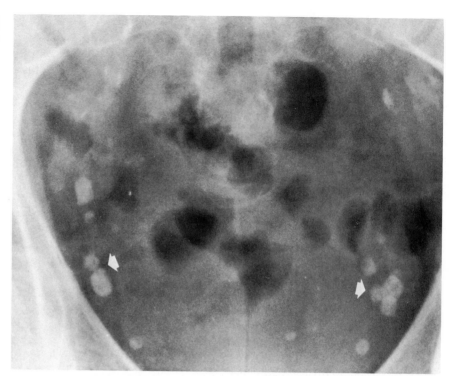

Fig. 73-92. Phleboliths. Note the characteristic position of these calcified venous thrombi **(arrows)** along the lateral walls of the pelvis.

Fig. 73-93. Diffuse calcification of lymph nodes lying along the course of the aorta and iliac arteries.

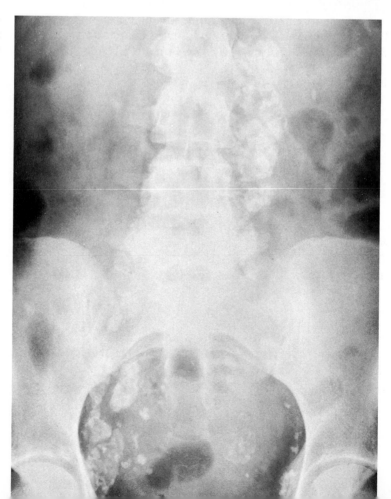

seldom found below the level of the ischial spines; in contrast, phleboliths usually occupy a position below the interspinous line.

Calcification of mesenteric and paravascular (aorta, iliac arteries) lymph nodes represents the effects of previous infection, usually histoplasmosis but occasionally tuberculosis or other chronic granulomatous disease (Fig. 73-93). This calcification is most frequently detected in the right lower quadrant or in the lower central part of the abdomen; it can occasionally be found to the left of the midline. A calcified mesenteric lymph node appears as a mottled density seldom more than 1 cm to 1.5 cm in diameter. Clusters of two or more nodes are often seen. A characteristic feature of calcified mesenteric lymph nodes is their movement over a fairly wide area on serial radiographs and on films made with the patient in different positions (supine and upright).

Residual contrast from a prior lymphogram can be demonstrated in para-aortic and pelvic lymph nodes. Serial radiographs demonstrating displacement of the opacified nodes can be a subtle sign of an expanding or recurrent neoplasm.

Eggshell calcific deposits accompanying similar lesions in the thoracic nodes have been reported in the lymph nodes of the para-aortic and subdiaphragmatic areas in two patients with silicosis.

ABDOMINAL WALL CALCIFICATION

Skin
  Soft-tissue nodules
  Scars
  Tattoo markings
  Colostomy/ileostomy stomas
Muscle
  Parasites
    Cysticercosis (pork tapeworm)
    Guinea worm
  Injection sites
    Quinine
    Bismuth
    Calcium gluconate
    Calcium penicillin
  Myositis ossificans
Soft tissue
  Hypercalcemic states
  Idiopathic calcinosis

Skin lesions on the abdominal wall (papillomas, neurofibromas, melanomas, nevi) can simulate intra-abdominal calcifications (Fig. 73-94). In most cases, however, these skin lesions appear as soft-tissue rather than calcific densities. Simple inspection of the patient is sufficient to eliminate any diagnostic difficulty. Calcification or ossification of old abdominal surgical scars can produce linear densities (Fig. 73-95). Tattoo markings and colostomy and ileostomy stomas sometimes present puzzling radiographic patterns.

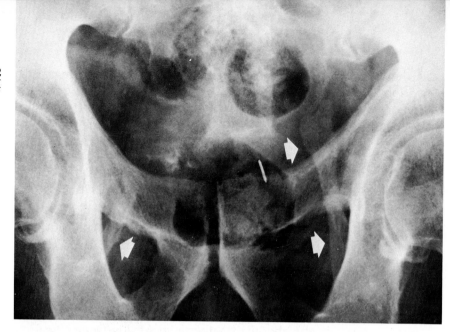

Fig. 73-97. Calcification of the sacrotuberous ligaments (arrows).

tion can resemble a ureteral calculus, close inspection should permit proper differentiation.

The iliolumbar, sacrotuberous (Fig. 73-97), and sacrospinous ligaments are sometimes calcified. Such calcification can represent a normal variant or be related to fluorosis.

MISCELLANEOUS CALCIFICATION

Ingested foreign bodies
Retained barium
Nonabsorbed cholecystographic contrast material
Suppositories
  Rectal
  Vaginal
Retained surgical sponges (gossypidoma)
Surgical gauze, drains, catheters, sutures

A variety of miscellaneous radiopaque densities can simulate calcification on abdominal radiographs. Ingested pills (Fig. 73-98), coins (Fig. 73-99), and marbles (Fig. 73-100), as well as unusual culinary delights such as chopped razor blades (Fig. 73-101), can appear radiographically as single or multiple calcium-like densities in the gastrointestinal tract. Indeed, the variety of foreign objects that are ingested appears to be unlimited (Figs. 73-102, 73-103, 73-104). In young children, irregular paint fragments (pica) in the gastrointestinal tract suggest lead poisoning (Fig. 73-105). Retained barium, especially in colonic diverticula (Fig. 73-106), and nonabsorbed cholecystographic contrast material (Fig. 73-107) can also appear as abdominal opacities. Rectal suppositories containing zinc oxide and various bismuth compounds can

tracheobronchial rests of esophagus, narrowing due to, 70, 71f
tracheoesophageal fistula(s). *See also* fistula, esophagorespiratory
congenital, 118–121, 119–121f
trauma
acute gastric dilatation due to, 293, 293f
adynamic ileus due to, 438
bile duct stricture due to, 847, 848f
diaphragmatic hernia due to, 164f, 165, 166f, 167f
duodenal dilatation due to, 406
esophageal intramural hematoma due to, 131–132
esophagorespiratory fistula due to, 123–124, 124f
fistulas, abdominal, due to, 946, 948, 949f, 950
pancreatic pseudocyst due to, 346
pneumoperitoneum due to, 916, 916f
to small bowel, regular thickening of small bowel folds due to, 469
Trichuris trichiura, infection with, multiple filling defect of colon due to, 728–729, 730f
"triple-bubble" sign, in jejunal atresia, 429, 430f
truncus arteriosus, persistent, extrinsic impression on thoracic esophagus due to, 38, 39f
tuberculosis
of adrenal, calcification due to, 1002, 1003f
anorectal, external gastrointestinal fistulas due to, 951
bile duct narrowing, due to lymph nodes involved by, 845, 846f
of colon
colocolic fistula due to, 941f, 942
narrowing due to, 645–646, 646f
single filling defect due to, 700
ulcerative lesions due to, 620, 620f
coned cecum due to, 586, 587f, 589, 589f
diaphragmatic elevation due to diaphragmatic paralysis caused by, 145
of duodenum
dilatation due to, 406
narrowing/obstruction due to, 392, 394f
postbulbar ulceration in, 331, 330f
thickening of folds in, 336, 336f
enteric-enteric fistulas due to, 941f, 942
esophagorespiratory fistula due to, 125
of esophagus
diffuse nodular lesions in, 136
narrowing due to, 83
ulceration due to, 59, 60f

of ileocecal valve, 561, 562f
liver calcification in, 955–956, 955f
pneumoperitoneum due to, 914
retrorectal space enlargement with, 782–784
simultaneous involvement of gastric antrum and duodenal bulb in, 320
of small bowel
dilatation with thickened folds due to, 461, 461f
generalized, irregular, distorted folds in, 485, 486f
separation of small bowel loops due to, 527, 528f
spleen calcification due to, 963, 955f
of stomach
filling defect due to, 256
gastric outlet obstruction due to, 283
narrowing due to, 210, 210f
thickened folds due to, 234
ureteral calcification due to, 989, 990f
tumefactive extramedullary hematopoiesis, of stomach, filling defect due to, 264f, 265
Turcot syndrome, multiple filling defects of colon due to, 718, 718f
typhoid fever
coned cecum in, 592, 593f
generalized, irregular, distorted small bowel folds in, 489, 489f
of ileocecal valve, 561
pneumoperitoneum due to, 914
toxic megacolon in, 759
ulcerative lesions of colon due to, 617–619, 617–618f

ulcer(s)
aphthoid
of colon, 609–610, 610f
of stomach, 198–199, 199f
benign, nonspecific
of colon, 635–637, 637f
narrowing due to, 651, 650f
single filling defects due to, 701, 701f
benign, solitary, of cecum, filling defect due to, 579–581, 580f
bile duct narrowing/obstruction due to, 844
"collar-button," 605, 606f, 611
of colon, 597–637
of duodenum
duodenal-renal fistula due to, 946–947. *See also* peptic ulcer disease
giant, 541–543, 541–543f
gastric. *See* gastric ulcer
marginal
enteric-enteric fistulas due to, 942, 275f

following gastric surgery for peptic ulcer disease, 193–194, 194–195f
peptic. *See* peptic ulcer disease
perforated, gas in biliary system due to, 871
postbulbar, 325–331
duodenal narrowing/obstruction due to, 391–392, 392f
extrinsic pressure on duodenum by, 359–360
widening of duodenal sweep due to, 350, 351f
of stomach. *See* gastric ulcer
"ulcer within an ulcer" appearance, in giant duodenal ulcer, 542, 543f
ulcerative colitis, 598–607
cancer of colon complicating, 666, 667f
clinical symptoms and course of, 599
colonic narrowing due to, 641–642, 641–642f
coned cecum in, 589, 589f
extracolonic manifestations of, 599–601, 600f
fistulas due to, 942, 944, 945f
of ileocecal valve, 561, 561f
large bowel obstruction due to, 744
pneumoperitoneum due to, 914
pseudopolyposis in
multiple filling defects due to, 723–726, 724–725f
single giant filling defect due to, 699, 699f
retrorectal space enlargement with, 782, 782f, 783f
terminal ileum in ("backwash" ileitis), 561, 561f, 589, 603, 603f
thumbprinting of colon in, 769, 769f
toxic megacolon in, 759, 760f, 761–763f
umbilical hernia, 894, 894–895f
umbilical vein, catheterization of, gas in portal veins due to, 878, 879f
urachus, calcification of, 992
uremia
gastric dilatation without outlet obstruction in, 295
thickening of duodenal folds in, 334–336
ulcerative lesions of colon due to, 625–627, 628f
ureter, calcification of, 988–990, 989f
ureteral colic, localized ileus in, 438, 439f
ureteral stone, appendicolith similar to, 974, 975f
ureterosigmoidostomy, colonic cancer complicating, 667, 668f
urethra, calculi in, 992, 993f

urinary retention, adynamic ileus simulating mechanical obstruction in, 442

urticaria, colonic, multiple filling defects in, 736f, 737

uterus
  fibroid of, calcified, 996, 997f
  gas gangrene of, 933, 934f
  tumors of, retrorectal space enlargement due to, 787

vagotomy
  duodenal dilatation due to, 406
  enlarged gallbladder in, 805
  gastric dilatation without outlet obstruction in, 295
  small bowel dilatation with normal folds in, 447–448, 448f

varices
  duodenal
    duodenal filling defects due to, 374, 374f
    extrinsic pressure on duodenum due to, 362
    thickening of duodenal folds due to, 339, 338f
  esophageal, 111–117
    filling defects due to, 99, 100f
  gastric
    filling defects due to, 256, 258f
    vs primary gastric fundus tumor, 305, 304f
    thickening of gastric folds due to, 232–233, 233–234f
  in small bowel
    multiple filling defects due to, 513

vas deferens, calcification of, 992f, 994, 994f, 995

venous plexus, pharyngeal, extrinsic esophageal impression due to, 28, 28f

ventral hernia, 894

villous adenoma. See adenoma, villous

volvulus
  cecal, large bowel obstruction due to, 745, 746f, 742f
  gastric
    gastric outlet obstruction due to, 286–287, 287–288f
    hiatal hernia with, 150, 151f, 152, 153f
  midgut, duodenal narrowing/obstruction due to, 389–390, 390f
  sigmoid, large bowel obstruction due to, 747, 748–749f
  small bowel obstruction due to, 425

vomiting
  esophageal intramural hematoma due to, 128–130
  esophageal rupture due to, 124, 125f, 129–130, 131f

Waldenstrom's macroglobulinemia, 516, 517f

water-siphon test, 51

Whipple's disease
  gas in bowel wall due to, 908
  generalized, irregular, distorted small bowel folds in, 477, 477f

sandlike lucencies in small bowel due to, 520, 521f
separation of small bowel loops in, 527, 529f
thickened small bowel folds with concomitant gastric involvement in, 524
thickening of duodenal folds in, 337, 339

Wilms' tumor, calcification in, 1003, 1004f

Yersinia enterocolitica
  coned cecum in, 592, 594f
  generalized, irregular, distorted small bowel folds in, 488, 488f
  sandlike lucencies in small bowel due to, 520
  ulcerative colonic lesions due to, 621, 622f

Zenker's diverticulum, 106–107, 107–108f

Zollinger-Ellison syndrome
  hypersecretion of acid in, thickening of gastric folds due to, 227, 226f
  postbulbar ulceration of duodenum in, 328, 329f
  small bowel dilatation with thickened mucosal folds in, 459–460, 460f
  thickened small bowel folds with concomitant gastric involvement in, 524, 525f
  thickening of duodenal folds in, 333, 334f

$\dfrac{125.^{00}}{65-11083} = \dfrac{1}{89}$

New 2nd Ed. Due - Aug., 1989